U0879000

北京大学医学教材

预防口腔医学

Preventive Dentistry

主　编　卞金有
副主编　王伟健
编　者　(按姓氏笔画排列)
王文辉　北京大学口腔医学院
王伟健　北京大学口腔医学院
卞金有　北京大学口腔医学院
朱　凌　北京大学口腔医学院
张博学　北京大学口腔医学院
陈霄迟　北京大学口腔医学院
杨圣辉　首都医科大学口腔医学院
荣文笙　北京大学口腔医学院

北京大学医学出版社

YU FANG KOUQIANG YI XUE

图书在版编目（CIP）数据

预防口腔医学 / 卞金有主编. —北京：北京大学医学出版社，2006. 3

ISBN 7-81071-633-6

Ⅰ. 预… Ⅱ. 卞… Ⅲ. 预防医学 – 口腔科学 – 医学院校 – 教材 Ⅳ. R780. 1

中国版本图书馆 CIP 数据核字 (2006) 第 011358 号

预防口腔医学

主　　编：卞金有

出版发行：北京大学医学出版社（电话：010-82802230）

地　　址：（100083）北京市海淀区学院路 38 号 北京大学医学部院内

网　　址：http://www.pumpress.com.cn

E-mail：booksale@bjmu.edu.cn

印　　刷：北京圣彩虹制版印刷技术有限公司

经　　销：新华书店

责任编辑：暴海燕　**责任校对**：杜悦　**责任印制**：郭桂兰

开　　本：787mm × 1092mm　1/16　**印张**：43　**字数**：1123 千字

版　　次：2006 年 3 月第 1 版　2006 年 3 月第 1 次印刷　**印数**：1-3000 册

书　　号：ISBN 7-81071-633-6/R·633

定　　价：69.90 元

序

长学制口腔医学专业双语教材编辑委员会邀请我为16本8年制口腔医学专业的教材写一个总序。我想所以邀请我写总序，也许在参加这16本教材的百余名教师中我是年长者，也许在半个世纪口腔医学教学改革和教材建设中，我是身临其境的参与者和实践者。

1952年我作为学生进入北京大学医学院口腔医学系医预班，1953年更名为北京医学院口腔医学系，1985年更名为北京医科大学口腔医学院，2000年更名为北京大学口腔医学院。历史的轮回律使我已是老教授又回到北京大学，这是高等学府名称的变更。新中国成立后年制改动得频繁，1949年牙医学系为6年，1950年毕业生为5年半，1951年毕业生为5年并招收3年制，1952年改为4年制，1954年入学的为4年制，毕业时延长一年实为5年制。1955年又重新定为5年制，1962年变为6年制，1974年恢复招生又决定3年制，1977年再次改为5年制，1980年又再次定为6年制，1988年首次定为7年制，2001年首次招收8年制口腔医学生，以上是年制的变更。

20世纪50年代初期，没有全国统一的教科书，都是用的自编教材。到50年代末全国有三本统一的教科书，即口腔内科学、口腔颌面外科学和口腔矫形学；到70年代除了上述三本教科书外增设了口腔基础医学的两本全国统一教材，即口腔组织病理学和口腔解剖生理学；80年代除了上述五本教科书外又增加口腔正畸学（口腔矫形学更名为口腔修复学）、口腔材料学、口腔颌面X线诊断学和口腔预防·儿童牙医学。那时口腔医学专业已有全国统一的九本教材；90年代把口腔内科学教材分为牙体牙髓病学、牙周病学、口腔黏膜病学三本，把口腔预防·儿童牙医学分为口腔预防学和儿童口腔病学，口腔颌面X线诊断学更名为口腔颌面医学影像诊断学，同期还增设有口腔临床药物学、口腔生物学和口腔医学实验教程。至此，全国已有15本统一编写的教材；到21世纪又加了一本䄂学，共16本教材。从以上学院名称的变更、年制的变换以及教材的改动，说明新中国成立后口腔医学教育在探索中前进，在曲折中前进，在改革中前进，在前进中不断完善。而这次为8年制编写16本教材是半个世纪口腔医学教育改革中付出巨大辛劳后的丰硕收获。我相信，也许是在希望中相信我们的年制和课程不再有变动，而应该在教学质量上不断下功夫，应该在教材的质量上不断再提高。

书是知识的载体。口腔医学教材是口腔医学专业知识的载体。一套口腔医学专业的教材应该系统地、完整地包含口腔医学基本知识的总量，应该紧密对准培养目标所需要的知识框架和内涵去取舍和筛选，以严谨的词汇去阐述基本知识、基本概念、基本理论和基本规律。大学教材总是表达成熟的观点，多数学派和学者中公认的观点和主流派观点。也正因为是大学教材，适当反映有争议的观点，非主流派观点，让大学生去思辨应该是有益的。口腔医学发展日新月异，知识的半衰期越来越短，教材在反映那些无可再更改的基本知识的同时，概括性介绍口腔医学的最新研究成果，也是必不可少的，使我们的大学生能够触摸到口腔医学科学前沿跳动的脉搏。虽然创造性不可能教出来，但是把教材中深邃的理论表达得深入浅出，引人入胜，激发兴趣，给予思考的空间，尽管写起来很难，但这是可能的，这无疑有益于培养大学生的创造性思维能力。

本套教材共有16本，是供8年制口腔医学专业的大学生用的。这16本教材为：口腔医学导论、口腔组织学与病理学、口腔颌面部解剖学、牙体解剖与口腔生理学、口腔生物学、口腔材料学、口腔临床药物学、口腔颌面医学影像诊断学、牙体牙髓病学、临床牙周病学、儿童口腔病学、口腔黏膜病学、口腔颌面外科学、口腔修复学、口腔正畸学、口腔预防医学。可以看出这16本教材既有口腔基础医学类的，也有临床口腔医学类的，还有介于两者的桥梁类性质的科目。这是一套完整的、系统的口腔医学专业知识体系。这不仅仅是新中国成立后我院第一套系统教材，也是1943年成立北大牙医学系以来的首次，还是实行8年制口腔医学年制的首部。为了把这套教材写好，编辑委员会遴选了各学科资深的教授作为主编和副主编，百余名有丰富的教学经验并正在教学第一线工作的教授和副教授参加了编写工作。他们是尝试着按照上述的要求编写的，但是首次难免存在不足之处，好在道路已经通畅，目标已经明确，只要我们不断修订和完善，这套教材一定能成为北京大学口腔医学院的传世之作！

张震康

2004年5月

前 言
Preface

预防口腔医学是口腔医学的一门分支学科。究其策略地位而言，是构成口腔科学三大支柱（基础口腔医学，临床口腔医学，预防口腔医学）之一。预防口腔医学又称口腔公共卫生或社会口腔医学，又是公共卫生或预防医学不可分割的重要组成部分。其纵横关联涉及的学科范围很广，体现了多学科的交叉与跨越。

预防口腔医学的发展对于增进公众口腔健康，进而提高生命质量具有举足轻重的作用。正因为如此，近半个世纪以来，在世界上不少国家和地区，由于开展了口腔健康促进活动，采取了口腔公共卫生措施，使人们的口腔卫生状况有了明显改善，同时，预防口腔医学也得到了迅速发展。而在尚未开展口腔公共卫生措施的国家和地区，人们的口腔健康状况正在恶化，预防口腔医学的发展也相对缓慢。近二十年来，在我国，无论在口腔公共卫生措施和方法的应用方面，还是在口腔预防医学的教学与研究方面，都得到了较快的发展与提升。例如，在卫生部领导下，制定了我国 2010 年口腔卫生保健工作规划；开展了全国爱牙日等口腔健康促进活动；学校和社区口腔卫生保健工作不断深入以及正在进行的第三次全国口腔健康流行病学调查等。

本教材的架构与内容既反映了当前本学科的国际发展状况，包括工业化国家和发展中国家的状况，又反映了当前本学科在国内的发展状况。因此，这本教材有以下几个特点：

1. 它是一次编写双语教材的尝试，有助于起到中英文双向交流的桥梁作用，是一种探索和创新；

2. 其内容涵盖着预防与社会口腔医学两个分支学科，并涉及医学与公共卫生领域，体现着一种整合。它已经超越了传统的生物医学范畴，纳入了社会医学的基本内容，但仍然遵循着基本理论，基本知识，基本技能的"三基"原则；

3. 各章节内容构思反映出编者们的各自特色，实难舍弃或补遗，只有兼顾科学民主与规范，各尽其力，各负其责；

4. 本教材在编排格式上有创意，既展现出双语随义同行，便于阅读，查找和联想，又有双语不同行互不干扰的明显区别。

主编遵循的原则是：在内容的筛选上，只提供科学证据与实践经验充分的，不提供陈旧与过时的；既借鉴工业化国家的经验，也借鉴发展中国家的经验；既展现科学的前沿（即使还有争议），又不采纳科学证据尚不充分以及还不成熟的。为同学和读者提供一个思维空间。因为本学科尚在发展之中。

这本教材虽专为长学制编写，但也适合于其他学制的大学生选用。主编希望它能成为一部启蒙教科书。尽管编者们尽了努力，主编又力图整合，也必有漏失之处，错误在所难免，还恳请读者予以批评指正，以求日后不断丰富与完善。

最后，主编要感谢各位编者的通力合作。在终稿审阅过程中，特别要感谢副主编和荣文笙博士的大力帮助，以及杨城大夫对图表的绘制和书稿格式采用电脑技术进行的统一编排，全书才得以告成。

主编　卞金有

目 录
Content

第四章　龋病预防与控制

第一章　导　论

Chapter I Introduction

概述 Overview

本章简要介绍预防口腔医学的理论基础，包括概念与定义，历史发展的四个时期：原始启蒙，科学基础形成与临床科学发展，预防口腔医学的产生与发展以及21世纪口腔健康科学的发展趋势与面临的挑战，最后部分简单叙述口腔卫生保健供给体制的形式、特点及其影响因素。

This chapter briefly introduce the scientific basis, including the concepts and definition; the four eras of its historical development: the original initiation, the basic science and chinical science, the emergence and development of oral health science in the 21st century, and its trends and challenges. The last part briefly describes the oral health care delivery systems, and its development, components, characteristics and influencing factors.

要点 Key points

- *Concepts of health and disease*
- *Definitions of pervente medicine, preventive dentistry, public health and dental public health, community dentistry.*
- *Determinants of health*
- *Goal and preventive strategies*
- *Guiding principles for future planning*
- *Factors influencing development of modern health care systems*

第一节　立论基础

Section 1 The Establishment of Scientific Basis

一、预防医学的哲学思维 The philosophical thought of preventive medicine

生命伦理学（bioethics）定义为根据道德价值和原则对生命科学和卫生保健领域内的人类行为进行系统的研究。生命科学（life science）是研究生命体和生命过程的科学学科，包括：生物学、医学、人类学和社会学。卫生保健是指对人类疾病的治疗和预防以及对健康的维护。

预防的目的是为保持一个人的健康状态而进行的任何干预。预防医学是以健康为中心，以预防为主体，以人群为主要研究对象，针对人群中健康与疾病的转化规律，以基础科学，流行病学，统计学与社会学基本原理为主要研究方法，通过临床预防，社会预防以及公共卫生实践，消除有害因素的影响，达到预防疾病的发生和控制疾病的发展，增进健康，提高生命质量的科学。预防医学已经经历了从个体到群体，从社会（社区）到人类（全球）的发展过程。

1. 医学与哲学 Medicine and philosophy

医学与哲学之间的关系是密切不可分割的。从医学发展史看，在两者的关系问题上存在着两种倾向：一种是经验主义的倾向。主要表现为一些医务工作者轻视理论思维，忽视哲学对医学的启发或辅助的作用。这种倾向有其认识上的原因，因为经验对一个医生确实很重要，当科学不发达时医生看病主要靠临床经验。在历史发展过程中，这种倾向因科学哲学中实证主义的产生和发展而得到了加强。在实证主义影响下，有的医生认为"哲学无用"。另一种是自然哲学的倾向。这种倾向是指用哲学的概念和理论演绎出医学的结论来。用推理来代替事实。这两种倾向反映了传统的临床医学模式是以经验与推理为基础。而以"证据为基础的现代医学的概念与模式是把疾病的防治干预，建立在有充分的科学证据的基础之上"。遵循客观证据是循证医学的本质所在，它正是以辩证唯物主义作为指导思想，表明了医学与哲学关系的相互作用。

2. 医学的研究对象 Subject for medical research

医学的研究对象是人。从医学研究的范畴考虑，人的含义包括病人和健康人，而且，随着医学的发展与医学使命的扩展，健康的人正越来越成为医学研究的对象。医学实践，作为一种独特的人类活动，其目的是保持和恢复人的健康。为了保持和恢复人的健康，就有必要对人是什么，人体又是什么，以及医学是什么，有一个大概的了解与认识。首先从人的科学概念出发，认为人是社会生物，为了解人的现代概貌，几乎所有的学科（约 800 种）都以人为研究对象。医学的贡献是对人进行规范性论证研究。人的本性是具有合二为一的生物与社会本性。而人的本质是一种社会人。根据人的生物社会本性把人分为两个子系统：一个是人的生物本性，即人的生命活动（生命质量），另一个则是人的社会本性，即人的个性，人的社会活动表现，两者之间相互联系、相互作用。

那么，从医学哲学的高度，又如何辩证地认识人体呢？应当把人体看作为一个多层次的等级系统。这个等级系统不仅包括人体以内的层次，例如，系统、器官、组织、细胞、细胞器、分子等，而且包括人体以外的层次。例如，人与人的关系、集体、社会、国家、全球生态圈。各层次系统之间相互作用，互为因果，构成人的实体基础。因此，人体又是身心统一体，处于社会关系影响之下。人生活在自然环境与社会环境中，而自然环境是经过社会改造了的，人的精神和行为大多是人对社会生活变化的反应。因此，人的机体是自然因素与社会因素的统一体。

医学是什么？医务工作者也不一定能直接给予明确的回答，因为他们只是从事某一个方面的医务工作，但是有一点共识，大家都清楚，那就是医学应该为恢复和增进人们的健康服务。而医学哲学工作者认为医学既是一种知识体系，又是一种人类活动，是艺术与科学，理论与实践的独特结合，是人文科学中最科学的，科学中最人道的，既非纯科学，又非纯艺术的学科。

总之，在为人的健康而进行的斗争中，医学依赖人体在正常状态（健康）和病理状态（疾病）下的活动规律，依赖人的个性表现，对人进行整体综合系统的研究。这是医学科学研究的突出特点。

3. 健康与疾病的概念 The concepts of health and disease

健康与疾病是医学哲学最基本的概念，也是最难以阐明的概念，至今还没有一个最终的解释。

(1) 健康的概念 (The concept of health) 关于健康与疾病的关系，许多人，包括医务工作者在内，认为健康就是没有疾病，有病就是不健康。凡是与健康不一致的都认为是疾病，这种传统的医学公理是健康的消极定义。健康应比不存在疾病有某种更积极的思想与内涵。现代医学已经抛弃了把重点放在治疗患者的传统，而趋向于预防和以群体为重点。世界卫生组织 (World Health Organization, WHO) 提出的健康定义是：个体在身体上，精神上和社会上的完好状态。

In 1946, the World Health Organization (WHO) introduced a paradigm shift in the definition, the WHO states that "Health is a state of complete physical, mental and social well-being and not merely the absence of disease and infirmity."

功能正常是健康概念的重要内容。功能是生物学的，而正常状态是统计学的。功能正常是机体健康的必要条件，它是以物种的共性为标准，而并非指特异功能。

健康是生态条件的函数——如果环境改变超出了机体所能适应的限度，就会导致机体与环境原有平衡的破坏，危及到健康。

真正积极的健康要领是帮助个人或集体，使生命质量达到最大限度发挥全部人类的潜力。所谓"生命质量" (quality of life) 是指健康与长寿的统一，它包括人的体质，素质以及人的社会活动，为社会创造财富，享有人生最大乐趣和幸福生活。

Quality of life (QOL) recognizes the value of an individual's health in the broader psychologic and social aspects of his or her life. The QOL construct considers patients' satisfaction with their present health state as well as their goals for the future. QOL is a multidisciplinary concept that includes survival or duration of life; the absence of impairment, disease, or symptoms; appropriate physical functioning, the absence of discomfort and pain; emotional functioning; social functioning associated with the performance of normal roles. Psychological functioning considers the effective and cognitive domain, in particular noting distress and well-being.

Functional health status is a critical dimension of QOL. Maintaining good function and preventing deterioration of function are primary goals.

1984 年，WHO 进一步解释了健康的概念：

健康是一个人或一组人能力的程度，一方面实现渴望与满足需要；另一方面，改变或适应环境。因此，把健康看作为一种生命的资源，而不是生活的目标，这是一种强调社会与个人资源，以及身体资本的积极概念。

A more recent WHO (1984) definition of health summarizes well the nature of contemporary understanding of the concept:

Health is the extent to which an individual or group is able, on the one hand to realize aspirations and satisfy needs; and on the other hand, to change or cope with the environment. Health is, therefore, seen as a resource for everyday life, not an object of living; it is a positive concept emphasizing social and personal resources, as well as physical capacities.

(2) 疾病的概念 The concept of disease

人类对疾病的认识比对健康的认识要早得多。

最早的疾病概念是一种本体论疾病观，认为疾病是独立存在的实体。随着医学的独立发展，形成了自然哲学疾病观，认为疾病是人体诸元素之间失去平衡。随着基础科学的发展，又形成了自然科学的疾病概念，认为疾病在本质上是一种生物过程，和健康一样，是生命的一种表现形式。

从 19 世纪到现在，疾病被认为是机体对致病因子有害作用的一种反应。在疾病过程中，一方面机体受到损害，发生紊乱，另一方面机体还有防御、适应与代偿的反应，是病理性反应与生理性反应共存的过程。临床症状是病症概念不可缺少的内容。

4. 健康的决定因素 The determinants of health

人类的健康受到各种因素的影响。1974年Blum提出假设，环境、行为与生活方式，卫生保健服务与人类生物学四大主要因素决定着一个人的健康状态，被称为关于健康状态决定因素的 Blum 模式。

（1）环境因素　环境因素包括自然环境与社会环境两个方面。个人是很难摆脱环境因素的，而环境状况决定着人类的健康水平。人类社会作为一个整体，不断作用于环境，改造着环境，尤其是社会环境。随着人类社会历史的发展，自然环境因素对健康的直接作用逐渐减弱，社会因素的作用则逐渐增强。自然环境对健康的影响和作用往往要通过社会环境为中介，才能作用于机体。自然环境条件相似，社会发展水平不同，或者社会生活环境，文化背景不同，人群的健康状况会有很大差异。人类活动使社会环境发生了巨大变化，同时也影响到自然环境，例如，森林破坏，水土流失，气候反常，环境污染等。

自然环境因素包括：物理、化学与生物学因素；社会环境因素包括：社会政治制度、经济发展水平、文化教育与科技发展水平、人口状况等。对人类健康产生根本影响的是社会经济发展水平。贫穷落后是健康的危险因素，社会法律、政治制度对健康的影响也十分明显。人口数量过多，素质过低，教育落后，就业困难，居住条件恶劣，食品供应不足等社会因素都可以是健康的危险因素；另一方面，有效的社会措施或健康教育与促进，可以帮助人们适应和克服不良社会因素的影响。

（2）行为与生活方式　行为与生活方式是指因自身行为所产生的影响健康的因素。不利于健康的行为是受社会心理因素的影响，包括无知愚昧的习惯势力，使自身健康受到自身行为的不必要的伤害。社会环境不同，对个人行为与生活方式的影响也不同，如一个人的受教育程度与个人行为习惯有很密切的关系。教育落后可以引发一系列的不良行为习惯，成为健康的危险因素，如吸烟，饮酒，不合理营养与饮食，缺少适当运动等。行为与生活方式是引起死亡与常见病的主要危险因素，这种影响在一次美国的调查中占48.9%，在中国的调查中占37%。行为与生活方式因素对健康的影响在我国有不断增大的趋势。

（3）卫生保健服务因素　卫生保健服务因素是社会因素中直接与健康有关的一个重要方面，包括预防服务和医疗与康复服务。医务人员缺乏预防意识，重治轻防，初级卫生保健不健全，经费缺乏和分配不合理或使用不当等都是不利于健康的危险因素。预防性服务是保护和促进健康的最有效的卫生保健措施。由于社会经济与文化发展不平衡，使许多行之有效的预防措施在许多地方未能很好地实施，而使许多疾病不能及时得到预防和控制。

（4）生物遗传因素　已知人类的遗传性缺陷和遗传性疾病近三千种，约占人类各种疾病的五分之一。有些不良遗传基因的传递将会增加人类有害基因的频率。先天性遗传缺陷是引发多种疾病的重要因素。而人的年龄、性别、特殊生理状况、某些生物因素对健康与疾病也有明显的影响。但是生物遗传因素只是影响人类健康的必要因素，而不是充分因素，疾病是否会发生以及发病的严重程度还要受到环境与行为因素的影响。总之，遗传、成熟与老化以及复合内因都是影响人类健康的生物遗传因素。

The Lalonde Report published in Canada in 1974 was influential in identifying four "fields" in which health could be promoted:

Genetic and biological factors which determine an individual's predisposition to disease;

Lifestyle factors in which health behaviours such as smoking contribute to disease;

Environmental factors such as housing or pollution;

The extent and nature of health services;

Dahlgren & Whitehead (1991) thus talk of "layers of influence on health" that can be modified:

Personal behaviour and lifestyles;

Support and influence within communities which can sustain or damage health;

Living and working conditions and access to facilities and services;

Economic, cultural and environmental conditions such as standards of living or the labour market.

二、预防医学的定义和内容 Definition and content of preventive medicine

1. 定义 Definition

预防医学是预防疾病，延年益寿，促进人体身心健康与效力的一门科学与艺术。它通过临床实践（医学的与口腔医学的）为个人与家庭服务，通过公共卫生实践为社会人群服务，通过全社会与每个人的行动达到预防和中止疾病的过程。

Preventive medicine is the science and art of preventing disease, prolonging life and promoting physical and mental health and efficiency for groups and communities by organized mass action - public health practice, and for individuals and families by private patient care - medical and dental practice to intercept the natural history of disease at any stage of its evolution.

从人的疾病发展史来看，疾病可以分为病理形成前期（prepathogenesis period）和病理形成期（period of pathogenesis）两个阶段。以慢性疾病为例，有助于认识预防医学的性质和特点，大多数慢性疾病通常都是由多种致病因素——致病因子（agent）、宿主（host）与环境因素（environmental factors）相互作用对机体产生疾病刺激（disease stimulus），在病理形成前期，疾病刺激物的产生与作用以及机体的防御反应之间的抗争需要经历一个相当长的时期才能逐渐显示出具有临床意义的症状，即进入病理形成期，但也可能中止或逐渐恢复正常。在病理形成期间，组织结构的病理改变是导致临床体征与症状的基础。在临床症状与体征日渐明显，疾病得以确诊之后，若不及时采取适当的干预措施，疾病将会进一步恶化，造成组织结构或形态缺陷，功能丧失，最终可能导致衰竭死亡。对疾病自然发展史的研究有助于探索预防对策。因此，预防医学是人类在与环境和疾病抗争的过程中形成的一门战略性综合医学学科。在预防医学的发展过程中，经历着以个人、群体和人类为对象的三个阶段。

From natural history of any disease of man, the developmental process of a disease could be divided into two stages: prepathogenesis period and the period of pathogenesis. Taking one example in the chronic diseases, it will be helpful to recognize the nature and characteristics of preventive medicine. Most of chronic diseases usually are interrelation among various causal agents - agent, host, and environmental factors to produce disease stimulus. It will take a relatively long time to make host and stimulus interaction, then gradually appear the clinical signs and symptoms at clinical horizon, it means entering into a period of pathogenesis. However, it is still a reversible phase, either in suspense or recovery to be normal status. During the pathogenic period, the tissue change is the basis of resulting in clinical signs and symptoms. While, the clinical symptoms and signs become evident increasingly, and the diagnosis of disease is identified, if there is no appropriate intervention followed in time, the disease will be getting worse. After then, it will further cause defect of tissue structure, or morphology, and function loss or disability. Finally, it could induce failure, even death. The study of natural history of disease is contributed to explore the strategy of prevention. Therefore, the preventive medicine is a strategical and comprehensive medical subject. In the developmental process of preventive medicine, it will go through three stages of individual, population and human being as subjects.

2. 内容 Content

预防医学是以社会人群为主要研究对象，用预防为主的策略思想，针对人群在疾病时的消长规律，采用基础科学（物理学、化学、生命科学），临床医学和环境卫生科学等的理论和方法来控制自然和社会环境因素对人群健康与疾病的作用规律，应用流行病学与卫生统计学等原理和方法，分析环境中主要致病因素对人群健康的影响，给予定量评价，并以此为依据，制定防治对策，通过公共卫生措施达到促进健康，预防疾病发生，控制疾病发展，防止伤残与死亡的目的。

3. 目标与策略 Goal and strategy

预防医学的目标是预防疾病的发生，控制病症的发展，康复机体的功能，保护和促进健康，正如 WHO 提出“使所有的人都尽可能地达到最高的健康水平”。

预防医学与临床医学相辅相成，但预防实践先于临床实践，防患于未然是公共卫生措施的理论与实践基础。按疾病自然发展史，预防措施可以从疾病发展的任何阶段介入，即预防贯穿于疾病发生前直到疾病发生后转归的全过程。根据各个阶段的特点与内容，划分为三级预防策略：

（1）一级预防或初级预防（primary prevention）处理病理形成前期过程，以病因预防为主，针对致病因素采取预防措施。强调自我保健，健康教育与促进，以及特殊的防护措施，即社区公共卫生措施，监测危险因素与疾病发展趋势等。

（2）二级预防（secondary prevention）已经进入病理形成期，但处于疾病的早期阶段，因此，早期发现，早期诊断，及时采取适当的治疗措施，阻止病理过程的进展，尽可能达到完全康复。

（3）三级预防（tertiary prevention）疾病已发展到严重和晚期阶段。防止伤残与康复功能为主要目的，如恢复器官的功能，尽可能恢复一定的生产能力和生活自理能力。

三、社会医学的发展 Development of social medicine

社会医学是随着人类社会的发展引起一系列的社会环境卫生与社会疾病问题，社会因素对人类疾病的发生与发展的影响为医学家们所重视而开始的。例如，古代中外医学家早就注意到人类健康与环境因素有关。《黄帝内经》中就有关于社会状况、居住环境、饮食起居的变化与疾病有关的论述。西方医学之父希波克拉底提出人的生活环境与健康有关。古罗马名医盖伦注意到社会环境和心理因素的致病作用。瑞士医生巴拉塞尔苏斯，意大利医生拉马兹尼深入社会，调查工作健康状况。19世纪中叶，法国医生盖林首次提出“社会医学”名词及其内容。德国医生塔尔曼、魏尔啸强调社会经济条件对健康与疾病的重要作用。19世纪末德国医生格罗帝扬提出了用社会观点研究人类疾病的一些重要原则。二次大战后德国把社会卫生学改为社会医学。20世纪40年代英国把公共卫生学改为社会医学。在前苏联、日本等国也有类似学科。

在20世纪30～40年代，中国的公共卫生包含着社会医学的部分内容。到50～70年代，形成了单独的保健组织学。80年代后正式发展为社会医学。社会医学的发展，既来自社会发展的实际需要，又来自医学哲学观念的更新和医学模式的转变。20世纪以来，大量事实说明健康和疾病与社会因素关系密切。人类防治慢性疾病的实践证明，预防医学必须从个体到群体，从临床到社会发展。社会医学的发展源于预防医学，又高于预防医学，它是预防医学发展深化的产物，又表明预防医学发展的新阶段，而社会医学向着更明确的社区医学方向发展，同时，超越了传统的公共卫生的范畴。正如英国牛津大学社会学教授赖尔（Ryle）认为的那样，整个公共卫生、工业卫生、社会卫生服务及公共医疗事业都属于社会医学。

1. **社会医学的定义** Definition of social medicine

关于社会医学的定义，各家陈述很多，但其核心类同。它主要是研究社会因素与健康、疾病的关系，研究和制定促进健康，防制疾病的社会措施。它是医学的一个分支。从医学角度，研究社会因素与疾病的发生、发展、治疗、预防的关系，研究社会因素与群体健康的相互影响以及与保护健康和促进健康的关系。

其研究对象是研究群体健康的社会过程，一定的社会规范对一定的群体健康的影响，以及社会变迁对群体健康状况的新变化和造成的卫生保健问题。同时研究城市和农村的保健问题，家庭环境对人健康的影响。在研究方法上，多采用社会学方法，如群体健康状况的抽样调查、问卷调查、社会统计、典型调查、观察—实验等，对影响群体健康的社会因素进行横向研究，适时作出“社区诊断”，并开出“社区处方”，采取相应的社会干预措施，通过全社会和全体居民的共同努力，以增进群体健康。

2. **社区医学和社区卫生保健** Community medicine and community health care

20世纪60年代，英国是第一个把社会医学应用到实际工作中去的国家。现时流行于英国的社区医学实际上是社会医学在社区服务方面的实践，也称为社区卫生保健。社区医学是社会医学的一部分。随着疾病谱的改变和群众对卫生保健的需求日益增加，社区卫生保健工作逐渐与流行病学，社会医学等学科结合，由于它更直接地立足于社区，面向社区，服务于社区全体居民，而成为专门确定和解决有关社区全民卫生保健问题的一门科学。它以社区为基础，开展社区医学教育实践，以及一系列的研究活动。作为社区医生，必须熟悉所辖社区的人口结构与发展动向，研究社区地理环境，社会环境，职业状况，文化信仰，生活方式等因素对社区卫生保健服务的影响，并评价其服务成效。现在，在英国等一些国家，社区医学已趋成熟，成为以流行病学与卫生统计学为重点，并包括其他学科在内的综合性学科，而社区卫生保健则主要是在了解社区人群的需要，应用“社区诊断”确定社区健康问题，并选择优先解决的重点问题制定社区卫生保健计划、选择适当策略、充分利用社区的有限资源、最大限度地促进社区人群的健康。

3. 公共卫生的发展 Development of public health

公共卫生是从解决城市的具体问题开始的，例如，古罗马的公共卫生事业无与伦比，城市大型输水管网、公共浴池、食品卫生以及体育活动等。

早期的公共卫生实践，从 17 世纪开始在英国称为济贫法，把重点放在当地社区的贫困人口上，在一个农业社会是很合理的途径，因为发病率很低，但是到 18 世纪中叶工业革命的出现，济贫法失效了，工业化实际上是一场群众性社会革命，人们开始从农村到城市集中，引起居住拥挤，疾病流行，那个时代的放任主义态度导致少数人拥有大量财富，而出现了中产阶层，而对多数人而言，日益可怕的贫困，济贫法只能缓解贫困，不能完全解决新的社会与健康问题。

口腔医学在美国早期公共卫生发展中并没有起到重要的作用。当人们不断地受到伤寒、白喉、霍乱、天花与胃肠道疾病大批死亡的时候，很少考虑到口腔健康。虽然早在 19 世纪中叶在牙科医生志愿的基础上建立了少数公共诊所，在许多年之中，公共口腔保健设施几乎并不存在。例如，直到 1919 年，美国公共卫生服务并没有在定期的基础上雇用牙科医生，慈善牙科诊所，如 Eastman， Forsyth， Guggenheim 及 Strong-Carterall 是在 1910 至 1930 年期间开设的。

Early public health practice in the colonies on the eastern seaboard naturally reflected the English experience. The so-called Poor Laws in England, dating from the 17th century, put the burden of caring for the disadvantaged on the local community, a rational enough approach in an agricultural society in which there was little mobility. But with the advent of the Industrial Revolution in the mid-18th century, the Poor Laws broke down, for industrialization was really a massive social revolution. Mass migration to the cities created overcrowding, disease, and epidemics, while the laissez-faire economic attitudes of the time led to great wealth for some, the emergence of a comfortable middle class, and appalling squalor for many. The Poor Laws, which dealt only with the relief of destitution, were not designed for these completely new kinds of social and health problems.

Dentistry did not play a significant part in the early development of public health in the United States. Oral health was of little concern at a time when the population was decimated periodically by typhoid, diphtheria, cholera, smallpox, and gastro-enteric diseases. Although a few public clinics were established on a voluntary basis by dentists as early as the mid 19th century, public dental care facilities remained almost nonexistent for many years. The US Public Health Service, for example, did not employ dentists on a regular basis until 1919, and philanthropic dental clinics such as Eastman, Forsyth, Guggenheim, and Strong-Carterall opened in the period from 1910 to 1930.

Ashton认为，19世纪中叶以来，在欧洲与北美的公共卫生与有组织的卫生保健分为三个活动阶段。现在，我们处于第 4 个阶段（Ashton，1993）。

第一阶段（1840～1900），由于工业化与快速城市化的特点影响，导致贫困人口生活状况恶化。那时公共卫生的主要成就在于环境卫生的改善，这个时期的医学与流行病学的成功在于调查涉及营养不良，不良卫生状况以及感染性疾病的因果关系。

第二阶段（1900～1930），看到了微生物学与免疫学方面的进展，在人群的基础上带来了个人预防。这个阶段还看到了妇幼福利的增长。

第三阶段（1930～1970），医学服务主要集中在医院，增加了医疗的复杂程度，削弱了公共卫生的作用。这个阶段也与主要感染性疾病的消失有关系。

第四阶段（1970～），亦称作新公共卫生，由于逐渐认识到治疗对于处理慢性生活方式疾病的局限性以及卫生保健费用的螺旋式上升，这个阶段发表了许多关于健康的新的见解与世界卫生组织人人享有卫生保健的概念紧密相关。

There have been three phases of activity in public health and organized health care in Europe and North America since the middle of the 19th century and we are now part of the fourth phase.

The first phase, 1840-1900, was characterized by industrialization and rapid urbanization leading to desperate living conditions for the poor. Public health achievements were principally those of sanitary reform. This was the time when medical and epidemiological approaches were successful in detecting causal relationships involving malnutrition, unhygienic conditions and infectious diseases.

The second phase, 1900-1930, saw advances in bacteriology and immunization bringing personal prevention on a population basis. This also saw the growth in maternal and child welfare.

The third therapeutic phase, from 1930 to 1970, was characterized by medical services shifting their principal focus to hospitals, increasing complexities of medical treatments and less emphasis on public health. This also coincided with the disappearance of the major infectious diseases.

The fourth phase, sometimes called the 'new public health' (Ashton, 1993) , had its origins in the growing awareness of the limitations of therapy to tackle chronic lifestyle diseases and the spiraling costs of health care. This led to the publication of new perspectives on health (Lalonde, 1974) , closely followed by the World Health Organization (WHO) Health for All concepts.

4. 公共卫生的概念 Definition of public health

公共卫生又称大众健康，在许多定义之中，最广泛被接受和引证的是 Winslow's 的定义。Winslow认为公共卫生是一门科学与艺术，它从环境卫生，传染病控制，健康教育，医疗与服务机构对疾病的早期诊断，预防与治疗，发展社会机构，保证每个人适当的生活标准诸方面，通过有组织的全社会努力，达到预防疾病，延年益寿，促进健康与提高工作效率，并且以这样一种方式组织社会福利事业，使每个公民都能享有生来就有的健康长寿的权利。

最近的公共卫生定义中，摆脱了不实际的理想主义，接受健康作为一种手段而不是结果的概念。1988年美国医学研究院的一份具有历史意义的报告中提出的定义，描述公共卫生机构的功能为：

①评估：定期收集与散发有关健康状况，社区健康需求与流行病学研究的资料；

②政策发展：在影响公共卫生决策事务中促进基础科学知识的利用；

③保障：通过各种途径提供必要的服务内容，达到双方同意的目标。

Public health too is not easy to define. Among the many definitions that have been formulated, Winslow's is the most widely accepted and quoted. Winslow defined public health as "the science and art of preventing disease, prolonging life, and promoting physical health and efficiency through organized community efforts".

Among the more recent definitions of the public health mission, one that moves away from starry-

eyed idealism and accepts health as a means rather than an end is: "fulfilling society's interest in assuring conditions in which people can be healthy". That seems to encompass everything from maintaining the stratospheric ozone layer to providing recreational facilities or dental care where needed. The landmark report from the Institute of Medicine, from which that last definition came, goes on to describe the functions of public health agencies as:

Assessment. The regular collection and dissemination of data on health status, community health needs, and epidemiologic studies.

Policy development. The promotion of use of the base of scientific knowledge in decision making on policy matters affecting the public's health.

Assurance. Assurance of the constituents that services necessary to achieve mutually agreed-upon goals are provided, either directly, by encouraging other entities, or by regulation.

公共卫生是以预防医学的概念、理论、措施、方法与技能为基础，针对预防疾病，促进群体健康而采取的社会性实践。这种社会实践通常称为公共卫生措施。它常常需要结合医学科学以外的多种相关学科的知识技能，如环境科学、社会学、行为学、教育学、经济学、伦理学与法学、心理学等，借以补充和完善其必须具备的知识结构，提高科学水平，还需要动员社会各界与社区成员的积极参与，确保公共卫生措施的有效实施并获得成功。

作为一项公共卫生措施，必须具备以下条件：

（1）实验室、动物试验与临床试验已提供了充分的科学证据，证明其效果肯定；

（2）同时已证明安全可靠，不会出现任何副作用，并已形成一套安全操作、监测与评价的规范程序；

（3）社区大多数人能从中获益；

（4）其成本投入最低，社区和人群都可以承担，可以接受。

Public health, in essence, determines the health sttus of the community; identifies populations potentially affected or at risk for a particular problem; analyzes the dimensions of the problem through the use of epidemiologic methodology; and then plans, implements, and evaluates the appropriate interventions.

5. 新的公共卫生 The new public health

在过去30年中，公共卫生的重点已经在改变。1977年世界卫生大会决议案的目的在于推动实现2000年世界上所有的公民能够达到允许他们从事社会与经济生产活动的健康水平。随着具体健康目标的确定，WHO出台了一系列的卫生政策文件。随后，许多国家制定了国家目标。公共卫生的重点之一是在城市或者学校机构内开展工作，促进建立健康的环境。其目的是加强社区的行动和提高个人健康保护的技能。

新公共卫生运动重新集中关注政治、经济与环境在当代社会中对健康的影响。因此，更加强调发展政策，创建促进健康的环境。

Over the last 30 years, the focus of public health has been changing (Dean, 1994). The 1977 World Health Assembly resolution added impetus with the aim that by the year 2000 all citizens of the world would attain a level of health permitting them to live socially and economically productive lives. Several health policy documents followed giving specific health goals, internationally presented by WHO (1981,

1985). The next step was the national setting of targets by many governments. One of the focuses in public health is to promote the establishment of healthy environments by working in settings such as cities or schools. The aim is to strengthen community action and develop personal skills for health protection.

The new public health movement has refocused attention on to the political economic and environmental influences on health within contemporary society. More emphasis in therefore placed upon developing a range of policy options to create a more health-promoting environment.

6. 预防的公共卫生途径 The public health approaches to prevention

Rose（1992）把公共卫生的策略途径分为全民途径和危险因素途径，全民途径针对全民；危险因素途径针对目标人群和高危人群。

Rose (1992) divides strategy approaches into two distinct groups: those aimed at the whole population and those in which certain sections of the population are identified, either as a group or as individuals. The first approach is known as the whole-population approach, and the second as the risk approach. The risk approach has two subdivisions. Where population subgroups are identified it is known as the directed or targeted approach and where individuals are identified it is known as the high-risk approach.

7. 预防口腔医学 Preventive Dentistry

预防口腔医学是口腔医学的重要组成部分，与口腔医学的各个领域都有着密切的内在联系，其重点汇集成口腔医学的预防领域。它的规范名称是“预防口腔医学”（preventive dentistry）。全国自然科学名词审定委员会（1992）公布的口腔医学名词中与预防有关的几个学科名词与国际上常用的名词基本一致。例如社区口腔医学（亦称社会口腔医学）（community dentistry），口腔公共卫生／公共卫生口腔医学（dental public health/public health dentistry），以及社会（区）口腔卫生（community oral health）。虽然在各个国家的口腔医学教育中，课程、教研室，以及教科书的名称各不相同，但是学科内容与范围大体相同。因此，它们的趋同性已经达成共识，可以把它们整合成为“通过有组织的社会努力，预防口腔疾病，延续口腔健康和提高生命质量的科学与艺术。

Preventive dentistry: that phase of dentistry concerned with the preservation of healthy teeth and the maintenance of oral structures in a state of optimal health for the longest period of time possible. It comprises: a. primary prevention, which includes fluoride therapy, diet control, plaque control, sealants, and pulp protection; b. secondary prevention (intervention), which includes operative dentistry, periodontics, orthodontics and other fields; and c. tertiary prevention (replacement), which includes fixed and removable prosthodontics.

Community dentistry, that branch of dentistry concerned with the distribution of dental and associated oral diseases, their causes, and the management of resources for their prevention and treatment.

Dental public health, the prevention and control of dental diseases and promotion of dental health through organized community efforts, including dental health education of the public, applied dental research, the administration of group dental care programmes, and prevention and control of dental diseases on a community basis, called also public health dentistry.

Therefore, these concepts could be integrated into a common recognized convergence, which may be defined as "the science and art of preventing oral disease, prolonging oral health and improving the quality of life through the organized efforts of society".

The terms "preventive dentistry", "community oral health", "community dentistry" and "dental public health" are essentially synonymous.

8. 口腔公共卫生的定义与任务 Definition and mission of dental public health

美国American Dental Association，ADA已经认可口腔公共卫生为口腔医学9大专业之一。美国口腔公共卫生委员会作为一个专业委员会建于1954年，从采纳了Winslow的公共卫生定义之后经过修正，口腔公共卫生的任务，反映在这个定义之中：它是通过有组织的社会努力，预防和控制口腔疾病，促进口腔健康的科学与艺术。口腔实践的方式是服务于社区而不是个人。它涉及公众的口腔健康教育以及研究和应用研究的发现，群体口腔保健的项目管理，通过一种社区途径预防与控制口腔疾病。在美国，像公共卫生一样，口腔公共卫生已经扩展到重点包括口腔保健提供系统及其对口腔健康状态的影响上。原因是发展可供选择的提供系统对公众健康的影响正逐渐增强。

口腔公共卫生是关系到促进全人口的健康，因此，其重点是在社区水平上采取行动。口腔公共卫生是针对影响口腔健康的因素，采取最有效的手段预防和治疗口腔疾病。

The American Dental Association, ADA has recognized dental public health as one of nine specialties of dentistry. The American Board of Dental Public Health (ABDPH), which is the regulatory agency for the specialty, was established in 1954. Dental public health's mission is set forth in the definition adopted by the ABDPH. It is a modification of the previously mentioned Winslow definition of public health. The ABDPH defined dental public health as.

The science and art of preventing and controlling dental disease and promoting dental health through organized community efforts. It is that form of dental practice that serves the community as a patient rather than the individual. It is concerned with the dental health education of the public, with research, with the administration of programmes of dental care for groups, and with the prevention and control of dental disease through a community approach.

Dental public health, like public health, recently has expanded its focus to include the dental care delivery systems such as dental health maintenance organizations, independent practice associations, point-of-service organizations, and preferred-provider organizations are having an increasing impact on the public's health.

Dental public health can be defined as the science and practice of preventing oral diseases, promoting oral health, and improving quality of life through the organized efforts of society.

The science of dental public health is concerned with making a diagnosis of a population's oral health problems, establishing the causes and effects of those problems, and planning effective interventions. The practice of dental public health is to create and use opportunities to implement effective solutions to oral health and health care problems in population.

Dental public health is concerned with promoting the health of the population and therefore focuses action at a community level. This is in contrast to clinical practice which operates at an individual level.

However, the different stages of clinical and public health practice are broadly similar.

Dental public health is a broad subject which seeks to expand the focus and understanding of the dental profession on the range of factors that influence oral health and the most effective means of preventing and treating oral health problems. Dental public health is underpinned by a range of related disciplines and sciences which collectively enrich the value and relevance of the subject.

9. 21 世纪公共卫生的挑战 Public health challenges for the twenty-first century

19 世纪末 20 世纪初，第一次公共卫生革命的成就集中于环境干预，以减少感染因子的影响。在20世纪后期，第二次公共卫生革命是减少慢性疾病引起的死亡与相关的行为危险因素。进入 21 世纪，需要发展更多的国际合作以对抗自然环境的威胁。

现在，英国政府已经把公共卫生作为其卫生策略的中心，正在制定和实施目的在于减少健康的不平等，以及社会、经济与环境为健康决定因素的政策，这一公共卫生策略将会直接影响到未来口腔保健服务的发展。

The first revolutionary public health achievement of the late nineteenth and early twentieth centuries focused on environmental intervention to reduce the effects of infectious agents. The second revolution, later in the twentieth century, was the progress in methods and interventions to reduce the toll of chronic diseases and related behavioral risk factors. Looking ahead as we enter the twenty-first century, an increasing need will develop for more inter-organizational cooperative intervention to counter the human-generated threats to our physical environment.

The present UK government has placed public health at the centre of its health strategy (department of health 1999) . Policies aimed at reducing health inequalities and addressing the social, economic, and environmental determinants of health are being developed and implemented. This public health agenda will directly impact upon the future development of dental services.

美国对未来口腔公共卫生的挑战提出了 9 点对策：

（1）达成共识，口腔健康不仅意味着牙齿的健康，还包括整个颅颌面部的健康；

（2）消除口腔医疗保健水平之间的差异；

（3）认识到口腔健康对全身健康和生命质量的影响；

（4）充分利用医疗保健资源，促进全民口腔健康；

（5）建立有效的口腔保健机构，满足全民口腔健康需要；

（6）制定行之有效的全国口腔健康计划，改善全民口腔健康状况；

（7）消除影响口腔健康的不良生活方式和行为；

（8）将循证医学应用于临床与公共卫生实践；

（9）在考虑成本效益的同时，确保医疗保健质量。

To achieve the recognition that dental/oral health means more than healthy teeth-it means the health of the entire craniofacial complex.

To close the gap between levels of medical and dental access to care and between untreated and undiagnosed medical and dental disease.

To better recognize that oral health can have a significant impact on the overall health and well-being of the U.S. population.

To increase the use of public-private partnerships to improve the nation's oral health.

To build an effective dental health infrastructure that meets the oral health.

To develop a viable, effective National Oral Health Plan to improve the oral health status of the entire U.S. population.

To more effectively influence lifestyle behaviors that negatively influence oral health.

To increase the use of evidence-based practice in both clinical dental practice and public health practice.

To prevent the potential that the implementation of evidence-based methodology will be used to control costs without sufficient concern for the quality of care.

10. 预防口腔医学在我国全民口腔保健中的作用 The Role of preventive dentistry in implementing oral health care for the Chinese population

21世纪是预防世纪，是全民保健时代，包括口腔保健。根据我国现有的以及可以预料到的未来口腔医疗保健资源的状况，要使全民都能享有最基本的口腔卫生保健，只有通过教育、研究与服务三个方面，加快发展预防口腔医学，即口腔公共卫生。

我国人口的主要口腔健康问题是口腔卫生差、龋病、牙周病。要解决这些最基本的问题，主要是加快发展预防口腔医学。

21 世纪我国预防口腔医学面临着十分严峻的挑战，表现在：

（1）龋病和牙周病依然普遍而又严重地威胁着全人口的口腔健康，影响着全身健康；

（2）龋病对儿童青少年以及老年人的危害正在加重；

（3）我国是世界上氟牙症、氟骨症危害严重的国家之一；

（4）不良生活方式对我国人民口腔健康的影响日益严重，如吸烟，酗酒，吸毒，监用药物，以及饮食无节制等不良生活方式导致某些口腔疾病出现上升趋势；

（5）人口老龄化带来的严重问题：我国人口已进入标准型老年结构，有1.3 亿以上的老年人。老年人的口腔健康问题比其他人群都严重，解决的难度也大；

（6）群众的口腔卫生知识与个人防护技能普遍缺乏，旧观念的制约很深；

（7）医务人员，包括口腔专业人员，在医务活动中受到传统生物医学模式的制约，重治轻防，还缺乏对预防口腔医学的正确认识；

（8）社会口腔健康保障机构，服务模式不能满足人民需要，其发展趋势使人担忧；

（9）经费、人员、设备等口腔保健资源严重匮乏，分布与利用极不合理。

发展我国口腔卫生保健事业的基本原则应该是：

（1）政府主导，社会参与；

（2）继续认真贯彻“预防为主”，“预防第一”的方针；

（3）根据大多数群众的最基本需求，强调防治结合；

（4）以自力更生的原则，实施“以治养防”的原则；

（5）开发潜在市场，提高需求水平，加强“以防促治”的力度；

（6）以循证管理为指导，加强项目管理与行政管理。

发展我国口腔卫生保健事业的策略与途径：

（1）全民途径 A population approach：全民途径有可能以相对低的成本达到减少危险因素

在人群中的影响力。在宏观水平上，主要依靠社会各部门之间的大力协作、共同参与计划，实施与评价。在微观上，促进学科之间的相互交叉融合，在各层人员之间加强协作与团队意识，共同努力。

（2）危险因素途径 A common risk factor approach：饮食、卫生、吸烟、酗酒、压力与意外事件等不仅是口腔健康的危险因素，也是主要慢性病的共同危险因素，通过此途径，动员口腔专业人员与全体医疗卫生人员都来关心和支持，促进口腔健康和全身健康。

（3）高危人群重点突破途径 A high risk approach：在口腔疾病的患者人群中有三分之一为高危人群，在一般人群中有三分之一为患病人群，高危人群对整个人群的健康有重要影响，需要提供特殊的防护措施。

11. 社区（会）口腔医学的定义与目标 Defination and objectives of community dentistry

社区口腔医学主要涉及社区健康促进，它是与群体有关的口腔医学的一个分支，是由社会科学与流行病学衍生而来的一种策略和手段，其目的是为了群体健康，发展社区诊断和计划实施的必要技术。

Community dentistry is mainly concerned with health promotion in the community and should be defined as; that branch of dentistry which is practiced in relation to populations and groups, which derives from the social sciences and epidemiology an awareness of the strategies and tactics required and which includes the development of the techniques necessary for population diagnosis, planning and implementation of measures for the benefit of the community.

社区口腔医学的目标为（1）全民健康促进；（2）发现并消除或控制社区存在的、不利于口腔健康、全身健康与生命质量的危险因素；（3）评估社区口腔保健需求；（4）通过①实施有效的防治措施；②在确定重点的基础上，配置所需资源；③评价社区口腔保健服务效果；④将口腔保健服务纳入整体卫生保健服务中；促进社区口腔健康；（5）为社区弱势人群提供医疗服务。

The objectives of community dentistry includes: health promotion for the entire population, the detection and eradication or control of those factors operating in the community which are inimical to oral health, general health, and well-being, the assessment of the needs for dental care of the community, the improvement of community oral health by: ① implementing effective preventive and therapeutic measures; ② deploying the available resources to meet the needs on the basis of priority; ③ the measurement of the effectiveness of present services and the planning of new services; and ④ the coordination and integration of dental services and health services, and providing treatment services to persons who do not have easy access to general practitioners.

第二节 发展简史

Section 2 Outline of Developmental History

根据美国牙医史学家Malvin E. Ring于1985年出版的《牙医学图解说明史》（Dentistry-An Illustrated History）及我国牙医史学家周大成著《中国口腔医学史考》（1991）及郑麟蕃等主编《中国口腔医学发展史》（1998）的记述，世界与中国的口腔医学发展史起源可以追溯到远古的旧石器时代，也就是100多万年以前，还没有文字记载的化石。距今约10万年以前的山顶洞人的颌骨上已发现有龋，距今约1万年至4千年前的新石器时代人头骨发现龋和严重牙周病。世界与中国有文字记载的历史约5千年。在中国，公元前约1400年殷墟甲骨文就有“疾齿”、“疾口”与“龋”的记载。自古以来，人类就已经受到牙病的折磨，并寻找各种方法来解除痛苦。1958年McGarvran，E.G发表的“公共卫生对医学工作者的挑战”以及“把社区看作公共卫生的一个病人”文章中，把健康科学的历史发展分成为4个时期：经验主义时代（从远古至1850年），基础科学时代（1850～1900年），临床科学时代（1900～1950年），以及公共卫生时代（1950年至今）。

从整个预防口腔医学发展过程来看，也大致可以分为4个时期：原始启蒙时代，或可称之为经验主义时代（公元前14世纪至公元1840～1850年）；理性发展时代，或可称之为科学基础形成与临床科学发展时代（1840～1949年或1850～1950年）；预防口腔医学诞生与发展时代（1949～2000年）；21世纪口腔健康科学的发展时代（2001年至今）。

一、原始启蒙时代 The original initiative era

公元前14世纪至公元1840年这一段漫长的时期，由于牙病的痛苦难忍，古人很自然就产生了各种预防牙病的意识与实践。例如：

1. 漱口 Mouthrinse

公元前1100年，西周《礼记》有“鸡初鸣，咸盥漱”的记载。可见当时就有了早起漱口的口腔卫生习惯。至公元25年《金丹全书》记载：“今人漱齿每以早晨，是倒置也，凡一日饮食之毒，积于齿缝，当于夜晚洗刷，则污垢尽去，齿自不坏，故云晨漱不如夜漱，此善于养齿者。今观智者，每于饮后必漱，则齿至老坚白不坏，斯存美之功可见矣。”这时已经开始认识到“饮食之毒，积于齿缝”应早晚洗刷和漱口，并且夜间洗刷比早晨重要。其后各个朝代，漱口已成为日常口腔卫生习惯。到宋代苏东坡著《东坡集》杂记中的《漱茶说》记有“每食已，辄以浓茶漱口，烦腻即去”……“缘此渐坚密，蠹病自已”。现在知道茶含有氟，有防龋作用。到清代光绪年间，已有漱口药方，供慈禧、光绪漱口。直至今日，漱口已成为普通百姓的口腔卫生习惯。

伊斯兰世界在穆罕墨德时代，把基本口腔卫生引入阿拉伯世界并与伊斯兰教结合，古兰经要求除了清洁身体与思想之外，还要求在祈祷前，每天进行5次清洗仪式，这种清洗包括每天3次或15次漱口。

From the very earliest times, humans have been plaqued by dental problems, and have sought a variety of humans to alleviate them, such as:

Mouth rinsing

At Muhammad's time in the 7th Century, he introduced basic oral hygiene into the Arab world by in corporating it into the Muslion religion, Islam teaches the importance of cleanliness of the body as well as the mind. Among other duties required by the Koran, ritual ablution five times a day before prayers is a compulsory obligation. This ablution includes rinsing the mouth three times or fifteen times a day.

2. 叩齿 Biting teeth

公元前500年汉墓中出土的简帛医书中的《养生方》记载“朝夕啄齿不齲”，“鸡鸣时叩齿三十下，长行无齿虫，令人齿坚”，“叩齿百遍，咽唾三次，常数行之，用齿不痛”。“叩齿”，“咽唾”可以增强嚼肌与唾液分泌的功能，似有一定的口腔保健作用。至隋唐以后仍提倡“叩齿”。

3. 齿垢、洁齿与揩齿 Dental calculus，cleansing teeth

公元前400年《黄帝内经》中的《素问·诊要经终论》曰：“齿长而垢”。唐代孙思邈（581～682年）《备急千金要方》的“齿痛论”记载：“每旦以一捻盐内口中，以暖水含，揩齿及叩齿百遍，为之不绝，不过五日，口齿即牢密”“凡人齿断不能食果菜者，皆由齿根露也，为此盐汤揩齿法，无不愈也。”这时已见“揩齿”之说。早在6世纪的南梁时代（公元502～557年），我国就首次出现药物牙膏，这是世界上最早的药物牙膏。至公元752年，王焘撰《外台秘要》中关于牙石及其刮除的记载：附齿，有黄色物，如烂骨状，名曰食床，凡疗齿看有此物，先以钳刀略去之，然后依方用药，其齿断内附着齿根者，形如鸡子膜，有如蝉翼缠著齿者，亦须细看之，不尔，甚齿断永不附着齿根也。”到公元900年，晚唐敦粕壁画中的“揩齿图”是国内最早的一幅口腔卫生行为记录。王焘在《外台秘要》中引自张文仲《千麻揩齿方》曰：“每朝杨柳枝咬头软，点取药揩齿”已有柳枝制刷记载。据说嚼木为刷刷牙的方法自汉代由印度传至中国。在印度，用菩提树枝揩齿。“揩齿”做法一种是用手指，另一种是嚼木为刷（chewing stick）。用一种齿木，菩提树或杨柳枝用牙咬成絮状，揩刷牙面。敦煌壁画中有一幅诏景福年间用柳枝制成的牙刷画图是世界上最早的资料。这种方法至今仍然在东南亚及非洲的一些落后地区流行，世界卫生组织曾在培训教材中作过介绍。

在伊斯兰世界的穆罕默德还介绍了一种称为Siwak（或者misswak）的原始牙刷用于洁牙。用一种萨尔瓦多桃树枝制成，其木质含二碳酸钠，鞣酸，还有其他收敛剂，对牙龈有益，称为中东“天然牙刷”。浸泡于水中一天，纤维散开形成牙刷，用来刷牙。还有许多传统的口腔卫生方法，例如用牙签剔牙去除食物残渣，或用手指按摩牙龈。

直到19世纪，穆斯林神学家ibn-Abdin描述在5种情况下仍应用穆罕默德时代的许多洁牙方法：①牙色变黄；②口腔味觉改变；③任何时候起床；④祈祷前；⑤洗礼前。

在公元500年左右，古印度医学家Charaka与Sushruta以及公元650年的一位外科学家Vagbhata都特别关注口腔清洁。Sushruta与Vagbhata都说需要去除牙石，并说“一个人早晨起床应刷牙”，他们用新鲜树枝制作成牙刷。这种树枝一般有点苦味，有收敛作用。

二千年多以前，希腊医生就熟悉印度除口臭的配方，在白酒中加入洋茴香，莳萝与没药。

最早的洁牙剂，特别是牙粉，源于古希腊。古罗马的牙粉配方中有动物的骨、蹄、角、蛋壳与海鱼，用收敛剂混合而成。

The Muhammad also recommended cleansing the teeth with a siwak (or misswak) a twig of the Salvadora persica tree, whose wood contains sodium bicarbonate and tannic acid as well as other astringents that have a beneficial effect upon the gum. A siwak twig about half an inch in diameter is soaked in plain water for twenty-four hours until the fibers have separated. The fibers were called "nature's toothbrush" or "the Middle Eastern toothbrush".

There are many more traditions of oral hygiene attributed to the prophet, including th the last century: ①when the teeth become yellowish; ②when the taste of the mouth changes; ③after arising from bed at any time; ④before prayer; and ⑤before ablutions. Of the first half of the first millennium A.D. Indian two great treatises, Charaka and Sushruta and another surgeon, Vagbhata, active about A. D. 650, giving special attention to oral cleanliness, and both Sushruta and Vagbhata speak of the need for removing calculus from the teeth, using for the purpose a special instrument with a flat, diamond-shaped end. Sushruta begins his chapter on general hygiene with the admonition, "Early in the morning a man should leave his bed and brush his teeth. Their toothbrush is made from a fresh twig whose end is frayed into fibers. It generally has a bitter taste and an astringent quality.

More than two millenniums ago, Greek doctors were familiar with Indian mouthwashes for bad breath. In Diseases of Women, Hippocrates describes an "Indian preparation" made by pounding together anise, dill and myrrh in white wine.

4. 植毛牙刷 Toothbrush with implanted bristles

公元 916 ～ 1125 年的辽代已有骨柄植毛牙刷。从内蒙赤峰县辽驸马墓的随葬品中见到两把骨制牙刷柄，与近代牙刷相似。到了宋代，用牛角制成器物，植上马尾，制成牙刷。宋代日本名僧道元禅师在其著作《正法眼藏》下卷"洗面"中有此记载：僧侣们除漱口之外，尚用剪成寸余之马尾，植于牛角制成的器物上，用以刷洗牙。国外的植毛牙刷到 17 世纪才有，据法国牙科学者福查德（Pierre Fauchard 1678 ～ 1761）在《外科牙医》一书中记载："现在的牙刷是用马尾做的"，可见欧洲使用植毛牙刷比中国晚 500 多年。

16世纪的英国牙刷使用还不普遍，虽然有些人用布缠绕手指洁牙，而用牙签在贵族与绅士中间流行。牙签主要从法国，西班牙与葡萄牙进口。

The toothbrush was apparently not in common use, although some cleaned their teeth by rubbing them with a cloth-wrapped finger, but using a toothpicks was fashionable among the nobility and gentry, who imported them from France, Spain, and Portugal.

5. 砂糖损齿 Sugar damaging teeth

唐初，孟洗（约公元621 ~ 714年）著《食疗本草》中记载：多食砂糖有损牙齿。北宋寇宗奭在其著作《本草衍义》中也记有"砂糖小儿多食则损齿"。而日本到1881年才有类似记载。又有日人丹波康赖撰《医心方》引用了我国医书 80 多种，其中《产经》云："小儿齿未易，密及饴糖，不易与食，令儿齿朽坏，虽易齿不坚。"说明早在公元七世纪就已知道食糖过多容易引起龋病。

16世纪英国牧师医生Andrew Boorde出版了一本最早的英国医学书，认为"牙是有感觉的骨，因此牙疼是非常疼的。"他的病人一定有严重的牙疼，当时上层与中层社会的人们膳食富含糖，他指出了牙疼与糖的关系。

In 16th century, a priest-physician. Andrew Boorde published one of the earliest English medical books, described "a tooth is a sensible bone, and therefore the toothache is an extreme pain". His patients must have suffered grievously from toothache, for the diet of the upper and middle classes, at least, was extremely rich in sugar. He proposed a relationship between toothache and sugar.

6. 刷牙 Toothbrushing

元代（公元 1281 年）的罗元益著《卫生宝鉴》提倡要早晚刷牙两次。忽思慧在《饮膳正要》中提出"清旦用盐刷牙，牙无齿疾"，另外还提出"凡清旦刷牙，不如夜刷牙齿疾不生。"

强调晚上刷牙的重要。到了明朝，帝王们的一些牙上都有楔状缺损，说明刷牙已成习惯。

7. 牙签 Toothpicks

我国使用牙签的历史更为久远。元代赵孟頫（1254～1322年）在《老态》一诗中叙述“食肉先寻剔牙签”。明代李时珍在《本草纲目》中记载：“柳枝去风消肿止痛，其嫩枝削为牙杖，剔牙甚妙”。《清代北京竹枝词》詠《柳木牙签》。清代牙签的种类很多，如银制挂式牙签等。

1570年英国女王Elizabeth收到一件装有6根金牙签还有“擦牙布”（tooth cloths）的礼物。莎士比亚在他的剧本里多次间接提到牙签。说明牙签是当时上流社会的一种时尚。

Elizabeth in 1570 received a gift of six gold toothpicks as well as “tooth cloths” edged in silver and black.

Shakespeare alludes to toothpicks many times in his plays. It indicated that toothpicks were a fashion in the upper class at that time.

8. 17 ～ 18 世纪的欧洲 Europe in the 17th ～ 18th century

17世纪，基础科学有了伟大的发现，这些发现成了现代医学的基础，但是医学实践仍然是迷信、无知、没有活力的。

英国医生、解剖学家 William Harvey 发现了血液循环，1628 年发表了他的发现，有效地创立了生理学。

解剖学的进展导致了另外两门科学的成长：比较解剖学与组织学。

显微镜的发明开创了一个科学研究的新世界。显微镜学家Anton Van Leeuwenhock（1682～1723）发现了牙本质小管和微生物，包括细菌，以及粘附于牙上的牙垢。他用显微镜证实了牙虫原来是大批存在的奶酪。17世纪期间大多数理发匠继续以各种名义提供牙科服务。但有证据表明在义齿修复方面有些实际进展。但就总体而言，17世纪的牙医学很少有发展，英国有个理发匠兼外科医生 Charles Allen 写过一本书“The Operator for the teeth”但没有新的内容。

During the seventeenth century, great discoveries in the fundamental sciences were made, discoveries that would form the basis of modern medicine, but medical practice still languished in superstition and ignorance.

Of paramount importance was the English physician and anatomist William Harvey’s discovery of the circulation of the blood. By demonstrating his findings, which were published in 1628, Harvey effectively established the science of physiology.

Progress in anatomy led to the growth of two other sciences: comparative anatomy and histology.

The invention of the microscope in the 17th century opened a new world for scientific study. The great early microscopist anton van Leeuwenhock (1682 ～ 1723) advanced knowledge immeasurably. Among Leeuwenhock’s findings of importance to dentistry were the tubules in the dentin and the microorganisms, including bacteria, that he found in the material alba adhering to the teeth. He effectively disproved that they were tooth worms by providing microscopically that they were identical to the maggots that infest overripe cheese.

But on the whole, dentistry made little progress during the 17th century. Evidence of this is found in the first book on dentistry published in English. Entitled The operator for the teeth which was authored by Charles Allen, but he gives us little that is new. Dentistry had to wait until the next century to become a true science.

18世纪，牙医学实践发生了的深刻变化，其推动力来自上个世纪的科学发现。牙医学最终成为一门独立的学科。

法国人，Pierre Fauchard 综合了西方牙医学，于 1728 年出版了《牙外科医生》。这本巨著包含了牙医学的所有领域，他所倡导的许多想法与操作，直到今天还有价值。他讨论了龋病，病因及其预防，并否定了虫牙理论，而相信龋病是“体液不平衡”的结果。他对牙周病的理解在那个时代是先进的，他深信洁牙与根面清创术能预防牙周病，大力倡导预防牙医学，推荐将漱口作为家庭保健的一部分，并提供许多配方。

英国外科学家John Hunter，早年从事牙医学实践，他的第一本主要出版物题目是《牙齿》。他对人的口腔与颌骨作了详细研究，叙述了人牙的自然史，说明其结构、生长发育、以及疾病。

总之，在口腔疾病预防的启蒙与早期发展阶段，不论在国内还是国外，已经开始发明并应用了多种原始的口腔卫生保健用品，如木制牙刷，植毛牙刷，牙签，漱口液等，以及口腔卫生方法，如早起漱口、刷牙、洁牙、叩齿、揩齿等，但是由于当时科学发展水平的限制，还不能确切地知道这些口腔保健方法的效果以及发病与防病的机制。

The 18th century unshed in profound changes in the practice of dentistry, the impetus for which came from the scientific discoveries of the proceeding century. Dentistry ultimately becomes an independent scientific discipline.

Modern dentistry owes its greatest debt to a remarkable Frenchman, Pierre Fauchard, who synthesized what was known in the West about dentistry and who presented it in an organized form so that all practitioners could benefit.

In 1723, he completed his epic work, Le Chirurgien dentiste, ou, traite des dents (The surgeon-dentist, or, Treatise on the Teeth) which was published in 1728.

In his great book Fauchard covered the entire field of dentistry, and many of the ideas and procedures he advocated or described are still current today. He discussed tooth decay, its causes and prevention and rejected the tooth worm theory; rather he believed that caries were the result of a "humoral imbalance".

Fauchard's understanding of periodontal disease was well in advance of his time. He was a firm believer in scaling the teeth and debridement of root surfaces to prevent gingival disease. A strong advocate of preventive dentistry, he recommended the use of mouthwashes as part of home care and gave many formulas for concocting them.

Another greatest English surgeon of the eighteenth century，John Hunter, who early in his career studied the practice of dentistry and made the teeth the subject of his first major publication. He made a detailed study of the mouth and jaws that culminated in the publication in 1771 of his first major work. The Natural History of the Human Teeth: Explaining their structure, use, formation, growth and diseases.

Hunter's book is remarkable for its exceptionally accurate plates and most of his statements on dental anatomy hold true today.

二、科学基础形成与临床科学发展时代 The basic science and clinical science era (1850 ~ 1950)

以社会经济发展与自然科学进步为基础，在西方，欧洲的文艺复兴运动推动了医学与口腔医学的发展。

1839 年，世界上第一本牙科期刊杂志——美国牙医学杂志（American Journal of Dental Science）创刊。由于两位著名牙科医生Hayden与Harris的努力，1840年美国马里兰州的Baltimore牙医学院成立，成为世界上第一所牙医学院。同时成立了世界上第一个全国性牙科医师学会。1859 年，美国牙医学会（American Dental Association，ADA）成立。

19 世纪后 20 年间，两项主要发现推动了牙医学专业的革命并指出了新的口腔医学途径，它们的影响扩展到口腔医学的教学、研究以及临床实践的各个方面，即Miller的关于龋病的化学细菌学说和氟化物的防龋作用。

1901 年，第一届国际牙科联盟（International Dental Federation， FDI）在英国剑桥召开。

Professional dentistry rests upon a three fold base: education, organization, and literature. During the years 1839 and 1840 in the United States the tripod of dental professionalism was established for the very first time anywhere and dentistry was elevated to the high level of excellence.

Due to the efforts of Hayden and Harris, in 1840 the first dental college in the world, the Baltimore College of Dental Surgery, was chartered by state of Maryland. Hayden was a professor of dental physiology and pathology, and president of the college, and Harris was a professor of practical dentistry and dean.

Hayden and Harris also collaborated to form the first nationwide association of dentists. In 1840, the American Society of Dental Surgeons was formed, the first national organization in world. In 1839, Chapin Harris, who long had foreseen the need for an authoritative dental periodical, was instrumental in founding the first in the world, the American Journal of Dental Science (ADJS) . In 1859, the American dental Association (ADA) was organized.

During the last two decades of the 19th century two major discoveries revolutionized the profession of dentistry and pointed the way to new paths, their effects extending into every aspect of research, teaching, and practice. They are Miller's chemo-bacerial theory and fluoride.

The first official meeting of the FDI was held in Cambridge, England, 1901.

1902 年，由德国 Ernst Jessen 医生建立的儿童口腔诊所可能是世界上第一个免费的儿童口腔诊所。但是，也有人认为1901年由New York， Rochester牙医学会成员建立的为特需儿童提供服务的儿童诊所是世界上第一个免费的儿童口腔诊所。

第二次世界大战时，美国政府对口腔医学的态度发生了深刻的变化。应招参军的美国年青人的口腔健康状况令人震惊。在首次招募的两百万男子中有五分之一的人不能满足口腔内存留有 12 颗牙齿的最低口腔标准。战后，美国、欧洲等西方国家作出了巨大的努力，来促进全民的口腔健康。

第二次世界大战之前，在美国公共卫生中没有口腔医生的位置。20 世纪 50 年代开始，口腔公共卫生这门学科在美国兴起。

The first free dental clinic for children in the world was probably the one established about 1902 by Dr. Ernst Jessen of Strassburg, Germany, and eventually taken over by the municipal government. Which was the first in the world is debatable. There is evidence that a clinic for children was set up in Camden, New Jersey, in 1899, but credit is usually given to a clinic established by the clinic to needy children.

World War II brought about profound changes in Americans' attitude toward dentistry. Citizens were shocked to learn from the office of the Surgeon General that the dental health of the nation's young men was truly deplorable. The selective Service System had adopted as a minimum dental standard that a potential recruit need have only twelve teeth - three pairs of matching incisors and three pairs of chewing teeth - to be accepted into the armed forces. Among the first two million men summoned for service, one out of five lacked even the minimum number, and dental defects constituted the chief cause for physical rejection for active duty. As a consequence, after the war the United States and European countries as well, made a vigorous effort to improve the dental health of the world's population.

During the 1950s the new field of public-health dentistry emerged in America. Before World War II, dentists had no established place on the public-health team, and scarcely any dental schools were teaching anything at all on the subject.

总之，在此期间，预防口腔医学的科学基础得到发展的重要原因是Dr. Miller在口腔微生物学方面提出的龋病化学细菌学说，以及氟化物防龋作用的发现。

20世纪初，西方现代牙医学开始传入中国。随着牙科诊所、牙科学校的建立，有关口腔卫生的刊物、宣传、展览、牙膏陆续出现，同期还开展了龋病、斑釉等调查工作。例如，1914年中西医学报登载有关口腔疾病，口腔卫生访谈的文章。1919年中国保牙会成立，中国卫生日报创刊。1926年上海生产的三星牌管状牙膏问世。1930年科普读物“家庭口腔卫生学”出版。1935年司徒博提出了“发展我国齿科医学事业，推行口腔卫生的计划”报告，同年上海牙医公会举办了第一届口腔卫生展览会。1936年对上海高桥小学学生进行了牙病调查。1936年调查了吸烟对牙齿与口腔组织的影响。1942年周大成在沈阳对农村学童龋蚀频度进行了调查。1944年郑麟蕃在北京调查了中小学生的口腔状况。1945年发表了贵州氟区斑釉调查。1945年上海又有药物牙膏消治龙（磺胺）问世。1947年朱端伯发表了氟与龋预防的文章。

上述这些事件的发生与出现都说明了具有一定科学基础的预防口腔医学也已在中国开始萌芽并逐渐发展。

三、预防口腔医学的诞生和发展时代 The emergence and development era of preventive dentistry（1950 ~ 2000）

自从1948年世界卫生组织成立以来，在其宪章中明确规定了其宗旨是“尽可能使人类达到最高的健康水平”，并明确阐述“健康是每个人的基本权利之一，不分种族、宗教、政治信仰、经济或社会状况”。规定了六个主要工作领域：卫生服务、人力开发、家庭卫生、疾病控制、环境卫生与协调、热带病生物医学研究。从50年代开始，把重点放在传染病、环境危害与营养缺乏的同时，建立了口腔卫生项目，以保持和促进全球人口达到可以接受的口腔健康水平为目标。在认识到充填治疗、拔牙与外科手术、冠桥与义齿修复并不能从根本上解决全球人口的基本口腔健康问题时，开始制定了总政策。在全球范围内开展预防和控制口腔疾病的项目与活动，最早支持在新西兰召开的氟化物研讨会以及在美国、加拿大等地开始的饮水氟化项目。组成了15个专家委员会作为WHO的专家咨询机构。60年代以来，组织专家制定了口腔健康调查基本方法（1-4版），国际疾病分类法在牙医学的应用（1-3版）。WHO自1969年以来建立了全球口腔资料库（Global Oral Data Bank， GODB），每年发布一次全球龋病流行趋势报告。在1975年与1978年的二次世界卫生大会上，通过了有关饮水氟化预防龋病的两项决议，向各成员国作出积极推荐。把12岁儿童的龋均不超过3作为一项指标纳入2000年人人享有卫生保健的指标体系中，并提出了2000年人人享有卫生保健的同时也享有口腔卫生保健。1978年，把社区牙周治疗需要指数（Community Periodontal Index for Treatment Need， CPITN）作为指数纳入口腔健康调查基本方法中。1979年，WHO与FDI联合提出了2000年全球口腔卫生保健目标的指标体系。在WHO提出的人体健康十大标准中，把口腔健康作为十大标准之一，并把它具体规定为“牙齿清洁，无龋洞，无痛感，牙龈颜色正常，无出血现象”。70年代以来，WHO口腔卫生处（Oral Health Unit）与FDI合作，组成了15个联合工作组（JWG），开展了广泛的合作研究。1970年WHO组成了一个由11个国家参加的口腔保健提供系统国际合作研究项目（ICS-I），并在70年代中陆续在各个国家进行了调查与资料收集工作，直到1985年才完成了整个调查工作并由WHO出版了《口腔卫生保健系统》的专项调查文集，其后又组织了由6个国家参加的ICS II项目，主要调查口腔健康结果（oral health outcomes），到90年代中期完成了整个调查报告。80年代以来，WHO的主要工作是开展社区预防并帮助发展中国家培训人员、建立机构，开展项目，统称为国际合作口腔卫生发展项目（international collaborative oral health development programme）。在1983年与1989年世界卫生大会的决议案中，确认把口腔卫生保健纳入初级卫生保健途径，作为其中一个组成部分。1982年在泰国清迈成立了WHO地区口腔卫生保健中心，开展了社区口腔保健模式的试点，尝试采用模拟操作培训基层口腔保健人员。不久，又在叙利亚大马士革成立第二个地区合作中心，开始了学校口腔健康教育的试点。直到20世纪末，WHO已在全球建立了38个口腔卫生保健合作中心和4个地区合作中心。

Since 1948, after the establishment of the World Health Organization (WHO) , the concept of health was defined by WHO in its constitution that “Health is a complete state of physical, mental and social well-being and not merely the absence of disease or infirmity.” And the goal of WHO set out in 1948 namely:” the attainment by all peoples of the highest possible level of health.”

It is appropriate to look at the contribution of WHO to achievement of these advances in last more than 50 years.

In the 1950s, the Oral Health Programme was established. The actual efforts were analyzed carefully in order to recognize the urgent problems and to develop a general policy for prevention and control of oral diseases.

20世纪50年代之后，预防口腔医学与口腔公共卫生在美国与欧洲国家迅速发展。从40年代开始，Michigan大学在Dr. Kenneth A. Easlick指导下首次开设了口腔公共卫生研究生课程，培训口腔公共卫生专家。今天，许多学院都在Michigan之后开设了高级学位课程。1954年，美国Oregon大学的Dr. D.M. Hadjimarkos进行了一次全国范围的调查，发现虽然有30所学院开设了公共卫生课程，但课时较少，只有5所学院有16学时的课程。1960年，Philip E. Blackerby，W.K. Kellogy基金会口腔医学部主任发表了一篇文章“为什么没有社会口腔医学学科？”他提出了一门与环境有关的口腔医学。从此，几乎所有的学院都采纳了这一观点。虽然学科名称不一样，如环境口腔医学、社区口腔医学、预防和公共卫生口腔医学、生态口腔医学等，但是他们的目标都是通过各种手段促进全民的口腔健康，包括临床服务、学校儿童的口腔检查以及公众的健康教育。1950 年建立了美国口腔公共卫生委员会，宗旨在于促进全民的口腔健康。

在战后的年代里，增加了“第三方支付费用”的方式，主要由保险公司提供支付基本口腔保健的费用。在60～70年代，许多联盟在劳资谈判协议中担保这样的口腔保健计划，到1980年几乎有 1 亿美国人在一定程度上纳入了口腔保险计划。

美国的口腔保健预付计划的经验完全不同于欧洲，在那里已有许多国家多年来存在着由政府资助的口腔保健。英国在第二次世界大战之后，首先采取社会化医疗保健计划，包括口腔保健。其他国家如挪威、丹麦只为学校儿童提供免费口腔保健，为成人提供政府保险计划。在法国，口腔保健纳入社会安全系统，偿还病人75%的花费。在德国有类似的政府经营的保险计划（包括 97% 的人口）。在丹麦与卢森堡，偿还 80% 的费用。卢森堡最近已采取了新的措施鼓励预防口腔医学，一个人如果每年都为预防保健的目的就诊，保险计划将支付全部的费用。瑞典也鼓励预防，1973 年的大众口腔保健法也增加了预防口腔医学的费用支付。

In 1954 Dr. D.M. Hadjimarkos of the University of Oregon made a nationwide survey and found that though thirty schools at that time included public health in their curriculum, in fact little time was devoted to it: only five schools allocated as much as sixteen hours to the subject.

The first graduate course of study in dental public health was established in the 1940s by the University of Michigan under the direction of Dr. Kenneth A. Easlick, a member of the faculty of the School of Public Health. Easlick trained other dental public-health specialists, and today a number of schools have followed Michigan's lead and established courses leading to advanced degrees in the field.

In 1960 Philip E. Blackerby, then director of the division of dentistry of the W. K. Kellogg Foundation, presented a paper before the American Association of Dental Schools entitled "Why Not a Department of Social Dentistry?" He envisioned a discipline that would relate dentistry to the environment, and since then almost all schools have taken up the idea, although the names they have given their departments are many and various, ranging from environmental dentistry, community dentistry, preventive and public-health dentistry, to ecological dentistry. They all, however, have as their objective the improvement of the dental health of the population by a variety of means, including clinics, examination of schoolchildren, and public-health education.

The establishment in 1950 of the American Board of Dental Public health has immeasurably aided in promoting dental health throughout the world. This country has been the undisputed leader in the field, and dentists of many other nations have come to American schools to gain knowledge and experience that they then have carried back to their homelands.

The decades that followed World War II also saw a great change in the means by which dental care is made available to the people of the United States and Europe in this country there has been a tremendous increase in group practices and clinics. No longer an almost exclusively one-man, one-office profession, dentistry in many areas is organized into groups of practitioners operating under one roof, who pool their skills for the patients' benefit.

Also beneficial has been the increase during the postwar years of "third-party payers." These are essentially insurance group plans that provide payment for basic, routine dental care, plus, in certain instances, more extensive dentistry at an additional premium. During the 1960s and 1970s many unions secured such dental plans in their collective-bargaining agreements, and by 1980 almost 100 million Americans were covered, to some degree, by a dental insurance plan.

The American experience with dental prepayment plans is quite different from that in Europe, where some form of government-sponsored dental insurance has existed in a number of countries for many years. Great Britain took the lead immediately after World War II with its socialized medicine plan, which included dental care. Other countries, such as Norway and Denmark, provide free dental care to schoolchildren only, offering government insurance plans to adults. In France, dental care is incorporated into the social security system, which reimburses the patient for 75 percent of his costs. Similar government run insurance plans are operative in West Germany (in which 97 percent of the population is enrolled) and in Denmark and Luxembourg, where patients are reimbursed for up to 80 percent of their costs. Luxembourg has recently pioneered a novel procedure to encourage preventive dentistry: if a person visits the dentist every year for preventive care, the insurance plan pays 100 percent of the charges. Sweden, too, fosters prevention, and its 1973 Law of General dental Health Insurance also ensure increased payment for preventive dentistry.

这一时期，另一个对全球口腔预防保健有深刻影响的权威机构是成立于1948年的美国国立牙科研究所（National Institute for Dental Research， NIDR）。NIDR成立后的头10年，主要是确认了社区饮水氟化防龋项目的安全、有效与经济。1956年在Grand Rapids的调查结果显示，儿童患龋率下降了60%以上，使饮水氟化项目取得了重大的科学突破，是口腔预防医学的一项革命，历史上第一次证明龋病是可以预防的。如今，饮水氟化已经得到了世界上150多个科学与卫生组织的认可，已有39个国家2亿1千万人在饮用氟化水。饮水氟化被称为是继饮水净化、牛奶巴斯消毒、免疫注射之后的第四次公共卫生革命。

60年代，NIDR的主要贡献是证实了龋病与牙周病都是感染性疾病。70年代NIDR的病毒学研究，如疱疹病毒等，获得了世界公认。并且在全美的氟水漱口示范项目、社会行为科学与口腔健康的关系等研究方面取得了进展。80年代又在细胞与分子生物学新技术方面有了新的发展。在流行病学调查与研究方面不断有新的发现。

After the establishment of the National Institute of Dental Research (NIDR) in 1948, the third of now 11 National Institutes of Health, progress moved more swiftly. The NIDR supported the major experiments and clinical studies that confirmed what for long had remained controversial theories: dental caries and the periodontal diseases are infectious disorders. They can be controlled by a variety of mechanical, chemical or surgical means. They can be prevented by regimens designed to clean, preserve, strengthen and protect teeth and gums.

中国预防医学的发展主要始于20世纪50年代。从牙医学向口腔医学的调整与发展也发生在这个时期。50年代初，预防牙医学曾作为一门课程在几所大学的牙医学系中讲授，在口腔医学迅速发展的阶段，由于受到当时前苏联教学模式的影响，预防牙医学不再作为一门课程，而并入口腔内科学范畴。但在50～60年代间，龋病与牙周病的社会调查、龋病病因学的研究、氟化物防龋的研究、在广州、东莞相继开始的饮水氟化防龋试点项目以及口腔医疗小分队在学校、厂矿、居民区与农村开展的普查普治与群防群治工作等还是取得了一定的进展。例如，1950年上海《大众医学》开始了口腔卫生宣传教育。1951年北京设立流动口腔保健站。1957年成立龋病牙周病全国调查委员会，制订统一调查标准。1958年姜元川编著了第一本《牙病预防学》专著，比较全面地阐述了牙病防治的原理与方法，提出了牙病预防学的学科性质是“自然科学与社会科学的结合”，对象是“群体口腔健康”，内容是“调查统计、实验研究、宣教推广三个类型，组成相互联系的一门完整学科……是口腔科方面的一种社会医学和预防医学”。尽管从现代预防口腔医学发展的水平看，在认识上、内容上与方法上还有欠缺与不完善之处，但对推动我国预防口腔医学的发展起到奠基的作用。此外，60年代还在龋病和牙周病的病因学，氟防龋作用等方面开展了研究，并对高氟地区的氟牙症流行状况进行了调查。70年代中，广州因饮水氟化一度出现氟牙症而引起学术争议。1975年在全国推广保健牙刷。开始了防龋涂料、变形链球菌与龋病关系的研究，分析了中国人的龋病患病状况。1980年，北京医科大学口腔医学系第一个成立了口腔预防科。

80年代以来，WHO开始帮助中国发展口腔保健项目。1981～1983年联合国开发署（United Nations Development Programme， UNDP）首先资助中国发展口腔预防项目，聘请WHO的巴姆斯（D.E. Barmes）和森特（C.T. Sundram）博士为项目顾问。1981年举办了首次全国高校教师培训班，引进了WHO的标准口腔健康调查方法、状况分析、口腔健康教育与疾病预防。1982年WHO与北京医科大学口腔系口腔预防科合作，首先开始了口腔健康捷径调查。同时把北京医科大学口腔医学研究所确定为中国第一个世界卫生组织预防牙医学研究与培训合作中心。同年，在卫生部领导下，由北京医科大学口腔预防科负责指导开始采用WHO标准方法进行了第一次全国学生龋病与牙周病流行学病调查，使中国的预防口腔医学开始逐步与国际接轨。1984年公布了调查结果。1985年得到了联合国儿童基金会（UNICEF）的资助，在部分地区开始了为期5年的学校儿童初级口腔卫生保健项目。同年，以山西运城为基地，开始探索中国农村社区口腔保健模式。1987年第一版高等口腔医学专业教材《口腔预防医学》正式出版。至此，全国已有5所高校成立了口腔预防教研室，口腔预防医学作为一门独立课程开始正式纳入教学课程中。同年，中华医学会口腔医学专业委员会口腔预防学组在天津第一次召开了全国口腔预防医学研讨会。1988年WHO西太平洋地区办事处在运城召开了本地区的口腔保健项目管理研讨会，并确定运城口腔卫生学校为WHO农村口腔保健合作中心。继1987年北京WHO／DANIDA口腔公共卫生培训班之后，1988年全国牙病防治指导组成立。1989年在北京举办了第二届国际预防牙医学大会，中国的预防口腔医学与世界展开了国际交流。同年9月以“爱牙健齿强身”为中心主题，开展了全国爱牙日活动。这一切有代表性的事件标志着预防口腔医学的科学基础与社会实践的结合已经在中国取得初步成效，并缩短了中国与世界的距离。

90年代以来，预防口腔医学在国内取得的主要进展是：制订了2000年我国口腔预防保健目标规划，完成了第二次全国口腔健康流行病学调查与报告，连续开展了11届全国爱牙日活动并对其社会影响进行了监测与评价。成立了中国牙病防治基金会，资助了一批口腔预防应用研究项目。1996年与1997年分别成立了中华预防医学会口腔卫生保健专业委员会与中华口腔医学会口腔预防医学专业委员会，同时举办了口腔预防保健最新进展国际学术报告会与第一届国际龋病预防学术研讨会，举办了非创伤性充填治疗技术（Atraumatic Restorative Treatment，ART）培训班。在预防口腔医学的教学方面，编著出版了第二版、第三版、第四版教材，许多高等与中等院校都单独开设了预防口腔医学课程，并开始探索社会实践的途径，以便使新一代口腔专业人员在知识、态度与技能方面具备从事社区口腔保健工作的能力。

Oral health status and trends in the Chinese population

During the period between 1949 and the mid 1980s, there were several hundred local oral health investigations on dental caries status in students, farmers, housewives, and minority groups.

As early as 1957, the Medical Scientific Committee of the Ministry of Health established a national committee for the investigation and statistical analyses of dental caries and periodontal diseases. The results found by this committee played a role in guidance, but were not widely applied due to statistical problems arising from too many items and details on the surveys.

By the early 1980s, the World Health Organization cooperated with the Research Institute of Stomatology, Beijing Medical University, and designated it as a first WHO Collaborating Centre for Research and Training in Preventive Dentistry in China. One of the prime missions of this centre was, and continues to be, to train dental personnel to serve as the backbone in teaching and research of oral prevention. In 1981, under the direction and participation of D.E. Barmes, chief dental officer of Oral Health Unit, WHO worked together with the staff of the Department of Preventive Dentistry, School of Stomatology, Beijing Medical University to undertake a survey in Beijing using WHO basic methods. In the same year, a training course for faculty members from key dental schools in China was held in Beijing, during which WHO basic methods for oral health epidemiologic surveys were introduced. In 1982, a first epidemiological survey for school children was carried out. These data demonstrated the oral health status of the Chinese population, the mean DMFT (weighted) was 0.67 at 12 years of age, which is a very low level according to the WHO standards; however, caries experience in the primary dentition at 7 years of age was moderate (72.66% with caries; mean DMFT, 3.7).

With respect to periodontal conditions as assessed by WHO standards, the average number of sextants with calculus was 2.43 (weighted) at 15 years of age, which was also low, and the average number of sextants with gingivitis was 2.83.

The Second National Oral Health Epidemiological Survey was completed in 1995, under the leadership of the Ministry of Health, and was conducted by the National Committee for Oral Health and financially supported by China Oral Health Foundation. The statistically analyzed data demonstrated that the mean DMFT was 0.88 (weighted) in children 12 years of age.

With respect to periodontal conditions, the percentage of calculus in children 15 years of age remained at a low level (67.91%) with a mean of 2.46 sextants per person, and the percentage of bleeding was 34.93%. The soft debris index was higher in all age groups and indicated poor oral hygiene.

In general, the data available from the two National oral health epidemiological surveys and other available local data indicated that the number of caries experiences appears to follow significant changes in lifestyle and improvement in living conditions. The general trend in dental caries prevalence, based on WHO standards, was still at a low or very low level. The single exception is the higher caries experience in the deciduous dentition; and its causes and influencing factors are unclear. It is estimated that a slow upward trend will continue if no community-based public health measures are taken. Periodontal conditions would not be significantly changed and oral hygiene status would probably be improved. Therefore, it seems necessary to regularly monitor oral health status.

Promotion of Oral Health

During the more than 30 years from 1949 to the early 1980s, there were only a few activities in public oral health propaganda and education. Since 1980, the International Children's Day has been defined as an oral health propaganda day in Shanghai. In 1982, Bai Chengping published the first issue of "Dental Care for Friends," and in 1987 a "Love Teeth Day" campaign was initiated in Lanzhou City. After the establishment of the National Committee for Oral Health (NCOH) in 1988, an announcement was made in an official document that nine government and nongovernment organizations jointly designated September 20 of each year for the Love Teeth Day. This 1989 announcement was based on a proposal by the older generation of experts. Since then, a massive campaign on Love teeth Day (LTD) and other oral health promotion programs and activities, such as oral health world, oral health promotion action, and New Long March for oral health have been implemented nationwide. Under the central slogan of "Love teeth, care for teeth, and be healthy and strong," a theme with a special slogan has been defined each year to guide each campaign through news and other mass media. Face-to-face consultations on the streets have been undertaken to transfer oral health knowledge, improve self-care skills, and to carry out oral examinations.

Although oral health promotion activities have affected about 50% of the population, they are still neglected in rural and remote areas, where lack of basic knowledge, ineffective toothbrushing, and poor oral hygiene are common.

Objectives, strategies, and measures for oral health

In the early 1980s, following the global goal of "health for all by the year 2000" and the basic approach of "primary health care" as defined by the WHO, after the establishment of the NCOH in 1988, a national goal of "primary oral health care for all by the year 2000," with its relevant indicators and strategies, was laid down.

Basic oral health care services were provided to children living in the kindergartens or schools

International cooperation and academic exchange

Since 1980 China has started to cooperate with WHO and other international organization in developing oral health programmes. The first collaborating project on research in oral health was supported by UNDP and technical consultation made by WHO from 1981 to 1983. The overall objective was to develop oral health care services, especially for children.

A national teachers' training course on oral health was conducted in 1981. WHO basic methods and standards on oral epidemioiogical survey, methodology on oral health education and promotion, and oral diseases prevention have been popularized through the course.

The first department of preventive dentistry in China set up in the school of Stomatology, Beijing medical university (BMU) in 1980. Since then, the Research Institute of Stomatology, BMU was designated as the first WHO collaborating centre for training and research in preventive dentistry in 1981.

In 1980's, several training courses in preventive dentistry and dental public health also sponsored by WHO regional office for the western pacific (WPR) were held in Beijing and other cities of China.

On the other hand, under the WHO's support, a few dental professionals participated some other training courses in oral epidemiology, dental public health and pit and fissure sealant in Malaysia, Thailand and New Zealand.

From 1985 to 1989, a5-year project entitled "primary oral health care for school children" sponsored by UNICEF, was conducted by the department of prevention, BMU. .There were two provinces and Beijing Municipality involved in the project. In 1987, a WHO/DANIDA training course in dental public health was introduced.

A WPR workshop on management of the oral health programme took place in Yuncheng WHO collaboration centre for rural oral health designated in 1988.

The Second World Congress on Preventive Dentistry, jointly sponsored by WHO, WHO Collaboration Centre in Beijing, and School of Stomatology, BMU, was successfully held in Beijing in 1989, and more than 300 participants from 29 countries and regions of the World participated.

四、21 世纪口腔健康科学的发展时代 The developmental era of oral health science in the 21st century

20世纪后半叶，口腔卫生保健最基本的进展之一是日益增强了它的科学基础。口腔健康与疾病预防的生物学机制方面的许多研究提供了大量的科学证据，进一步认清了龋病和牙周病这两大主要口腔疾病的性质。毫无疑问，所有这些已使口腔卫生保健的各个方面发生了巨大变革，其结果是使得相对狭隘而又主要集中在技术工艺方面的牙医学变成为科学基础广泛、社会功能更强大的生物医学学科——口腔健康科学。

21世纪，人们对口腔健康的需要与期望更多、更高。他们把口腔健康看作为口腔幸福，它的内涵已远远超出了传统的“口福”概念。没有口腔疾病和保持最佳的口腔功能状态，以这种方式维护一个人的最高自尊与最佳人际关系。

人类的口腔除了口腔的疾病外，还是许多感染性疾病的传播途径和不健康因素的载体。例如，精神压力、烟酒及其他毒物，某些地方习俗都可能有损于口腔和全身健康。因此，促进口腔健康信息的传播，防止有害因素对正常口腔功能及全身健康的伤害，应纳入 21 世纪口腔健康的目标之内。

适量氟化物防龋措施的应用，已经使龋病大幅度下降。如果采取全面的预防措施，将会使儿童与成人的龋病继续下降，至少到 2025 年时 50 ～ 60 岁的人会出现龋病减少的状况。对龋病的对策主要是预防和控制，而不是治疗。有些群体对危险因素更敏感，或者较多暴露于危险因素之中，对这些危险因素需要有进一步的研究和认识。

当我们迈进21世纪时，最终消除龋病和牙周病这两大口腔疾病不仅合理，而且可能。因为没有其他健康学科能像预防口腔医学那样，如此快地取得巨大成果。现代的知识虽不能消除，但也足以控制龋病。在某些工业化国家已阻止了导致牙齿丧失的牙周病，而且牙科研究继续在产生新的材料技术，新的诊断与治疗方法以及广泛的预防措施，以较好的方式为公众提供这些产品与服务，将会取得丰硕成果。

One of the fundamental advances in oral health care has been the increasing emphasis on its scientific basis. Research has done much to clarify the biological mechanisms involved in oral health and the prevention of disease, and to increase understanding of the nature of the two main oral diseases, caries and periodontal disease. Undoubtedly, this has revolutionized all aspects of oral health care. As a result, a primarily technical profession with a relatively narrow focus has adopted a more appropriate role as a broadly and scientifically based biomedical discipline: dentistry has become oral health care - oral health science.

Oral health is the well-being of the oral cavity, including the dentition and its supporting structures and tissues - the absence of disease and the optimal functioning of the mouth and its tissues, in a manner which preserves the highest level of self-esteem and interpersonal relationships. Retention of functional teeth is clearly the foundation of this state, high quality replacement being the second choice in maintaining adequate oral health and well-being.

Oral health problems negatively affect the quality of human life. Maintaining the most desirable levels of oral health and function, within the context of healthy lifestyle practices, is the goal for now as well as for the longer term.

Positive oral functions include eating (masticating, tasting, swallowing, digesting) communicating orally (speaking, singing, kissing, etc.), breathing, and presenting a pleasing appearance; all of these contributing substantially to one's self-esteem and ability to engage in satisfying interpersonal relationships.

However, the oral cavity may also serve as a vehicle for unhealthy, sometimes stress-related, habits such as the use of tobacco, alcohol and other toxic substances. In addition, some local customs may also be harmful to oral and general health. The need to disseminate health-promoting information to limit these harmful practices which reduce proper function should be included in oral health objectives for the 21st century.

Dental caries: preventive measures, especially exposure to appropriate levels of fluoride from a variety of sources, have brought about a dramatic decline in the prevalence of dental caries in industrialized countries over the past few decades. In countries that have access to a full range of preventive measures, caries will continue to decline in children and adults, at least to 50-60 years of age by 2025. In the long term, it is anticipated that caries management will be transformed into a prevention and control, rather than a therapeutic problem.

Periodontal diseases: periodontal health is improving in some industrialized countries, especially for age groups below 60 years of age.

Where improvement has occurred, it is believed that better oral hygiene has played a key role. As hygiene continues to improve, and decline to very low levels by 2025.

As we approach the 21st century, the eventual goal of virtually eliminating the two main oral diseases appears not only to be reasonable, but also probable for a large majority in most populations. Perhaps no other health discipline has realized such a quick and dramatic result from efforts in prevention. Current knowledge is sufficient to control, if not eliminate, caries. Periodontal diseases have already ceased to be a major cause of tooth loss in some industrialized countries. Moreover, dental research continues to yield a rich harvest of new and better materials and techniques, new diagnostic methods and treatments, and a broad array of preventive options, and better ways to deliver these products and services to the public.

口腔保健提供方面的重大改变或发展趋势，现时还难以认清。然而，健康服务，包括口腔保健，全球趋于私有化发展的趋势。在工业化国家已经如此，有迹象表明，发展中国家也会这样。许多国家都在进行卫生保健经费新体制的尝试或实施。

工业化国家的口腔保健项目中，已减少了治疗，增加了对保健的重视。更关注预防与确定可能发病的高危人群。发展中国家有众多的保健提供体制，从西方式的私人开业与很少比例的国立机构，到由卫生部提供的妇幼保健所与学校的预防项目，或者由正规或非正规人员提供的急诊保健，主要是成人拔牙。

一方面是更多的学校开展系统预防与治疗，以及初级卫生保健服务；另一面是给传统体制施加压力，用高科技、修复产品来取代预防，显然这在质量、成本以及接受等方面并不恰当。发展中国家面临着口腔专业人员大量流向工业化国家的问题。在我国，则是大量流向发达地区、改行、私人开业。工业化国家的大学生、研究生教育方面已有大的改变。特别是欧洲重视教育过程，以及卫生人员的标准化培养。

在工业化国家，人们逐渐认识到健康牙列对生命质量的价值，口腔保健（专业与自我保健）成为生活方式的一部分。寻求口腔保健服务的人口在增加，为预防目的就诊的人群在增加（检查、洁治），同时因出现症状就诊的人数在减少。

1. 制订口腔卫生保健规划的指导原则 Guiding principles for future planning

公共卫生机构在制订口腔卫生保健规划时，首先要结合现有的资料，同时遵循下列指导原则：

（1）口腔健康是全身健康、维持正常机体功能以及提高生命质量的基础；

（2）口腔卫生保健人员要关注全身健康并参与到维护全身健康的活动中；

（3）口腔卫生保健人员的类型、数量以及分布必须与需要、质量、成本以及可及性保持一致的水平才能达到所期望的口腔健康状况；

（4）计划、卫生保健措施以及健康项目应该针对人群或环境中存在的问题；

（5）研究、评价与教育是口腔健康继续发展的基础；

（6）卫生专业人员必须终生不断学习；

（7）维护和促进口腔健康应采取最经济的方式，并与服务的质量和服务的可及性相一致；

（8）预防比治疗更为可取；

（9）尽可能地调动个人的积极性来促进和维护个人口腔健康；

（10）龋病与牙周病是可以预防和控制的；

（11）社区预防方法应有个人或自我保健的支持，在有些情况下是更为有效的；

（12）口腔卫生保健应当是综合卫生保健的一部分。

Guiding principles for future planning

Most public health organizations and agencies are involved in future planning for the short-term, e.g., goals for the next decade, five-year work programmes and budgets, etc. however, the development of guidelines and recommendations for a longer range future is not so common nor simple. While data regarding current trends and advances are (hopefully) objective, the extrapolation of those data into a picture of the future, and the planning for that future, can be highly subjective. To minimize this subjectivity, before making recommendations, the members of the group first agreed on a set of guiding principles - standard precepts of oral public health which are not constrained by time or circumstances. It is the understanding, acceptance, and application of these principles which form the basis for sound recommendations for the future.

(1) oral health is an essential part of general health, human function and the quality of life;

(2) oral health care providers should be prepared and motivated to consider general health, and should participate in the provision of general health care;

(3) the type, number and distribution of oral health care personnel should be maintained at levels consistent with need, quality, cost and access necessary to achieve desired oral health status;

(4) planning, health care practices and educational programmes should be appropriate for the population or situation in question;

(5) research, evaluation and education are essential for the continued advancement of oral health;

(6) learning must continue throughout the career of the health professional;

(7) oral health status should be improved and maintained in the most economical manner consistent with quality and access;

(8) prevention is preferable to treatment as a general rule;

(9) individuals should be motivated to do as much as possible for themselves to achieve and maintain oral health;

(10) caries and periodontal diseases can be prevented and controlled;

(11) community methods of prevention should be supportive of individual and personal care and in some situations is more efficient;

(12) oral health care should be provided in the context of comprehensive care.

2. 世界卫生组织促进21世纪口腔健康的途径 The approach of continuous improvement of oral health in the 21st century

在世界上除少数地区外，慢性疾病与创伤是健康的首要问题。快速改变的疾病谱与变化中的生活方式有紧密联系，它包括富糖膳食，吸烟，酗酒等。口腔疾病与这些生活方式因素也高度相关。口腔疾病在所有人群中的患病率都较高，在弱势群体中，其疾病负担更大，必然会影响到生命质量。WHO防制慢性病的全球策略增加了共同危险因素途径是防制口腔疾病的一种新策略。

2000年，第53届世界卫生大会推荐“把重点放在与多种疾病有联系的共同的、可以预防的、与生活方式有关的危险因素方面（如不健康的膳食，吸烟），包括口腔健康。”

WHO正在建立口腔健康信息系统以便监测全球口腔疾病与危险因素的发展趋势。WHO评价了 2000 年 WHO / FDI 的全球口腔健康目标的完成情况，并开始制订新的 2020 年的目标。目的是为不同水平的卫生政策制订者提供一个框架，其目标主要着眼于全球水平，鼓励地方采取行动。

Chronic diseases and injuries are the leading health problems in all but a few parts of the world. The rapidly changing disease patterns throughout the world are closely linked to changing lifestyles, which include diets rich in sugars, widespread use of tobacco, and increased consumption of alcohol. In addition to socio-environmental determinants, oral disease is highly related to these lifestyle factors, which are risks to most chronic diseases as well as protective factors such as appropriate exposure to fluoride and good oral hygiene. Oral diseases qualify as major public health problems owing to their high prevalence and incidence in all regions of the world, and as for all diseases, the greatest burden of oral diseases is on disadvantaged and socially marginalized populations. The severe impact in terms of pain and suffering, impairment of function and effect on quality of life must also be considered. Traditional treatment of oral diseases is extremely costly in several industrialized countries, and not feasible in most low-income and middle-income countries. The WHO Global Strategy for Prevention and Control of Non-communicable Diseases, added to the common risk factor approach is a new strategy for managing prevention and control of oral diseases.

The new public health is no longer oriented to single diseases. The Common Risk/Health Factor approach (CRHFA) distinguishes between actions aimed at reducing "risk factors" and actions promoting "health factors". The strategy includes efforts to improve health by reducing risks, promoting health and strengthening possibilities to cope with "given" risk factors - creating supportive environments reducing the negative effects of certain risk factors and facilitating behaviour changes. A major benefit of the Common Risk/Health Factor approach is the focus on improving health conditions in general for the whole population and for groups at high risk. It thereby reduces social inequities.

The 53rd World Health Assembly (resolution WHA 53.17) endorsed to the formulation of a global strategy for prevention and central of these non-communicable diseases. Priority is given to diseases linked by common, preventable and lifestyle related risk factors (e.g. unhealthy diet, tobacco use) , including oral health.

At WHO, information systems are being established for the surveillance of global trends in oral disease and risk factors. The main surveillance tool is called STEPS (STEP-wise approach to surveillance) . WHO Oral Health Programmes recently assessed the accomplishment of the WHO/FDI goals for oral health by the year 2000. The formulation of new WHO goals has been initiated. It aims to provide a framework for health policy makers. The goals and targets are not intended to be prescriptive. By being focused broadly on the global level, it is hoped that it will encourage local action in the spirit of the United Nations Development programmes report: "Think globally act locally". This, the document will provide an instrument for local and national health care planners specify realistic goals and standards for oral health to be achieved by the year 2020.

根据我国人民现时的口腔疾病患病状况与发展趋势，现有的以及可以预料到的未来口腔医疗保健资源的状况，要想使全民都能享有最基本的口腔卫生保健，只有通过教育，研究与服务三个方面加快发展预防口腔医学与社会口腔医学，即口腔公共卫生。

联合国人口年鉴（1994）有一篇为“口腔保健评价”的专题文章指出：全球 80% ~ 85% 的人口无口腔保健，15% 的人享有急诊和基本保健，其中只有 1% ~ 2% 的人享有优质口腔保健。大多数经济学家都同意，医疗性保健在现代化国家里对全民的健康贡献很小。英国著名口腔公共卫生学家Sheiham教授指出，传统的口腔医疗性保健只对社会口腔健康状况的改善起到微薄的作用。

发展预防口腔医学的战略意义在于：（1）加强预防口腔医学是降低主要口腔疾病的发病率，失牙率和提高群体口腔健康水平及生命质量最有效、最经济的战略措施；（2）预防口腔医学是促进社会经济持续发展、社会文明发展以及提高综合国力的有力保障。2010年“人人享有初级口腔卫生保健”标志着 21 世纪我国全民口腔保健时代的开始。

总而言之，推动学科发展的动力来自群众的需求。通过科学研究提供充分的证据发展循征口腔保健，用于社会实践，促进全民口腔健康，减少社会不公平性，提高全民的生命质量是21世纪我国预防口腔医学发展的方向。

第三节　口腔卫生保健供给体制
Section 3 Oral Health Care Delivery Systems

一、简介与背景 Introduction and background

口腔保健供给体制（或称提供系统）的组织机构与职能能够满足人们的口腔保健需求时，则为健全的体制。这个体制必须有效地教育和培训人员、提供口腔保健服务、进行成本效果分析，必须适应它所服务人群的不断变化的需要。

口腔保健提供系统是一个复杂的组织，它有一个不断变化的过程。口腔医学是其中很小的组成部分，其本身是整个社会福利系统的一部分。口腔医师需要了解卫生保健提供系统的基本要素。

世界上存在着不同的卫生保健系统。现代卫生保健系统的性质反映出其社会已经形成的价值观。在美国大部分是私人或私立组织提供卫生服务。我国的卫生保健系统是由国家控制和公共经费支持的。

A dental care delivery system is efficient when its structure, organization, and performance satisfy the dental needs of the population it serves in the best way possible. This requires efficiency in the education and training of its dental manpower, as well as in the production, distribution, consumption, and financing of dental services. To remain efficient over time, a dental care delivery system must adapt to the changing needs of the population it serves.

Health care systems are complex organizations that are in a constant process of change and evolution. Dentistry is one very small component of the wider health care system, which is itself part of the overall social welfare system within society. Dentists, as health professionals, need to understand the basic elements of the health care system within which they are working.

Modern health care systems and the health professionals providing care within them have a long history of evolution and development. Across the world different systems of health care have emerged, linked to the social and political changes within each country. Historically only the wealthy had access to doctors, but gradually systems of care developed for a wider range of groups in society, often due to concerns over political instability and the fitness of army recruits (Mays 1991) .

The nature of modern health care systems largely reflects the values and priorities of the societies in which they have developed. In the US a largely privately funded and organized health system operates, based upon the notion of individual responsibilities. In total contrast, health services in countries such as Cuba or China are state controlled and publicly funded. These systems are based upon a concept of collective benefit.

二、影响现代卫生保健系统发展的因素 Factors influencing development of modern health care systems

影响卫生保健系统的发展与变化的主要因素有：疾病谱的改变、社会人口状况改变、公众的要求与期望、专业人员的培养、高科技的发展、国际事务全球化、政府的卫生政策与改革项目等。

Factors influencing development of modern health care systems are changing patterns of disease, socio-demographic changes, public demands and expectations, professional development, high technology, international affairs-globalization, and government health policy and reform programmes.

三、卫生保健体制的组成 Components of health care systems

Gift等提出了卫生保健体制的组成包括：机构、职能、人员、经费投入、支付方式、以及目标人群。

1. 机构 Structure

组织机构通常存在三个基本保健水平：

初级水平：当地的综合与常规服务，它是公众与系统之间第一个接触点，例如，全科医生、药师、口腔全科医生等。在我国则是乡村医生，一般只能提供最基本的初级卫生保健服务。

二级水平：在医院机构内由专业人员提供的服务，如，区综合医院。在我国，则是乡镇卫生院或社区卫生保健中心，一般由执业医师提供常见病的防治服务。

三级水平：为最高的临床机构，常常是教学与研究机构，例如，大学的附属医院。在我国的农村地区则是县医院以上的各级医院。

Gift et al. (1997) have suggested the following approach:

Structure: how is the system organized?

Functions: what does the system aim to achieve?

Personnel: who works in the system?

Funding: how is the system funded?

Reimbursement: how are the health professionals paid?

Target population: who does the system provide care for?

The organization and structure is one of the most complex and dynamic components of the system. However three basic levels of care often exist within a system:

Primary: local general and routine services, which are the first point of contact between the public and the system; for example, general practitioners, pharmacists, general dental practitioners.

Secondary: specialist services provided in hospital settings; for example, district general hospital.

Tertiary: centres of clinical excellence, which are often teaching and research institutions; for example, university hospitals.

2. 职能 Functions

按传统的医疗模式，卫生服务的目的是为患者提供治疗。现在逐渐认识到大多数的治疗效果有限，取而代之是为全民提供保健。

在卫生保健服务中，除提供治疗外，还有其他职能，如社区健康教育与促进、流行病学调查、研究、服务质量监控、人员培训等。

Traditionally，health services following the medical model have aimed at curing disease in sick patients. It is now increasingly recognized，however，that few cures or "magic bullets" exist，and indeed many treatments have only limited effectiveness（Cochrance 1972). Instead，a core function of medicine is to provide care and support for individuals suffering from chronic conditions to improve their quality of life（McKeown 1979).

Although the provision of treatments is the dominant activity with in health services，other functions are also performed to a lesser extent. These include: preventive advice to patients; health promotion within the community; epidemiological surveying; population screening; research; quality assurance and review; training; and personnel.

3. 人员 Personnel

在卫生服务机构内，雇用各种不同的人员。Friodson概括出卫生专业人员的主要特征：必须具备执业资格；专业技能要求高；具备行业自治与自律；遵循执业医师道德规范等。

A range of different personnel are employed within health services. What distinguishes health professionals from the other staff employed within health services? Friedson (1970) has developed a core set of defining characteristics of the professions:

Tasks are highly skilled and require specialized knowledge;

Registration provides a monopoly of their field of work;

Professions have enjoyed considerable autonomy and self-regulation;

A code of ethical practice prevents malpractice and exploitation of the public.

4. 经费投入 Funding

用于卫生服务方面的经费投入逐年增加已成为政府主要考虑的问题。卫生服务资金的主要来源包括税收、保险以及个人。

Spending on health services has been rising steadily in most industrialized countries for many years. The basic sources of funding for health services are taxation, insurance, and individuals.

5. 支付方式 Reimbursement systems

卫生服务的支付方式有很多种。主要有：

按项目付费：按医生提供的每项服务内容支付；

人头费：按医生提供服务的病人数目支付；

工资：按医生年薪支付；

按期支付：按合同支付。

A range of different methods have been developed to reimburse health professionals for their services. Systems of reimbursement can become very complex when a mixture of different methods of payment are utilized. Essentially there are four basic systems of payment:

Fee for item: practitioners are paid a fee for each item of work they provide.

Capitation: payment is based upon the numbers of patients the practitioner has registered under their care.

Salary: employers pay an annual income for the services provided by practitioners.

Sessional arrangements: a set fee is agreed in a contract between employer and practitioner.

6. 目标人群 Target population

为全人口提供卫生服务是一个基本原则。根据需要，不同卫生保健服务针对不同的人群。

Based on an assessment of particular needs or characteristics of potential users, different services within the system may also be targeted at groups within the population.

四、卫生保健体制的完善 A good health care system

Maxwell（1984）提出了评价卫生保健体制的标准如下：

效果：这个系统提供的治疗与保健是否达到了预期的结果与效益。

效率：在这个系统中资源是否被很好地利用。

可及性：需要的人是否能利用这个系统并从中获益。

公平性：每个公民是否有同等的机会。

社会可接受性：服务是否能达到社会人群的不同期望。

与需要相关性：所提供的服务是否与人群的需要匹配。

Maxwell (1984) has developed a useful set of criteria to evaluate the quality of a health care system:

Effectiveness: do the treatments and care provided in the system produce desired outcomes and benefits?

Efficiency: how well are the resources used within the system?

Accessibility: can individuals in need use and benefit from the system?

Equity: does the service provide a fair system for accessing care and are the outcomes of use equal across groups of users?

Social acceptability: does the service strive to accommodate the characteristics and expectations of diverse social groups across society?

Relevance to need: is there a good match between the needs of the population and the services offered?

五、口腔卫生保健的组织原则与提供模式 The principles of organization and models of oral health care delivery system

1. 口腔卫生保健供给系统 The Oral health care delivery system

世界上不同的口腔卫生保健系统有不同的历史根源。直到19世纪，在欧洲和美国，才有口腔卫生保健机构的注册和人员的培训。学校保健系统始于20世纪早期。20世纪龋病在工业化国家的快速增长，以及口腔材料与设备的改进影响着口腔卫生保健系统的发展。

在发展中国家，大多数没有单独的口腔卫生保健供给系统，口腔卫生保健供给系统是医疗保健系统的一部分。

口腔卫生保健系统应能适应人口结构、口腔疾病谱、口腔疾病与相关的其他系统疾病的变化，同时反映社会政治、经济结构的变化，以及国家政策法规和支付系统的变化。

Oral health care systems throughout the world have different historic roots. Dentistry as an established independent occupation was not widespread until the 19th century when oral health care became more organized with licensing and training in Europe and the USA. School care systems began early in the 20th century in several countries. During the 20th century, there was a rapid increase in dental caries in industrialized countries as well as improvements in dental therapeutics, materials and equipment. These factors, combined with expectations of medical and dental professionals, influenced the organization of systems of care as well as the structure and process of dental practices.

In some developing countries, there is no unique, separate system of oral health care and community health care workers are trained to respond to a variety of social, medical and dental conditions. In many countries the oral health care system is an integral part of the medical system and may be perceived to be a subspecialty of medicine. In others, systems evolved separately from medicine and remain unique systems for terms of whether the system is integrate with social, educational and employment institutions in the society. Similarly, the organization of oral health education of the public has emerged uniquely in different countries in response to dominant societal pressures.

Oral health care systems have been dynamic, responding to changes in population demographics; patterns of oral diseases; impact of oral diseases in relation to other systemic diseases; and, most importantly, to changes in social, political or economic structure and societal norms as reflected in national policies, legislation, regulations and payment systems.

口腔卫生保健供给系统具有以下特征：谁为谁提供什么服务，在什么场所，用什么资源，通过什么支付机制；以及有什么效果。通常一种口腔卫生保健供给系统只具有一种或两种特征，如新西兰卫生保健供给系统是以学校为基础、雇用牙科护士提供服务；英国是国家卫生服务；美国则是私人开业提供服务。每一种系统都有它自身的特征。现存的口腔卫生保健供给系统面临着政策、组织机构与资源之间不协调的问题。

Oral health care systems worldwide can be described by policy, organization, payment mechanisms and outcomes. They are characterized by the following parameters: who provides what services/functions for whom; in what locations; with what resources; with what payment mechanisms; and with what effects. Often an oral health care system is described on the basis of only one or two characteristics, perhaps reflecting what is most unique to that country. For example, the New Zealand system if often characterized as a school-based system employing dental nurses; the British system is described as a fee-for-service private practice system. However, each system should be understood for all its characteristics. Many of the current challenges to oral health care systems are based on incongruencies evolving between policy, organizational structures and resources.

2. 政策与目标 Policies and objectives

口腔卫生保健供给系统的目标范围可以从预防未来的口腔疾病到治疗现有的疾病以及处理和消除急诊、疼痛与创伤。也可以从发现新的预防和治疗口腔疾病的方法到改进现有的预防或治疗技术，阻止疾病的发展。

口腔卫生保健供给系统受到社会政策的影响。制订政策要与口腔卫生保健供给系统的目标相适应。制订政策应该考虑到哪个年龄组是重点，接收什么样的保健，由谁提供保健，以及在什么地方提供保健。

At the very basis of the system of oral health care are the goals and objectives - the purposes and expected outcomes of care. Objectives of oral health care systems range from preventing future oral diseases, to treating existing diseases, to managing and eliminating emergencies, pain and trauma, or a combination of any of these.

Systems of oral health care are influenced by societal policies and have policies of their own that affect the organization of the system and services provided. National policies influence which age group is emphasized, what types of care are received, who provides the care and where the care is provided.

3. 组织 Organization

什么样的口腔卫生保健系统与由政策确立的资源导致一个正式的组织。这样的组织有一个机构，还有各个组成部分的协调与质量控制策略，如研究，教育／培训与保健提供。一般来说，供给系统的组织用一种医学模式来叙述，限于与牙学院，临床诊所，个人开业以及直接与政策，报酬或提供口腔卫生保健有关的口腔卫生保健专业人员。最近，综合社区／公共卫生模式已经得到的赞赏超过了医学模式。于是，在其他国家开展的这些活动，口腔卫生保健的提供包括社区水平的活动，如与糖食品消耗政策实施有关的促进，建立规范并实施，如那些与烟草消耗，停止社区饮水氟化；在产前与婴儿诊所的口腔健康教育与提供氟化物治疗。采用这种扩人的模式，药师，医生，护士，学校教师，饮水工作监督者变成为口腔卫生保健提供系统的一部分。同样地，工作场所，医院，护理家庭与机构是开展保健活动的适当场所。然而，用这种广泛的口腔卫生保健提供系统的定义说明我们叙述，评价和改善保健组织的能力非常有限。

六、发展中国家的卫生保健体制 Health care systems in developing countries

许多发展中国家依据欧洲国家的社会福利模式来发展自身的卫生保健体制。在建立卫生保健系统的过程中，除了缺乏物质资源之外，还面临着卫生专业人员短缺的问题。解决的办法是培养中级水平的卫生保健工作者。有些国家按初级卫生保健的途径建立它们自己的卫生保健系统。

在发展中国家，口腔卫生保健服务有两种途径：合理的与传统的。合理的口腔卫生保健服务是建立在调查分析，制订计划，合理使用资源的基础上。传统的口腔卫生保健服务是建立在培训专业人员的基础上。

经济模式的改变影响到口腔卫生服务体制的变化。

柏林口腔健康联合宣言（Oral Health Alliance，1992）中确定了发展口腔卫生服务的框架，包括减少不公平性，减少依赖性，鼓励社区参与，建立合作伙伴，采取口腔健康促进和预防策略等。

不论采取哪一种方式来组织口腔卫生保健供给系统，都必须由国家承担费用。这是对一个国家承诺健康为基本人权的一种检验。21 世纪对口腔医学来说这也是一种挑战。

Many developing countries, unsurprisingly, opted to develop health care systems based on the social welfare models emanating from Europe at the time of their independence.

To a large extent, the conflicts of transposing a western medical model-based system in general health care to developing countries have been echoed in oral health care systems.

Two approaches to the development of oral health care and services. Out of this history there have arisen two competing models on which the organization of oral health care has been based in developing countries: the rational and the traditional.

The rational development of services and practices is based on carefully gathered and analyzed quantitative and qualitative data, which are then translated into strategic and operational plans (including patient treatment, education and research) , based on scientifically sound principles and the availability of resources. The other is based on tradition and is usually found in the training institutions.

The purpose of an oral health care system is to influence the population's way of life so that oral health is promoted or maintained, and oral disease prevented; and to provide adequate treatment to those members of the population affected by oral disease so that disease is arrested at an early stage and loss of function is prevented. These two functions, in the context of the PHCA, apply no matter whether the service is in a developing or developed country. Using these functions as a basis, principles have been established to guide the development of oral health services or programmes in the Oral Health Alliances Declaration of Berlin (Oral Health Alliance, 1992) . These principles hold for developing and developed countries alike and provide a framework for rational consideration of the role of governments; reducing inequalities; underdevelopment; dependence; empowerment; community involvement; partnerships; oral health promotion; preventive strategies; ethics; personnel preparation; rights of health workers and the scientific basis of oral health strategies.

All preventive avenues need to be explored, in particular those that can be sustained within the society and culture of the country, for whichever route is taken in organizing oral health care it is clear that even where the state accepts responsibility for funding (and in some cases also providing) oral health services there will only be a commitment of funds if the procedures and programmes are effective and efficiently run. The problem is that any funds available for the health sector are likely to be small and, for oral health, infinitesimal. This will be a test of the world's commitment to health as a fundamental human right. It will also be the challenge to dentistry in the coming millennium.

小结 Summary

通过本章学习，主要应了解预防医学，预防口腔医学和未来口腔健康科学的发展，各种口腔卫生保健供给体制的形成与发展，熟悉健康与疾病的概念及其发展，健康的四大决定因素，人类疾病发展史与三级预防策略，社区口腔卫生保健，新公共卫生运动，掌握发展口腔卫生保健的策略与途径。

思考题 Review questions

1. To discuss the concept of health and its development
2. To describe the determinants of health and oral health
3. How does the life style influence on health and oral health?
4. What is dental public health and its challenges in the 21st century?
5. To describe the factors influencing health care systems

参考文献 References

1. Daly Blanaid, et al. essential dental public health. Oxford University Press, 2002
2. Gluck George M., et al. Jong's Community dental health, 5th edition. Mosby, 2003
3. Pine Cynthia M. Community oral health, Wright, 1998
4. James Morse. Dunning Principles of dental public health, 4th edition. Harvard University Press, 1986
5. Kathy Vaigt. Geurink Community Oral health practice for the dental hygienist. W. B. Saunders Company, 2002
6. WHO/UNICEF, Alma-Ata 1978. Primary health care. WHO, Geneva, 1978
7. Sheiham Aubrey. Improving oral health for all: focusing on determinants and conditions. Health Education Journal (2000) 59, 351-363
8. Murray JJ. CBE, et al. the prevention of Oral Diseases, 4th edition Oxford University Press
9. WHO. Oral Health for the 21st century. WHO/ORH, Geneva, 1994
10. Bian Jinyou. A Review of Preventive Dentistry in China: The past 50 years. The Chinese Journal of dental Research June, 2001, Vol.4. No. 2: 27-34
11. Petersen. P.E. The World Oral Health Report 2003. Community Dentistry and Oral Epidemiology. Vol. 31 Supplement 1, 2003
12. Malvine E. Ring. Dentistry. An Illustrated History. Harry N. Abrams, Inc, publishers, New York, 1985
13. 周大成. 中国口腔医学史考. 人民卫生出版社, 1991
14. 郑麟蕃等. 中国口腔医学发展史. 北京医科大学／中国协和医科大学联合出版社, 1998
15. 顾学箕. 预防医学. 上海科学技术出版社, 1991
16. 马伯英. 中国医学文化史. 上海人民出版社, 1994
17. 卡斯蒂廖尼著. 程之范主译. 医学史上、下册. 广西师范大学出版社, 2003
18. 邱仁宗等. 医学的思维和方法. 人民卫生出版社, 1985
19. Burt/Eklund. Dentistry, dental Practice and the Community. 4th edition W, B. Saunders Company, 1992
20. WHO Technical Report series 782. monitoring and Evaluation of Oral Health. WHO, Geneva, 1989

（卞金有）

第二章　口腔健康流行病学
Chapter II Oral Health Epidemiology

概述 Overview

本章介绍了口腔流行病学的基本概念、定义、作用及其发展。着重阐述口腔流行病学的基本原则和研究方法；流行病学研究中的偏倚及其控制。重点介绍口腔健康调查的基本原则和方法。

In this chapter，the basic concepts, definition and role of oral epidemiology and its development are introduced. The basic principles and methodologies of oral epidemiology and how to do quality control for the bias are explored and oral health survey is clarified in detail.

要点 Key points

- 口腔流行病学的定义 Definition of oral epidemiology
- 口腔流行病学的作用 Role of oral epidemiology
- 口腔流行病学基本原则 Basic principles of oral epidemiology
- 口腔流行病学研究类型和方法 Methodologies of oral epidemiology
- 口腔健康调查 Oral health survey

第一节　概　述
Section 1 Overview

一、流行病学的定义和发展 The definition and development of epidemiology

流行病学是人类在与疾病作斗争的长期实践过程中，为认识、描述人群疾病与健康，预防和控制疾病以及促进健康，在不断积累实践经验与发展研究方法的基础上，逐渐形成和发展起来的一门学科。它既是一门共同的基础学科，又是介于医学和公共卫生学之间的一门桥梁学科。

目前国内外教科书对流行病学的定义是：

流行病学是研究人群中疾病或健康状态的分布及其影响因素，并研究防制疾病及促进健康的策略和措施的科学。

Epidemiology is a central medical science that studies of the distribution and determinants of health-related states or events in specified populations, and the application of this study to control of health problems.

Epidemiology is defined as the study of the health and disease in populations, and of how these states are influenced by heredity, biology, physical environment, social environment, and ways of living.

18世纪以前相当漫长的时期内流行病学尚未形成，但人们生活在社会、经济、文化不发达的情况下已逐渐自发地有了防病的要求和管理疾病的办法及措施。流行病学方法仅限于对病情的描写和记载，没有什么系统分析，形成了流行病学的原始萌芽。17 世纪的 Samuel Pepys 利用死亡者名单描述和记录了 1665 年发生在英国伦敦的鼠疫大流行。1775 年 Percival Pott 第一次科学地描述了在烟囱清扫工人中高发的职业病——阴囊癌。

1848 ~ 1854 年，在病原微生物没有被发现以前，英国内科医生 Snow 关于伦敦霍乱流行的调查就揭示了该传染病的流行特点和规律。Snow 利用霍乱病死者名单，以标点地图的方法显示了死亡的地域分布现象及其规律，分析出共用污染的饮用水是疾病传播的途径，以此推论其病原可能为某种活的物质，经采取关闭水厂等措施控制了发病。Snow 成功的调查分析和控制疾病流行成为流行病学史上不朽的里程碑。

19世纪流行病学的早期发展成果仍然具有现实指导意义：在揭示了艾滋病的流行特点和规律后，在社会公众中进行健康教育，预防和控制其传播，继而在1983年首次确认了艾滋病毒，这也是流行病学的工作成果。

目前流行病学的研究已从对疾病的研究，发展到对健康及其相关问题的研究。人类的健康关系到人的机体、精神与社会的完好状态。任何对健康产生影响的因素，如生活环境条件、生活方式与习惯、精神状态与思想观念、文化生活、生产劳动与社会活动，以及卫生条件与医疗保健服务保障等，都已成为现今流行病学研究的课题。探索与健康有关的各种因素，制定完善的卫生规划与策略选择，以及卫生保健服务效果评价，流行病学在这些方面都发挥着至关重要的作用。

Epidemiology was learned and practiced empirically long before it was named. It was from the more rational study of these epidemics that epidemiology evolved to its present form. Samuel Pepys, who wrote vivid chronicles of life in 17th-century London, used the Bills of Mortality, the forerunner of modern death certificates, to measure the onset and decline of a plague epidemic in London in 1665. Percival Pott's treatise of the chimney Sweep's Cancer, in 1775, described the unusually high occurrence of scrotal cancer among chimney sweeps, which is one of the first scientific descriptions of an occupational hazard.

In 1848～1854, John Snow, a medical practitioner in the Soho of London, went so far to control an outbreak of cholera by the application of his epidemiologic conclutions. His investigation took place some years before the germ theory of disease was understood, so Snow began by trying to identify the features common to those who died from the disease. After mapping out the residences of those who had died, his subsequent enquiries disclosed that all of the victims had used water from the same source. That source, in the days before indoor plumbing, was a pump in Broad Street. Snow reached the rational conclusion that something in the water was responsible for the spread of the disease. Snow's method of controlling the epidemic, still without knowing its cause, was to persuade the authorities to remove the pump handle. The epidemic soon subsided.

Snow's subsequent investigations on the relations between cholera and the source of water supply are epidemiologic classic.

The results of the patiently executed research of 19th-century workers such as Snow still benefit present-day society. Their work continues today: the understanding of the mode of transmission of the human immunodeficiency virus, and its translation into public health education to prevent AIDS, followed remarkably quickly on the first identification of the virus in 1983. That, too, is epidemiology.

二、口腔流行病学的定义 Definition of oral epidemiology

口腔流行病学是流行病学的一个分支，即用流行病学的原则和方法，研究人群中口腔健康与口腔疾病分布的规律及其影响因素，为探索病因及其影响因素，制定口腔健康目标和规划，选择疾病防制策略和效果评价提供依据的科学。

1. 国际口腔流行病学的发展 The development of oral epidemiology over the world

在西方，口腔流行病学起源于20世纪初。1901年在美国的科罗拉多州，年轻牙医McKay发现当时在该地流行着一种以往牙医书上从未提到过的疾病，患者表现为牙面上有白色的条纹或棕黄着色，他称为棕色牙釉。在当时美国西北大学牙科学院Dr Black院长的帮助下，对科罗拉多州的一些地区进行了流行病学调查，结果显示，这些带有斑纹牙的患者主要生活在一些湖泊周围，他们取湖泊水作为饮用水。1916年发表的研究报告将这种疾病定名为斑釉牙（mottled teeth），认为斑釉牙的发生与饮用水有关。1931年美国科学家终于发现引起斑釉牙的饮用水中氟元素的含量远高于普通饮用水，从而找到引起斑釉牙的原因是氟。

在研究斑釉牙的同时，科学家们发现斑釉牙流行的地区，患龋率低，认为氟有预防龋病的作用。为证明斑釉牙与龋病的关系，1931 年美国学者 Dean 开始对美国斑釉牙流行程度不同的市、镇进行流行病学研究。结果发现在两个未发现斑釉牙的城镇中，无龋儿童少；而在两个斑釉牙高发的城镇中，无龋儿童多。后来 Dean 又对美国 21 个城市 7257 名 12 ～ 14 岁的儿童做了流行病学调查，观察龋病、斑釉牙和饮水氟含量的关系。结果证实随着饮水氟含量增加则龋病患病率降低，饮水氟含量在1mg/L时龋病患病率降低最大，氟牙症患病率最低，从而证实了氟与龋病和氟牙症三者之间的关系。这些研究推动了口腔医学的进步，同时也发展了口腔流行病学。

Oral epidemiology was developed at the early of the 20th-century in the world. Dr Frederick McKay who arrived in Colorado in 1901, the year following his graduation from the dental school. He soon noticed that many his patients, particularly those who had lived in the area all their lives, had a permanent stain on their teeth which was called the stain 'mottled enamel'. Dr McKay got help from Dr Green Vardiman Black, Dean of the Northwestern University Dental School in Chicago to define the geographical area of the stain - the endemic area. The result of the investigation led they to believe that something in the water supply was responsible for mottled enamel in 1916. To look for traces of rare elements - those not usually tested for. The spectrographic analysis was run and that fluoride was present in the water was noted in 1931.

At the same time, the fact was discovered that caries experience was no higher in mottled teeth. The study of the relationship between fluoride concentration in drinking water, mottled enamel, and dental caries was assigned to Dr H. Trendley Dean in 1931. The result of the research was clear that caries experience in Macomb and Quincy was more than twice as high as that in Galesburg and Monmouth. This study paved the way for a much larger investigation of caries experience of 7257 12-14 year-old children from 21 cities in four states. The results show clearly the association between increasing fluoride concentration in the drinking water and decreasing caries experience in the population. Furthermore this study showed that near maximal reduction in caries experience occurred with a concentration of 1 mg/L F in the drinking water. At this concentration fluoride caused only sporadic instances of the mildest forms of dental fluorosis of no practical aesthetic significance in 1942.

2. 我国口腔流行病学的发展 The development of oral epidemiology in China

我国有记载的最早的口腔流行病学调查是在 1936 年，黄仁德对上海市高桥区的小学生检查牙。1944年，姜元川对“成都市小学生第一恒臼齿之研究”。1957年卫生部龋病牙周病全国性统计调查委员会首次制定《关于龋病、牙周病全国统计调查规定》，以后在 50 ~ 60 年代姜元川先后发表了《龋病在社会人群中的自然分布状况》、《龋病年龄因素之规律性》、《龋病的社会性调查》等文章，揭示了龋病患病与年龄性别等的关系，为探索国人龋病流行规律提供了一定的科学依据。

1983年在卫生部的领导下，在我国首次采用WHO的标准方法进行全国中、小学生的口腔健康调查（The first national oral health survey）。调查涉及全国 29 个省、市、自治区，调查人数131340人，调查对象的年龄为7、9、12、15、17岁。调查的内容包括龋病、牙周病、氟牙症和四环素牙。调查采用分层抽样的方法，全国共调查232个点。这次调查为我国制定2000年口腔健康目标提供了科学依据。1988 年栾文民等参照 WHO 标准方法对北京市 2191 名老年人进行口腔检查，分析了老年人的口腔健康状况。

1995年在卫生部和全国牙病防治指导组的领导下，我国开展了第二次全国口腔健康流行病学调查（The second national oral health survey），这次调查涉及 11 个省、市，共调查 140712 人，调查采用分层、不等比、多阶段、整群抽样的方法，并应用了WHO推荐的指数年龄组与基本调查方法（第三版）及美国国立牙科研究院（NIDR）的根面龋调查方法，调查年龄分别为 5、12、15、18、35 ~ 44、65 ~ 74 岁，内容包括龋病、牙周病、氟牙症、口腔卫生状况、戴义齿和需义齿以及无牙颌情况。这次调查还增加了问卷调查的内容，以了解我国人民的口腔卫生知识、态度、实践、习惯和观念，探索口腔疾病的发展因素。

2005 年开展了第三次全国口腔健康流行病学调查（The third national oral health survey），此次调查将涉及 30 个省、市和自治区，采用多阶段分层等容量随机抽样的方法，调查了解全国城乡 5、12、35 ~ 44、65 ~ 74 岁年龄组人群的口腔健康状况及影响因素，监测患病趋势和评估口腔卫生需求。为监测和评价 2010 年我国口腔健康目标提供信息支持。

三、口腔流行病学的作用 The role of oral epidemiology

1977 年第 30 届世界卫生大会（World Health Assembly， WHA）提出了“2000 年人人享有卫生保健”的全球战略目标，为实现这个目标，流行病学将在实施与评价方面起到重要作用。1989 年第 42 届世界卫生大会又强调应用流行病学方法监测和评价这个目标的进展，此后流行病学的应用受到越来越多的重视。口腔流行病学主要用于：

1. 描述人群口腔健康与疾病的分布状况 To describe the epidemic distribution of oral health and diseases in the population

口腔流行病学可用于对人群口腔健康状况进行描述，横断面调查是描述性口腔流行病学最常用的方法。它可以通过对一个地区人群在一定时间内的某种或某些口腔疾病进行调查，获得该地区特定人群某种或某些口腔疾病的患病情况和分布特点。如这些疾病在年龄、性别、职业、种族、文化、经济、习惯等方面的分布情况，用于与其他地区人群或不同时期人群进行比较和评价。1995年我国完成的全国第二次口腔健康流行病学调查，其结果对我国人群的口腔健康状况做了描述，通过这个调查了解到现时我国龋病、牙周病、牙龈炎、氟牙症和牙列缺失等口腔疾病的患病情况和特点，口腔卫生状况、龋病治疗状况和义齿修复等情况，这些情况对全面评估我国城市和农村居民口腔健康状况，制定防制疾病的策略和措施提供了确实可靠的依据。

2. 研究口腔疾病的病因和影响流行的因素 To study the determinants of oral diseases and to identify the epidemic factors

用横断面调查的方法难以研究疾病的病因，但通过横断面调查可以提供某种或某些疾病的流行因素线索，形成危险因子假设，然后用分析性流行病学的研究方法对该危险因子进行验证，借以判断该疾病可能的病因。如果需要再采用其他的研究方法，如流行病学实验和多种实验室的方法，有时还可结合临床研究，综合这些结果，可有助于进一步揭示该疾病的病因因素。如 1962 年 Keyes 对龋病的病因归纳为三因素即细菌——宿主——食物，是用流行病学方法与实验室研究结果为依据提出的。

3. 用于研究疾病预防措施并评价其效果 To study preventive measures for oral diseases and to evaluate the effectiveness

口腔流行病学也可用于口腔疾病预防措施和预防方法的研究，并对其效果进行评价。一种新的预防方法或预防措施，在取得大量非实验流行病学研究的证据之后，可用流行病学实验方法对其效果进行检验，通常是把受试人群随机分配到干预组或对照组，并在实验过程中采用盲法或双盲法。经过一定的试验周期，比较两组人群的发病差异。这样可检验新的预防措施的防病效果。1945 年 Ast 等为了观察饮水氟化对龋病的预防作用，在美国的 Newburgh 和 Kingston 两个镇进行了为期十年的流行病学社区干预试验研究，在 Newburgh 镇通过供水系统加入适量氟使水氟浓度达到 1mg/L，而距 Newburgh 镇仅 30 公里的 Kingston 镇作为对照区，水氟浓度仍保持0.1mg/L水平，十年后对两镇儿童的龋病患病情况进行调查，结果发现，Newburgh镇儿童龋病患病率明显下降，而Kingston镇儿童的龋病患病率有所上升，说明饮水氟化能有效降低患龋率，这项研究结果与其他同期研究结果一样，为以后各国开展饮水氟化提供了充分的科学依据。

对于已经应用的预防措施和预防方法，其效果可用口腔流行病学方法进行评估，以确定这些措施是否可供选择应用。1982 年 Driscoll 对含氟漱口液（900mg/LF^-）用于学龄儿童后的防龋效果进行评价，连续观察 30 个月，发现降低患龋率 22%，证明含氟漱口液对龋病预防同样有效。

4. 监测口腔疾病的发展趋势 To surveillance the trends of oral diseases in the population

口腔流行病学还可用于口腔疾病发展趋势的监测。口腔疾病的流行常受到多种因素影响，如行为与生活方式、环境、卫生保健服务状况等，这些因素的改变常会导致口腔疾病流行情况的变化。WHO在1969年建立了全球口腔数据库，每年发布一次全球口腔疾病（龋病和牙周病等）流行趋势的报告。一些国家为了解本国口腔疾病的流行趋势，制定了口腔疾病的监测措施，尤其是工业化国家，如美国从60年代开始，先后在国家健康统计中心（NCHS）和美国国立牙科研究院的领导下，定期组织全民口腔健康流行病学调查，每5年一次，从调查结果分析龋病和牙周病的发展趋势、评价预防保健措施的效果、人们自我口腔保健意识增强的程度。日本也开始积极进行口腔疾病的监测，据日本厚生省报告，每六年进行一次口腔疾病的流行病学调查，最近一次调查在1993年。我国的全国性口腔健康调查在1949年以后共进行了三次：1983年的全国学生龋病、牙周病的抽样调查；1995年的第二次全国口腔健康流行病学调查；2005年的第三次全国口腔健康流行病学调查，这三次调查对了解我国人民的口腔疾病的现状和发展趋势有重大意义。

5. 制定口腔卫生保健规划并评价其进展 To plan and evaluate oral health care services and its process

口腔流行病学调查的结果是各级卫生行政部门制定口腔健康目标、规划口腔保健措施的主要依据。我们国家疆土宽广，各地区情况很不平衡，经济状况、卫生保健状况、生活习惯、地理环境以及气候条件等相差很大。这种状况使卫生行政部门在制定口腔健康目标和规划时，必须有大量确切的调查资料作为依据，根据这些信息，卫生行政部门可制定一定时期的口腔健康目标规划，这些目标应具有很强的针对性，尽可能量化并切实可行。同时，为了实现这些目标，卫生行政部门还必须提出具体的口腔保健策略措施，合理地分配各种资源，以期在规定的实施期限结束时评价达标的程度。

6. 对社区和人群口腔健康作出诊断 To diagnosis the situation of oral health for the community

以发病率、患病率以及相关指数衡量口腔疾病的分布状况，对社区和人群口腔健康作出诊断。这种研究有助于发现需要采取社区干预的口腔健康问题，有助于确定这些口腔健康问题的相对重要性和需要优先考虑的问题，同时发现那些需要特殊口腔保健的易感人群。

采用口腔流行病学方法可对目标规划的实施效果进行评价。一般一个目标规划制定后，在实施之中，应有中期评估，以确定所制定的目标能否达到。如果发现期限结束时达到该目标有困难，则在中期就应对目标进行适当调整，使其更切合实际。

第二节　口腔疾病的流行病学
Section 2 The Epidemiology of Oral Diseases

一、口腔疾病的流行趋势 The trends and distribution of oral diseases

2003年世界卫生组织口腔健康状况报告指出，尽管全球口腔健康状况取得巨大进步，但世界各国特别是发达国家和发展中国家的弱势群体仍存在许多问题。龋病和牙周病一直是全球口腔健康的主要问题。目前，世界各国及一些国家和地区内部的口腔疾病分布以及严重程度差异显著。大量流行病学调查资料表明，社会行为因素和环境因素在口腔健康和口腔疾病中起着重要作用。

Despite great achievements in the oral health of populations globally, problems still remain in many communities around the world - particularly among underprivileged groups in developed and

developing countries. Dental caries and periodontal diseases have historically been considered the most important global oral health burdens. At present, the distribution and severity of oral diseases vary in different parts of the world and within the same country or region. The significant role of socio-behavioural and environmental factors in oral disease and health is demonstrated in a large number of epidemiological surveys (WHO 2003) .

描述口腔疾病的流行趋势不能不先提到指数。指数（Index）表明某种现象变动的程度。在口腔流行病学中，指数是起到指标或指示作用的标识，常用一组序数作代码并加上某种记分标准来说明口腔疾病在个体或群体中的表现程度，用数值级差作标准，测量和比较疾病的扩展范围和严重程度。在口腔流行病学研究中已经应用了多种指数作为评价预防措施、个人家庭保健以及临床实验效果的指标。

理想的指数具有以下特点 The properties of an ideal index are:

①有效性 Validity.

②可靠性（重复性好）Reliability.

③客观性以及简单易学 Clarity, simplicity, and objectivity.

④可量化便于统计分析 Quantifiability.

⑤灵敏度 Sensitivity.

⑥可接受性，能被检查对象接受 Acceptability.

The index must measure what it is intended to measure, so it should correspond with clinical stages of the disease under study at each point.

The index should be able to measure consistently at different times and under a variety of conditions.

The criteria should be clear and unambiguous, with mutually exclusive categories. Ideally, it should be readily memorized by an examiner after some practice.

The index must be amenable to statistical analysis, so that the status of a group can be expressed by a distribution, mean, median, or other statistical measure.

The index should be able to detect clinically - relavant but small shilfts, in either direction, in the condition.

The use of the index should not be unnecessarily painful or demeaning to the subject.

二、口腔疾病的分布状况 Distribution of oral diseases

口腔疾病的分布是指观察口腔疾病在人群中的发生、发展和消退状况，描述口腔疾病在不同时间、不同地区和不同人群中的频率与分布的现象。这是流行病学研究的起点和基础。

研究分布状况的意义在于：研究疾病的流行规律和探索病因的基础。因为疾病的分布特征受病因所左右，所以它可以提供病因线索，即提出研究的问题和假设。对分布状况的描述可以帮助认识疾病流行的基本特征，这是临床诊断的重要依据和信息。对分布规律及其决定因素的分析可以提供科学依据，有助于制订疾病防治规划和口腔保健策略与措施。

主要口腔疾病的流行趋势和分布状况分别在第七、八、九章里描述。

三、病因和病因推断 The cause and diagnostic testing

口腔流行病学研究中的病因和病因推断就是分析流行病学的指导架构和评价标准，对因果关系的形成和准确认识研究结果具有重要意义。病因的概念是流行病学的基本组成部分，判定病因的相关准则主要有以下几点：

判定病因的相关准则 Selected criteria for a causal relationship

1. 时间顺序 Temporal sequence

如果怀疑病因X引起疾病Y（X→Y），则X必须发生于Y之前，这就是前因后果的时间顺序。在确定前因后果的时间顺序上，实验和队列研究最佳，病例对照研究和生态学研究次之。

2. 相关强度 Strength of association

一般说来，关联的强度越大， 该关联为因果的可能性就越大。一个强关联如果是混杂因素所致，该混杂因素与疾病的关联将更强，因此这种混杂就容易识别出来，而相对弱的关联则可能是未识别的偏倚所致。关联强度的测定根据资料的性质或来源可分为：优势比OR（病例对照研究），相对危险度RR（队列研究）等反映分类资料的关联指标。

3. 剂量—反应关系 Dose-response relationship

针对资料的性质不同，“剂量—反应关系”有等级相关系数和积差相关系数等反映相关（关联）的指标。例如进食甜食的量和频率增加，龋病的相对危险度增加。

4. 分布一致性 Consistency of association

实际上是利用群组资料反映的生态学相关，既暴露与疾病在不同群组之间表现为共同变动关系。例如吸烟与牙周病的相关系数。

5. 生物合理性 Biological plausibility

病因与疾病的关联逻辑符合主观和客观的评价。

The concept of causation is an essential part of epidemiology. Some of the criteria that have been suggested and may be used to establish a causal relationship are given.

To be causal, an exposure must precede the occurrence of the disease. Demonstration of this temporal sequence requires longitudinal study.

In valid studies, the stronger the association between exposure and outcome, the more likely it is that the association is causal.

If an exposure is causal, then the risk of disease should be related to the degree of exposure: a dose-response relationship.

If there is a good number of studies on whether an exposure is a cause of a disease, and if all of them produce fairly similar positive results, it is more likely that the factor is causal.

The association must make biologic sense from our knowledge of the disease. It follows that the better understood a disease is, the more stringent this criterion can become.

（一）病因的概念 Concept of cause

病因的概念是流行病学的基本组成部分，流行病学中病因的概念是符合概率论的因果观的，流行病学的病因常称为危险因素（risk factor），也就是说病因是使疾病发生的概率即危险升高的因素。病因是自然界客观存在的，其中有些是直接病因（direct cause），有些是间接病因（indirect cause）；有的是主要病因（primary cause），有的是辅助病因（auxiliary cause）；它们形成了复杂交错的联系——病因网。在病因中也可分为必要病因（necessary cause）和充分病因（sufficient cause）。必要病因就是指引起某种疾病发生不可或缺的因子。但是，有了必要病因，不见得一定会出现该病因所引起的疾病。例如，糖被认为是龋病的病因，但不是充分病因，因为需要区分糖的种类和进食糖的频率以及进食方式。并不是每个人吃糖都会患龋病，若要确定龋病易感者，可能还需要考虑菌斑类型和菌斑量，致龋微生物的基因分型，釉质矿化程度以及氟化物摄入情况等。虽然确定一种疾病的全部相关病因是不可能的，但是对具有相似已知病因的人群可以确定共同危险因素。充分病因是由几种因素共同组成而非单一因素。所谓充分病因，就是导致疾病发生的最低限度的条件，或是辅助必要病因致病的不可缺少的因素。

（二）病因的推断 Diagnostic testing of cause

流行病学病因研究过程可分为三个部分：根据病因模型设想可能的病因；描述性研究提出病因假设，分析性研究验证假设；根据病因综合判定标准作出判断。1987年，世界卫生组织在我国召开了一个专家委员会，讨论了病因研究的有关问题并制定了病因研究和鉴定的一般程序。

1. 建立假设 Establishing hypothesis

通常采用描述性流行病学方法（如横断面研究、历史性回顾研究、疾病监测资料和生态学研究等）描述疾病的三间分布。依据疾病的三间分布特点，并比较病区与非病区的不同，从中发现与疾病有关的现象或因素，再采用下面的逻辑推理方法建立病因假设。

2. 验证假设 Testing hypothesis

病因假设建立后，应用分析流行病学方法（如病例对照研究、队列研究或实验流行病学）验证假设因素和疾病的相关性，从相关研究中进一步探索其因果关系以验证假设。病例对照研究是比较病例人群与对照人群危险因素的暴露比例是否具有差异及其程度；队列研究是比较危险因素的暴露组与非暴露组的发病率是否具有差异及其程度。

3. 证实假设 Evidencing hypothesis

通过病例对照研究和队列研究等对病因假设进行初步验证后，一般需要通过流行病学实验研究来加以证实。实验方法可以人为控制某些因素，它不仅可以控制已知是重要的混杂因素，而且也能控制尚未认知的混杂因素。

表 2-1 流行病学的病因推断

检验结果 Result	疾病 Disease	无病 No disease	合计Total
阳性 Positive	真阳性 TP	假阳性 FP	TP + FP
阴性 Negative	假阴性 FN	真阴性 TN	TN + FN
合计 Total	真阳性 + 假阴性 TP + FN	假阳性 + 真阴性 FP + TN	All

灵敏度 Sensitivity: 患病人群检验为阳性率 TP/（TP + FN）

特异度 Specificity: 无病人群检验为阴性率 TN/（FP + TN）

阳性预测值 Positive Predictive Value: 检验为阳性者患病的几率 TP/（TP + FP）

阴性预测值 Negative Predictive Value: 检验为阴性者不患病的几率 TN/（FN + TN）

假阳性率 False-Positive Rate: 检验为阳性者不患病的几率 FP/（FP + TN）

假阴性率 False-Negative Rate: 检验为阴性者患病的几率 FN/（TP + FN）

近年来，口腔医学领域开展了多项疾病预测研究，尤其是龋病研究。关于龋病预测研究，目前认为患龋既往史是预测患龋与否的最好指标，而细菌类、酶类或其他生物学方法作为龋病预测指标尚没有足够的可信度。

In dentistry, various predictive tests have been developed through the years, especially for caries. It is concluded that there was little at that time in the way of bacteriologic, enzymatic, or other biologic tests that predicted caries with a sufficient degree of reliability. The best predictor of future caries was past caries experience, a result consistently found in more recent studies.

第三节　口腔流行病学的研究类型

Section 3 Types of Oral Epidemiological Studies

流行病学研究按照其性质可分为观察法、实验法及理论研究等。观察法就是研究者从描述性流行病学方法发展到分析性与实验性流行病学方法的应用。研究者没有控制暴露的能力，尽管能控制混淆因素，但不能随机分配暴露，只能客观收集人群有关暴露或疾病资料，评价暴露与疾病的联系。这种方法是流行病学研究的主要方法，如描述性流行病学、分析性流行病学。实验法与观察法不同，实验者具有控制实验条件的能力，并能控制其他混淆因素评价暴露与疾病的联系。这种方法是实验流行病学方法。理论研究是对疾病的病因、宿主和环境之间的联系所做的假设得到了反复验证之后，用数学公式阐明疾病流行的规律，提出数学模型，用于研究预防措施的成本效益和流行病学预测。

Having described the terminology in oral epidemiology, it is now possible to apply that understanding to categorize types of studies. Although the distinctions are not always clear-cut, epidemiological research can be categorized according to whether the primary focus is on describing the distributions of disease or on analyzing its determinants (Table 2-2).

表 2-2　口腔流行病学的研究类型

描述性研究方法	Descriptive studies
观察性研究方法	Observational studies
病例报告	Case reports
病例分析	Case series
相关性研究	Populations (correlational studies)
横断面调查	Cross-sectional surveys
分析性研究方法	Analytical studies
观察性研究方法	Observational studies
病例 - 对照研究（不匹配和匹配）	Case-control studies (unmatched and matched)
队列研究（前瞻性和历史性）	Cohort studies (prospective and historical)
实验性研究方法	Experimental studies
干预实验	Intervention studies
临床试验	Clinical trials

一、描述性研究方法 The descriptive studies

描述性流行病学（descriptive epidemiology）是流行病学中最常用的一种，它对疾病或健康现象在人群中的分布以及发生、发展的规律作客观的描述。这种研究的作用是描述某种现象在人群中的分布和发生发展规律；提出病因假设。描述性流行病学主要有下面几种。

1. 横断面研究 Cross-sectional study

又称现况调查，调查目标人群中某种疾病或现象在某一特定时点上（较短的时间内）的情况。它的作用在于了解疾病的患病情况和分布特点，以便制定预防措施和为研究病因提供线索。我国最近进行的第三次全国口腔流行病学调查就属于横断面研究。

In cross-sectional studies we can look at distributions of variables within the sample. Cross-sectional designs are suitable to describe variables and their distribution patterns. Cross-sectional studies can also be used to look for potential associations, but to decide which variables are risk factors and which are outcomes depends on the hypotheses of the investigator, rather than on the study design. Concerning constitutional factors such as age, sex and race, the decision is easy because they cannot be altered and therefore are generally predictors. For most variables, however, the decision is more difficult.

2. 纵向研究 Longitudinal study

又称“疾病监测”，即研究疾病或某种情况在一个人群中随着时间推移的自然动态变化。也就是对一组人群定期随访，两次或若干次横断面调查结果的分析。它的作用在于动态地观察疾病或某种现象的演变情况及其原因分析。如对一小学某个班级学生的龋病发病情况进行定期检查，以观察龋病在这个班级学生中的变化情况并分析其原因，如斯里兰卡茶叶工人牙周病自然史研究，就属于这种研究。

To study the patterns of the diseases or the state in the defined sample of subjects that is a series cross-sectional study of the same population observed at two or more points in time. It is used to draw inferences about changing diseases patterns over time.

A longitudinal project of major importance was the 15-year study of periodontitis among 480 tea workers in Sri Lanka. The group studied had virtually no dental treatment of the type found in developed countries, so the data reflected the natural history of periodontitis. Based on tooth loss and interproximal attachment levels, it was concluded that some 8% demonstrated rapid progression, 81% moderate progression, and 11% no progression beyond gingivitis. This study provided important evidence for demonstrating the range of susceptibility to periodontitis.

3. 常规资料分析 Routine data-sets analyzing

又称历史资料分析，即对已有的资料或者疾病监测记录做分析或总结。如病史记录、疾病监测资料等。如研究某市居民拔牙原因，可研究该市若干医院近5年的病历资料，经统计分析可找出不同年龄组牙齿丢失最主要的原因，如因龋病、牙周病、外伤、修复需要等原因而拔除病牙。这种研究结果可为开展口腔保健工作提供必要的信息。

Historical data-sets analysis is to review the data or the record for evaluation. For example, The causation of extraction (caries, periodontal diseases, traumatic and orthodontics) can give the information for oral health care.

二、分析性研究方法 The analytic studies

分析性流行病学（analytic epidemiology）的研究方法就是对所假设的病因或流行因素进一步在选择的人群中探索疾病发生的条件和规律，验证病因假设。主要有病例－对照研究（case-control study）和队列研究（cohort study）。

病例—对照研究的特点是观察时间短、需要研究的对象少，适合研究一些病程较长的慢性病和一些比较少见的疾病。又由于它一次可研究多个因素，尤其适合那些原因未明疾病的研究。但由于病例－对照研究是对过去因素的回顾性调查，所以准确性较低，可靠性较差，回忆偏倚较大。因此要求严格设计、实施和客观评价，减少与控制偏倚发生。

Case-control studies are, like cohort studies, designed to assess the association between an outcome, usually disease, and an exposure. Case-control studies are also called case-referent studies to stress that the controls do not serve as control in the same sense as the unexposed group in cohort studies. The major characteristic that distinguishes a case-control study from cohort study is that the selection of study participants is based upon their disease status and not exposure status. Cases are selected from among those persons who have the disease of interest and non-cases from those who have not. The general principle involved is that the likelihood of a case being included in the study must not depend on whether that case was exposed to the risk factor of interest. Non-cases are chosen independent of exposure, and the cases and non-cases are examined to assess association between exposure and disease. In an optimally designed case-control study, cases are selected from a clearly defined population, sometimes called the study base or source population and the non-cases from same population. The basic design of a case-control study is shown in table 2-1 (Pine 1997).

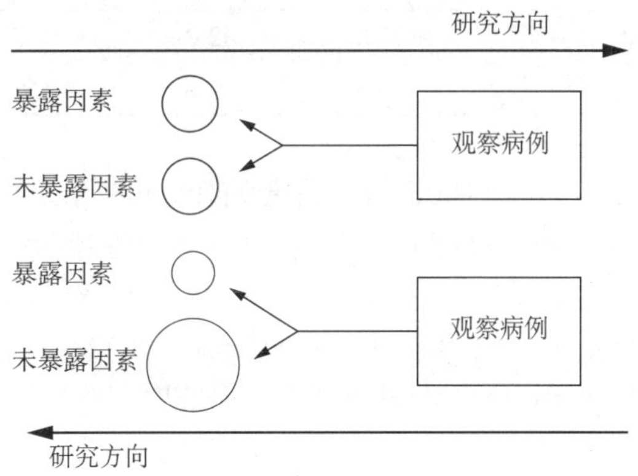

图 2-1 病例对照研究的设计模式图 Schematic presentation of the design of a case-control study

如果病例组有暴露史者的比例（a/m_1）统计学上显著高于对照组（b/m_2），则提示暴露因素与疾病有联系，可能是因果关系。病例 - 对照研究的方法如下：

在应用病例—对照研究时，①首先需确定危险因子，提出病因假设。病因假设可以来源于以往文献复习，或来源于横断面流行病学调查提供的线索，也可来源于临床医疗实践；②然后确定病例组与对照组的配比方式，一般配比方式有两种：一是组间配比，也就是混杂因子（confounding factor）在两组间的频数分布基本相等。所谓混杂因子就是会夸大或缩小研究因素与疾病之间真实联系的一些因素。最常见的如年龄、性别，文化程度等。另一配比方式是配对，即给每个病例挑选一个或数个混杂因子相同或相近的对照；③确定配比之后再确定病例组与对照组的人选，病例组的人选可从医院中患该病的对象中取，也可从流行病学调查时发现的病人中选取，对照组的人选可从医院中未患该病的人中挑选，也可从社会上挑选，但不管是病例组或对照组的研究对象，他们的诊断必须明确，应有统一的诊断标准与暴露的标准，防止错分，尽量减少两个组的选择偏性，不然会影响调查结果；④然后设计调查表，调查病例组与对照组对象以往的暴露史，资料收集可采用直接询问、通信、查阅记录等方式；⑤最后将收集到的资料用统计学的方法进行分析。一般用相对危险度（Relative Risk，RR）或比数比例（优势比）（Odds Ratio，OR）或归因危险度（绝对危险度Attributable Risk，AR）作为暴露与疾病之间关联强度的统计量，然后通过成组资料相对危险度的显著性检验及其可信限计算，以推断疾病与危险因子之间的关系。

例如：1997年上海市叶玮等应用病例－对照研究的方法，调查幼儿猖獗性龋的危险因素。他们采用组间配比的方法，将400名2～5岁患猖獗性龋的幼儿作为病例组，401名患非猖獗性龋的幼儿作为对照组。两组中不同年龄和性别的比例无显著差异。调查采用向父母发放问卷的方法，内容包括婴儿时期喂养方式、补充食品种类、口腔卫生习惯、日常饮食、父母受教育程度等。资料收集采用双盲法。结果如下：

表 2-3　猖獗性龋与摄入甜食的关系

组别	喂奶时加糖（人数 %）		吃甜食习惯（人数 %）			P 值
	是	否	不吃	1～2 次 / 天	＞3 次 / 天	
病例组	57.8	42.2	6.5	45.6	47.9	＜0.05
对照组	40.8	59.2	15.6	56.4	28.0	

以上结果表明患猖獗性龋幼儿在用奶瓶喂奶时加糖和平时吃零食的比例均显著高于对照组，推断甜食可能是引起幼儿猖獗性龋的原因。

群组研究的特点是只要暴露组与对照组可比性较好，资料准确完整，则研究结果准确度高，可以获得不同暴露强度与疾病的关系。也可以观察一种暴露因素与多种疾病的关系。但由于群组研究属前瞻性研究，研究时间较长，尤其对慢性病的观察费时更多，需要大量的人力物力，所以常在病例 - 对照研究获得较明确的危险因素后用于进一步验证病因假设。

Cohort study, also called follow-up studies or longitudinal studies, are observational studies where measurements are made more than once on the members of the cohort. In a cohort study we choose or define a sample of study subjects who do not have the outcome of interest at the beginning of the follow-up; or they have the potential to develop new disease, e.g. in caries studies, subjects have or will be erupting surfaces at risk. The objective of a cohort study is to compare the incidence of disease among those exposed to a factor with the IR among those not exposed to this factor in order to assess whether this exposure influences the outcome. As we collect information about the total person-time, i.e. the amount of time contributed by the participants, during the follow-up and about the outcome, we can calculate the incidence of the disease or condition of interest.

例如：Sullivan 等从 1947 年起在澳大利亚两所饮食结构不同的学校研究饮食与龋病的关系，一组是澳大利亚新南威尔市州学校儿童，另一组是社会经济状况差的农村Hopewood House儿童。前者的饮食结构与普通的澳大利亚学校学生类似，后者的饮食特点为：儿童自出生后到开始添加食品从不吃肉及精制糖，主食一般为未经烹调的蔬菜及含麸面包，如莴苣、黄瓜、白心菜、黑面包加奶油及蛋黄以及水果等。追踪15年，观察二所学校年龄社会经济状况相同的学生口腔健康状况与饮食的关系。

表2-4 澳大利亚Hopewood House和新南威尔士州学校儿童龋均（1952～1956年）

年龄（岁）	Hopewood House 儿童 DMF		州学校儿童 DMF	
	均数	SD	均数	SD
6	0	0	0.99	1.38
7	0.14	0.46	2.31	1.70
8	0.24	0.66	3.22	1.91
9	0.41	0.84	4.44	2.32
10	0.38	0.82	5.28	3.08
11	0.61	1.28	6.98	4.10
12	1.08	1.9	9.32	5.33
13	1.06	1.78	10.7	5.15

资料来源：Marthaler（1967）

表2-4显示，不管哪一个年龄，Hopewood House儿童的龋均都低于州学校儿童。而Hopewood House儿童的全身健康状况与牙萌出时间和州学校儿童基本一致。说明改变饮食与龋病密切相关，增加糖摄入可增加龋病发生。

三、实验性研究方法 The experimental studies

实验性研究方法是流行病学的主要研究方法之一。即使用人工手段以干预某一疾病的自然分布规律，探索某一因素是否为流行因素或某一措施是否有效。

The Experimental Study based on epidemiological principles and designed to test the hypothesis that a particular agent or procedure favorably alters the natural history of a disease.

实验流行病学（experimental epidemiology）又称为流行病学实验（epidemiological experiment）或现场实验（field trial）或干预实验（intervation study /trial），是指在研究者的控制下对人群采取某项干预措施或施加某种因素或消除某种因素以观察其对人群疾病发生或健康状态的影响，它有两个重要特点：①是实验法而非观察法；②要求设立严格的对照观察，即研究对象随即分配到不同的组，而非自然形成的暴露组与非暴露组。

对于流行病学实验的分类迄今尚无权威的定论，也无公认的分类原则。不过，一般根据不同的研究目的和研究对象等特点可以分为三大类：现场实验（field trial）、社区干预实验（community intervention trial）和临床实验（clinical trial）。临床试验的本意是以病人作为研究对象的试验，但是随着流行病学试验方法的不断发展，其实际内涵要广泛得多，既包括病人，又包括健康人群。例如，某种口腔保健药品或用品，某种含氟牙膏或某种牙刷的临床试验，通常是在一定的选择人群中进行，以观察其实际功效与安全性。欧洲社会医药产品标准临床试验指南（1990～1991）关于临床实验的定义：医药产品的临床试验意味着对人类作为受试者，不论是病人或非病人志愿者所进行的任何系统地研究，为了发现或者检验、研究产品的作用或者确定其任何副作用，或者研究产品的吸收、分布、代谢与排泄，以查明其效果与安全性。

社区干预实验是现场试验或临床实验的一种扩展。接受某种预防措施的基本单位可以是整个社区，或社区的某一有代表性人群。

在现场实验与社区干预实验中，研究者关心的不是疾病的后果，而是如何预防疾病的发生。例如饮水氟化，观察龋病发生状况的改变。其研究人群有健康者或可能患某种疾病的高危人群所组成。

流行病学实验的应用范围日益广泛，尤其是口腔预防保健方面，其主要用途有四个方面：①预防措施的效果与安全性评价；②评价某种新药，新方法或新制剂的效果，新保健品新技术与相反事件；③探讨疾病的病因；④医疗保健措施质量成本效果，成本效益评价。

另有一种类似流行病学实验的方法称为“类实验”或“准实验”（quasi-experiment，或semi-experiment），其不同之处在于：①由于实际情况不允许，对研究对象不作随机分配；②研究对象数量较大，范围较广；③不设对照组或可设对照组，但不随机分组。

例如饮水氟化或食盐氟化、牛奶氟化项目预防儿童龋病的研究，可以选择一个社区人群为实验组，而选择另一个同质社区人群作为对照组。

实验流行病学研究也是一种前瞻性研究，它与群组研究的不同之处在于根据随机化原则进行分组，并需要对研究对象采取某种干预措施，而群组研究仅根据研究对象原来的暴露状况进行分组，除进行观察外，不采取任何措施。由于这种研究方法是在严格控制的实验条件下进行的，所以验证假设的可信度较高，是评价预防措施的好方法，是人群医学研究中常用的工具，用途相当广泛。

口腔医学中的临床试验和社区试验 Clinical trial and community trial in dentistry

In medical terminology, clinical trials are carried out among patients, frequently hospital inpatients, and field trials are carried out with people in the community who may not necessarily be patients. This medical model dose not transfer well to dentistry, where the definition of a patient is less clear-cut. The term clinical trial tends to be loosely applied in dentistry to both types study, so we will use it when describing research principles common to both strict clinical trials and field trials. We will use the term field trial (sometimes called a Community Trial) only when specific reference to a field trial is needed.

A clinical trial is a controlled experimental study of group comparison, based on epidemiologic principles and designed to test the hypothesis that a particular agent or procedure favorably alters the natural history of a disease. The group receiving the agent of regimen under study is the test group, sometimes called the experimental or study group, whereas the comparable group not subject to the agent or regimen is the control group. Clinical trials compare 2 or more segments of are a single population, divided into groups that are essentially similar (in distribution of age, sex, race, socioeconomics, disease experience) . The aim is to make the only difference between the groups the fact that the test group receives the agent under study and the control group does not.

Much of the basis for preventive procedures in dentistry has come from clinical trials, although the quality of trials described in the dental literature varies from excellent to poor. The reader can judge the validity of a trial by determining how closely the report adheres to certain principles in its conduct.

试验研究设计的主要内容或步骤，包括以下几个方面：

1. 确定目标人群 study subjects

制定受试者的入选与排除标准，并严格按标准选择，如观察窝沟封闭的防龋效果，应选择窝沟龋易感儿童为受试对象；如观察牙膏抗牙石的效果，应选择牙石易形成者作为受试对象。受试者依从性好，愿意自始至终参加并遵守有关规定。

This should be determined by the purpose of the trial. If the purpose is to test the efficacy of a particular agent (i.e. whether it works) , then it deserves the most favorable conditions to show that it dose work. For that reason, the project should be conducted with subjects who are selected for their susceptibility to the disease. This means that a population of a specific age range is usually chosen deliberately, as many oral diseases are age-associated. Sex, race, socioeconomic status, and geographic location are other factors that can be included in the choice of a study population for efficacy trials. If the purpose is to assess the effectiveness of an agent under everyday conditions, however, then broad community population, those with varying degrees of the disease under study, should be chosen. Confusing the purposes of trials can lead to the error of generalizing from efficacy trials with special populations with unusual disease distributions, such as some institutionalized people, to the general population.

2. 确定受试样本量 Sample size

依据定义，事件在一般人群中的发生率高低，试验组与对照组之间差异的大小程度；检验的显著性水平和单尾或双尾检验。样本量过小，检验效能偏低，所得结论不可靠，反之，样本量过大，则会造成不必要的人力、物力、财力与时间的浪费。可以参考一定的样本量计算公式进行计算。

Loss of subjects during a prospective clinical trial is a fact of life and must be planned for. If the numbers of subjects in the groups are not big enough to begin with, at the end of the trial the researcher will be left with too few subjects to be able to show, by statistical logic, whether it is likely that an observed difference between the groups is real or a chance result. The result may then be that a real difference cannot be detected, and an agent that in fact is effective will not seem to be so. This issue relates to data analysis and the conclusions from the trial.

3. 试验组与对照组的可比性 Comparability of study and control groups

正确的分组是保证可比性的关键之一，目的是减少偏倚，增加试验结果的准确性。正确的分组方法应遵循随机化的原则，随机化的目的是保证试验组和对照组样本有相似临床特征和可能影响效果的因素。完全随机分配可先将样本编号，再利用随机数字表等方法分组。区组随机分配可将总的样本数按进入研究的时序分成若干组。分层随机分配可根据不同类别的因素将样本先分为若干层，然后在层内随机分配样本至试验组和对照组。

The randomized trial (随机试验) , always the most elegant design, is one in which group similarity is achieved by random allocation of subjects to the study and control groups. Random allocation means that subject has an equal chance of being assigned to either study or control group. Statistical probability is such that the assumption can then be made that the groups differ from each other only in terms of the agent under study. Uncontrolled variables influencing the outcome are likely to affect subjects in both groups equally.

Nonrandomized trial designs (非随机试验设计) are not uncommon in the dental literature. Although they are weaker than randomized designs, sometimes practical considerations dictate their use. For example, a school system taking part in a caries preventive trial may insist that there be no control group because school administrators want all participating children to receive a benefit. In such cases a before-and-after design (sometimes called historical controls) can be used. In this design, children are examined at the beginning of the trial, the agent or regimen is applied, and then cross-sectional groups of children of similar ages are examined periodically until the completion of the trial. Differences between caries status at the beginning and the end of the trial are then judged for children of similar age or grade levels. The weakness in this design is that uncontrolled change could take place during the trial to invalidate results. For example, in a trial of a fluoride mouthrinse, children in sixth grade at the completion of a 3-year trial may have brushed with a fluoride toothpaste more often than did the sixth-graders examined at the beginning. Without a true control group, it is impossible to tell if beneficial outcomes were due entirely to the mouthrinse or at least in part to the additional toothpaste use. Before-and-after trials are more properly called demonstrations, intended to "demonstrate" the value of accepted preventive measures. The greatest threat to the validity of a before-and-after design comes from sociodemographic change in the population under study during the period of the trial.

4. 对照组的安慰剂应用 Use of a placebo in the control group

A placebo is a material or formulation like the test product but without the active ingredient, such as a toothpaste that feels and tastes like fluoride toothpaste but contains no fluoride. The purpose of using a placebo in a trial is to have subjects unaware of whether they are in test or control group (a blind study), so hat their dental health behavior will not be consciously or unconsciously affected by group allocation. Bias, systematic although usually unconscious error, also can affect examiners. Examiners who expect a product to be effective may unconsciously apply stricter criteria for caries in a control group if they know which children are in which group. When neither participants nor examiners know the group allocations, the trial is double-blind.

5. 实施的监控 Control of operational procedure

试验现场的选择是有一定条件的，不是任意的。①受试地区或单位目标人群在受试期间保持相对稳定，流动性小，以保证试验能顺利进行；②受试人群的疾病发病率符合方案要求；③受试单位有一定的卫生保健机构与人员，帮助组织联络工作；④有关领导理解支持，群众接受。

开放试验可用于对改变生活方式（如饮食、口腔卫生习惯、吸烟）等干预效果的观察。盲法试验又可分为单盲、双盲或三盲。单盲的受试者不知道自己的组别；双盲法是研究者与受试者都不知道受试者组别；三盲法还包括资料收集、监督与分析者也不知道。其中双盲法比较常用。

应制定统一的措施、方法与标准，这种措施、方法和标准应体现在受试对象纳入、排除时，也应该体现在对结果的评判上。检查人员应经过校正试验，合格上岗。

An efficacy study, designed to answer the question of whether a particular agent or regimen works, has to give the test agent every chance. Susceptible populations are chosen for the trial, but in addition, the researchers need to be sure that the agent is used as prescribed. If it is a professionally applied agent or a treatment regimen, the protocol must specify precisely how the agent will be used, for how long, how often, at what concentration, and by whom. A placebo, or positive control, would be applied agent is being tested, such as a mouthrinse, the protocol should call for the agent to be used under professional supervision. It is the researchers' task to ensure that the protocol is adhered to throughout the course of the study.

In an effectiveness trial, the agent/treatment can be used as it normally would. That means that professionals are given instructions in use of a procedure, or participants are given the rinse to take home and use as instructed. There is less certainty in an effectiveness trial that the material has been used as intended, but part of the aims of an effectiveness trial is how the material works under "real lift" conditions. In operational control, as in other aspects of a trial, the purpose of the study must be kept in mind.

6. 检查诊断的可靠性 Reliability in diagnosis

Examiners in trials must record disease (at the second and subsequent examinations) that has developed over a relatively short time. This requirement forces the examiner to diagnose disease at an early stage of its development, which increases the risk of error. In caries trials, the most troublesome form of error is that a lesion classed as carious at the first round of examinations may be classified as sound in subsequent examinations, a negative reversal, more commonly referred to just as a reversal. Reversals are virtually unavoidable in any form of sequential diagnosis, although they should remain a fairly small proportion of all diagnoses.

The validity of trial results depends heavily on the reliability of the examiner. This factor is usually referred to as intraexaminer reliability, the ability of an examiner to record the same conditions the same way over time. Most examiners with training and experience develop an acceptable degree of intraexaminer reliability. Reliability between different examiners, interexaminer reliability, is often more difficult, even when they train together from the same written criteria. Ideally it is best to use one well-qualified examiner, but large-scale studies often require that more than one examiner should undergo a period of training to bring their diagnostic standards as close together as can possibly be managed. This training procedure is referred to as standardization. Where one of the group is the "gold standard" examiner and the training is to enable other examiners to record similarly, term calibration more accurately describes the exercise.

7. 试验周期 Duration of the trial

根据试验的目的决定试验观察期限，如氟防龋效果观察，至少应持续2年，一般为2～3年。牙周病预防措施的效果观察可以为6周到18个月。

Clinical trials must be continued long enough to permit detection of new disease or extension of lesions already present during the period of the trial. For caries trials, the minimum duration is usually 2 to 3 years, although precise timing depends on the purposes of the trial. The longer the trial, the more expensive, so trade-offs are required. The Federation Dentaire Internationale (FDI) suggested in 1977 that trials of plaque-inhibiting agents could be as short as 8 - 21 days, but that guideline was for plaque measurements only. The American Dental Association (ADA) requires plaque-inhibiting agents that seek the association's seal of approval to demonstrate gingivitis reduction as well; it requires such trials to be at least 6 months long. The FDI in its 1977 report, also recommended that studies of calculus-

preventing agents should last 90 days for supragingival calculus and longer for subgingival calculus.

8. 重视医学伦理 Ethical considerations

Humans taking part in clinical trials must give informed consent (知情同意书), which means a written acceptance that the participant understands the conduct of the trial and the nature of any risks involved. Authors should certify that the study protocol has been accepted by their institution's Institutional Review Board (IRB), which any institution conducting research is required to maintain. If the study includes vulnerable populations (e.g., children, illiterate or mentally retarded people), extra explanations are usually required. Additional explanation for how the rights of participants have been safeguarded may also be needed if the study is conducted in a developing country that dose not have the rigorous standards for human subject protection that developed nations have. (Burt 1999)

第四节　流行病研究中的偏倚及其控制

Section 4 The Bias and its Control in Epidemilogical Studies

在流行病学研究中，无论采用何种研究方法都应尽量保证研究结果与客观实际状况相一致。但由于各种因素的影响，研究结果与客观实际往往存在差异，有时甚至会得出完全错误的结果。造成这种差异的原因有两个，即随机误差和偏倚。随机误差是因抽样所产生的差异，一般可以通过统计学方法予以估计和评价。偏倚是指随机误差以外的误差，即系统误差。流行病学研究中的偏倚种类较多，应深入了解和认识并在研究过程中尽量加以避免和控制，从而保证研究结果的真实性。

一、偏倚的类型 Types of bias

偏倚一般分为三大类，即选择偏倚（Selection bias）、信息偏倚（Information bias）和混杂偏倚（Confounding bias）。

1. 选择偏倚 Selective bias

选择偏倚是指被选择进入研究的研究对象与未被选择进入研究者特征上的差异所造成的系统误差。选择偏倚在确定试验组和对照组的样本时很容易产生，也可产生于资料收集过程中的失访和无应答等。在各类流行病学研究中选择偏倚均可发生，以在病例对照研究与现况研究中最常见。

（1）选择偏倚 Selective bias

在调查过程中样本人群的选择不是按照抽样设计的方案进行，而是随意选择，由于调查对象的代表性很差，破坏了同质性，使调查结果与总体人群患病情况之间产生的误差，称为选择性偏倚。如用医院病例说明人群患病情况，显然有误差。

（2）无应答偏倚 Unresponsive bias

无应答偏倚实际就是漏查。在随机抽样时，属于样本人群中的受检者，由于主观或客观原因未能接受检查，如未接受检查的人数达到抽样人数的30%，应答率仅有70%，结果就难以用来估计总体的现患率。

（3）选择偏倚的控制 Control of selective bias

- 研究者对在整个研究中可能会出现的各种选择偏倚应有充分的了解和掌握；
- 严格掌握研究对象的入选和排除标准；
- 在研究中采取相应措施，做好组织工作和教育宣传工作，尽量使研究对象积极配合。

Many types of bias can destroy the internal validity of a study, but it is common to put them into one of three categories: selection bias, information bias and confounding.

In a descriptive, for example dental caries, can be biased for several reasons. The sample we study may not be representative of the population we wish to describe. If that is the case, our estimate of the amount of dental caries in the population will not be correct, and we talk about selection bias. In most studies we do not get information from all members of our sample. For various reasons some people do not wish to participate and a response rate as low as 80% is not common. Since the non-responders and the responders usually differ with regard to the factors we wish to study there may be bias in our study. This bias cannot be reduced by increasing the sample size. It may happen that we have information about some characteristics of the non-responders that may allow us to speculate remains speculative. In a cohort study, the major potential selection bias is loss to follow-up, and certain types of people are more likely than others to drop out. Selection bias is of particular importance in case-control studies where we select the cases and non-cases in a setting in which the exposure has already occurred. For example, we may decide to use existing (prevalent) cases at the onset of the study regardless of duration of their disease or decide to use newly diagnosed (incident) cases, if the use of prevalent cases can lead to a biased conclusion.

2. 信息偏倚 Information bias

信息偏倚又称观察偏倚（observational bias），是指在研究的实施过程中从研究对象获得的信息时所产生的系统误差。信息偏倚在各类流行病学研究中均可发生，可来自研究对象和研究者自身，也可来自器械设备等。

（1）测量偏倚 Detective bias

因检查器械等造成的测量偏倚在龋病、牙周病流行病学研究中，各指数的应用是基于临床检查。因此，检查器械不规范，现场工作条件差，如光线不足等，都可造成系统误差。如检查龋病时，按WHO口腔健康调查要求使用CPI探针（第四版）与使用5号尖探针（第三版），结果就会有很大差异。

（2）回忆偏倚 Recall bias

回忆偏倚是指在询问疾病的既往史和危险因素时，研究对象常常因时间久远，难以准确回忆而使回答不准确，这在病例对照研究中最常见。

（3）报告偏倚 Reporting bias

报告偏倚是指由研究对象有意夸大或缩小某些信息所导致的误差。有时调查对象对询问的问题不愿意真实回答，使结果产生误差。如在调查个人收入情况时，常常得不到真实的回答。又如在调查口腔卫生习惯时，一些没有刷牙习惯的人有时不愿实说，而使记录不属实。

（4）信息偏倚的控制 Control of information bias

按研究规定使用标准检查器械，并保持稳定的环境条件。在研究设计中尽量提供可能的回忆目标，对一些敏感的问题采用间接询问法，对象转移法等技术以保证信息的可靠。

Information bias (or misclassification) can occur when there are errors in obtaining the required information. The misclassification may be differential or non-differential. When the error in classification of exposure or disease status is independent of the level of the other variable, the misclassification is called non-differential. Non-differential misclassification may occur in a case-control study if the participants' recollection of exposure is not related to whether the participants have the disease or condition of interest or not. The participants may answer a question about the exposure with a socially acceptable but inaccurate response. Consider a case-control study of periodontal disease in which the exposure of interest is poor oral hygiene. Redardless of disease status, respondents may overreport the measures they take to increase their oral cleanliness because they know that good oral hygiene is much more socially acceptable. What happens when this kind of non-differential misclassification occurs is that the differences between the study groups are blurred as illustrated in 表 2-5

表 2-5 Non-differential misclassification in a hypotherical case-control study of the association between poor oral hygiene and periodontal disease

The study		
	Poor hygiene habits	Good hygiene habits
Periodontal disease	100	50
No periodontal disease	50	100
	Odds ratio= (100 × 100) / (50 × 50) =4.0	
The study	Poor hygiene habits	Good hygiene habits
Periodontal disease	80	70
No periodontal disease	40	110
	Odds ratio= (80 × 110) / (40 × 70) =3.1	

In this case, the association we observe between the exposure, poor oral hygiene and periodontal disease will less than an unbiased estimate. In general, non-differential misclassification tends to introduce bias towards the null hypothesis. We will underestimate the association between exposure and disease or maybe find no association at all.

Two common types of differential information bias are often referred to as recall bias and interviewer bias. Recall bias results from the participants' ability to recall previous events and exposure. Mothers of children with a cleft palate may well recall previous exposures better than other mothers. Recall bias is a possibility in case-control studies where people have to remember something in the past. Interviewer bias may occur when an interviewer knows the research objectives. The interviewer may explore the responses from the cases more thoroughly than those from non-cases and may even unknowingly send subtle signals by body language or voice. Therefore, it is desirable to blind the interviewers to the research hypothesis, although this way be impossible in a case-control study. The terminology og bias in relation to the type of study and misclassification of exposure and outcome can be summarized as in 表 2-6 (Pine 1997).

表 2-6 Bias in relation to type of study

	Exposure/risk bias	Disease/outcome
Case-contral studies	Information bias	Selection bias
Cohort studies	Selection bias	Information bias

3. 混杂偏倚 Confounding bias

混杂偏倚或称混杂（confounding），是指在流行病学研究中，由于一个或多个混杂因素的影响，掩盖或夸大了研究因素与疾病之间的联系，从而使两者之间的真正联系被错误的估计。

（1）混杂因素 Confounding factors

混杂因素又称混杂因子或外来因素（extraneous factor），是指与研究因素和研究疾病均有关，若在比较的群组中分布不均，可以掩盖或夸大因素与疾病之间真正联系的因素。

（2）混杂偏倚的控制 control of confounding bias

①限制 Restriction　针对某一或某些可能的混杂因素，在研究设计时对受试者的入选条件给予限制。实行限制后可得到同质的研究对象，以防止可能出现的混杂偏倚。这样可以对研究因素与疾病间的关系作出比较准确的估计。但也可能使受试者对总体的代表性受到影响，从而研究结论的外推受到一定限制。

②匹配 Maching　匹配是指在为指示研究对象选择对照时，使其针对一个或多个潜在的混杂因素与指示研究对象相同或接近，因而消除混杂因素对研究结果的影响。匹配在实验性研究和非实验性研究设计中均可应用。

③随机化 Randomization　指以随机化原则，使研究对象以同等的几率被分配在各处理组中，从而使潜在的混杂因素在各组间分布均匀。随机化方法主要用于实验性研究，但多用于临床试验研究。

④统计处理 Statistics　混杂偏倚在资料分析阶段也可以通过一定的统计处理方法加以控制。如使用 Mantel-Haenszel 分层分析方法和多因素分析方法等。

Confounding refers to the mixing of the effects of an extraneous variable with the effects of the exposure and disease or condition of interest. Confounding can be illustrated as in figure 2-2. D is the effect or outcome, E is the exposure and C a potential confounder. A confounder must be an independent risk of disease and it must be associated with both the exposure and the disease under study, but it must not be a link in the causal chain between the exposure and the disease.

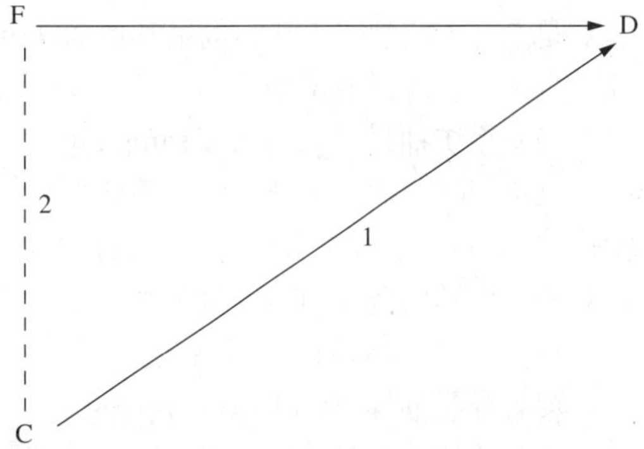

图 2-2　Schematic presentation of confounding where C is confounder (s), E is exposure and D is disease or outcome

We know that plaque is a risk factor for the development of periodontal disease. However, smoking seems to be a risk factor too, and we know that smoking is associated with poorer oral hygiene. An unadjusted estimation between the presence of plaque and periodontal disease will therefore re-

flect the population's smoking habits too, because there will be more individuals with poor hygiene among the smokers than non-smokers. Smoking will be a confounder.

第五节 口腔健康调查

Section 5 Oral Health Surveys

口腔健康调查是口腔流行病学研究中最常用的一种方法，就是在一个特定的时间内收集某人群口腔疾病和口腔健康的频率、流行强度、分布及流行规律的资料，是一种横断面调查。对了解某人群的口腔健康状况；掌握口腔疾病的流行特征；揭示影响口腔疾病发生的因素及发现口腔疾病的流行趋势，以及为进一步开展口腔健康流行病学研究和制定口腔保健工作规划提供科学的依据。

1. 普查 Mass examination

普查是指在特定时间范围内，一般为 1 ~ 2 天或 1 ~ 2 周。对特定人群中的每一个成员进行的调查或检查，又称全面调查。普查可以有不同的目的，有的是为了早期发现并及时治疗一些疾病。有的是为了了解疾病的患病状况与分布，为制定具体防制计划提供依据，或作为社区人群试点的基线资料。普查的最大优点是能发现调查人群中的全部病例并给予及时治疗，或用作项目开发的依据。但普查的应查率要求在95%以上，漏查率太高会使结果正确性差。最大缺点是这种调查需要的工作量大，成本高，所以只能在较小范围内使用，如计划在一所或几所学校或某个社区开展的口腔保健活动，在此之前可使用普查以准确获得疾病的基线资料。

2. 抽样调查 Sampling survey

为查明某病或某些疾病在某个国家或某个地区的现患情况或流行强度，多用抽样调查的方法。所谓抽样即从目标地区的总体人群中，按统计学随机抽样原则抽取部分人作为调查对象，这个程序称为抽样。被抽到的人群称为样本人群。抽样调查是用样本人群调查的结果，推断总体人群的现患情况。前提条件是抽取的数量足够大，调查的数据可靠，这种调查方法的优点为：省时间、省劳力和省经费，且所得资料同样具有代表性。抽样的方法有：

（1）单纯随机抽样 Simple random sampling

是最基本的抽样方法，也是其他抽样方法的基础。它是按一定方式以同等的概率抽样称单纯随机抽样。可以使用抽签的方式，也可以使用随机数字表来抽取样本。

（2）系统抽样 Systematic sampling

又称间隔抽样、机械抽样。将抽样对象按次序编号，先随机抽取第一个调查对象，然后再按一定间隔随机抽样。如一个学校有 1000 名学生，根据调查要求只需抽取 100 名学生作为调查对象，抽样比例为 10%。抽样可先对学生编号，可先在 1 ~ 10 号学生中随机抽取一个号，然后每隔 10 个编号抽取一个学生。

（3）分层抽样 Stratified sampling

先将总体按某种特征分成若干个“层”，即组别或类型等，再在每个层中用随机方式抽取调查对象，再将每个层所有抽取的调查对象合成一个样本，称分层抽样。常用的分层类别有年龄、性别、居住地、文化程度、经济条件等，将调查人群分成若干组。还可分成等比例（即按比例）和不等比例（即最优分配）两种分层随机抽样。

（4）整群抽样 Cluster sampling

是以整群为抽样单位，从总体中随机抽取若干群为调查单位，然后对每个群内所有对象进行检查。如：欲知道 20 所小学 10000 名学生的患龋率，抽样比例定为 20%。由于学生太多，且分散在 20 所学校内，用单纯随机抽样的方法太麻烦，此时可随机抽取 4 所学校，再对抽到的学校学生全部进行调查，这样组织比较方便，适用于群体间差异较小的调查单位。

（5）多级抽样 Multistage sampling

又称多阶段抽样。在进行大规模调查时，常把抽样过程分为几个阶段，每个阶段可采用单纯随机抽样，也可将以上各种方法结合起来使用。我国第二次口腔健康流行病学调查就是采用这种方法，称为分层，不等比，多阶段，整群抽样法。

一、调查的设计 The design of survey

1. 目的 Objectives

口腔健康调查是用于收集某人群口腔健康状况和治疗需要的资料以监测患病水平和种类的变化，借此评价现有口腔保健服务的适宜性和有效性，并依据需要安排或调整口腔保健服务和人员培训方案。通过调查得到的资料也可用于监测口腔保健服务的效果。

Oral health surveys are used to collect information about the oral health status and treatment needs of a population, and subsequently, to monitor changes in levels and patterns of disease. In this way, it is possible to assess the appropriateness and effectiveness of the services being provided and plan or modify oral health services and training programmes as needed. The information obtained using the survey can also be used to monitor aspects of the effectiveness of oral care services.

口腔健康状况调查的目的可以概括为以下 5 点：

（1）查明口腔疾病在特定时间内的发生频率和分布特征及其流行规律。

（2）了解和分析影响口腔健康的有关因素。

（3）为探索病因，建立和验证病因假设提供依据。

（4）选择预防保健措施和评价预防保健措施的效果。

（5）估价治疗与人力需要。

2. 口腔疾病的特点 Special characteristics of oral diseases

在某些情况下，调查人员可以得到卫生统计人员对设计调查方案的指导和建议。但是，口腔疾病特殊的流行病学特征使得常见口腔疾病的调查方案和样本设计与传统调查方法有所不同。对口腔主要常见疾病即龋病和牙周病的调查应考虑以下特点：

（1）与年龄密切相关，随着年龄增长，其患病率和严重程度增加。

（2）可发生于所有人群，但患病率和严重程度不同。

（3）龋病具有不可逆性（指已形成龋洞者），现况调查的数据既有目前发病状况，也包括过去患病状况。

（4）处于不同社会经济发展水平和环境状况的人群，其龋病患病水平不同。

（5）对每位受检者的多项检查按统一标准进行，如龋病以牙为单位，牙周病则以口腔的6个区段为单位。

（6）需要在口腔健康调查中常规收集的其他重要资料也要包括在调查表中。但是，对口腔非常见病的进一步研究则需要采取不同的调查设计。

In some situations, investigators will have access to the advice of an expert in health statistics who might be able to provide guidance on planning a survey. However, particular features of the epidemiology of oral diseases have permitted the development of an approach to sample design and survey planning for the most common oral diseases that is different from traditional sample designs. The special considerations concerning the two major oral diseases - dental caries and periodontal diseases - are as follows:

The diseases are strongly age-related, as there is often an increase in severity and prevalence with increased age.

The diseases exist in all populations, varying only in severity and prevalence.

One of the diseases, dental caries, is irreversible (at the cavitation level used in the methods described here) and thus information on current status provides data not only on the amount of disease present, but also on previous disease experience.

There is extensive documentation on variation of profiles of dental caries for population groups with different socioeconomic levels and environmental conditions.

Many observations are made in standard measurements for each subject, e.g. for each tooth in the case of caries and for the six sextants of the mouth in the assessment of periodontal diseases.

Other important information which needs to be collected routinely in oral health surveys is also included in the assessment. It should be noted, however, that in-depth studies of the less common oral diseases require different survey designs.

二、调查的组织实施 The organizing and implementing of survey

1. 调查的组织工作 Organizing the survey

（1）准备调查方案 Preparing a survey protocol

It is important to prepare a written protocol for the survey, which should contain the following information:

- *Main objective and purpose of the survey*
- *A description of the type of information to be collected and of the methods to be used*
- *A description of the sampling methods to be used*
- *Personnel and physical arrangements*
- *Statistical methods to be used in analyzing the data*
- *A provisional budget*
- *A provisional timetable of main activities and responsible staff*

（2）调查获得批准 Obtaining approval from the authorities

Permission to examine population groups must be obtained from a local, regional or national authority. For example, if schoolchildren are to be examined, then the school authorities should be approached, the purpose of the survey explained and their approval obtained. In some instances, written permission from parents must be given before children can be examined. It is the responsibility of the local organizer of the survey to ascertain local practices regarding consent. The survey organizer should also notify the health authorities, since it may be necessary to time the survey to fit in with other health-related activities. This applies particularly when adult populations are to be surveyed.

It is important to provide the dental profession and oral health administrators in the area with details of the survey. Officers of dental societies and local dental practitioners can often help in gaining the cooperation of the community for the survey, and of any their patients who may be included in the sample.

(3) 调查经费预算 Budgeting

A budget for the survey should be prepared, which should include all the resources required, including personnel, to carry out the survey. Basic oral health survey can often be conducted as part of the duties of dental public health workers, and may be undertaken with only minor additions to existing budgets.

(4) 调查实施计划 Scheduling

One of the most important aspects of survey planning is the preparation of a schedule for data collection. If this is not done, examining personnel may waste time, waiting for subjects to arrive, or be otherwise unnecessarily delayed.

The planner can estimate from the preliminary survey, or from previous experience, how much time, on average, each examination will take. As a guideline, a basic examination of a child usually takes about 5～10 minutes, while a complete examination of an adult may take between 15 and 20 minutes. Daily and weekly schedules can then be prepared. These should be made available to survey personnel, as well as to school and health authorities. The schedules should allow for some flexibility so that unexpected delays do not cause major upsets in the survey timetable.

Reliable observations and consistent judgments are important in surveys. Since fatigue contributes significantly to inaccuracy and inconsistency, it is unwise to make the schedule too demanding. For example, if classes of 25-30 children in several schools are to be examined by one examiner, the planning schedule should include time for:

- *Introducing the examining team to the school director and class teachers concerned;*
- *Choosing an appropriate place to carry out the examinations in each school, and setting up equipment;*
- *Examining one class of 12-year-olds;*
- *Providing a brief oral report to the school director; and*
- *Traveling to the next school.*

(5) 调查报告 Survey reporting

It is appropriate, and often essential, to report the survey findings to local authorities. The report may be a simple summary of the number of subjects examined and the observations of the examiner. This can usually be delivered personally, on the spot. A full technical report will require more time to prepare, but sent as soon as it is complete.

2. 调查的实施工作 Implementing the survey

基本工作 General work

(1) 调查点的组织联系

The organization of a survey must commence well before the date on which it is intended to start examinations. It is necessary to contact persons in authority in the institutions or organizations where people will be examined.

(2) 建立调查工作日志

The organizer of the survey should maintain a logbook in which the location of each day's examinations, the number of persons examined, and information about each survey location are recorded. Occasionally, observations made and impressions formed at this time can have an important bearing on later assessment of survey results. If these are not clearly described at the time of observation, they will be forgotten or confused.

(3) 调查前的练习

For investigators planning their first oral health survey, it is helpful to examine two classes of 12-year-old children in local primary schools as a preliminary exercise. This will give the survey personnel an opportunity of working together and of identifying and discussing any organization or technical problems that may arise. The calibration of the examiners and training of the recording clerks can be performed at the same time.

(4) 当地氟源状况

A sample of drinking-water should be collected at each examination site and sent for analysis of fluoride content. Clean polyethylene bottles of 25-30 ml capacity should be used for this purpose. They should be rinsed in distilled water prior to rinsing twice with the water to be sampled. The bottles should then be filled, closed firmly and clearly labeled with a permanent ink pen, giving the date of collection, location and source of the water. In many countries, it is possible to obtain fluoride analysis services through public health and/or water supply departments.

In addition, information should be gathered on:

♦ *sources of fluorides available to the survey population, other than water (e.g. salt, tablets and milk);*

♦ *levels of usage of topical fluorides especially dentifrices and/or other products likely to have an impact on dental caries.*

(5) 检查器械的准备与消毒

Sufficient numbers of instruments should be available to avoid the need to interrupt examinations while used ones are sterilized. Generally, a minimum of 30 mouth mirrors and 30 periodontal probes per examiner should be provided, as this will permit instruments to be sterilized while the others are being used.

Used instruments should be placed in disinfectant solution, then washed and drained well before sterilization. Current national recommendations and standards should be followed for both infection control and waste disposal.

Examiners are responsible for maintaining adequate infection control in survey procedures. During their training, it should be emphasized that with proper use of dental mirrors and the periodontal probe, all areas of the oral cavity can be fully examined without the need for digital manipulation of the oral tissues, hence reducing the risk of cross-infection. The use of disposable masks and gloves and the wearing of protective glasses are recommended.

3. 调查项目与表格 Catalogue and assessment form of survey

（1）调查项目 Items

调查项目即调查涉及口腔健康状况的主要内容，这应根据调查目的来确定。一般可将调查项目分为三类：一类是直接反映口腔健康状况的信息，如龋病、牙周病、口腔卫生状况等，这些项目将用于调查以后的统计分析。另一类是背景状况信息，如受检者姓名、性别、年龄、学校名、受检者编号等，这些项目部分用于统计分析，部分用于信息管理；还有一类为问卷调查项目，如与口腔健康有关的知识、态度、行为习惯与生活方式。

选择调查项目必须慎重，应选择那些与调查目的有关的项目，保证把时间和精力集中于必要的调查。但也不能遗漏任何有关的项目，开展一次口腔流行病学调查常会花费大量人力、物力、财力，尤其开展大规模的口腔流行病学调查，常会涉及许多省市，动员很多人员参加，政府投入相当大的经费，这种调查常常难以在短期内重复，一旦在设计时遗漏某些重要项目，将会失去很多有价值的信息，带来很难弥补的损失，因此在设计时须考虑周全。根据设计的不同调查内容，可将调查项目具体分为一般项目、健康状况项目和问卷调查项目。

1）一般项目 General information

包括受检者的一般情况，如：姓名、性别、年龄、职业、民族、籍贯、文化程度、经济状况、宗教信仰、出生地区、居住年限等信息，这些项目常常反映疾病分布的差异，调查以后将这些项目与健康状况项目结合分析，有可能会发现某种口腔疾病的流行特征。一般项目常列入口腔流行病学调查表的第一部分，可通过询问或从户口本上获得。

2）健康状况项目 Oral health status

包括各种口腔疾病，是口腔健康状况调查的主要内容，根据调查目的而定。最常用的调查项目如龋病、牙周病、牙列状况等，其他如氟牙症、釉质发育不全、口腔黏膜状况、颞颌关节状况等。我国第二次口腔健康流行病学调查所确定的调查项目包括冠龋、根龋、牙周状况、口腔卫生状况、义齿和无牙情况等。

3）问卷调查项目 Questionnaire

除上述一般项目的内容外，主要包括口腔卫生知识、态度与信念，行为与实践等方面的具体内容，如：个人口腔卫生、牙刷和牙膏的选择、刷牙习惯、饮食习惯、预防意识与就医行为等。

（2）调查表格 Assessment form

口腔健康状况调查项目确定后，应根据具体调查项目设计调查表。根据不同的目的确定的调查项目应设计不同的调查表。本节主要以第三次全国口腔健康调查表为例作简单介绍。根据表中列出的调查项目有：一般情况、口腔黏膜、牙列状况（龋齿）、牙周状况、氟牙症、义齿修复情况和需要立即处理及安排治疗的情况说明等项目（表 2-7）。具体检查的项目有以下五项：口腔黏膜、牙列状况（包括冠龋和根龋）、牙周状况（包括牙龈出血、牙石、牙周袋深度、附着丧失）、氟牙症、义齿修复状况。

下面就调查表中这些项目的填写作一说明。

姓名________ ID号(1) □□□□□□□□□□□□ (12)

户口类型 城=1 乡=2 □ (13) 性别 男=1 女=2 □ (14) 职业(15) □□ (16) 民族(17) □□ (18)

受教育年限(19) □□ (20) 出生日期(21) □□□□□□□□ (28)

检查日期(29) □□□□□□□□ (36) 检查者编号 □ (37)

口腔黏膜

状况			部位	
0	无异常		0	唇红缘
1	恶性肿瘤（口腔癌）		1	口角
2	白斑	(38) □□ (41)	2	唇
3	扁平苔藓		3	唇沟
4	溃疡（阿弗他、疱疹、创伤性）	(39) □□ (42)	4	颊黏膜
5	急性坏死性龈炎	(40) □□ (43)	5	口底
6	念珠菌病		6	舌
7	脓肿		7	硬腭/软腭
8	其他（详细说明）		8	牙槽嵴/牙龈
9	不作记录		9	不作记录

牙列状况

					55	54	53	52	51	61	62	63	64	65				
		18	17	16	15	14	13	12	11	21	22	23	24	25	26	27	28	
冠龋	(44)	□	□	□	□	□	□	□	□	□	□	□	□	□	□	□	□	(59)
根龋	(60)	□	□	□	□	□	□	□	□	□	□	□	□	□	□	□	□	(75)
					85	84	83	82	81	71	72	73	74	75				
		48	47	46	45	44	43	42	41	31	32	33	34	35	36	37	38	
冠龋	(76)	□	□	□	□	□	□	□	□	□	□	□	□	□	□	□	□	(91)
根龋	(92)	□	□	□	□	□	□	□	□	□	□	□	□	□	□	□	□	(107)

冠根龋符号

乳牙	恒牙冠		恒牙冠	
A	0	无龋	0	无龋
B	1	有龋	1	有龋
C	2	已充填有龋	2	已充填有龋
D	3	已充填无龋	3	已充填无龋
E	4	因龋缺失	6	残根
X	5	因其他原因失牙	7	种植牙
F	6	窝沟封闭	8	牙龈无萎缩，牙根未暴露
G	7	桥基牙、特殊冠或贴面，种植牙	9	不作记录（缺失牙、或无法检查的牙根）
X	8	未萌牙		
N	9	不作记录		

表 2-7 第三次全国口腔健康调查表

牙周状况

		18	17	16	15	14	13	12	11	21	22	23	24	25	26	27	28	
牙龈出血	(108)																	(123)
牙石	(124)																	(139)
牙周袋	(140)																	(155)
附着丧失	(156)																	(171)

		48	47	46	45	44	43	42	41	31	32	33	34	35	36	37	38	
牙龈出血	(172)																	(187)
牙石	(188)																	(203)
牙周袋	(204)																	(219)
附着丧失	(220)																	(235)

牙龈出血

0 无
1 有
9 不作记录
X 缺失牙

牙石

0 无
1 有
9 不作记录
X 缺失牙

牙周袋

0 无
1 牙周袋4～5mm（龈缘在第一个黑区内）
2 牙周袋≥6mm（龈缘超过第一个黑区的上限）
9 不作记录
X 缺失牙

牙周附着丧失

0 0.3mm
1 4～5mm（釉牙骨质界在第一个黑区内）
2 6～8mm（釉牙骨质界在两个黑区之间）
3 9～11mm（釉牙骨质界在第二个黑区内）
4 ≥12mm（釉牙骨质界超过第二个黑区的上限）
9 不作记录
X 缺失牙

义齿修复状况

0 无义齿
1 单桥（一个固定桥）
2 多桥（多个固定桥）
3 局部义齿
4 桥和局部义齿
5 总义齿
6 非正规固定桥
9 不作记录

	上颌	下颌	
(237)			(238)

需要立即处理和安排治疗的情况说明

有=1
无=0

☐ (239)

表格类型

原始表=1
复查表=2

☐ (240)

1）调查表及其所列项目都必须使用标准代码，否则调查资料就难以进入计算机标准程序进行统计。即使调查表中某些项目的资料没有被收集或记录，某些项目不适合于所检查的人群，代码亦须保持不变。表内未使用的项目，用代码9填写在相应的栏目，表示不作记录。

2）凡属于方案中规定不作检查的项目，表内方格可以空着，否则表内各项方格都必须有英文字母或阿拉伯数字。

3）表格内代码填写必须清晰、规范，如零应写成“0”。如连续几个牙位的检查符号相同时，则中间可以用直线代替，但直线两侧符号必须一致。如：

0 ———————————— 0

4）表格的设计为便于以后计算机进行处理，各栏旁边均有记录代码的说明。每栏都编有一识别符号（圆括号内的小数字），该代码代表计算机程序上的一个位置。为了减少错误，所有进入计算机的数字必须填写清楚，有的数字常易混淆，如1和7，2和4，6和0，为了避免混淆和保证统计结果准确，数字应按下列方式以印刷体书写：

1 2 3 4 5 6 7 8 9 0

采用字母作代码时，例如记录乳牙牙列状况的检查结果，必须用大写字母如下：

A B C D E

根据国际牙科联盟两位数字系统，两位数字代表特定的牙齿，第一位数字代表口腔的象限，第二位数字代表牙位。在确定某一牙齿的位置时，建议首先读出象限的代号，然后读代表牙位的数字，如右上侧第二切牙（12）读“一、二”，不读“十二”；左下第三磨牙（38）读“三八”不读“三十八”。

三、指数与标准 Indices and criteria

根据调查目的确定使用的指数和调查标准。标准不一致可导致所收集的资料缺乏可比性，因此在调查设计中首先要根据目的确定调查标准。

1. 龋病的调查标准和常用指数 The criteria and index for dental caries

冠龋的诊断标准是：牙的窝沟或光滑面有底部发软的病损，釉质有潜在损害或沟壁软化者即诊断为龋。对于釉质上的白斑、着色的不平坦区、探针可插入的着色窝沟但底部不发软及中到重度氟牙症所造成的釉质上硬的凹陷，均不诊断为龋。

根龋的诊断标准是：用CPI探针在牙根面探及软的或皮革样的损害即为根龋。

Sound crown:

A crown is recorded assound if it shows no evidence of treated or untreated clinical caries. The stages of caries that precede cavitation, as well as other conditions similar to the early stages of caries, are excluded because they cannot be reliably diagnosed. Thus, a crown with the following defects, in the absence of other positive criteria, should be coded as sound:

- *white or chalkly spots;*
- *discoloured or rough spots that are not soft to touch with a metal CPI probe;*
- *stained pits or fissures in the enamel that do not have visual signs of undermined enamel, or softening of floor or walls detectable with a CPI probe;*
- *dark, shiny, hard, pitted areas of enamel in a tooth showing signs of moderate to severe fluorosis;*

- *lesions that, on the basis of their distribution or history, or visual/tactile examination, apear to be due to abrasion.*

Decayed crown:

Caries is recorded as present when a lesion in a pit or fissure, or a smooth tooth surface, has an unmistakable cavity, undermined enamel, or a detectably softened floor or wall. The CPI probe should be used to confirm visual evidence of caries on the occlusal, buccal and lingual surfaces. When any doubt exists, caries should not be recorded as present.

Decayed root:

Caries is recorded as present when a lesion feels soft or leathery to probing with the CPI probe.

记录龋病患病状况常用的指数有龋失补指数、患病率、龋病发病率与根龋指数，分述如下：

（1）恒牙龋失补指数 DMF index

恒牙龋失补指数是检查龋病时最常用的指数，该指数是由Klein等于1938年研究龋病分布时提出的，其主要依据是牙体硬组织已经形成的病变不可能再恢复为正常状态，将永远留下某种程度的历史记录。

龋失补数用龋（Decayed）、失（Missing）、补（Filled）牙数（DMFT）或龋失补牙面数（DMFS）表示。“龋”即已龋坏尚未充填的牙；“失”指因龋丧失的牙；“补”为因龋已做充填的牙。作为个别病人统计，DMF指数是指龋、失、补牙数或牙面数之和，而在某人群中的DMF指数为这个人群的平均DMF牙数或牙面数，通常可称之为龋（牙）均（DMFT）或龋面均（DMFS）。

成年人因牙周病而失牙的几率较高，因而统计成年人龋失补牙数时有可能将因牙周病丧失的牙也计算在内。因此，按照世界卫生组织的记录方法，检查30岁以上者，不再区分是龋病还是牙周病导致的失牙，其失牙数按口腔内实际丧失牙数计。

（2）乳牙龋失补指数 dmf index

乳牙龋失补指数指乳牙的龋（d）失（m）补（f）牙数（dmft）或龋失补牙面数（dmfs），龋补定义与恒牙龋相同，计算因龋丧失的牙数须与生理性脱落的乳牙区分，不应以患儿或家长的回忆为依据。世界卫生组织计算失牙的标准是：9岁以下的儿童，丧失了不该脱落的乳牙，如乳磨牙或乳尖牙，即为龋失。或用龋拔补牙数（deft）或龋拔补牙面数（defs）为乳牙龋指数。“拔”指因重度龋坏，临床无法治疗已拔除的乳牙。也可用龋补牙数（dft）或龋补牙面数（dfs）说明人群中乳牙的患龋情况表2-8。

表 2-8　龋失补牙数和牙面数使用方法

	DMFT/dmft	DMFS/dmfs
一颗近中殆面患龋的牙	D(d) = 1	D(d) = 2
一个牙面有充填体另一牙面有原发龋的牙	D(d) = 1	D(d) = 1 F(f) = 1
一个牙面上既有原发龋又有充填体的牙	D(d) = 1	D(d) = 1
可疑龋	不记分	不记分
一颗龋失牙	M(m) = 1	后牙龋失 M(m) = 5 前牙龋失 M(m) = 4

资料来源：杨是主编《口腔预防医学》（第二版）

(3) 龋均(DMFT)和龋面均(DMFS)

龋均指受检查人群中每人口腔中平均龋、失、补牙数。龋面均指受检查人群中每人口腔中平均龋、失、补牙面数。龋均和龋面均的计算公式如下：

$$龋均=\frac{龋、失、补牙之和}{受检人数}$$

$$龋面均=\frac{龋、失、补牙面之和}{受检人数}$$

虽然龋均和龋面均都反映受检查人群龋病的严重程度，但两者反映人群龋病严重程度的敏感性是不同的。相比之下，DMFS较为敏感。一颗牙如有3个牙面患龋，用DMFT计分则为1，而用 DMFS 计分则是 3，客观上放大了计分值。

(4) 患龋率 Prevalence

患龋率指在调查期间某一人群中患龋病的频率，人口基数以百人计算，故常以百分数表示。患龋率主要用于龋病的流行病学研究，如比较和描述龋病的分布，探讨龋病的病因和流行因素等。计算公式如下：

$$患龋率=\frac{患龋病人数}{受检人数}\times 100\%$$

评价患龋状况时，必须参考龋病发病率，DMF 指数等才能作出较全面的评价。

(5) 龋病发病率 Incidence

龋病发病率通常是指至少在一年时间内，某人群新发生龋病的频率。与患龋率不同的是仅指在这个特定时期内，新龋发生的频率。计算公式如下：

$$龋病发病率=\frac{发生新龋的人数}{受检人数}\times 100\%$$

例：1985年检查某班15岁学生50人，其中患龋病者35人，龋失补牙数为：D=70，M=2，F=8，龋失补牙面数为：D=210，M=10，F=16；2 年后再对这 50 名学生检查，发现其中 10 名学生有新的龋损，患新龋的牙数为15，牙面数为18，计算这班学生在1985年的龋均、龋面均、患龋率以及 2 年后龋病发病率如下：

表 2-9 1985 年的龋均、龋面均、患龋率以及 2 年后龋病发病率

1985 年	龋均	=(70+2+8)/50 = 1.60
	龋面均	=(210+10+16)/50 = 4.72
	患龋率	= 35/50 × 100% = 70%
1987 年	龋病发病率	= 10/50 × 100% = 20%

这一指标在口腔流行病学中应用最为广泛，例如估计龋病流行强度，描述龋病的分布特

点，探讨疾病发生因素，评价预防措施效果，以及前瞻性研究等。

（6）龋充填构成比 Proportion of FT in DMFT

龋充填构成比是指一个人群的龋、失、补牙之和中已充填的龋所占的比重，常用百分数表示。如果已充填牙存在继发龋，此牙面仍算作龋，不计为已充填的牙。龋充填构成比可用于反映地区口腔保健工作的水平，也可反映充填这些龋齿所需要的工作量。其计算公式为：

$$龋充填构成比=\frac{受检人群已充填牙数}{受检人群龋、失、补牙数之和}\times 100\%$$

（7）根龋指数 Root caries index

根龋常发生在中老年人牙颈部，多见于牙龈退缩后，发生在牙根面的龋和因牙根面龋而做的充填。平时所用的患龋率和龋均难以表达牙龈退缩与根面龋的关系。Katz于20世纪80年代提出根龋指数（root caries index， RCI），将牙龈退缩引入其中，其计算方法如下：

$$根龋指数\ (RCI)=\frac{根龋数}{牙龈退缩牙数}\times 100\%$$

根龋指数也就是根患龋率，其中根龋数包括患根龋的牙数和因根龋而充填的牙数。牙龈退缩数指牙龈退缩的牙数。

例如：对一名老年人做口腔健康检查，发现该名老年人口腔中牙龈退缩的牙有50个，其中患根龋的牙5个，因根龋而充填的牙5个。该名老年人的根龋指数是：

$$根龋指数(RCI)=\frac{5+5}{50}\times 100\% = 20\%$$

（8）无龋率 Caries-free rate

无龋率指全口牙列均无龋的人数占全部受检查人数的百分率。这里的无龋人数指根据明确的诊断标准，这些人口腔中没有龋，没有因龋而拔除以及没有因龋而充填的牙。无龋率主要用来表示一个地区人群中某些年龄组的口腔健康水平和预防措施的成果，如5～6岁儿童乳牙无龋率。计算公式如下：

$$无龋率=\frac{该年龄组全口无龋的人数}{受检年龄组人数}\times 100\%$$

2. 牙周健康状况的指数和标准 Periodontal indeces and criteria

与已稳定应用50余年的龋病DMF指数相比，多数牙周病的指数仅对牙周组织某一部分的改变作出评定，这些指数在短时间内修改多次。虽然目前应用的一些指数是40年前提出的，但已经数次修改。下面仅介绍几种流行病学调查常用的牙周病指数。

In the world, most of the survey provides considerable detail and depth. The results could be applied in the process of planning for periodontal care.But internationalcomparison is difficult to perform because of the different, often elaborate methods applied.Some of these studies provide indepth details, which are of great value for the researcher, but superfluous to the public health decision-maker: more details do not always assist in making decisions.

In contrast to the stability of the DMF index for caries over 50-year period, the philosophical basis for measuring periodontal disease has changed several times over a short time.

The separate clinical measures now used for gingivitis and periodontitis were first described 40 years ago, although some measures based on molecular biology are emerging at the end of the 20th century.

牙周健康状况常用指数：

(1) 简化口腔卫生指数 Oral Hygiene Index-Simplified， OHI-S

Greene 和 Vermillion 对他们两人在 1960 年提出的口腔卫生指数（Oral Hygiene Index，OHI）加以简化，使之更易操作的基础上于1964年提出的。两者的区别在于OHI需检查全口28颗牙，评价12个牙面（每个区段选择覆盖软垢、菌斑与牙石最多的1个唇面，1个舌（腭）面），而 OHI-S 只检查 6 个牙面（16，11，26，31 的唇（颊）面，36、46 的舌面）。简化口腔卫生指数包括简化软垢指数（Debris Index-Simplified， DI-S）和简化牙石指数（Calculus Index-Simplified， CI-S）。简化口腔卫生指数可以用于个人，但主要用于人群口腔卫生状况评价。

The OHI-S has had wide use in surveys. It is quick and practical, although its lack of sensitivity makes it less useful in the individual patient than in a group. The OHI-S scores caculus and plaque together, both supragingivally and subgingivally.

1）检查方法　检查软垢以视诊为主，根据软垢面积按标准记分，当视诊困难时，可用镰形探针自牙切缘1/3处向颈部轻刮，再根据软垢的面积按标准记分。检查牙石时，将探针插入牙远中面龈沟内，然后沿龈沟向近中移动，根据牙颈部牙石的量记分。将每个牙面软垢或牙石记分相加，即为个人简化口腔卫生指数。将个人简化口腔卫生指数相加，除以受检人数，即为人群简化口腔卫生指数。

2）记分标准　软垢指数 DI（Debris Index -Simplified， DI-S）（图 2-3）

0 = 牙面无软垢

No debris on the surface of the teeth

1 = 软垢覆盖面积占牙面 1/3 以下

Debris covered less than one third of the surface of the teeth

2 = 软垢覆盖面积为牙面 1/3 与 2/3 之间

Debris covered between one third and two third of the surface of the teeth

3 = 软垢覆盖面积占牙面 2/3 以上

Debris covered more than two third of the surface of the teeth

牙石指数 CI（Calculus Index -Simplified， CI-S）（图 2-4）

0 = 龈上、龈下无牙石

No calculus

1 = 龈上石覆盖面积占牙面 1/3 以下

Calculus covered less than one third of the surface of the teeth

2 = 龈上石覆盖面积占牙面 1/3 与 2/3 之间，或在牙颈部有散在龈下石

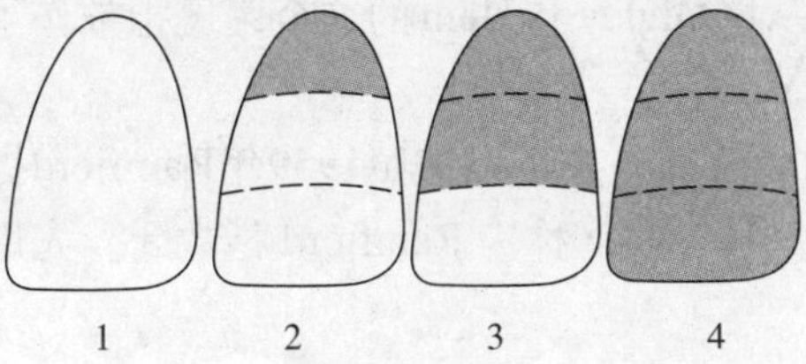

图 2-3 软垢指数

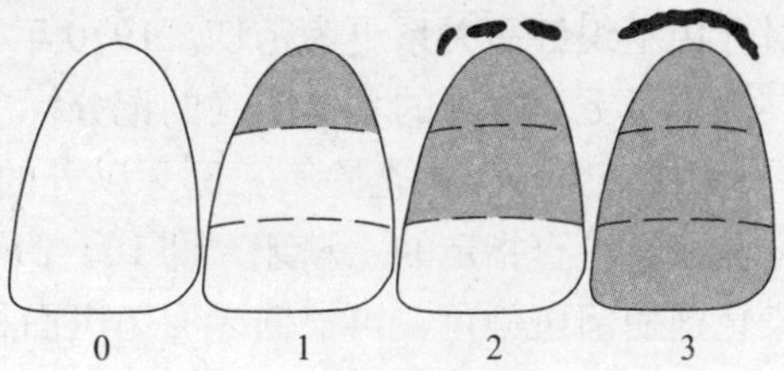

图 2-4 牙石指数

Calculus covered between one third and two third of the surface of the teeth

3 = 龈上石覆盖面积占牙面 2/3 以上，或在牙颈部有连续而厚的龈下石

Calculus covered more than two third of the surface of the teeth

（2）菌斑指数 Plaque index（PLI）

菌斑指数由 Silness 和 Löe 在 1964 年提出，根据牙面菌斑的厚度记分而不根据菌斑覆盖面积记分。用于评价口腔卫生状况和衡量牙周病防治效果。

The principal difference between the PLI and the OHI-S approach is that the PLI scores plaque according to its thickness at the gingival margin rather than its coronal extent, a measure claimed to be more valid.

1）检查方法　用视诊结合探针的方法检查，检查时用探针轻划牙面，根据菌斑的量和厚度记分。菌斑指数可检查全口牙面，也可检查选定的几颗牙。每颗牙检查4个牙面，即近中颊面、正中颊面、远中颊面以及舌面。每颗牙的记分为 4 个牙面记分之和除以 4，个人记分为每颗牙记分之和除以受检牙数。

2）记分标准（图 2-5）

0 = 龈缘区无菌斑

No plaque in the gingival area

1= 龈缘区的牙面有薄的菌斑，但视诊不可见，若用探针尖的侧面可刮出菌斑

A film of plaque adhering to the free gingival margin and adjacent area of the tooth, the plaque may be recognized only by running a probe across the tooth surface

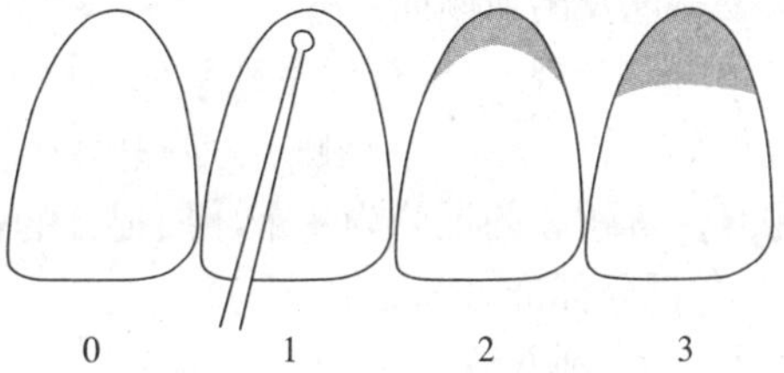

图 2-5 菌斑指数

2 = 在龈缘或邻面可见中等量菌斑

Moderate accumulation of soft deposits within the gingival pocket, on the gingival margin and/or adjacent tooth surface, which can be seen by the naked eye

3 = 龈沟内或龈缘区及邻面有大量软垢

Abundance of soft matter within the gingival pocket and/or on the gingival margin and adjacent tooth surface

（3）改良菌斑指数 Turesky modified Quigley-Hein plaque index

Quigley和Hein在1962年提出了菌斑指数的记分标准，提出的依据是他们认为牙颈部的菌

斑对牙周组织健康关系更为密切。1970年Turesky等对Quigley和Hein的这个菌斑指数作了修改，提出了更为客观的具体明确的记分标准。

1）检查方法　检查除第三磨牙以外的所有牙的唇舌面，也可以按照1959年Ramfjord提出的方法，只检查指定的六颗牙，即16、21、24、36、41、44，称为Ramfjord指数牙。先用菌斑染色剂使菌斑染色，再根据牙面菌斑面积记分。

2）记分标准（图2-6）

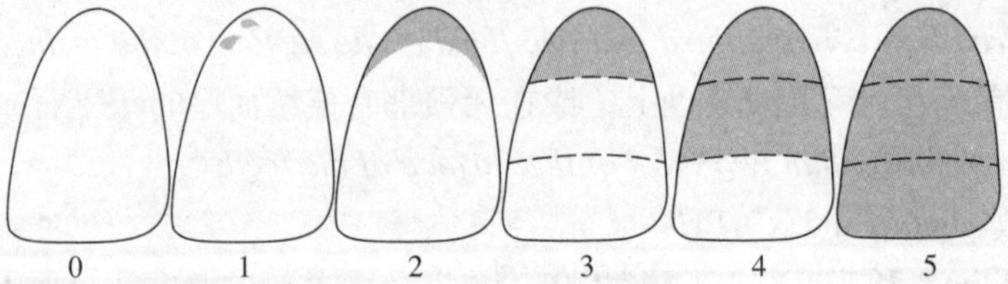

图2-6　QT改良法

0= 牙面无菌斑

1= 牙颈部龈缘处有散在的点状菌斑

2= 牙颈部菌斑宽度不超过1mm

3= 牙颈部菌斑覆盖宽度超过1mm，但在牙面1/3以下

4= 菌斑覆盖面积占牙面1/3与2/3之间

5= 菌斑覆盖面积占牙面2/3以上

（4）牙龈指数 Gingival index（GI）

牙龈指数为Löe和Silness于1967年修订的。该指数只观察牙龈情况，检查牙龈颜色和质的改变，以及出血倾向。

1）检查方法　检查使用钝头牙周探针，结合视诊和探诊。检查全口或几颗选定的牙。须检查每颗牙的牙龈，将牙龈分为近中唇（颊）乳头、正中唇（颊）缘、远中唇（颊）乳头和舌侧龈缘。每颗牙的记分为4个牙面记分的平均值，每人记分为全部受检牙记分的平均值。

2）记分标准（图2-7）

0= 牙龈健康

Normal gingival

1= 牙龈轻度炎症：牙龈的色有轻度改变并轻度水肿，探诊不出血

Mild inflammation - slight change in color, slight edema. No bleeding on probing.

2=牙龈中等炎症：牙龈色红，水肿光亮，探诊出血

Moderate inflammation - redness, edema, and glazing. Bleeding on probing.

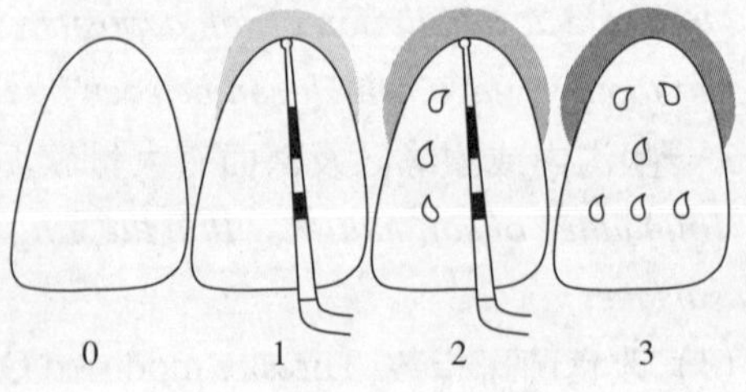

图2-7　牙龈指数

3= 牙龈严重炎症：牙龈明显红肿或有溃疡，并有自动出血倾向

Severe inflammation - marked redness and edema. Ulceration. Tendency to spontaneous bleeding.

对于群体牙龈炎的流行程度，可按以下标准估计：

（5）龈沟出血指数（Sulcus Bleeding Index, SBI）

牙龈炎时，一般都有红肿现象，但龈沟出血则是牙龈炎活动期的表现，因此Mühleman和Son认为根据龈沟出血情况对牙龈进行评价更能反应牙龈炎的活动状况。据此，1971年Mühleman和Son提出了龈沟出血指数。

表 2-10　群体牙龈炎的流行程度

牙龈指数	牙龈炎流行程度
0	无流行
0.1 ～ 1.0	轻度流行
1.1 ～ 2.0	中度流行
2.1 ～ 3.0	重度流行

1）检查方法　检查用视诊和探诊相结合的方法，所用探针为钝头牙周探针，检查时除观察牙龈颜色和形状外，还须用牙周探针轻探龈沟，观察出血情况。检查龈沟出血指数前，一般不能检查菌斑指数，因染色剂使用后，会影响龈沟出血情况的辨别。

2）记分标准

0= 龈缘和龈乳头外观健康，轻探龈沟后不出血

1= 龈缘和龈乳头呈轻度炎症，轻探龈沟后不出血

2= 牙龈呈轻度炎症，有颜色改变，无肿胀或水肿，探诊后点状出血

3= 牙龈呈中度炎症，有颜色改变和轻度水肿，探诊后出血，血溢在龈沟内

4= 牙龈呈重度炎症，不但有色的改变，并且有明显肿胀，探诊后出血，血溢出龈沟

5= 牙龈有颜色的改变，明显肿胀，有时有溃疡，探诊后出血或自动出血

Sulcus Bleeding Index (SBI)

Critertia:

0 = Healthy appearance of papillary gingival (p units) and marginal gingival (m units) , no bleeding on sulcus probing.

1 = Apparently healthy P and M showing on change in colour and no swelling, but bleeding from sulcus on probing.

2 = Bleeding on probing and change of colour caused by inflammation. No swelling or macroscopic edema.

3 = Bleeding on probing and change in colour and slight edematous swelling.

4 = (1) Bleeding on probing and change in colour and obvious swelling.

(2) Bleeding on probing and obvious swelling.

5 = Bleeding on probing and spontaneous bleeding and change in colour, marked swelling with or without ulceration.

（6）社区牙周指数 Community periodontal index（CPI）

WHO推荐使用CPI指数为牙周病流行病学诊断标准，判断牙龈出血、牙石和牙周袋深度。1987年在世界卫生组织出版的口腔健康调查基本方法第3版中采纳了Ainamo等提出的社区牙周治疗需要指数（CPITN），这个指数的特点是不仅反映牙周组织的健康状况，也反映牙周的治

疗需要情况，且操作简便，因此被世界卫生组织采纳，推荐作为牙周病流行病学调查指数。1997 年口腔健康调查基本方法第 4 版对社区牙周治疗需要指数作了修改，取名社区牙周指数(Community Periodontal Index, CPI)。这个指数操作简便，重复性好，适合于大规模的口腔流行病学调查。

1）检查方法　社区牙周指数需借助特殊器械在规定的牙位上检查。

①检查器械: 使用世界卫生组织推荐的CPI牙周探针（图 2-8）。探针尖端为一小球，直径为 0.5mm，在距顶端 3.5 至 5.5mm 处和距顶端 8.5 至 11.5mm 处为两段黑色涂没的区域。

在牙周检查时 CPI 探针的作用是：①检查牙龈出血情况，顶端小球可避免探针头部过于尖锐而刺伤牙龈组织导致出血，而误诊为牙龈炎；②探测龈下牙石；③探测龈沟或牙周袋的深度，探针刻度在3.5mm至5.5mm处的黑色区域便于测定牙周袋深度。探针刻度在 8.5mm 至 11.5mm 处的黑色区域便于测定附着丧失。

Community periodontal index CPI is recommended by WHO for diagnoses of periodontal diseases. Three indicators of periodontal status are used for this assessment: gingival bleeding, calculus and periodontal pockets.

A specially designed light CPI probe with a 0.5 mm ball tip is used, with two black bands between 3.5 to 5.5 and 8.5 to 11.5 from the ball tip.

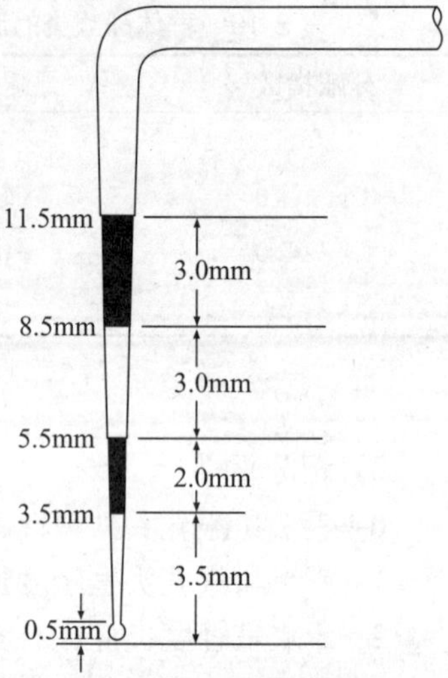

图 2-8　CPI 探针

②检查项目：CPI 检查内容为牙龈出血、牙石和牙周袋深度。

③检查方法：以探诊为主，结合视诊。检查时将CPI探针轻缓地插入龈沟或牙周袋内，探针与牙长轴平行，紧贴牙根。沿龈沟从远中向近中移动，作上下短距离的颤动，以感觉龈下牙石。同时查看牙龈出血情况，并根据探针上的刻度观察牙周袋深度。CPI探针使用时所用的力不超过 20g，过分用力会引起病人疼痛，有时还会刺破牙龈。

Using the probe as a “sensing” instrument to determine pocket depth and to detect subgingival calculus and bleeding response. The sensing force used should be no more than 20 grams. The lightest possible force that will allow movement of the probe ball tip along the tooth surface should be used.

检查指数牙将口腔分为 6 个区段，即：

17-14	13-23	24-27
47-44	43-33	34-37

检查每个区段的指数牙，20岁以上者需检查以下 10 颗指数牙的牙龈出血、牙石和牙周袋情况：

17 16	11	26 27
47 46	31	36 37

20 岁以下，15 岁以上者，为避免第二磨牙萌出过程中产生的假性牙周袋，只检查6颗指数牙：

16	11	26
46	31	36

15 岁以下者，因相同原因，也只检查以上 6 颗指数牙，并且只检查牙龈出血和牙石情况，不检查牙周袋深度。

WHO 规定，每个区段内必须有 2 颗或 2 颗以上功能牙，并且无拔牙指征，该区段才做检查。成年人的后牙区段，有时缺失一颗指数牙或有拔牙指征，则只检查另一颗指数牙。如果一个区段内的指数牙全部缺失或有拔牙指征时，则检查此区段内的所有其余牙，以最重情况记分。每颗指数牙的所有龈沟或牙周袋都须检查到。每个区段两颗功能牙检查结果，以最重情况记分。以 6 个区段中最高的记分作为个人 CPI 分值。

2）记分标准（图 2-9）

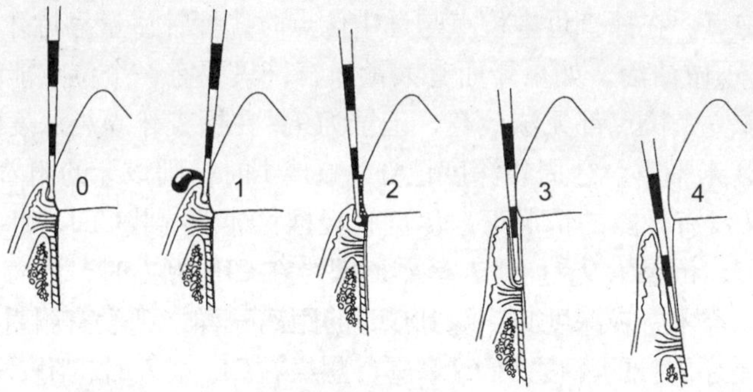

图 2-9　CPI 标准

0= 牙龈健康

Healthy

1= 牙龈炎，探诊后出血

Bleeding observed, directly or by using a mouth mirror, after probing.

2= 牙石，探诊可发现牙石，但探针黑色部分全部露在龈袋外

Calculus detected during probing, but all of the first black band on the probe visible

3= 早期牙周病，龈缘覆盖部分探针黑色部分，龈袋深度在 4 ～ 5mm

Pocket 4-5 mm (gingival margin within the first black band on the probe)

4= 晚期牙周病，探针黑色部分被龈缘完全覆盖，牙周袋深度在 6mm 或以上

Pocket 6 mm or more (the first black band on the probe not visible)

X= 除外区段（少于两颗功能牙存在）

Excluded sextant (less than two teeth present)

9= 无法检查（不记录）

Not recorded

例：①男性，成年人，用CPI标准检查其 10 颗指数牙的牙周组织后，结果记录为：

4	2	3
2	2	×

说明他的右上区段至少一颗牙有深牙周袋。左上区段至少一颗牙有浅牙周袋。上下中区段和右下区段至少各有一颗牙有牙石。左下区段由于 2 颗功能牙已不存在，为除外区段。

②女性，12岁。用CPI标准对其6颗指数牙检查后，结果记录为：

0	1	0
1	0	1

说明她的上颌左右侧及下中区段牙周健康。下颌左右侧及上中区段患牙龈炎。

以上两例个人CPI记分，前者为“4”，后者为“1”。

(7) 牙周附着丧失 Loss of attachment，(LOA)

牙周附着丧失是指釉牙骨质界（CEJ）到牙周袋底的距离。

1）临床检查 每颗牙齿检查6个位点，唇颊面的近中点、正中点、远中点，舌腭面的近中点、正中点、远中点。在探查近中位点与远中位点时，探针尽量靠近牙齿的邻面接触点。在进行LOA检查前，不做洁治。如果牙面有大量牙石，只要有一个位点能够检查，则以该点的检查结果记录。如果6个位点都无法检查，记录为9。在探查牙周袋深度的同时记录附着丧失的情况。牙齿的CEJ未暴露，牙周袋深度记分为0或1时，则该牙的附着丧失记分是0。深牙周袋但牙齿的CEJ又没有暴露的情况下，尽量轻轻推移牙龈寻找CEJ，计算附着丧失程度。如果仍然找寻不到CEJ，记录为9。CEJ未暴露，龈缘在CEJ冠方时，附着丧失＝牙周袋深度－龈缘到CEJ的距离，若牙周袋深度与龈缘到CEJ的距离一样，则没有附着丧失。龈缘与CEJ一致时，附着丧失即是牙周袋的深度。CEJ暴露，龈缘在CEJ根方时，附着丧失＝牙周袋深度＋龈缘到CEJ的距离，按图示方法检查。

2）记分标准

0——附着丧失0～3mm（未见釉牙骨质界并且牙周袋记分为0或1；CEJ可见，在第一段黑区下限）

1——附着丧失4～5mm（CEJ在第一段黑区内）

2——附着丧失6～8mm（CEJ在第一段黑区上限和第二段黑区下限之间）

3——附着丧失9～11mm（CEJ在第二段黑区内）

4——附着丧失12mm或以上（CEJ超过第二段黑区上限）

9——不作记录（大量牙石覆盖牙面、残根或有不良修复体而无法检查）

X——缺失牙

附着丧失记分图示（图2-10）：

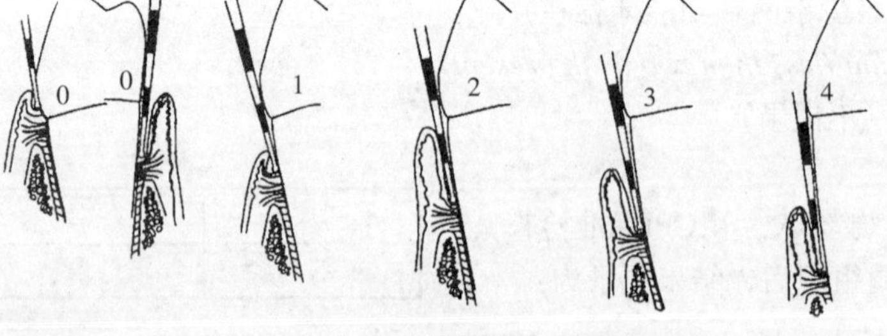

图2-10 附着丧失记分

3. 氟牙症的指数和标准 The criteria and index of dental fluorosis

氟牙症损害常表现为牙列中对称出现、分布于牙面的水平纹理斑块，WHO推荐的氟牙症诊断标准为Dean氏指数，以釉质表面光泽度、颜色改变程度、缺损程度和侵犯面积作依据。氟牙症的评价采用Dean分类法（图2-11～图2-16），根据牙釉质颜色、光泽和缺损的面积来确定损害的程度。从每个人的牙列中找到受损害最重的两颗牙记分，如两牙受损程度不同，则根据较轻的一颗牙记分（表2-11）。

Fluorotic lesions are usually bilaterally symmetrical and tend to show a horizontal striated pattern across the tooth. It is recommended that Dean's index criteria be used. The recording is made on the basis of the two teeth that are most affected. If the two teeth are not equally affected, the score for the less affected of two should be recorded.

表2-11　社区氟牙症指数分类系统标准 Criteria for community dental fluorosis index（CFI）

分类（加权）	标　　准
正常（0） Normal	釉质表面光滑，有光泽，通常呈浅乳白色 The enamel surface is smooth, glossy and usually a pale creamy-white colour
可疑（0.5） Questionable	釉质半透明度有轻度改变，可从少数白纹斑到偶见白色斑点。临床不能诊断为很轻型，而又不完全正常的情况 The enamel shows slight aberrations from the translucency of normal enamel, which may range from a few white flecks to occasional spots
很轻度（1） Very Mild	小的似纸一样白色的不透明区不规则地分布在牙齿上，但不超过唇面的25% Small, opaque, paper-white areas scattered irregularly over the tooth but invoving less than 25% of the labial tooth surface
轻度（2） Mild	牙釉质的白色不透明区更广泛，但不超过牙面的50% The white opacity of the enamel of the teeth is more extensive than for code 2, but covers less than 50% of the tooth surface
中度（3） Moderate	牙齿的釉质表面有明显磨损，棕染，常很难看 The enamel surface of the teeth show marked wear and brown stain is frequently a disfiguring feature
重度（4） Severe	釉质表面严重受累，发育不全明显，以至可能影响牙齿的整体外形。有几颗缺损或磨损区，棕染广泛。牙齿常有侵蚀现象 The enamel surfaces are badly affected and hypoplasia is so marked that the general form of the tooth may be affected. There are pitted or worn areas and brown stains are widespread; the teeth often have a corroded appearance

资料来源：WHO1997

说明：

正常（图2-11）：釉质呈浅乳白色，半透明，表面平滑有光泽。在发育期因营养障碍或患病引起的釉质发育不全不能诊断为氟斑牙。

可疑（图2-12）：可疑类型是牙釉质从正常到很轻型的过渡型，既不属于正常又不能划分为很轻型。釉质上的白色程度浅，有时呈云雾状。

很轻（图 2-13）：釉质上的白色程度较明显，呈纸白区。经常在前磨牙或第二磨牙牙尖顶端有 1 ～ 2mm 的白色不透明区，包括尖牙尖端经常出现的小的点状白色区。

轻度（图 2-14）：牙釉质上白色不透明区范围更加扩大，但覆盖面积不超过牙面的 50%。

中度（图 2-15）：釉质表面大部分受累而变色，常有细小的坑凹状缺损，多见于唇颊面。如发生在后牙，牙面常出现磨损，颜色改变更明显，呈黄褐色或棕色，影响美观。但此型的划分并不是根据颜色的改变。

重度（图 2-16）：釉质表面全部受损，坑凹状缺损明显，牙冠失去正常外形且脆性增加，可因咀嚼或外力而致牙折，染色深，对美观和功能都有严重影响。

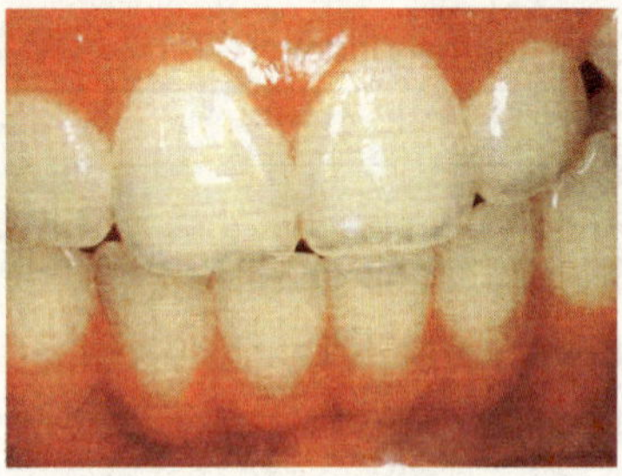

图 2-11　氟牙症图

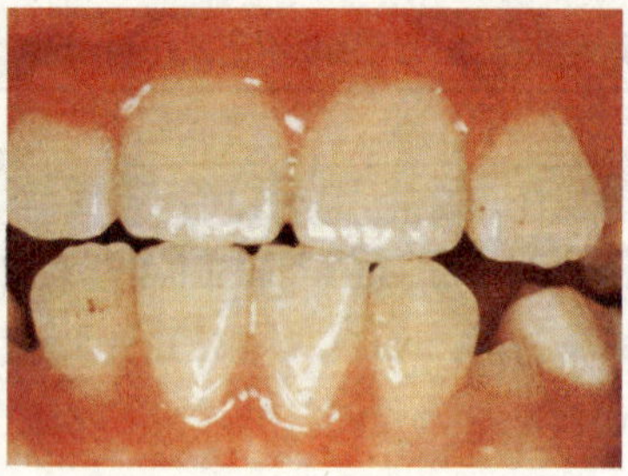

图 2-12　氟牙症图

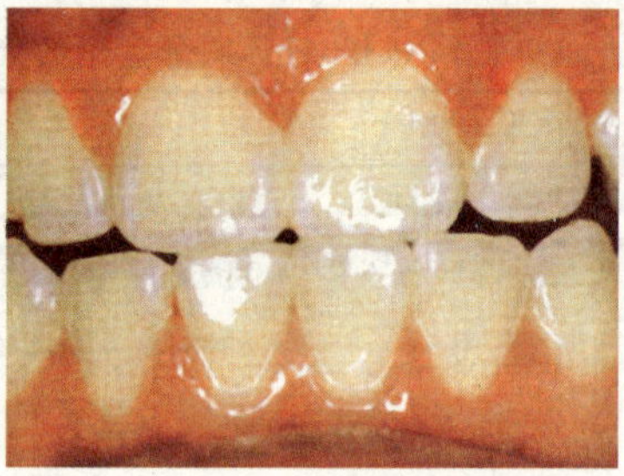

图 2-13　氟牙症图

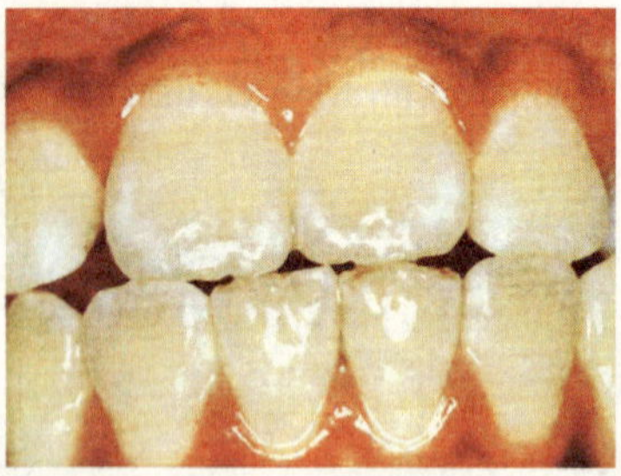

图 2-14　氟牙症图

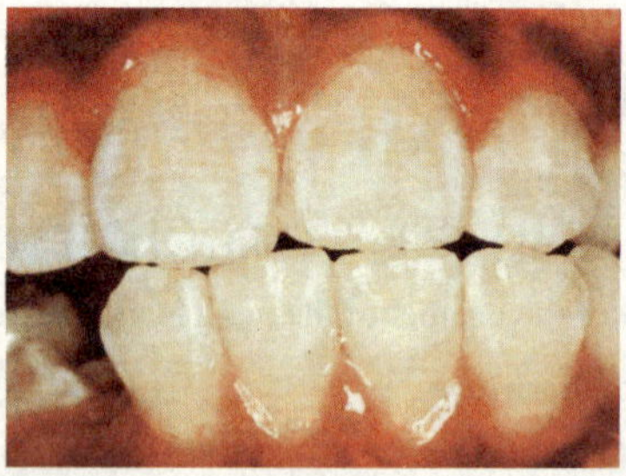

图 2-15　氟牙症图

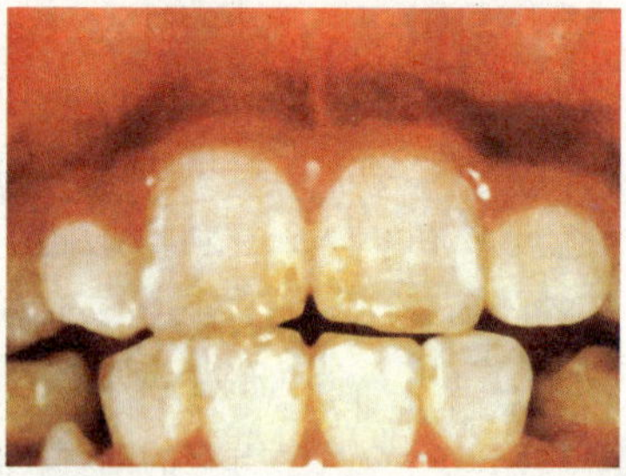

图 2-16　氟牙症图

根据以上氟牙症的分类记分系统，可以换算出社区氟牙症指数（community dental fluorosis index, Fci），计算公式如下：

$$\text{Fci} = \frac{(n \times W)}{N} \times 100\%$$

N 为总人数，n 为每一种人数，W 为每一种加权。

$$\text{氟牙症指数 Fci} = \frac{(0.5\times\text{可疑人数})+(1\times\text{很轻人数})+(2\times\text{轻度人数})+(3\times\text{中度人数})+(4\times\text{重度人数})}{\text{受检人数}} \times 100\%$$

例如：为了解某地氟牙症流行情况，检查 110 名当地居民，结果如下：

表 2-12　110 名某地居民氟牙症流行情况

氟牙症加权记分	人数	加权总和
0	50	0
0.5	25	12.5
1	15	15
2	10	20
3	5	15
4	5	20
合计	110	82.5

$$氟牙症指数\ Fci = \frac{82.5}{110} = 0.75$$

考虑到Dean指数在应用过程中尚存在不足（可疑和很轻程度不易区分，中度以下区分不细等），1984 年 Horowitz 等提出了氟牙症牙面指数（TSIF）用于临床。分类标准见下表（表 2-13）：

表 2-13　氟牙症牙面指数分类标准 Criteria for tooth surface index of fluorosis（TSIF）

分类（记分）	标准
0	釉质正常，没有氟牙症表现 Enamel shows no evidence of fluorosis
1	釉质表面有不超过冠部唇面1/3面积的纸样白色不透明区域，包括只有前牙切缘和后牙牙尖部位的白色不透明区域 Enamel shows definite evidence of fluorosis, namely, areas with parchment-white color that total less than one-third of the visible enamel surface. This category includes fluorosis confined only to incisal edges of anterior teeth and cusp tips of posterior teeth (“snowcapping”)
2	釉质表面纸样白色不透明区域超过冠部唇面 1/3，不超过 2/3 的面积 Parchment white fluorosis total at least one-third of the visible surface, but less than two-thirds
3	釉质表面纸样白色不透明区域超过冠部唇面 2/3 的面积 Parchment-white fluorosis total at least two-third of the visible surface
4	釉质表面有纸样白色不透明区域并有着色（由黄至棕黑） Enamel shows staining in conjunction with any of the preceding levels of fluorosis. Staining is defined as an area of definite discoloration that may range from light to very dark brown
5	釉质表面有散在的缺损区和着色 Discrete pitting of the enamel exists, unaccompanied by evidence of staining of intact enamel. A pit is defined as a definite physical defect in the enamel surface with a rough floor that is surrounded by a wall of intact enamel. The pitted area is usually stained or differs in color from the surrounding enamel
6	釉质表面有连片的缺损区和着色 Both discrete pitting and staining of the intact enamel exist

续表

分类（记分）	标准
7	大面积的釉质缺损可改变牙外形并常伴有棕染 Confluent pitting of the enamel surface exists. Large areas of enamel may be missing and the anatomy of the tooth may be altered. Dark-brown stain is usually present

（Horowitz 1984）

表 2-14　TF 氟牙症指数分类标准 Clinical Criteria and Scoring for the TF index of fluorosis

分类（记分）	标准
0	吹干后的釉质表面仍显示正常的半透明状 Normal translucency of enamel remains after prolonged air-drying
1	釉质横脊上有细小白斑纹 Narrow white lines corresponding to the perikymata
2	光滑面和窝沟部位 Smooth surfaces: More pronounced lines of opacity that follow the perikymata. Occasionally confuence of adjacent lines Occlusal surfaces: Scattered areas of opacity < 2mm in diameter and pronounced opacity of cuspal ridges
3	光滑面和窝沟部位 Smooth surfaces: Merging and irregular cloudy areas of opacity. Accentuated drawing of perikymata often visible between opacities Occlusal surfaces: Confluent areas of marked opacity. Worn areas appear almost normal but uaually circumscribed by a rim of opaque enamel
4	光滑面和窝沟部位 Smooth surfaces: The entire surface exhibits marked opacity or appears chalky white. Parts of surface exposed to attrition appear less affected Occlusal surfaces: Entire surface exhibits marked opacity. Attrition is often pronounced shortly after eruption
5	光滑面和窝沟部位 Smooth surfaces and Occlusal surfaces: Entire surface displays marked opacity with focal loss of outermost enamel (pits) <2mm in diameter
6	光滑面和窝沟部位 Smooth surfaces: Pits are regularly arranged in horizontal bands <2mm in vertical extension Occlusal surfaces: Confluent areas <3mm in diameter exhibit loss of enamel. Marked attrition
7	光滑面和窝沟部位 Smooth surfaces: Loss of outermost enamel in irregular areas involving <1/2 of entire surface Occlusal surface: Changes in the morphology caused by merging pits and marked attrition
8	光滑面和窝沟部位 Smooth surfaces and Occlusal surface: Loss of outermost enamel involving >1/2 of surface
9	光滑面和窝沟部位 Smooth surfaces and Occlusal surface: Loss of main part of enamel involving with change in anatomic appearance of surface. Cervical rim of almost unaffected enamel is often noted

（Thylstrup and Fejerskov 1978）

此后又有 Pendrys（1990）提出了氟牙症危险指数（fluorosis risk index FRI），但常用的多是 CFI 指数和 TSIF 指数。

鉴别诊断

在调查和诊断氟牙症时，要注意鉴别非氟牙症的釉质异常的临床表现。以下几种情况应鉴别诊断：①釉质钙化不全（enamel hypocalcification）和釉质发育不全（enamel hypoplasia），在牙列上的分布有明显的发育年代特征，患牙的其他部位釉质正常。氟牙症牙的其他部位釉质则常受累。当釉质钙化不全和釉质发育不全合并氟牙症时，以其他部位釉质表现分度；②四环素牙（tetracycline pigmentation tooth），多牙本质受累，釉质表面有光泽，半透明度存在，常全牙冠呈黄灰或灰褐色；③非氟性斑（non-fluoride enamel opacity），见于一个或数个牙冠部的白色或米黄色斑块，其边缘清楚很少对称，在强光下垂直观察更明显。氟牙症常为多个牙，左右对称，条纹沿釉质生长线散布，边缘不清，在强光下垂直观察不明显，而沿切线观察更清楚；④色素附着（extraneous pigmentation），可被刮除，氟牙症则刮不掉；⑤脱矿性斑（demineralized enamel opacity），形状和程度与牙菌斑有关，常在牙的龋病好发部位。

4. 牙颌异常的指数和标准 The criteria and index of dentofacial anomalies

1997 年 WHO 根据牙颌异常的不同类型，推荐采用牙美观指数（Dental aesthetic index DAI），一般用于 12 岁以后的年龄组作为流行病学调查的记分标准，介绍如下：

（1）前牙和前磨牙缺失这一标准包括前牙和前磨牙缺失。检查上下颌牙弓切牙、尖牙和前磨牙的缺失情况，记录缺失牙数。了解所有前牙缺失原因是否因美观原因而拔牙，如果缺牙后间隙已关闭，或该牙位恒牙未萌出乳牙仍滞留，或缺失的切牙、尖牙和前磨牙已被固定修复替代，则不能作为缺失牙记录。

（2）切牙段拥挤两侧尖牙之间的间隙不足以容纳4颗切牙正常排列，切牙扭转或错位于牙弓之外。按以下标准记分：

0= 不拥挤

1= 一段拥挤

2= 两段拥挤

对于 4 颗切牙排列整齐而有 1 颗或 2 颗尖牙错位的情况，则不作为切牙拥挤记录。若有疑问，以低标准记分。

（3）切牙段出现间隙上下牙弓左右尖牙之间的间隙超过容纳4颗正常切牙的需要，则出现间隙。如果一颗或多颗切牙的邻面没有牙间接触，此段记录为切牙有间隙。对于乳牙刚脱落恒牙即将萌出而出现的间隙，不记录为切牙间隙。切牙段出现间隙按以下标准记分：

0= 无间隙

1= 一段有间隙

2= 两段有间隙

若有疑问，以低标准记分。

（4）中切牙间隙过宽指两颗上颌恒中切牙之间，在正常位接触点出现数毫米的间隙。可按两中切牙近中面之间最短的距离（mm）记录。

（5）上下颌前牙排列最不规则指前牙扭转、错位排列于正常牙弓之外。用CPI探针测量最大排列相邻牙之间不规则部位的距离。测量时探针与𬌗面平行，与正常牙弓线垂直，探针的顶端置于最舌向突出或扭转的牙的唇面，根据 CPI 探针的刻度，可以估算出牙不规则的毫米数，以最短（mm）距离记分。排列不规则可以有前牙拥挤或者不拥挤，如果 4 颗切牙正常排列的间隙足够且仍有牙扭转或错位，按前牙排列最不规则记分，不按切牙拥挤记分。如果存在侧切牙远中面排列不规则也应记录（图 2-17）。

（6）上前牙覆盖指在正中颌位测量切牙间的水平距离。测量时，CPI 探针与𬌗平面平行。测量上前牙覆盖时，测量最突出的上切牙唇-切边缘至相应下切牙唇面之间的距离；测量下前牙覆盖时，测量最突出下切牙的唇-切边缘至相应上切牙唇面之间的距离，以最接近的毫米数作为最大前牙覆盖的记分。如果所有的上颌切牙缺失或反𬌗，则不作为上前牙覆盖记录。对刃𬌗记录为0。任何下前牙向前或向唇侧突出于上前牙，即为反𬌗，记录为下前牙覆盖。应以最接近的毫米数记录最大的下前牙覆盖（下颌前突），或反𬌗。下切牙扭转造成的一部分切缘在唇侧（反𬌗）、而另一部分在舌侧的情况不作为下前牙覆盖记录（图 2-18）。

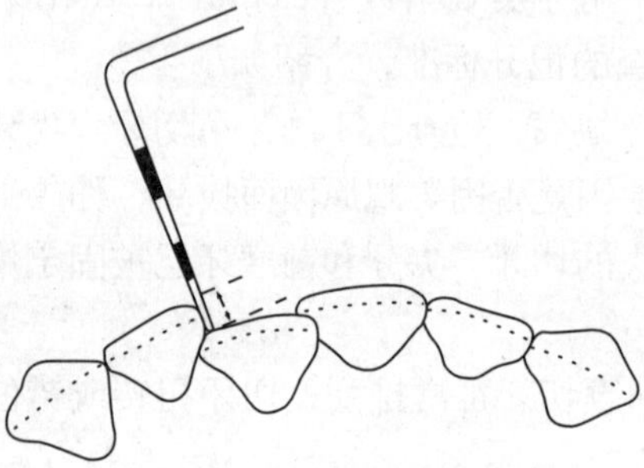

图 2-17 前牙排列不规则的测量方法

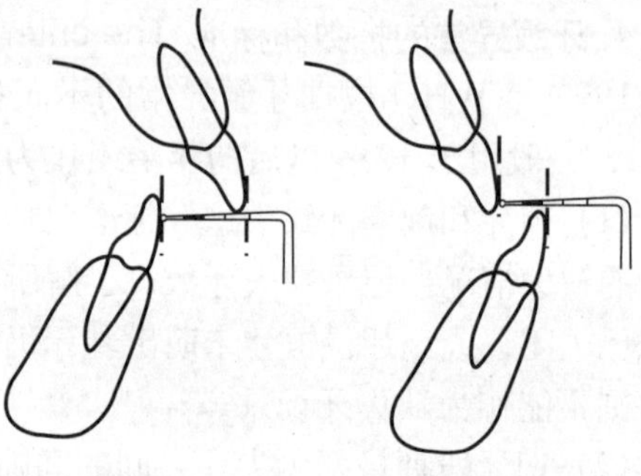

图 2-18 前牙覆盖的测量方法

（7）前牙开𬌗指相对应的任何前牙之间出现无垂直性覆盖，可用CPI探针按下图表示的方法，测量开𬌗的程度，以最接近的毫米数记录对应的上下切牙切缘之间最大的距离 (mm) (图 2-19)。

（8）磨牙前后错位关系通常依据上下颌第一恒磨牙的关系进行测量。如果由于一颗或二颗第一恒磨牙缺失、未完全萌出或因为广泛龋坏或充填物不能依据磨牙前后关系测量，则可测量恒尖牙和前磨牙的关系。根据咬合时左右两侧出现的偏差情况，仅以正常磨牙关系的最大偏差记分（图 2-20）。记分标准如下：

0= 正常

1= 半个牙尖，下颌第一恒磨牙与正常𬌗关系相比，向近中或远中错位半个牙尖

2= 一个牙尖，下颌第一恒磨牙与正常𬌗关系相比，向近中或远中错位一个牙尖

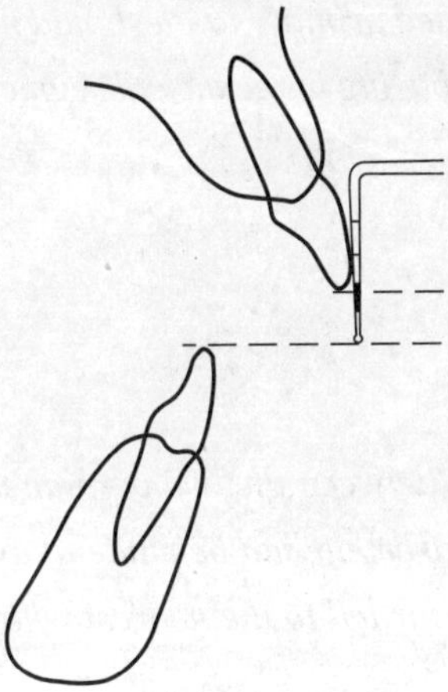

图 2-19 前牙开䓘的测量方法

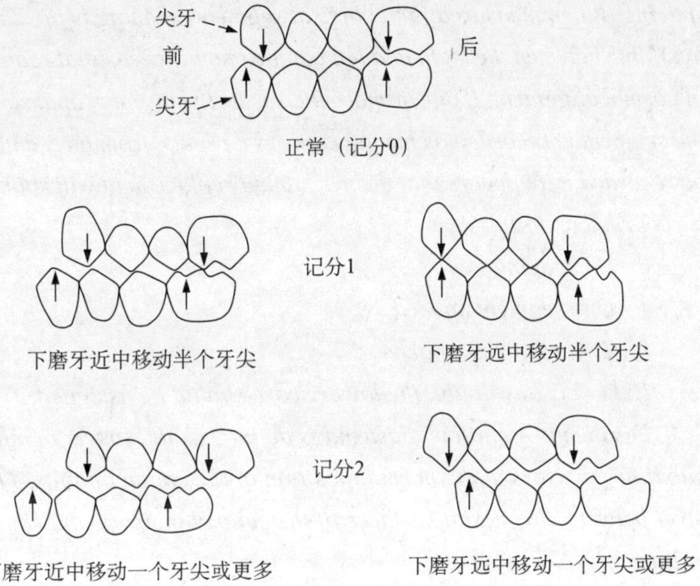

图 2-20 磨牙前后错位关系的测量方法

It is recommended that this index be used for age groups in which there are no longer primary teeth, usually from 12 years. The codes and criteria are as follows.

Missing incisor, canine and premolar teeth: The number of missing permanent incisor, canine and premolar teeth in the upper and lower arches should be counted. This should be done by counting the teeth present, starting at the right second premolar and moving forward the left second premolar. There should be 10 teeth present in each arch. If there are less than 10, the difference is the number missing. A history of all missing anterior teeth should be obtained to determine whether extractions were performed for aesthetic reasons. Teeth should not be recorded as missing if spaces are closed, if a primary tooth is still in position and its successor has not yet erupted, or if a missing incisor, canine or premolar tooth has been replaced by a fixed prosthesis.

Crowding in the incisal segments: Both the upper and the lower incisal segments should be examined for crowding. Crowding in the incisal segment is the condition in which the available space between the right and left canine teeth is insufficient to accommodate all four incisors in normal alignment. Teeth may be rotated or displaced out of alignment in the arch. Crowding in the incisal segnments is recorded as follows:

0 - No crowding

1 - One segment crowding

2 - Two segments crowding

If there is any doubt, the lower score should be assigned. Crowding should not be recorded if the four incisors are in proper alignment but either or both canines are displaced.

Spacing in the incisal segments: Both the upper and lower incisal segments should be examined for spacing. When measured in the incisal segment, spacing is the condition in which the amount of space available between the right and left canine teeth exceeds that required to accommodate all four incisors in normal alignment. If one or more incisor teeth have proximal surfaces without any interdental contact, the segment is recorded as having space. The space from a recently exfoliated primary tooth should not be recorded if it appears that the permanent replacement will soon erupt. Spacing in the incisal segment is recorded as follows:

0 - No spacing

1 - One segment spaced

2 - Two segmenst spaced

If there is any doubt, the lower score should be assigned.

Diastema: A midline diastema is defined as the space, in milimetres, between the two permanent maxillary incisors at the normal position of the contact points. This measurement can be made at any level between the mesial surfaces of the central incisors and should be recorded to the nearest whole millimeter.

Largest anterior maxillary irregularity: Irregularities may be either rotations out, or displacements from, normal alignment. The four incisors in the upper arch should be examined to locate the greatest irregularity. The site of the greatest irregularity between adjacent teeth is measured using the CPI probe. The tip of the probe is placed in contact with the labial surface of the most lingually displaced or rotated incisor while the probe is held parallel to the occlusal plane and at right angles to the normal line of the arch. The irregularity in millimeters can then be estimated from the markings on the probe. It should be recorded to the nearest whole millimeter.

Irregularities may occur with or without crowding. If there is sufficient space for all four incisors in normal alignment but some are rotated or displaced, the largest irregularity is recorded as described above. The segment should not be recorded as crowded. Irregularities on the distal surface of the lateral incisors should also be considered, if present.

Largest anterior mandibular irregularity: The measurement is the same as on the upper arch except that it is made on the lower arch. The greatest irregularity between adjacent teeth on the lower arch is located and measured as described above.

Anterior maxillary overjet: Measurement of the horizontal relation of the incisors is made with the teeth in centric occlusion. The distance from the labial-incisal edge of the most prominent upper incisor to the labial surface of the corresponding lower incisor is measured with the CPI probe parallel to the occlusal plane. The largest maxillary overjet is recorded to the nearest whole millimeter. Maxillary overjet should not be recorded if all the upper incisors are missing or in lingual crossbite. If the incisors occlude edge to edge, the score is zero.

Anterior mandibular overjet: Mandibular overjet is recorded when any lower incisor protrudes anteriorly or labially to the opposing upper incisor, i.e. is in crossbite. The largest mandibular overjet, or crossbite, is recorded to the nearest whole millimeter. The measurement is the same as for anterior maxillary overjet. Mandibular overjet should not be recorded if a lower incisor is rotated so that one part of the incisal edge is in crossbite but another part of the incisal edge is not.

Vertical anterior openbite: If there is a lack of vertical overlap between any of the opposing pairs of incisors, the amount of openbite is estimated using a CPI probe. The largest openbite is recorded to the nearest whole millimeter.

Antero-posterior molar relation: This assessment is most often based on the relation of the permanent upper and lower first molars. If the assessment cannot be based on the first molars because one or both are.

四、调查方法 Survey methods

1. 捷径调查 Pathfinder survey

世界卫生组织向全球各国推荐的口腔健康调查方法是捷径调查。

捷径调查采用的是一种分层整群抽样技术，目的在于既涵盖有不同病变程度的最重要的年龄组，也可确定任一样本点标准指数年龄组的调查人数。

Pathfinder survey used is a stratified cluster sampling technique, which aims to include the most important population subgroups likely to have differing disease levels. It also proposes appropriate numbers of subjects in specific index age groups in any one location. In this way, reliable and clinically relevant information for planning is obtained at minimum expense. The method is suitable for obtaining the following information:

- *The overall prevalence of the common oral diseases and conditions affecting the population;*
- *Variations in disease level, severity and need for treatment in subgroups of the population. This enables groups in special need of services to be identified.*
- *Age profiles of oral diseases in the population to enable care needs for different age groups to be determined, to provide information about severity and progression of disease, and to give an indication as to whether the levels are increasing or decreasing.*
- *Pathfinder survey can be either pilot or national, depending on the number and type of sampling sites and the age groups included.*

A national pathfinder survey (全国性捷径调查) incorporates sufficient examination sites to cover all important subgroups of the population that may have differing disease levels or treatment needs, and at lest three of the age groups or index ages. This type of survey design is suitable for the collection of data for the planning and monitoring of services in all countries whatever the level of disease, availability of resources, or complexity of services. In a large country with many geographical and population subdivisions and a complex service structure, a larger number of sampling sites is needed. The basic principle of using index ages and standard samples in each site within a stratified approach, however, remains valid.

The following method is recommended as a general guideline for basic oral health survey for the planning, monitoring and evaluation of oral care services.

The number and distribution of sampling sites (调查样本点) depend upon the specific objectives of the study. Sampling sites are usually chosen so as to provide information on population groups likely to have different levels of oral disease. The sampling is usually based on the administrative divisions of a country - the capital city, main urban centers, and small towns and rural areas. In countries where there are different geophysical areas, it is usual to include at lest one sampling site in each area type.

If there are several distinct ethnic groups in the population with known, or suspected, differences in levels of oral disease, it may be necessary to include separate samples of each of these groups in the main subdivisions for the survey. However, maximum use should be made of available knowledge about variations between the different groups in order to limit the number of additional subsamples needed. Once the different groups are decided upon, application of random sampling of subjects within the groups is desirable.

The assistance of local health administrators can be very useful when the final decision is made as to which population subgroups are significant for the study and should be represented in the final sample. For a national pathfinder survey, between 10 -15 sampling sites are usually sufficient. If, however, there are large urban centers in the country, it may be necessary to locate several additional sampling sites in at lest two cities.

2. 试点调查（预调查） A pilot survey

为了在调查前初步了解被调查群体患病特点，制定调查计划，有时须先进行试点调查，WHO 推荐先对有代表性的 1 ~ 2 个年龄组少数人群进行调查，通常为 12 岁年龄组，加另一个年龄组，以获得少量的参考资料，以便制定调查计划。

A pilot survey is one that includes only the most important subgroups in the population and only one or two index ages, usually 12 years and one other age group. Such a survey provides the minimum amount of data needed to commence planning. Additional data should then be collected in order to provide a reliable baseline for the implementation and monitoring of services.

五、样本含量 Sample size

1. 指数年龄和指数年龄组 Index ages and age groups

WHO 提出的口腔健康捷径调查推荐采用指数年龄和指数年龄组：5 岁适用乳牙检查，12 岁、15 岁、35 ~ 44 岁和 65 ~ 74 岁适用恒牙检查。其中 12 岁为全球性龋病监测指数年龄，对该疾病趋势进行国际性比较和监测。

The following ages and age groups are recommended in the pathfinder survey by WHO: 5 years for primary teeth and 12, 15, 35-44 and 65-74 years for permanent teeth. 12 years has been chosen as the global monitoring age for caries for international comparisons and monitoring of diseases trends.

5 years. Where it is practical and feasible, children should be examined between their 5th and 6th birthdays. This age is of interest in relation to levels of caries in the primary dentition which may exhibit changes over a shorter time span than the permanent dentition at other index ages. In some countries 5 years is also the age at which children begin primary school.

Note: In countries where school entry is later, e.g. at 6 or 7 years, these ages can be used, though the mean age should be reported with the results. In these older age groups, missing primary incisor teeth should not be scored as missing because of the difficulty in differentiating between primary incisors lost due to exfoliation and those lost because of caries or trauma.

12 years. This age is especially important as it is generally the age at which children leave primary school, and therefore in many countries, is the last age at which a reliable sample may be obtained easily through the school system. Also, it is likely at this age that all permanent teeth, except third molars, will have erupted. For these reasons, 12 years has been chosen as the global monitoring of disease trends.

In some countries, however, many school-age children do not attend school. In these circumstances, an attempt should be made to survey two or three groups of non-attenders, from different areas, in order to compare their oral health status with that of children attending school.

15 years. At this age the permanent teeth have been exposed to the oral environment for 3-9 years. The assessment of caries prevalence is therefore often more meaningful than at 12 years of age. This age is also important for the assessment of periodontal disease indicators in adolescents. In countries where it is difficult to obtain reliable samples of this age group, it is usually to examine 15-year-olds in two or three areas only, e.g. in the capital city or other large town, and in one rural area.

35-44 years (mean = 40 years) . This age group is the standard monitoring group for health conditions of adults. The full effect of dental caries, the level of severe periodontal involvement, and the general effects of care provided can be monitored using data for this age group. Sampling adult subjects is often difficult. Samples can, however, be drawn from organized groups, such as office or factory workers. Use may also be made of readily accessible groups, e.g. at a market, to obtain a reasonably representative sample in situations taken to avoid obvious bias, such as sampling patients at medical care facilities.

65-74 years (mean = 70 years) . This age group has become more important with the changes in age distribution and increases in life-span that are now occurring in all countries. Data for this group are needed both for planning appropriate care for the elderly and for monitoring the overall effects of oral care services in a population. Examination of representative members of this age group is often not as difficult as for the previous age group, as elderly people are more likely to be found in or near their homes, or in day centers or institutions, and can therefore be examined during the day. Nevertheless, care should be taken to sample adequately both house-band and active members of this age group.

2. 样本含量 Sample size

每个特定年龄组的样本数量为每个抽样点取25～50个样本，具体依据口腔疾病的预测发病情况和严重性而定。

例：捷径调查中每个指定年龄和年龄组的样本设计：

城市：首都或大城市 4 个抽样点（4 × 25 = 100）

两个大城镇各 2 个抽样点（2 × 2 × 25 = 100）

农村：不同地区的 4 个村镇各 1 个抽样点（4 × 25 = 100）

合计：12 个抽样点 × 25 名受检者 = 300 人

如果将这种整群分布应用于调查人群的 4 个指定年龄，样本总量应为 4 × 300 =1200。

该样本设计可以确定城乡之间的显著性差异，在某些情况下也可以区分首都或大城镇中处于不同社会经济水平的各组间的差异。调查结果还可以用于发现疾病程度远高于或低于全国平均水平的地区。

每个点取25人男女各半，仅适用于调查估计龋病和牙周病患病水平低或很低的人群。对于已知患病水平为中或高的地区，例如12岁组无龋率仅5%～10%或更低，每个点应取40～50个受检者。

如果人群患龋水平未知，则需要在调查开始之前进行估计。快捷有效的方法是，将一组受检者按是否有龋进行划分。如果20%以上的儿童无龋则患龋水平为低；如无龋率在5%～20%之间为中度患龋水平；如无龋率低于5%为龋病高度流行。这种估计可用于指导确定样本量和完成调查方案。

The number of subjects in each index age group to be examined ranges from a minimum of 25 to 50 for each cluster or sampling site, depending on the expected prevalence and severity of oral disease.

An example of a sample design for a national pathfinder survey for each index age group is as follows:

Urban: 4 sites in the capital city or metropolitan area (4 × 25 = 100)

2 sites in each of 2 large towns (2 × 2 × 25 = 100)

Rural:1 site in each of 4 villages in different regions (4 × 25 = 100)

Total: 12 sites × 25 subjects = 300

If this cluster distribution is applied to four index ages in the population under study, the total sample is 4 × 300 =1200.

Such a sample design permits the identification of significant differences between urban and rural groups and, in certain situations, between different socioeconomic groups in the capital city or large towns. Areas where the disease prevalence is either much higher or much lower than the national average may also be identified from the results of such a survey.

A total of 25 subjects, with approximately equal numbers of females and males, is sufficient only in populations where caries and periodontal disease levels are estimated to be low or very low. In populations where these disease levels are known to be moderate or high - e.g. the percentage of caries-free 12-year-olds is 5%-10% or lower - the standard size for each sample should be 40～50 subjects.

If the level of dental caries in the population is unknown, it will be necessary to estimate the level of disease before starting a survey. A rapid and effective way of estimating the prevalence of caries in a population is by classifying a group of subjects as caries-free or not. If more than 20% of the children in the class are caries-free, the caries prevalence is low; if 5%～20% are caries-free, the prevalence is moderate; and if fewer than 5% are caries-free, the prevalence is high. This estimate of prevalence may then be used as a guide when deciding on standard sample size and when completing the protocol.

另外，样本含量的确定也随所采用的流行病学方法类型不同而不同，依据调查对象的变异情况、患病率大小、要求的精确度和把握度大小而定。一般来说，调查对象变异大、患病率低、调查者对调查要求的精确度和把握度大，所需的样本含量就大，反之则小。现况调查样本含量估计也可用以下公式：

$$N = \frac{t^2 PQ}{d^2} \tag{1}$$

t=1.96，为方便起见设 t 值为 2。d 为允许误差，N 为受检人数，P 为某病预期现患率，Q=1-P，当允许误差 d=0.1P 时，则

$$N = \frac{(2)^2 PQ}{(0.1P)^2} = \frac{4PQ}{0.01P^2} = 400 \times \frac{Q}{P} \qquad (2)$$

$$K = K \times \frac{Q}{P}$$

K 值是根据研究项目的允许误差大小而确定，当允许误差为 10%（0.1P）时，K=400，当允许误差为 15%（0.15P）时，K=178，当允许误差为 20%（0.2P）时，K=100。下表（表 2-15）根据不同的允许误差和预期现患率计算出需要的样本含量。

表 2-15　不同预期现患率和允许误差时的样本含量

预期现患率	允许误差		
	0.1P	0.15P	0.2P
0.05	7600	3382	190
0.075	4933	2193	1328
0.10	3600	1602	900
0.15	2264	1009	566
0.20	1600	712	400
0.25	1200	533	300
0.30	930	415	233
0.35	743	330	186
0.40	600	267	150

资料来源：陆培廉主编《预防医学》

例：为了解某市 12 岁学生患龋情况，准备开展一次口腔健康调查，从既往资料中，已知该市 12 岁学生恒牙患龋率为 52.1%，要求抽样误差为 10%，需要调查的人数为：

公式：$$N = K \times \frac{Q}{P}$$

今 P = 52.1% = 0.521

Q = 1 − P = 0.479

K = 400

代入公式：N = 400 × 0.479/0.521 = 368

需要调查 370 名学生。

六、调查质量的控制 Quality control of survey

1. 检查者的培训与标准统一 Training and calibrating examiners

Although examiners may differ in their assessments of the oral health status of individuals, they should be in close agreement in assessing the status of population groups. When an epidemiological survey is undertaken by a team, it is essential that the participating examiners be trained to make consistent clinical judgments. There are two main reasons for variability of clinical scoring:

- *The difficulty in scoring the deferent levels of oral diseases, particularly dental caries and periodontal diseases;*
- *Physical and psychological factors, such as fatigue, fluctuations in interest in the study, and variations in visual acuity and tactile sense. All these affect the judgement of examiners from time to time and to different degrees.*

The objectives of standardization and calibration are:

- *To ensure uniform interpretation, understanding and application by all examiners of the codes and criteria for the various diseases and conditions to be observed and recorded.*
- *To ensure that each examiner can examine consistently.*

When the survey is to be conducted by a group of examiners, it is necessary to assess the consistency of each examiner (intra-examiner reproducibility) and also the variations between examiners (inter-examiner reproducibility) . The experienced epidemiologist who has been trained in accordance with the recommended methodology for oral health survey should be employed as a trainer and calibrator. Training in the criteria usually takes 2 days with a further 2-3 days for calibration. It is desirable to have an interval of at lest a few days between training and calibration to allow the examiners time to assimilate knowledge of the indices and practice the procedures.

The subjects should be pre-selected so that they possess, collectively, the full range of conditions expected to be assessed in the main survey. By comparing the results of the two examinations, the examiner will be able to obtain an estimate of the extent and nature of the diagnostic variability. If the variability is large, the examiner should review the interpretation of the criteria and conduct additional examinations until acceptable consistency is achieved. In gegeral, agreement for most assessments should be in the range of 85%~95%. If certain examiners consistently produce significantly different results from majority, and attempts to correct their performance fail, they should be excluded from the survey team. It should be made clear to all potential examiners, before the examination begin, that ability to standardize examination results is not a measure of clinical skill.

2. 重复试验 Duplicate examinations

Examiners may change the way they apply diagnostic criteria during the course of a series of examinations. To allow detection and correction of this tendency, it is advisable for each examiner to perform duplicate examinations on 5%~10% of the sample (no less 25) in the main survey. As far as possible, the examiner should not be able to identify the subjects who are re-examined, or know that a subject has been examined previously, since this information may affect the thoroughness or quality of the duplicate examination. It is recommended that duplicate examinations are conducted at the beginning (i.e. immediately after calibration), about half-way through the survey, and at the end of the survey.

Assessment of reproducibility

Inter- and intra-examiner consistency can be assessed in a number of ways, the simplest being the percentage of agreement between scores, e.g. the percentage of subjects allocated the same score by two examiners. However, in the case of caries, if the prevalence of disease is low, this method dose not give an accurate measure of reproducibility. A more reliable way of assessing overall agreement between examiners is the Kappa statistic. The Kappa statistic relates the actual measure of agreement with the degree of agreement which would have occurred by chance. The Kappa score can be calculated from the table below (表 2-16) .

表 2-16 Kappa 值计算表

检查者	参考检查者		
	正常	龋	合计
正常	a	c	$a+c$
龋	b	d	$b+d$
合计	$a+b$	$c+d$	$a+b+c+d$（N）

a =两名检查者都认为是正常的牙数

b =参考检查者认为是正常而检查者认为是龋的牙数

c =参考检查者认为是龋而检查者认为是正常的牙数

d =两名检查者都认为是龋的牙数

公式：

$$K = \frac{P_o - P_e}{1 - P_e}$$

P_o =两名检查者观察一致的比例，即 $(a+d)/N$

P_e =预期偶然出现一致的比例，

$$P_e = \frac{(a+c)\times(a+b)+(b+d)\times(c+d)}{(a+b+c+d)^2}$$

当完全同意时，K=1，完全不同意时，K=0。K 值> 0.8 表明一致性为优，0.6 ~ 0.8 为良，0.4 ~ 0.6 为中。

When there is total agreement, K = 1. When there is total disagreement, i.e. a + d = 0, then K = 0. A score of kappa value over 0.8 indicates good agreement, 0.6 ~ 0.8 substantial agreement and 0.4 ~ 0.6 moderate agreement.

附：口腔健康调查的工作程序和内容（图 2-21）

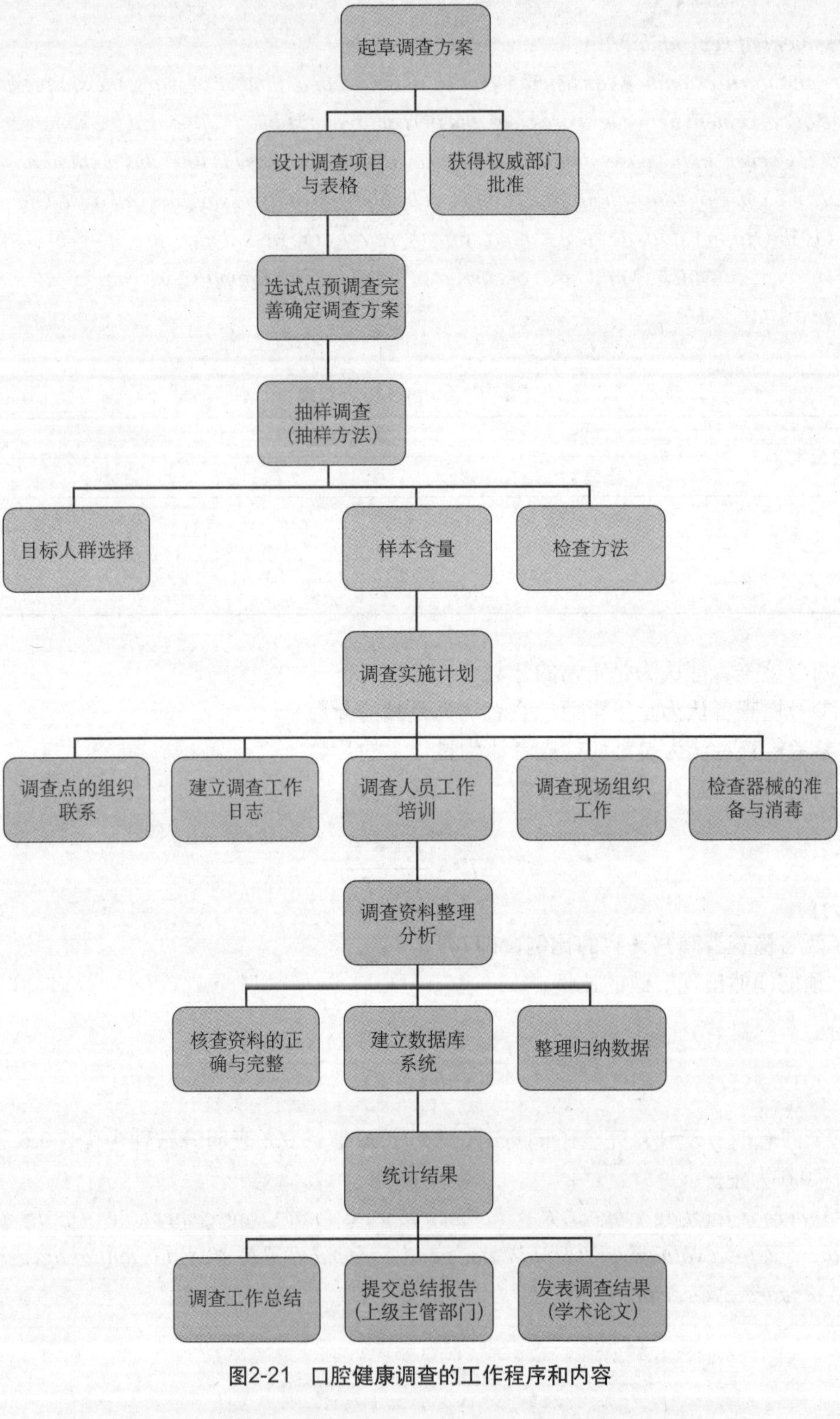

图2-21　口腔健康调查的工作程序和内容

World map on dental caries, 12 years, July 2003, WHO

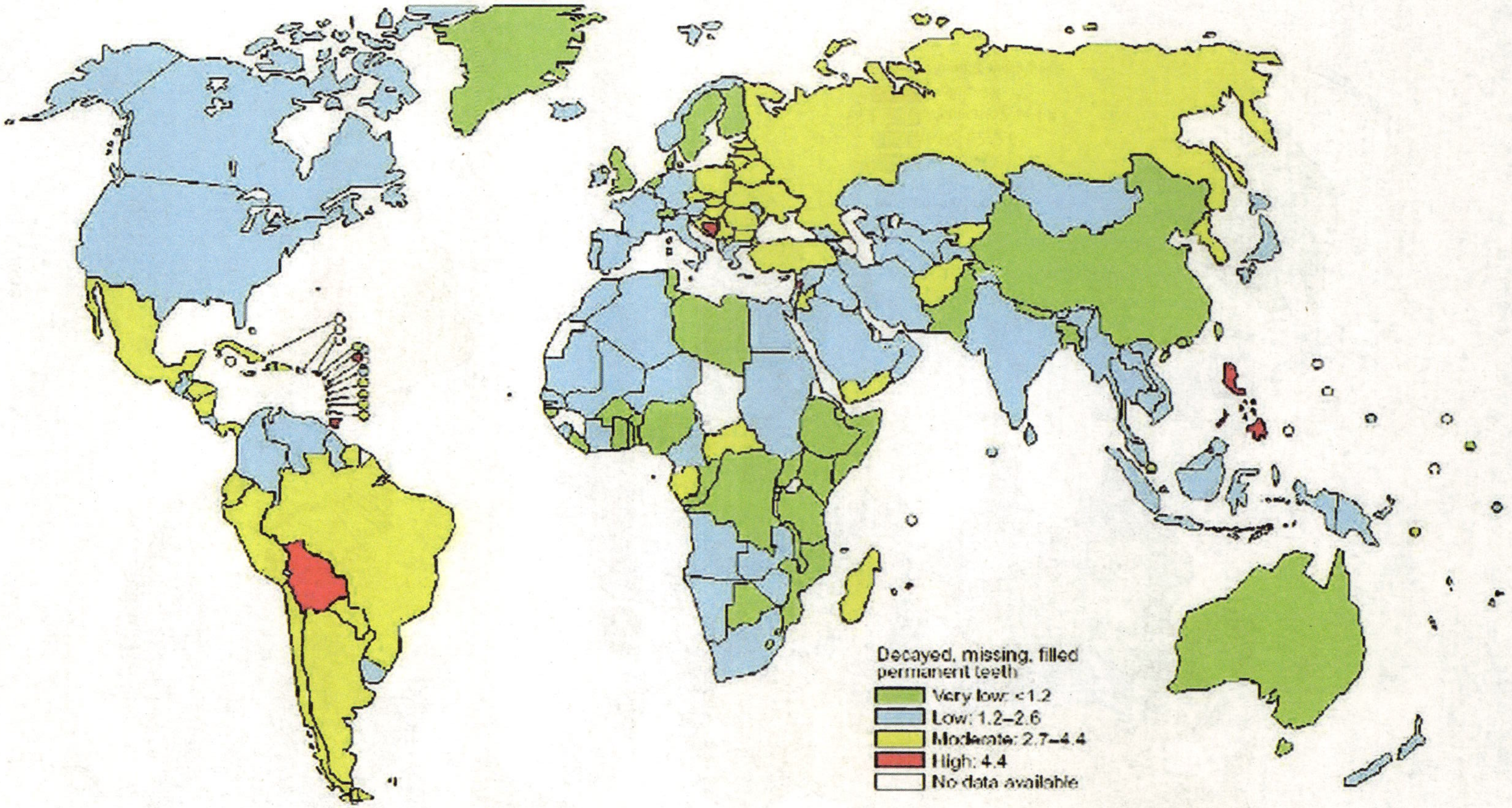

The designations employed and the presentation of material on this map do not imply the expression of any opinion whatsoever on the part of the World Health Organization concerning the legal status of any country, territory, city or area or of its authorities, or concerning the delimitation of its frontiers or boundaries. Dashed lines represent approximate border lines for which there may not yet be full agreement.

WHO 03.176

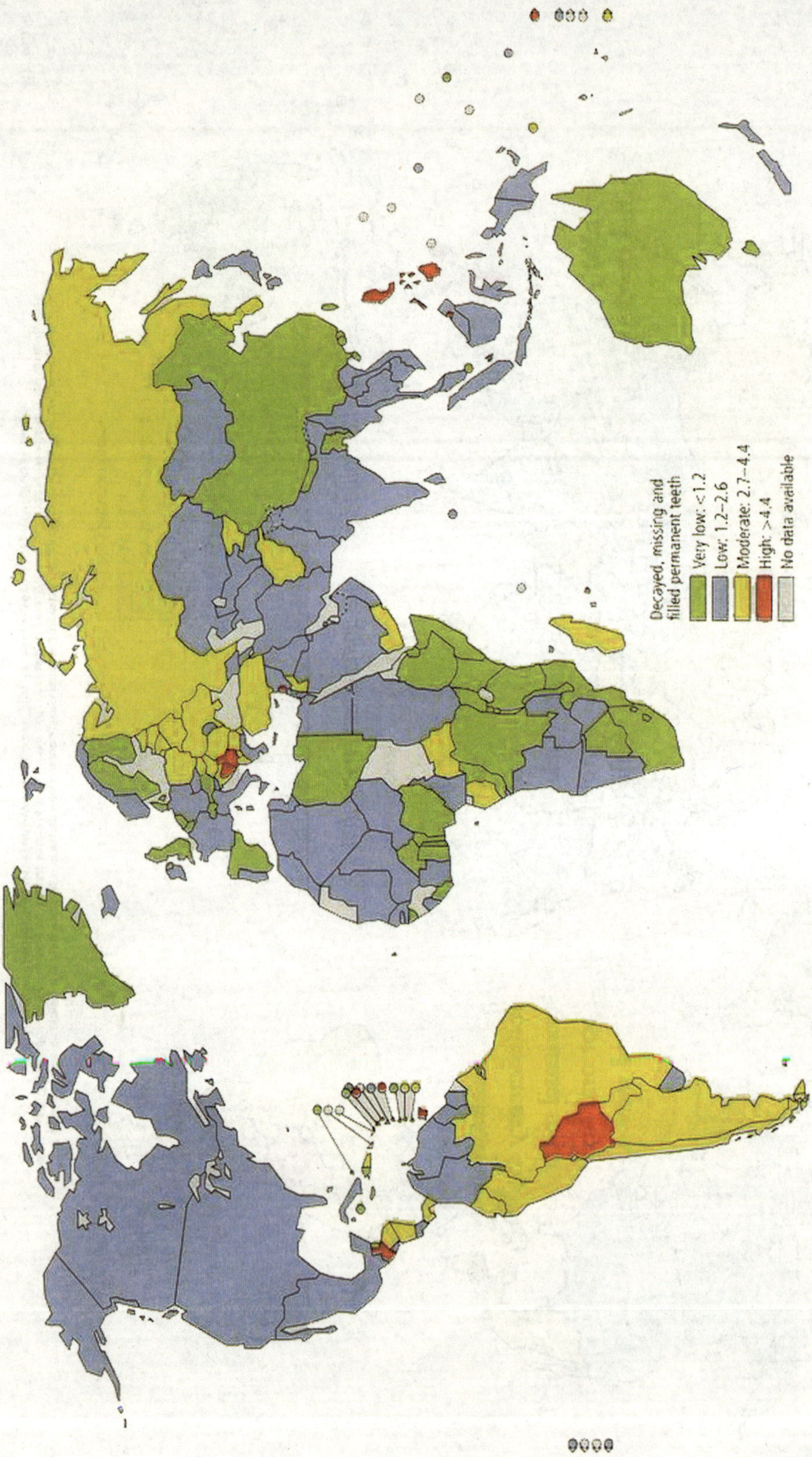

Fig. 1. **Dental caries levels (Decayed, Missing and Filled Teeth (DMFT) index) among 12-year-olds worldwide, December 2004,WHO**

（王伟健）

第六节 口腔健康问卷调查
Section 6 Questionnaire Survey for Oral Health

口腔健康问卷调查是口腔健康调查的方法之一，并且越来越受到重视。问卷调查一般以标准化的（standardized）、间接的（indirect）或直接的（direct）、书面（written）的访问调查为特点。在口腔医学领域访谈（interview）和问卷（questionnaire）的应用由来已久。访谈甚至可能是临床问诊内容的一部分。医生的提问不是预先设计好的，使用的词语、询问的内容、问题的顺序等因人而异。在问卷调查中，采用标准化的方法提问十分重要，因为经过标准化的问卷提供的数据提高了可重复性。

Less structured interviews may be useful in a preliminary survey, where the purpose is to obtain information to help in the subsequent planning of a study rather than facts for analysis, and in intensive studies of perceptions, attitudes, motivations and affective reactions.

在社会学研究中，问卷调查属于定量研究（quantitative research）方法。在行为学研究中，“问卷（questionnaire）”通常指自填问卷，而由访谈者使用的问题提纲不称作问卷。为简化概念，在本书中“问卷”指访谈问卷（highly structured interview）和自填问卷（self-administered questionnaire）。

In questionnaire survey, a standardized technique may be used, the wording and order of the questions being decided in advance. This may take the form of a highly structured interview, in which the questions are asked orally, or a self-administered questionnaire, in which case the respondent reads the questions and fills in the answers by himself (sometimes in the presences of an interviewer who 'stands by' to give assistance if necessary).

在口腔公共卫生领域，口腔健康问卷调查的基本目的是为采取公共卫生行动收集信息，提供依据。通常问卷调查的策划者意识到了需要解决的问题，因而决定进行针对性的调查研究，设计调查方案。设计良好的调查计划应该保证调查结果具有现实意义，甚至可能引起科学界更加广泛的关注。

一、问卷的类型 mode of a questionnaire

根据问卷调查实施的方式，可以将问卷分类。不同类型的问卷适用的被调查对象和条件不同。调查设计者应该根据调查目的和可以得到的资源条件，选择适当的类型。还要注意到不同类型的问卷所获得的信息质量不同。

邮寄问卷（mail questionnaire）：邮寄问卷要求受访对象具有一定的文化程度，邮寄问卷虽然花费低，但是其回收率往往不高，而且也不能保证回应者和不回应者之间没有差异（实际上他们之间往往存在差异）。

发送问卷（delivery questionnaire）：调查者派人将问卷送给被选定的调查对象，待被调查者填答完后再派人收回问卷。适用于集体的有组织的调查对象。通常回收率高，节省费用，回收迅速、整齐。但是调查对象相对集中，调查范围比较狭窄，回答质量较低。因为被调查者之间往往互相询问、互相影响，回答结果容易失真，甚至可能出现请人代答的现象。

电话访谈（phone interview）：电话访谈在发达城市的社区比较容易进行，但是不能涵盖没有安装电话和上班工作没有在家的人群。除一些比较特殊的研究外，电话访谈很难在发展中国家进行。

面对面的访问(personal interview or face to face interview)：面对面的访问经常用于社区调查和临床研究，由受过培训的调查员根据统一设计的问卷向被调查者当面一对一地提出问题，然后由调查者根据被调查者的口头回答填写问卷。回收率和有效率高，但访问问卷调查费人、费时、费钱，只适用于较小的调查范围。

这里，前面两类可以统称作自填问卷（self-administered questionnaie)，后面两类可以统称作访谈问卷（highly structured questionnaire)。

此外，标准问卷（standardized questionnaire）是指经过设计研究并普遍使用的问卷，通常有统一的评分和分析方法。

近年来计算机辅助访谈（computer-aided interviewing）有明显的发展。高技术的应用使得某些多选项和需要跳跃的问题变得简单易行。特别是一些涉及个人隐私的问题，被调查者会更愿意用计算机回答。但是，尽管能够编写程序设置检错控制，由敲击键盘失误带来的错误率还是高于在纸上填写答案。有些纸上填写的答案出现错误可以在以后的录入过程中根据逻辑关系加以纠正，计算机记录的答案使得研究者失去了这一改错机会。同时，在使用计算机辅助访谈的调查，也必须准备一定数量的印刷问卷，以备发生意外情况。

二、问卷设计 The Design of Questionnaire

问卷是采用问卷调查法收集信息的主要工具。问卷的设计是资料质量的主要保证，在很大程度上决定着问卷调查的回答质量、回复率、有效率，乃至整个问卷调查的成与败。由此可见，科学地设计问卷，在问卷调查中具有至关重要的意义。

（一）问卷设计前要明确的要素（the factors to be clarified before the design of a questionnaire）

在开始设计问卷之前要首先明确以下几点，否则问卷的设计就会是盲目的。

首先要明确的问题是调查研究目的和要解决的最主要的问题。明确的调查目的是问卷设计的基础。调查研究的设计者对所要研究的问题的发现可能来源于他们对某些状况的了解和思考，可能来自对某事的好奇心，来自于直觉或者由自身和他人的经验推理论证得出。很多灵感还可以来源于对文献的阅读。

其次要建立研究假设。明确需要什么数据来接受或者拒绝研究假设，由此指导对问卷的设计。这里需要指出的是，问卷设计过程不是收集别人用过的问卷或问题，从中挑选感兴趣的问题，做适当修改或增减，组合起来成一个新的问卷。问卷的设计是一个由理论到概念，由概念到问题，由问题组成问卷的过程。问卷所收集的信息是用来论证研究假设所必需的。

要确定资料收集的方式。根据调查目的、研究对象和可获得的资源决定采取哪种方式收集资料。问卷调查从来都是受到客观条件制约的，最理想的资料收集方法往往是最费时费力、客观上不可能实现的。所以需要综合考虑社会结构、经济环境、政策支持、组织条件等各方面的因素，找出条件允许的最好的方法。

要有分析计划和框架图，以免遗漏重要内容。分析计划不能到资料收集完成之后才产生，而是在调查开始之前制定，要包括在调查计划中。

明确可利用的经费和资源。任何调查都会受到可以获得的资源的限制，调查的难度和规模要根据所获得的经费最后确定。

确定目标人群。通常考虑被调查者的年龄、性别、种族、语言、传统习惯、陌生人（没有丈夫的陪同，妻子能否接收访谈），最重要的是受试对象能否按照我们所希望的回答问题。

（二）问卷的一般结构（the structure of a questionnaire）

问卷一般包括前言、主体和结束语三个组成部分。

前言，是对调查目的及有关事项的说明，主要作用是引起被调查者的重视和兴趣，争取他们的支持与合作。前言内容一般包括：调查目的和意义，对被调查者的要求，问卷调查的匿名性和保密原则，回复问卷的时间和方式，以及主办调查单位、组织或个人的身份等。前言的语言要谦虚、诚恳、平易近人，文字简洁、准确、有可读性。

主体，包括调查的问题、回答的方式及说明等。它是问卷的主要组成部分，将在后几节中专门论述。

结语，可以是简短的几句话，对被调查者的合作表示真诚的感谢；可以稍长一些，顺便征询对问卷调查本身的看法和感受。有的问卷可以不要结语，但前言和主体却是不可缺少的部分。

如果是访问问卷，在结束语后面还应有以下内容：

问卷编号：　　　　访问员姓名：

访问时间：　　年　月　日　时　分至　时　分

对被访问者回答的评价：可信　　，基本可信　　，不可信

复核员姓名：　　　　复核时间：　年　月　日

（三）问卷设计的一般原则（General principles of questionnaire design）

1. 预先确定采用问卷的类型

由问卷的类型决定了将由谁来填写或记录对问题的答案。在实际问卷调查中大体可以分为由被调查者自己填写和由调查员提问并填写两类。由于问卷的填写者不同，问卷的问题设计、版式和遣词造句都会有所区别。

The choice between a self-administered questionnaire and a highly structured interview may not be an easy one. The use of self-administered questionnaires is simpler and cheaper; such questionnaires can be administered to many persons simultaneously (e.g. to a class of schoolchildren: and, unlike interviews, can be sent by post. On the other hand, they demand a certain level of education and skill on the part of the respondent; people of a low socio-economic status are less likely to respond to a mailed questionnaire. Face-to-face or phone interviews have many advantages. A good interviewer can stimulate and maintain the respondent's interest, and can create a rapport and atmosphere conductive to the answering of questions.

2. 明确调查对象特点

当以面对面提问的方式搜集资料时，应该假定所得到的答案是可靠和有效的。不过答案的可靠性和有效性常常受到被访者提供正确答案的能力和意愿所左右。而被访者对问题字句的了解，有无所需的资料，以及访问环境等都会影响到作答的能力。一般人对涉及个人不愉快经

历，敏感性或尴尬问题，都会不大愿意作答。特别是在不适当的访问环境，或对访问的保密性有所怀疑时，困难更大。当设计搜集意见的问题时，应留意答案容易受到措辞、问题重点以及结构等影响。这些问题属主观性，要由作答者凭主观作答，因此与客观性问题不同，一般难有外在准则可供判断其有效性。因此问卷设计必须严谨。此外，问题设计者要肯定措辞对所有的被访者而言都有相同意义。

3. 问卷内容围绕调查目的

问卷的问题一定要针对调查的主要问题，涉及范围不要过大，不要试图捎带搜集研究范围以外的资料，这会造成问卷过长。问题越多，费用亦会增高，而且访问时间会延长，使被访者和调查员都觉得不耐烦，影响答案的可靠性。因此，问卷设计者要根据调查目的严格剔除那些非绝对必要的问题。

4. 措辞要清楚、精确

用词过于简略或含糊是导致答案不准确或无效的主要原因。

例1：“请问你有多大年纪？”回答者可能以农历或是以公历计算，又可能以足岁或虚岁回答问题。如果变为问（公历或农历）出生日期或者身份证号码的生日编号就会获得更加准确的信息。

例 2：“上周你去过口腔医院吗？”当被调查者回答“去过”时，可能是指：

a. 到医院去检查过牙齿（没有治疗）

b. 到医院去接受了牙医的治疗

c. 到医院去咨询牙齿问题

d. 到医院去见一个朋友

如果这个问题改问“上周你接受了牙科治疗吗？”（假设这是提问的目的）就更加清楚。

双重否定的问法，会造成被调查者的迷惑，应该避免。

例：“你是否不认为使用含氟牙膏不是预防龋齿的好方法？”应改问：“你认为使用含氟牙膏是不是预防龋齿的好方法？”

5. 使用适当的语言

问卷中的语言应该适合被调查者的水平，尽可能地使用当地的日常用语和口语，包括在适当时候采用方言、俚语和行内常用语，以保证各种类型的被访者都能明白问卷中的问题，提高答案的准确度。在文化背景不同的研究中，应该把原始问卷翻译成当地语言或者方言，同时有必要让语言学家再翻译回原来的语言，以便核查有无误解的地方。

采用外语问卷，或采纳外语问卷个别问题时，要小心考虑问题的内容和提问方式，看是否适用于本地社会文化，必要时应先做适当修改。当问卷从外国语言翻译成本地语言后，为检验翻译工作做得是否妥善，一个可行的方法是请另外的翻译人员再从本地语言翻译回外国语言，比较两份外语问卷有没有明显差别，特别是文字意义方面的不同。如差异较大，就要改善或者重新翻译。

尽量避免使用医学术语和缩写。学术语言是问卷显得晦涩难懂，使被调查者产生回答问题的心理反感或畏难情绪。

还要注意语言的表达方式。一定要避免引导性问题，如问“您是否认为刷牙比用牙签能更有效清洁牙齿？”应该改为“刷牙和用牙签，您认为哪个方法能更有效清洁牙齿？”

（四）问题的排列（the array of questions）

问题的排列组合方式是问卷设计中的另一个主要问题。一般来说问题的排列要便于被调查者顺利回答问题，便于调查后的资料整理和分析。常用的排列方法有：

按问题的性质和类别排列；

按问题的复杂程度和困难程度排列；

按问题的时间顺序排列；

总之，问题的排列要有严密的逻辑性。但有些情况下，需要做非逻辑的排列。如，为了避免形成回答的定势，有意打乱一些问题的逻辑关系。检验性问题也应该打破问题的类别顺序。对于面对面的访问问卷，问题的排列应该便于问卷调查员与被调查者的交流，便于开始访问，推进访问和结束访问。例如第三次口腔健康流行病学调查所用的问卷就是从“请问您有多少颗真牙？”这个简单直观问题开始提问，便于问卷调查员开始与被调查者交流，继续提问其他复杂、深入的问题。关于个人社会背景的问题通常放在最后，避免在问卷的开始涉及过多个人隐私，使被调查者拒绝继续回答问题。

（五）问卷的长度（the lenth of a questionnaire）

多数专家认为问卷的理想长度是回答时间需半个小时，或者更短，半个小时到 45 分钟也可以勉强接受。然而再长的问卷就会有适得其反的效果。有经验的调查员可以使受访者回答1个小时的问题，特别是在开放式的问卷中，但这终归是少数，而且费用很高。目前大部分的调查员都是经过特殊培训的半专业人员，访问时间长就会导致他们的劳累，从而增加信息偏倚。

Length of questionnaire must be presumed to affect the morale of both interviewer and respondent, and probably also refusal rates and the quality of the data; these are unknown quantities unless special efforts are made in the pilot survey to estimate them. The difficulty again is to develop any general principles. Perhaps the lonely certainty is that the shorter the questionnaire the better the interviewer and respondent will like it, which is about as useful as saying that the bigger the sample the more precise will be the results. Both statements are unexceptionable, but neither suffices as a guide for action. An enormous sample may be desirable but financially out of reach; a short questionnaire may suit the respondent but not the purpose of the enquiry (nor does it necessarily suit the interviewer; too short a questionnaire gives little chance to create ;rapport' and secure full co-operation).

（六）确保资料机密

问卷调查的组织者一定要关注被访者所提供资料的隐私性。调查员应向被调查者清楚解释调查目的不是描述样本中个别人士的具体情况，而是要获得有关总体的统计资料。因此每一个个别受调查者决不会被识别出来，调查结果只会以集体概括的形式发表，如统计图、表等。有了这样的保证，被访者会较愿意合作和提供真实答案。

我们国家统计法的颁布为政府统计搜集资料的机密性提供了保障。调查的组织者，可参考下列一些办法，保障调查资料的机密性：问卷上只用密码识别被调查者；拒绝向任何外界组织和人士提供个别被访者的具体资料；得到的资料经适当处理和存档后，销毁所有问卷；供分析用的电脑储存文件不能有被访者的姓名和地址；所发布的统计表，表内采用的分类要避免个别被调查者的资料能被推算出来。

三、问题和答案的设计 The Design of Questions and Answers

为调查问卷写出问题很容易，但是设计好每一个问题却十分不易。这需要技巧和经验，需要周密的思考和实践的检验。一个问题由于提问方式不同，答案可以差异很大。例如：回答不能行走的老年人的比率可以从3%到16%不等，因为对这个问题的问法有“能否走一个街区或400 米”；“能否在没有帮助下行走或不需要完全停下来歇一会儿”；“行走是否需要借助拐棍”等。

（一）问题的种类（the category of questions）

用于口腔健康调查的问卷涉及的问题大致可以分为四类：

背景问题，主要是被调查者个人的基本情况。如性别、年龄、民族、文化程度、婚姻状况、职业、职务、职称、收入、宗教信仰、党派团体等。有时还要包括被调查者家庭的基本情况，如家庭人口数、家庭类型和收入等。

事实或行为方面的问题，包括已经发生和正在发生的客观情况。如：“过去的一年里您去医院看过几次牙？”“您现在口腔里带有假牙吗？”等等。

观念、态度方面的问题，如：“您认为有必要每年检查牙齿吗？”等。总之，凡是涉及到主观世界状况的问题，都属于这一类。

检验性问题，如：在问卷前先问到：“您今年的年龄是　　？”在问卷的后面再问：“您哪年生第一个孩子？”“当时有多大年纪？”这类问题一般由两组问题组成，安排在问卷的不同位置，通过互相检验了判断答案的真实性。

上述四类问题中，第一类问题是任何问卷都不可缺少的。背景问题是对被调查者分类的客观指标，是对不同类型的被调查者进行对比分析的主要依据。其他三类问题，依据调查的目的、内容可以取舍。如：口腔卫生行为调查主要涉及第二类问题，口腔健康观念主要涉及第三类问题。只有比较复杂的调查才需要设计检验性问题。

（二）问题的结构（the structure of a question）

封闭型问卷（close-ended structured questionnaire）：是指将问题的一切可能的答案全部列出，由被调查者从中选取一种或几种答案作为自己的回答，不能做这些答案之外的回答。

封闭型的结构问卷有以下优点：围绕研究目的展开，针对性强；容易操作；回答形式统一；提前编码，便于分析；分析所花费的时间少。

封闭型的结构问卷主要用于医学研究。

开放型问卷（open-ended questionnaire）：是指对问题的回答不提供任何具体答案，由被调查者自由填写。

开放型问卷主要用于人类学和社会学的研究，医学研究中也可能有开放型问题，但应该越少越好。有些问题需要受试对象自由发挥，然而又容易跑题。调查完成后需要对所得的答案重新进行编码，分析起来费时。

（三）封闭形问题答案的格式（the answer format to a closed question）

封闭形问题的答案常见以下几种：

1. 两项式（a dichotomous choice）

即只有两个答案可供选择，有“是”或者“否”、“同意”或者“不同意”、“有效”或者“无效”两个相反的答案，这类的问题通常还需要有“不知道”这个选项。这种回答方式适用于互相排斥的两择一类型的问题。

例：您的性别？（请在适用的（　）内打✓）

男（　）；女（　）

2. **多个备选答案（multiple choice of items）**

允许从给出的答案中选择两个以上的答案，可以指定可以选择几个，也可以允许任意选择多个。这类结构的问题选项往往需要一个全否定的选项，以保证超出选项范围的答案有答案可选。如：例题中的“以上都不是”选项。

例：您通过什么途径获得口腔保健的相关知识（请在您选择的项目后“□”内打✓，可以选三项）

老师　□

父母　□

朋友或者周围的人　□

电视、广播　□

报刊、杂志　□

牙科医生、护士　□

其他医护人员　□

以上都不是　□

3. **被选答案有等级关系（a rating scale）**

要求受试对象在两个极端（如“坏”对“好”；“同意”对“不同意”）之间选择合适的答案。

例：坏 1 2 3 4 5 6 7 好

同意 1 2 3 4 5 不同意

这种分类方法较复杂，可能会有很多受试对象看不明白。

4. **数值型答案（a numerical answer）**

例：“您的年龄　　（请填上相应的数值）”。

根据调查的目的不同，问题的格式还可以有更多的变化。

（四）编码（the coding format）

问题的答案应该包括受试对象所有可能的回答，而且经常需要包括“不知道”、“有时”“可能”等类似的答案。如果能够在编码的时候就对答案进行分度，在统计时就会节省很多时间。

如“你通常每天刷几次牙？”的答案可以设计成：

4、2 次或 2 次以上 / 天；　3、1 － 2 次 / 天；2、<1 次 / 天；1、不知道；0、从不刷牙

每个问题答案的设计都应该保持相互独立不重叠。每个问题都应该有编码，不能有空白，空白往往意味着遗漏或者跳跃。因此所有需要跳跃的问题（如，对于没有孩子的父母回答孩子的年龄）最好编码为“9”或者 “99”，代表没有适合的答案。

有些问题需要设计“多级串联”的形式，以便使每个问题都很简单，便于编码。如：

您近一年内有没有去医院看过牙？

没有　□ 1 跳到“问题 10”

有　　　　您是否还记得最后一次为什么看牙？
　　　　　不记得　　　　□2　　　　跳到“问题10”
　　　　　记得　　　　　　　　您有没有得到牙医关于刷牙方法的指导？
　　　　　　　　　　　　　　　　　没有　　　　　□3
　　　　　　　　　　　　　　　　　不知道　　　　□4
　　　　　　　　　　　　　　　　　有　　　　　　□5

四、质量控制 Quality Control

（一）问卷的信度（Reliability of questionnaires）

问卷的信度又称可重复性（reproducibility or repeatability）。信度反映对同一个问题获得相同答案的可能性。在纵向调查中问卷的信度就更加重要，因为这样的研究需要测量的是研究对象在一段时间之后对某一问题回答的变化。任何问卷调查对信度的控制不可能获得完全的信度，但是可以把变异降低到合理的水平。

Reliability refers to the consistency of a measure of a concept. The following are four prominent factors involved when considering whether a measure is reliable:

稳定性（stability）决定所测量的变量答案是否随着时间、地点不同而变异。如果所获得的答案保持稳定，我们就可以相信这个测量结果，说明被调查者对问题的回答没有因时间、地点的变化受到影响。

This means that, if we administer a measure to a group and then readminister it, there will be little variation over time in the results obtained.

内部信度（internal reliability），指的是问卷中相关联的问题所获得的答案是否一致。如果在同一个问卷中的不同位置设计意义相同，但表述不同的两个或几个问题，比较所获答案是否一致。常用的测量问卷内部信度的指标是Cronbach α系数。其取值范围是1到0.1表示完美的内部一致性，0表示没有内部一致性。一般数值达到0.8被认为可以接受。也有作者接受0.7水平的内部一致性。

The key issue is whether the indicators that make up the scale or index are consistent— in other words, whether respondents' scores on any one indicator tend to be related to their scores on the other indicators.

调查者之间一致性（inter-observer consistency）。进行大规模调查时，需要不只一个调查员参加，很可能不同调查员对同一问题和调查对象所作出的结论不一致。所以对调查员的选择和培训十分重要。

重复可信度（reproducible reliability）。测量方法是调查结束后间隔一定的时间，从研究对象中随机抽取一小部分受试对象再做相同的问卷，测其可靠性。一般多用事实型的问题来测量，因为态度或者观点不稳定，可能会随时间的变化而变化，当然知识水平的变化也可能是研究的结果。

（二）问卷的效度（Validity of questionnaires）

问卷的效度是指问卷的测量指标是否能够准确检测相应的变量。评价问卷的效度有不同的方法，其中有些方法依靠主观判断，如对表达效度和内容效度的评价。还有些方法基于对所获得数据的检查，包括对准则效度、趋同和区分效度、结构效度、预测效度等的评价。口腔健康调查问卷的效度评价主要有以下几个方面：

表面效度（face validity）对于一项新的测量指标这是最起码的要求，或者说问卷中的问题必须准确表达该问题所指向的变量。就问卷中的问题是否表达了想要检测的概念，征求有经验的专家意见可以判断其表达效度。

People, possibly those with experience or expertise in a field, might be asked to act as judges to determine whether on the face of it the measure seems to reflect the concept concerned. Face validity is, therefore, an essentially intuitive process. No measure should be used unless its validity has been appraised——a reasonable degree of face validity is a sine qua non. Sometimes the results of previous tests of validity are available. These may be helpful, but is important to realize that the validity of a measure may differ in different groups or populations or in different circumstances. This possibility of differential validity should always be kept in mind——it is often advisable to test validity in different subgroups of the study population.

内容效度（content validity)，如果问卷所调查的某一变量是由复合指标组成的，评价这类变量的内容效度是看测量指标是否包括了变量的各组成部分。和表达效度相似，内容效度评价是否将对概念的定义有效地转化成了问卷中的问题。

A composite scale for measuring satisfaction with dental care, for example, should specifically include attitudes to all important features of dental care, such as the way dentists and nurses relate with patients, the technical quality of care, convenience, cost, the efficacy of care, continuity of care, the physical environment, and the availability of facilities and care providers; questions about specific aspects are more likely to tap dissatisfaction than general questions.

认同效度（consensual valisity),如果一组专家一致认定对变量的测量是有效的，那么该测量就具有了认同效度。但是应该指出，不同的专家组的观点可能相去甚远，从而是认同效度改变。

准则效度（criterion validity)，评价准则效度的最好方法是找到标准测量，最理想的标准是“真值”，或者事实。问卷中的某些问题可以通过其他相关的事实调查来评价其准则效度。如，临床记录可以作为标准判断受试对象的回答是否真实，如：被调查者在过去的1年里到医院接受牙科治疗的病案可以用来判断其回答就医次数的真实性。

趋同和区分效度（convergent and discriminant validity)，趋同效度是将新的测量和其他对相同变量的测量比较。这一效度通常用于评价复合测量变量。但是如果两者比较的相关性过高，那么设计新的测量的必要性有可能受到置疑。另一方面，这种比较的相关性不够强，又被称作区分效度，即两个测量的变量不是紧密相关。

建构效度（construct validity)，是评价某个测量与其他相关测量的关系在多大程度上符合所研究的理论假设。检验建构效度的一个方法是看某一测量的组建区分度。

预测效度（predictive validity)， 当一种测量是用于预测未来事件发生的，那么这类事件的发生与否就是对这一测量最好评价。

（三）预实验（pre-test）

预实验就是对问卷进行预调查。选择与研究对象相似，但不是研究对象的少数人群进行问卷调查，根据预实验的结果进一步修订问卷。即使使用标准问卷也应该进行预实验，并要计算信度系数。

（四）培训调查员（training of interviewers）

必须精心选择调查员，并要经过一定的培训，保证不同的调查员采用统一的方式进行，以减少偏倚。在研究过程中调查员是资料收集的骨干。不应该在调查员的身上节省经费，调查员的自觉性和责任感和对调查员的监督同样重要（role-playing is as essential as is supervision）。

同时要培训调查员对自己所获得的信息保守秘密，有吃苦耐劳的精神，保持乐观、向上的积极态度，遵循指导原则等。此外还要坚持对调查员的监督(一人监督 4 － 6 个调查员)。

每天的工作结束后监督者都要仔细检查问卷，查看有无漏答、错答或者回答不完善者，如果有应该及时纠正，必要时找回受试对象重新回答。所有的问题的回答经过核对、确认无误后给予编码。

（五）尽量减少无回应（reducing the rate of nonresponse）

调查者应采取各种措施，尽量减少拒答者的数目。进行访问之前，调查负责人应该事先致函样本抽中的被调查者，说明调查目的和将派调查员造访。进行大规模的调查时，广泛宣传工作更为重要。调查如采用访问方式，应特别训练调查员如何避免拒答。例如在首次访问时发觉时间不合适（如住户正在吃饭），那么，调查员就应在较适当的时间再次造访。

若能在信函中说明调查的应用价值，将较容易取得被抽中的被调查者的合作。表明调查是由有声誉的机构主办，往往帮助更大。主办机构的良好声誉在邮寄问卷调查中，效用特别显著。调查的保密性，包括不用词句方式记录资料，通常可消除被访者对其所提供资料的用途可能产生的疑虑。一般问卷都是以较简单和不会引起疑虑的问题开始，以免被访者因面对尴尬问题而立即中止回答问题。

在访问时，被访者如“不在”，调查员都会“再访”(callback)。调查员如无法接触到被调查者，通常都会按计划进行三至四次的再访，每次再访应在不同的时间（白天或黄昏）进行。再访无疑会增加经费开支，因此应该适可而止。如调查员刚好在邻近地区工作，可进行更多再访。当样本指定的被调查者不在时，可能的话调查员应通过其家人预约访问时间，这可增加成功访问的机会。

进行电话访问时，再访问就容易得多，所以再访的次数也较上门访问的次数多。

用邮寄问卷方式进行调查时，与再访工作相似的是“跟进工作”follow-up。例如再寄出邮件鼓励没有回答者作答。此外还可采用混合的方法，即是当被调查者没有利用邮递回复时，派出调查员上门访问。

一般，调查者都应尽可能减少无法接触者和拒答者的数目。总而言之，足够的宣传工作，明确介绍主办机构及清楚证明调查员身份，事先知会样本中被调查者等等措施都会有帮助。此外要重视妥善安排再访及跟进，尽力劝说不愿合作的被调查者参与。

（六）搜集无回应者的特性（collecting attributes of non-respondents）

对没有应答的调查对象进行回访可以有效减少失访率。回访的时间应该选择调查对象最可能在家的时间。对于初次拒绝参加的调查对象也应该进行回访，也许能得到他们的支持与合作。虽然经过调查员的不断努力，但无回应者的数目有时仍不容忽视。在这种情况下，需以适当方法帮助调整调查的结果。这时，取得一些无回应者的特性资料很有用处。

其中一种调整无回应的方法，是需要研究者掌握所有样本单位（不论有无作答）的某些共有资料。例如某样本按基本单元处于农村、市郊或城市而划分为不同的地理区域。如这是个等概率样本，则调整方法是按不同区域的无回应率的高低而配以不同的权数；即以n(h)/r(h)加权到h区域的作答者。其中n(h)是样本大小，r(h)是已完成调查的样本单位数目。这样的调整使各个区域已完成调查单位的样本分布与整体样本分布吻合。这是利用对每区的作答者 进行加权的方法 代表无回应者。

（七）对回收资料的处理（data processing）

首先对调查的进度，必须有适当的控制。过于紧张的工作日程会导致现场调查工作的质量下降。控制个别访问员的质量也同样重要。这可以通过多种方式进行。常见的是由高级或指导人员再访或复核个别访问员所负责的部分样本单位。同时通过现场的文本校正程序，检查资料有无遗漏或明显错误。若情况允许尽量在现场弥补遗漏，纠正错误。

当访问完成，问卷填写完后，问卷必须经过处理才能把资料输入电脑。对未预先编码的问卷项目需要逐条编码。例如“职业”、“行业”的分类便是典型的烦琐、复杂编码工作，需小心控制质量。开放式问题的编码也如是。

抄录、编码、键盘输入或扫描录入等工序均会有人为错误出现，必须部分或全部复核，严格控制质量。当资料已输入电脑并存档后，需要进行电脑的校订工作，找出资料中矛盾和错误的条项（例如一个年仅六岁的人有祖父的身份等），并按已定的规则，更改此类条项。

（朱　凌）

第七节　龋病流行病学

Section 7 The Epidemiology of Dental Caries

一、龋病流行状况和趋势 The trends and distribution of dental caries

1. 世界龋病流行状况和趋势 The trends and distribution of dental caries in the world

世界各国龋病患病率差别悬殊，为了衡量各国或各地居民患龋情况，世界卫生组织（WHO）规定龋病的患病水平以12岁儿童龋均作为衡量标准（表2-17）。

表2-17　WHO龋病流行程度的评价指标（12岁）

龋均（DMFT）	等级
0.0 ~ 1.1	很低
1.2 ~ 2.6	低
2.7 ~ 4.4	中
4.5 ~ 6.5	高
6.6 以上	很高

Dental caries is still a major oral health problem in most industrialized countries, affecting 60% ~ 90% of schoolchildren and the vast majority of adults. It is also most prevalent oral disease in several Asian and Latin American countries, which it appears to be less common and less severe in most African countries. Figure 1 highlights the dental caries experience among 12-year-old children in the six WHO regions in the year 2000, based on the DFMT Index, which measures the lifetime experience of dental caries in the permanent dentition. Currently, the disease level is high in the Americans but relatively low in Africa. In light of changing living conditions, however, it is expected that the incidence of dental caries will increase in many developing countries in Africa, particularly as a result of a growing consumption of sugars and inadequate exposure to fluorides.

The caries decline observed in many developed countries (Fig .) was the result of a number of public health measures, coupled with changing living conditions, lifestyles and improved self-care practices. In some countries this positive trend could deter action to further improve oral health, or to sustain achievements. It might also lead to the belief that caries problems no longer exist at lest in developed countries, resulting in precious resources currently available for caries prevention being diverted to other areas. However, it must be stressed that dental caries, as a disease, is not eradicated but only controlled to a certain degree. (WHO 2003)

2. 中国龋病流行状况和趋势 The status and trends of dental caries in China

由于我国幅员辽阔，地理环境和气候条件等存在着很大差异，所以不同地区患龋情况相差较大。根据 1995 年第二次全国口腔健康流行病学抽样调查结果，我国 11 个省市所调查的 5、12、15、18、35 ~ 44、65 ~ 74 岁 6 个年龄段的龋均分别是 0.01、1.03、1.42、1.60、2.11 和 2.49（DF 均数）。将 12 岁年龄龋均与 WHO 的标准对比，可见我国患龋情况仍处于很低水平。与1983年我国第一次口腔流行病学调查结果相比，患龋情况略有上升趋势，1983年12岁加权龋均为0.67，1995年12岁加权龋均为0.88。所调查的11省市中大部分省市患龋情况有下降趋势，如北京、上海、天津、山东、湖北、四川。部分省市患龋情况却有上升，如甘肃、云南、辽宁和广东（表 2-18）。

表 2-18　我国 11 省市 12 岁年龄儿童恒牙龋均（加权）

地区	龋均（1983）	龋均（1995）
北京市	1.41	0.98
上海市	1.17	0.96
天津市	1.41	1.02
甘肃省	0.36	0.87
山东省	0.69	0.59
云南省	0.46	0.88
辽宁省	0.76	1.29
浙江省	1.22	1.46
湖北省	0.90	0.51
广东省	0.91	1.65
四川省	0.57	0.37
总计	0.67	0.88

资料来源：《第二次全国口腔健康流行病学抽样调查》（1995）

龋病在不同地区的分布与该地区的水氟含量和经济情况有一定的关系。水氟含量高的地区，患龋率较低。经济发展情况对龋病发病也有一定影响，在所调查的11个省市中经济发展较快些的广东省、辽宁省和浙江省等患龋程度有明显上升，而甘肃省、四川省仍处于很低水平，这反映出经济发展快慢对龋病发病可能有一定的影响。在经济发展更快的直辖市如北京市、上海市和天津市显示患龋情况有好转，这可能与这些城市的口腔健康教育水平、居民口腔卫生习惯的改变以及含氟牙膏的推广使用等有较多的联系。但是对于这种关系的确切程度与影响机制仍应作深入研究。

二、龋病流行特征及其影响因素 The epidemic characteristics of dental caries and its risk factors

龋病流行特征常受到多种因素的影响，人体氟摄入量与饮食习惯对龋病患病情况有密切关系。

1. 氟摄入量 The amount of fluoride intake

人体氟的主要来源是饮水，患龋率一般与水氟浓度呈负相关。据我国1983年全国中、小学生龋病、牙周病抽样调查结果说明，无论在南方或北方，水氟浓度在0.6～0.8mg/L时，龋均及患龋率最低，氟牙症率在10%左右，无中度氟牙症发生，当水氟浓度高于0.8mg/L时，氟牙症率直线上升，低于此浓度时，龋均、患龋率上升。由此说明，我国水氟浓度在0.6～0.8mg/L较适宜。在氟污染地区，人体氟的来源不同于非氟污染区，除水源性氟污染型外，其他如燃煤引起的气源性氟污染型，虽然当地的饮水氟浓度低，但龋均和患龋率却不高，居民总氟摄入主要通过呼吸道及消化道，可超过最大安全限量的几倍至十几倍，重病区居民氟牙症患病率可达90%以上，我国有少数地区属于这种情况。

2. 饮食与营养 The diet and nutrition

流行病学研究表明，糖的摄入量、摄入频率及糖加工的形式与龋病有密切关系。最典型的例子为日本、挪威和英国在第二次世界大战中及战前、战后的调查资料显示，糖的消耗量和患龋率的相互联系密切。战前日本，平均每人每年糖的消耗量为15公斤。6～9岁儿童患龋率为90%，大战期间，每人每年糖的消耗量减少到1公斤以下，患龋率下降50%～75%，1962年每人每年糖的消耗量增加到12～15公斤，患龋率回升。Toverud研究挪威的患龋情况，6～12岁儿童每人每年糖的消耗量由战前15公斤减少到10公斤时，5年内7岁儿童患龋率从65%降低到35%。同时还发现，吃糖的频率和糖加工形式的不同，与患龋率有关，如加工成粘性的蜜饯食品等更易致龋。

The suggestion that a deficiency of vitamin D was a causative factor in subsequent hypoplasia and development of dental caries dates from 1934, and was most likely influenced by contemporary findings on the importance of vitamins in human health.

The limited epidemiologic evidence thus favors the conclusion that severe, chronic malnutrition during infancy can predispose people to later dental caries. This situation is found in countries where malnourishment during early childhood is common but where there is later exposure to cariogenic foods; the malnutrition itself dose not produce caries without the later cariogenic challenge. In developed nations, this degree of severe malnutrition is seen only in unusual circumstances.

Vipeholm 流行病学试验研究：

Probably the best-known attempt to conduct an experimental study on the effect of tiet on dental caries in humans was the Vipeholm study, conducted in Sweden between 1945 and 1952. The study was conducted in a mental institution, and by today's standards is considered unethical because it gave high quantities of sugars to people unable to give their consent to this regimen. Its conclusions have profoundly influenced the way we view the role of sugars in dental decay. The study design was complicated and not free of flaws. Briefly, inmates of the institution were divided into groups with controlled consumption of refined sugars that varied in amount, frequency, physical form, and whether they were taken with or between meals. The extremes of intake were from (a) no added sugars at all in one group to (b) daily between-meal consumption of 24 sticky toffees, each of which was too large to be swallowed and so had to be sucked and chewed, in another. The differences in caries incidence between the groups were pronounced. Some of the conclusions from Vipeholm can be challenged in light of more recent research, but they are listed in Table-because of the historical importance of the study.

Vipeholm 流行病学试验研究的结论（1945 ~ 1952）

Surgar consumption increases caries activity.

The risk of increased caries activity is greater if the sugar is in sticky form.

The risk is greatest if the sugar is taken between meals and in a sticky form.

The increase in caries under uniform conditions shows great individual variation.

The increase in caries disappears upon withdrawal of sticky foodstuffs from diet.

Caries can still occur in the absence of refined sugar, natural sugars, and total dietary carbohydrates.

3. 致龋菌的传播 The transmittion of cariogenoic bacterias

龋病常在家族之中流行，同一家族成员之间会以相似的形式传播。父亲或母亲如果是龋病易感者，他们的子女常常也是龋病易感者。这种情况究竟源于遗传基因一致还是由于生活习惯相同目前尚无定论。但有许多专家从研究两代人口腔中致龋微生物相同的发现中推测，龋病在家族之中流行很可能与生活习惯导致龋微生物传播有关。母亲在喂养婴幼儿时，口腔中的致龋微生物被传播至她们的子女，致使她们的子女也具备了龋病易感性，但这种在母婴之间的传播关系在父子之间很少发现。

Familial tendencies are seen by many dentists and have been demonstrated by research. However, these studies do not pin down whether such tendencies have a genetic basis or whether they stem from bacterial transmission or continuing familial dietary or behavioral traits. Husband-wife similarities clearly have no genetic origin, and intrafamilial transmission of cariogenic flora, especially from mother to infant, is accepted as a primary way for cariogenic bacteria to become established in children.

Dental caries has been described as a carbohydrate-modified bacterial infectious disease, in which a cariogenic diet selectively favors cariogenic bacteria. It is a transmissible disease, usually passed along from mother to child.

三、乳牙龋流行特征及其影响因素 Epidemic trends of caries and its risk factors in primary teeth

学龄前儿童易患龋，乳牙萌出后不久即可患龋病，以后患病率逐渐增高，在3岁左右患龋率上升较快，至5～8岁乳牙患龋率达到高峰，6岁左右恒牙开始萌出，乳牙逐渐脱落，患龋率逐渐下降。

婴幼儿龋Early Childhood Caries（ECC）也称为奶瓶龋或喂养龋 baby bottle caries or nursing caries

The holding of the sweetened liquids in contact with the teeth for hours at a time, often while the child was sleeping, was assumed to be the prime causative factor. That etiology is clear in some instances, although it is now understood that broader use of cariogenic diets can also be involved.

Prevalence in the developed countries is estimated at between 1% and 12% of the infant populations, but in highly affected groups it can be as high as 70%. In US, a cursory visual inspection of children aged 12 to 23 months in the survey of 1988-1991 found a 2% prevalence, with most cases in children of Mexican-American heritage. It is more prevalent in low-SES populations, or where infants are being cared for by persons with little education. It has been associated with lower-than average growth among affected infants, and children with condition seem to be at greater risk for caries in the permanent dentition later in life. These latter observations may reflect chronically poor and cariogenic diets rather than direct cause and effect.

It is confirmed that a better understanding of the social and cultural factors involved among the population groups most affected is clearly needed if the prevalence of early childhood caries is to be seriously reduced.

四、恒牙龋流行特征及其影响因素 Epidemic trends of caries and its risk factors in permanent teeth

乳恒牙替换后，处于年轻期的恒牙尚未矿化完全，亦容易患龋病。如第一恒磨牙，又称六龄齿，易患龋，所以12～15岁是恒牙龋病的易感时期，因此患龋率又开始上升，此时加强年轻恒牙的防龋措施十分重要。25岁以后由于牙釉质的再矿化，增强了牙对龋的抵抗力，使患龋情况趋向稳定。

1995年第二次全国口腔健康流行病学抽样调查的恒牙龋结果显示，患龋率随年龄增加而增高；除5岁组外，城市患龋率高于农村；女性患龋率均高于男性。12岁组窝沟龋均与光滑面龋均之比为9：1。

1. 年龄 Age

Caries used to be considered a childhood disease, Mean DMF scores increase with age, a perception that arose in days of greater caries severity when most susceptible surfaces were usually affected by the time a child reached adulthood. Adults of all ages can develop new coronal lesions, and caries has to be viewed as a lifetime disease. Even the disease distribution seen in youth, is seen in the elderly. In populations where caries experience is severe, the disease atarts early in life and is common in the young. A more even occurrence of new lesions throughout life is characteristic of a lower community attack rate.

2. 性别 Gender

Females have usually demonstrated higher DMF scores than males of the same age, although this finding is not universal. When observed in children, the difference has been attributed to the earlier eruption of teeth in females, but this explanation is hard to support when the differences are seen in older age groups. A treatment factor is more likely to be affecting the differences. In US, the national survey data indicated that males usually have more untreated decayed surfaces than females, and females have more restored teeth. Females visit the dentist more frequently, so this observation is perhaps to be expected.

3. 社会经济状况 Socioeconomic status

Socioeconomic status (SES) is a broad measure of an individual's background in terms of such factors as education, income, occupation, and attitudes and values. SES is a vital measure in many health studies because it is so closely correlated with many health-related characteristics.

五、根面龋流行特征及其影响因素 Epidemic trends of root caries and its risk factors

进入中老年时期后，由于牙龈退缩，牙根暴露，加之个人口腔卫生较差，根面上常有牙菌斑堆积，容易引起根面龋。此时患龋率可能再次快速上升，所以50岁以后老年人的患龋情况比较严重，是继牙周病之后造成老年人失牙的又一个重要原因。

根据1995年第二次全国口腔健康流行病学抽样调查的结果，35～44岁组和65～74岁组根面龋均分别为0.07和0.39；有牙人中根面龋均分别为0.07和0.43；牙龈萎缩者中根面龋均分别为0.08和0.45；男女性别之间差别不大，65～74岁组城市根面龋均略高于农村。35～44岁组有3.96%根面龋患者需要治疗，65～74岁组有17.03%根面龋患者需要治疗。

In the developed countries, general awareness of root caries grew only in the early 1980s, when it became clear that older adults were keeping more teeth than they used to. Subsequent studies have confirmed that root caries is highly prevalent among older persons in developed countries. In the survey of US in 1988-1991, the prevalence of root caries among American adults aged 18 or more was 25.1%. Prevalence rose to more than 50% in men aged 65 or more, and in women aged 75 or more. Prevalence varies in more localized surveys according to the age and nature of the population seen. It was 71% in a group of adults aged 50 and higher in Ontario, Canada, while in an Australian population aged 60 or more it was 27%. In New England, prevalence among community-dwelling adults age 70 or more was 52%, with 22% of lesions being untreated. Prevalence in Scandinavia was estimated to be almost 100% among dentate adults aged 60 or more. Other localized surveys in parts of the United States and Canada have found that incidence can range from 0.3 to 0.6 surfaces per person per year, depending on the population seen.

Root caries, by definition, is strongly associated with the loss of periodontal attachment. Other correlates that have been found associated with root caries are primarily socioeconomic, such as years of education, number of remaining teeth, use of dental services, oral hygiene levels, and preventive behavior. An important risk factor is also the use of multiple medications among the elderly, a common practice in nursing homes that can promote xerostomia. People who suffer from coronal caries also seem likely to be at risk of root caries when gingival recession occurs, and root caries is not nearly as common in high-fluoride areas as it is in low-fluoride communities. Smokers exhibit more root caries than nonsmokers, and prevalence tends to be inversely related to the number of teeth remaining. (Burt 1999)

六、龋病危险性预测与评价 Prediction and assessment of caries risk

Dental caries is an infectious, transmissible disease. The development of a clinical carious lesion involves a complicated interplay among a number of factors in the oral environment and the dental hard tissues.

龋病危险性预测的原则 Principles of caries risk prediction

Some basic principles have to be followed for successful and cost-effective caries prediction, caries prevention, and caries control:

The higher the risk of developing caries for most of population, the more significant the effects of one single preventive measure and the stronger the correlations between one single etiologic or modifying risk factor and the risk for caries development.

In populations in which only a minority of the people will develop new carious lesions, it is necessary to use accurate risk predictive measures to select at-risk individuals and introduce needs-related combinations of caries-preventive measures, in other words, a "high-risk strategy".

In most child population today, accurate caries risk predictors are useful. However, the dilemma is that no method will guarantee that 100% of the selected high-risk individuals are "true" high-risk individuals. The percentage of "true" high-risk individuals among the selected group of high-risk individuals is termed sensitivity of the risk predictive method. Similarly, methods are used to select nonrisk or low-risk individuals. The percentage of "true" nonrisk or low-risk individuals is termed specificity of the predictive method used.

第八节　牙周病流行病学

Section 8 The Epidemiology of Periodontal Diseases

一、世界牙周病流行状况和趋势 The epidemic trends of periodontal diseases in the world

More than 70% of adults in all parts of the world have some degree of gingivitis or periodontitis. WHO's data suggested that although gingivitis and calculus are more prevalent and severe in developing countries, there are fewer global differences in the prevalence of severe periodontitis.

不同国家和地区的牙周病患病情况有很大差别，世界卫生组织以 15 岁少年的牙石平均检出区段数，作为牙周状况的评价标准，以便于不同国家或地区之间进行人群牙周健康状况的比较（表 2-19）。

表 2-19 WHO 牙周状况评价标准（15 岁）

牙石检出平均区段数	等级
0.0 ~ 1.5	很低
1.6 ~ 2.5	低
2.6 ~ 3.5	中
3.6 ~ 4.5	高
4.6 ~ 6.0	很高

Globally, most children have signs of gingivitis and, among adults, the initial stages of periodontal diseases are prevalent. Severe periodontitis, which may result in tooth loss, is found in 5% ~ 15% of most populations. Aggressive periodontitis, a severe periodontal condition affecting individuals during puberty that leads to premature tooth loss, affects about 2% of youth.

In industrialized countries, studies show that smoking is a major risk factor for adult periodontal disease, responsible for more than half of the periodontitis cases in this age group. Risk decreases when smokers quit, and the prevalence of periodontal disease has decreased in countries experiencing reductions in tobacco use.

To summarize the data on age and periodontitis, on average, a greater extent of LPA (loss of periodontal attachment) among older than younger persons, Pockets and subgingival calculus have a less direct relationship with age in cross-sectional data, indicating that the apparent increase of LPA with age is more a lifetime accumulation of effects rather than great suscepbility in the older years. Limited longitudinal data suggest that LPA increase rapidly with age among the 7% to 15% of any population susceptible to serious disease, and to a lesser extent among the majority that exhibits moderate disease. Those susceptible to serious disease exhibit LPA and bone loss when young, often in the teenage years.

Surveys of periodontal conditions usually show that men have poorer periodontal health than women. This has long been observed, and is still the case in the most recent national survey in US. There is little evidence to suggest different susceptibility to periodontitis among different races. No consistent relationships with race or ethnicity when persons of the same age and oral hygiene status were compared.

Gingivitis and poorer oral hygiene are clearly related to lower SES (socioeconomic status) , but the relationship between periodontitis and SES is less direct. The widely observed relation between SES levels and gingival health is a function of better oral hygiene among the more educated, and a greater frequency of dental visits among the more dentally aware and those with dental insurance. SES is a complex and multifaceted variable that can include a variety of cultural factors, and it is virtually impossible to remove the effect of SES as a confounder in the race/ethnicity relationships.

二、中国牙周病流行状况和趋势 The epidemic trends of periodontal diseases in China

据我国第二次口腔健康调查结果显示，15岁少年牙石检出率为67.91 %，牙石平均检出区段数为2.06，牙石检出的平均区段数为2.06。35～44岁和65～74岁中老年的牙周炎患病率分别为14.82%和22.4%。

根据世界卫生组织的标准，我国属于低度流行地区，但是，牙石检出率较高，15岁组为67.91%，因此，从牙周病患病的百分比来看，我国各地区中、小学生牙龈出血与牙石检出率还普遍较高，其中有些省市则更高，如北京、上海、广东、湖北、辽宁等（表2-20，表2-21）。

表2-20 全国城乡青少年牙周2项指征检出率（1995）

年龄（岁）	受检人数	牙龈出血		牙石	
		人数	率（%）	人数	率（%）
12	23452	8921	38.04	12202	52.03
15	23452	8191	34.94	15927	67.91
18	23452	7264	30.97	18431	78.59

资料来源：《第二次全国口腔健康流行病学抽样调查》（1995）

表2-21 5个省市15岁少年牙周2项指征检出率（1995）

省市人数	受检人数	牙龈出血		牙石	
		人数	率（%）	人数	率（%）
北京	2132	1086	50.94	1630	76.45
上海	2132	1123	52.67	1689	79.22
广东	2132	981	46.01	1418	66.51
湖北	2132	864	40.53	1819	85.32
辽宁	2132	935	43.86	1746	81.89

资料来源：《第二次全国口腔健康流行病学抽样调查》（1995）

资料说明，牙周病在我国人群中普遍存在，评价人群牙周病的流行状况，不仅要看平均牙石区段数，而且还要考虑其患病率。

在我国，农村牙周病的流行情况比城市严重，根据第二次全国口腔健康流行病学抽样调查结果，除65～74岁组以外，12、15、18、35～44岁4个年龄组的牙石平均检出区段数农村均高于城市。这种情况与受检人群口腔卫生状况有关。这次流行病学调查显示，用软垢指数对12、15、35～44岁年龄组人群做检查，在这3个年龄组中软垢指数记分为5的百分率，城市分别为38.56%、29.35%和29.69%，农村分别是42.95%、32.97%和44.12%，由此可见，不论城市还是农村，所有年龄组软垢指数都较高，同时，农村均高于城市。

牙周病患病率随年龄增长而增高。5～6岁就可能患牙龈炎，以后随年龄增长，部分牙龈炎逐渐发展成牙周炎，牙龈炎患病率逐渐下降，但牙周炎患病率逐渐上升。全国第二次口腔健康流行病学抽样调查对牙周病的调查采用CPI指数，依据牙龈出血、牙石、浅牙周袋和深牙周袋记分，从结果可以看出，牙龈出血百分率以12岁年龄最高，以后逐渐降低。牙石检出率从12岁开始逐渐上升，至35～44岁时为最高峰，65～74岁老年人因牙缺失，牙石检出率有所下降，所有被调查人群的牙石检出率均处于很高水平。牙周袋检出率也随年龄增加，老年人最

高。年龄与牙周病患病程度的关系呈现以上相同的趋势。(表 2-22)

表 2-22 全国 12 ~ 74 岁年龄组不同 CPI 记分的百分率（%）

年龄（岁）	CPI 记分				
	0	1	2	3	4
12	31.01	16.3	52.03	—	—
15	21.58	10.41	67.72	0.22	0.00
18	14.82	6.5	77.98	0.64	0.03
35 ~ 44	2.85	1.69	81.89	11.15	2.06
65 ~ 74	0.63	1.42	61.06	17.86	4.26

资料来源：《第二次全国口腔健康流行病学抽样调查》(1995)

据全国第二次口腔健康流行病学抽样调查结果显示（表 2-23、表 2-24），在受检者中，6个区段均健康的人数百分比除65～74岁组外，均为女性高于男性，而各年龄组中牙石检出平均区段数和检出率男性均高于女性，男性分别为1.63、1.29和1.44，女性分别为1.60、1.19和1.21。另外，牙周病在性别之间的这种分布与吸烟也有关系，据统计，我国吸烟的人数男性远多与女性。

表 2-23 全国 12 ~ 74 岁各年龄组不同性别牙周健康区段人数百分率比较（1995）

年龄（岁）	性别	受检人数	百分比（%）
12	男	11726	30.02
	女	11726	32.00
	合	23452	31.01
15	男	11726	19.87
	女	11726	23.3
	合	23452	21.58
18	男	11726	13.12
	女	11726	16.51
	合	23452	14.82
35 ~ 44	男	11726	1.94
	女	11726	3.76
	合	23452	2.85
65 ~ 74	男	11805	0.69
	女	11647	0.43
	合	23452	0.56

表 2-24 全国 12 ～ 74 岁年龄组不同性别牙石平均区段数（1995）

年龄（岁）	性别	牙石 均数 S.D	牙石 检出率（%）
12	男	1.43	1.82
	女	1.34	1.76
	合	1.38	1.79
15	男	2.18	2.04
	女	1.95	1.96
	合	2.06	2.01
18	男	2.76	2.09
	女	2.48	2.04
	合	2.62	2.07
35 ～ 44	男	4.17	1.89
	女	3.73	1.96
	合	3.95	1.94
65 ～ 74	男	2.84	2.14
	女	2.61	2.12
	合	2.72	2.14

三、影响牙周病流行的因素 Tha Risk factors of periodontal diseases

除以上地区、时间、年龄、性别以及民族等因素外，牙周病的患病情况还受到其他因素如口腔卫生习惯、吸烟和营养的影响。

The prevalence of periodontitis is also influenced by therisk factors such as oral hygiene, smoking, and nutrition.

1. 口腔卫生 oral hygiene

虽然全身健康状况会影响牙周病发病，但口腔卫生状况与牙周病有直接关系。口腔卫生好，也就是菌斑清除彻底，牙龈炎低，牙周状况就好；反之，口腔内菌斑很多，牙石堆积，牙龈炎则不能避免。如果这种情况持续存在，就会引起牙周炎。口腔卫生与龈炎和菌斑的关系见图 2-9。可见连续数天不刷牙，菌斑和牙龈记分迅速上升，刷牙后菌斑和牙龈记分很快下降。

2. 吸烟 smoking

吸烟是牙周病的高危因素之一，吸烟者牙周病患病危险高于不吸烟者。烟瘾不大者，牙周病的危险性比不吸烟者高2倍，烟瘾大者其危险性高7倍，尤其是严重牙周炎。吸烟者牙菌斑、牙石堆积增多，牙槽骨吸收加快，牙龈炎症、牙周炎症加重。Sheiham 调查了 706 名北爱尔兰人和 2004 名英格兰人，吸烟者平均牙周指数分别为 4.33 和 3.98，不吸烟者分别为 3.56 和 3.02，说明吸烟可促进牙周病发病。从加重牙周病的严重程度看，吸烟对牙槽骨丧失、牙松动和牙周袋加深有剂量反应作用，吸烟次数越多，时间越长，牙周病越严重。

在我国，吸烟方式主要有水烟、纸烟和旱烟3种方式。吸水烟时烟雾通过水的过滤，降低了热量和烟雾中有毒物质对牙龈组织的刺激作用；吸纸烟时由于纸烟末端有一段过滤头，也可有一定的过滤作用；但是没有一种是安全的。吸旱烟由于缺乏对烟雾和热量的过滤，烟草中的尼古丁等有毒物质直接刺激牙龈黏膜，对牙周病的危害更大。

有研究报道，当人们吸烟史在10年以下时，患牙周病的概率是不吸烟者1.3倍，当吸烟史为16～20年时，患牙周病的概率是不吸烟者8.0倍，这是由于牙周组织受到的破坏具有累积作用，吸烟史越长，牙周组织的患病情况越严重。

3. 营养 nutrition

口腔卫生状况可以影响牙周组织健康，然而也有一些人虽然长期口腔卫生差，但其牙周组织却并没有明显破坏。相反，有些患者口腔卫生保持得相当好，非常注意自我口腔保健，却患有严重的牙周病。这说明除了口腔卫生状况之外，还有其他影响牙周健康的因素，例如，营养状况是影响牙周组织对致病因素抵抗力的重要条件之一。

人体需要的营养包括碳水化合物、脂肪、蛋白质、纤维和矿物质，这些营养成分为牙周组织的代谢、修复和维持正常功能所必需。营养缺乏将造成牙周组织功能降低。蛋白质缺乏可使牙周结缔组织变性，牙槽骨疏松；还可影响抗体蛋白合成，免疫能力下降；维生素与牙周组织胶原合成有关，它们的缺乏会造成牙周组织创伤愈合困难。总之，营养是维持牙周组织健康的必要条件之一，营养不良可使牙周组织对口腔局部刺激因素的抵抗力降低，因而易患牙周病。

4. 系统性疾病 systemic deases

一些全身的系统性疾病也是牙周病的影响因素。系统性疾病常伴有组织缺损和某些机能下降，或肌体免疫调节能力减退。使牙周组织或易于发生炎症，或伤口难于修复，最终产生牙周病。在系统性疾病中比较得到公认的影响牙周组织的疾病是糖尿病。有研究表明，糖尿病患者牙周组织内一些炎症细胞活跃，炎症介质增多，使牙周组织受到破坏；同时牙周组织的修复功能也有所减弱，易于产生牙周病。对于这类病人，如果能够控制糖尿病的发展，就可能显著减轻牙周病的症状。

第九节　其他口腔常见疾病的流行状况

Section 9 The Epidemiological Status of other Common Oral Diseases

一、失牙 Tooth loss

Tooth loss, especially total tooth loss or edentulism, is the dental equivalent of death. In many developing countries, access to oral health services is limited and teeth are often left untreated or are extracted because of pain or discomfort. Throughout the world, losing teeth is still seen by many people as natural consequence of ageing. While in some industrialized countries there has been a positive trend of reduction in teeth loss among adults in recent years, the proportion of edentulous adults aged 65 years and older is still high in some countries. (WHO 2003)

二、氟牙症 Dental fluorosis

氟牙症（dental fluorosis）是牙在发育期间，长期接受过量的氟，使成釉细胞受到损害，造成牙釉质的发育不全。氟牙症又称斑釉牙（mottled enamel）。首先是在我国三国时代（公元223～262）嵇康《养生论》中的“齿居晋而黄的描述”，其后是1901年美国的eager在意大利的那不勒斯移民团中发现的当时称为“局部性釉质缺损”到20世纪初由美国学者Mekay等人把斑釉牙描述为“科罗拉多棕色条纹”，从此开始了系列研究。1916年他与Black将它定名为斑釉牙。1931年Churchill揭示了这种疾病与氟的关系。1934年Dean提出了估计斑釉牙严重程度的指数，分为正常、可疑、很轻度、轻度、中度、较重度与重度7类。1935年Dean等人提出将此分类法作为社区斑釉牙指数用作流行病学调查。1942年Dean修改了指数，减少了分类数，发展成为社区氟牙症指数记分系统，从0到4，至今仍为WHO所采用。

Dental fluorosis is a permanent hypomineralization of enamel, characterized by greater surface and subsurface porosity than in normal enamel, that results from excess F reaching the developing tooth during developmental stages . Excess F available to the enamel during maturation disrupts mineralization and results in excessive retention of enamel proteins.

1942年Dean等发表了饮水氟浓度与氟牙症率和氟牙症指数之间关系的调查结果，是一项经典研究，其主要结果摘录于表2-25内。

表2-25 水氟与氟牙症（白种儿童）

地区	检查人数	氟牙症率(%)	氟牙症指数	饮水氟浓度(mg/L)	氟牙症分类(%)						年龄（岁）
					正常	很疑	很轻	轻度	中度	重度	
Michigan City, Ind	236	0.0	0.01	0.1	97.5	2.5	0.0	0.0	0.0	0.0	12～14
Lima, Ohio	454	2.2	0.09	0.3	84.1	13.7	2.2	0.0	0.0	0.0	12～14
Elgin, ILL	403	4.2	0.22	0.5	60.5	35.3	3.5	0.7	0.0	0.0	12～14
Kewanee, ILL	123	12.2	0.31	0.9	52.8	35	10.6	1.6	0.0	0.0	12～14
Joliet, ILL	447	25.3	0.46	1.3	40.5	34.2	22.2	3.1	0.0	0.0	12～14
Colorado prings,Colo	404	73.8	1.3	2.6	6.4	19.8	42.1	21.3	8.9	1.5	12～14
Lubbock, Tex	189	97.8	2.7	4.4	1.1	1.1	12.2	21.7	46	17.9	9～12
Bauxite, Ark	26	100.0	3.4	14.1	0.0	0.0	3.9	3.9	38.5	53.8	14～19

资料来源：Dean等（1942）

氟牙症指数表示一个地区人群氟牙症的流行状况的严重程度，根据社区氟牙症指数的范围，1946年Dean把社区氟牙症指数记分作为有公共卫生意义的指征，并把氟牙症在一个地区的流行情况分为6类。

社区氟牙症指数的公共卫生意义是，一个地区的氟牙症指数在0～0.4范围内，发生率＜10%，属于正常范围。氟牙症指数在0.4～0.6为许可范围，很轻度＞10%，＜35%。当指数超过0.6时，很轻度＞35%，＜50%，中度＜35%，即为氟牙症流行，需采取公共卫生措施，以降低氟牙症患病率。上例氟牙症指数为 0.75，属轻度流行地区，应采取除氟措施。

表 2-26　Dean 规定的社区氟牙症指数的公共卫生意义（1946）

公共卫生含义	氟牙症指数范围
阴性	0 ~ 0.4
边缘性	0.4 ~ 0.6
轻度	0.6 ~ 1.0
中度	1.0 ~ 2.0
重度	2.0 ~ 3.0
极重度	3.0 ~ 4.0

1995 年我国进行第二次全国口腔健康流行病学抽样调查，采取 Dean 分类法检查氟牙症。所调查的十一省市水氟浓度从 0.1mg/L < 5mg/L 不等，12 岁氟牙症指数为 0.17、患病率是 6.89%，15 岁氟牙症指数为 0.18、患病率是 7.27%，均属于正常范围。

美国的调查资料显示（1986 ~ 1987），青少年氟牙症患病率为 22.3%（范围从 9 岁年龄组 25.8% ~ 17 岁年龄组 18.5%）。年龄越低患病率越高的趋势提示氟牙症患病率将逐年高。

Prevalence among children was reported as 22.3%, ranging by age from18.5% of 17-year-olds to 25.8% of 9 -year-olds. This higher prevalence in the younger children hints that prevalence might still be increasing, and more recent data do not refute that possibility. Almost all of the fluorosis recorded was the mild / very mild variety. (USA 1986 ~ 1987)

（一）流行特征 Epidemic characteristics

1. 地区分布 Distribution of geographic location

氟牙症的流行具有明显的地区性，其发病与当地水、土壤、空气中的含氟量过多密切相关，氟含量过高，氟牙症则流行。氟牙症是地方性氟中毒的早期指征，饮用水是摄入氟的一个最大来源，一般认为饮水氟含量以0.8 ~ 1mg/L为适宜浓度，超过这个浓度将引起氟牙症的流行。有的地区饮水中氟含量明显高于正常浓度，如我国的西北、华北、东北等一些地区，水氟浓度普遍超过3mg/L。在我国一些高氟煤矿区，土壤和空气中的氟含量很高，这些地区即使水氟浓度很低，但由于燃高氟煤烘烤粮食造成气源性氟污染，居民从其他途径摄入过多的氟，也会产生氟牙症，甚至氟骨症。如三峡地区调查资料显示，调查区人口 447 万，氟牙症患病者 150 万人，典型重病区氟牙症患病率为 90%，氟骨症为 40%。又如 1977 年湖北恩施地区防疫站调查湖北沫抚区发现，饮水含氟量为 0.12mg/L，由于当地居民用石煤烘烤玉米，石煤含氟量为 717.3mg/kg，玉米含氟量为 84.2mg/kg，居民食用这些玉米引起氟牙症。

2. 城乡分布 Distribution of the urban and rural areas

氟牙症在城乡居民中都可发生，但第二次全国口腔健康流行病学抽样调查结果显示，农村患病率高于城市，12 岁组分别是城市 5.21%、农村 10.23%，15 岁组城市 4.81%、农村 12.16%。城市与农村的差异，可能源于饮用水不同，城市居民以自来水为主，含氟量受到控制。农村居民饮用水较杂，如果饮用含氟量较高的深井水和河水，患病率就会上升。

3. 年龄分布 Distribution of ages

胎盘对氟有一定的屏障作用，过量的氟难以通过胎盘屏障，所以乳牙较少发生氟牙症，但氟量过高则会透过胎盘屏障，乳牙也可能会患病。慢性氟中毒主要损害恒牙，6岁以后恒牙逐渐萌出，氟牙症的患病率逐渐升高，至12岁左右恒牙全部萌出，造成不可逆转的危害，此后氟牙症患病率维持一个相对稳定的水平。中年以后因龋病或牙周病可能导致恒牙逐渐脱落，患病率才开始下降。

4. 性别分布 Distribution of sex

氟牙症在男女性别上未发现显著不同。

5. 牙位分布 Distribution of tooth position

Moller等的调查报告提出受氟牙症影响最严重的是前磨牙，Murray等调查显示受白垩釉质影响最大的是牙的颊（唇）侧面，上颌牙所受影响为下颌的2倍，其中上中切牙受影响最大。

（二）危险因素 risk factors

1. 饮水氟浓度高 High F concentration in water

Fluoridated water is a risk factor; it was documented long ago that even around 1.0 mg/L F in the United States, 7% to 16% of children born and reared in the area exhibit mild and very mild dental fluorosis in the permanent dentition. This degree of prevalence was recorded at a time when drinking water was virtually the only source of exposure to F. Even small changes in F concentrations in drinking water can lead to considerable change in fluorosis prevalence and severity.

2. 燃煤污染 Burning coal pollution

在我国贵州省及周边地区由于传统生活习俗，造成燃高氟煤烘烤粮食形成气源性氟污染，引起氟牙症流行。据贵州省疾病控制中心报告， 全省目前有氟斑牙患者1000余万人，氟骨症病人64万人， 8～12岁儿童氟斑牙患病人数110万人， 有1900万人正受到威胁。 是我国地氟病病情最重、病人数最多的省份。

3. 工业污染 Industry pollution

The principal sources of pollution are industries and mining. The fluoride content in the air in some factories can reach a level as high as 1.4 mg/m^3 and in the neighbourhood of such factories a level of 0.2 mg/m^3 in air may be attained. This has occurred in the past in industrialized countries, and , unless strong controls are ad hered to, is likely to occur in developing countries pursuing a policy of industrialization without proper environmental safeguards.

4. 补充氟过量 Over F supplements

Regardless of F supplements' role in preventing caries, there is now strong evidence that supplements are a risk factor for mild-to-moderate fluorosis. Case-control studies in nonfluoridated areas of New England have found that exposure to F supplements during the first 6 years of lift, together with higher socioeconomic status, significantly increased the risk of developing fluorosis. Later research found the risk to be extremely high when supplements were used in fluoridated areas, a clearly inappropriate procedure.

5. 多重氟暴露 Multiple F exposure

Exposure to multiple sources of fluoride can be beneficial or undesirable. It can be beneficial in the sense that fuller advantage is being taken of the several ways in which fluorides act to prevent caries, but it can also increase the potential for fluorosis. Some multiple exposure is controlled, as when a dentist applies fluoride gel to a caries-susceptible patient who is using a fluoridated toothpaste, but some exposure, for example to fluoride in food and drinks, is not. It is uncontrolled exposure to fluoride, sometimes from unsuspected sources, that is the principal public health concern. Periodic assessment of total fluoride intake in a population, as well as regular monitoring of fluorosis prevalence and severity in children, enables the public health administrator to determine whether further action is called for. (WHO 1994)

三、口腔癌 Oral cancer

The prevalence of oral cancer is particularly high among men, the eighth most common cancer worldwide. Incidence rates for oral cancer vary in men from 1 to 10 cases per 100,000 inhabitants in many countries. In south-central Asia, cancer of the oral cavity ranks amongst the three most common types of cancer. However, sharp increases in the incidence rates of oral/pharyngeal cancer have been reported for several countries and regions such as Denmark, Germany, Scotland, central and Eastern Europe and, to a lesser extent, Australia, Japan, New Zealand and USA.

In Asia, the age standardized incidence rate of oral cancer per 100,000 population ranges from 0.7 in China to 4.6 in Thailand and 12.6 in India. The high incidence rates related directly to risk behaviors such as smoking, use of smokeless tobacco (e.g. betel nut or miang chewing) and alcohol consumption. In Thailand, for example, the prevalence of smoking is about 60%, betel nut chewing 15% while alcohol consumption is 35% (WHO 2003) .

In US, like other cancers, oral cancer is usually expressed as a proportion or rate. The age-adjusted rate of years of life lost from oral cancer, for example, dropped from 23.1 per 100,000 populations in 1970 to 19.9 per 100,000 populations in 1985. Five-year survival rates are also useful cancer; a 5-year survival rate of 67%, for example, means that 67% of persons who had the condition diagnosed 5 years ago are still alive (Burt 1999).

在我国以舌癌、颊黏膜癌、牙龈癌、腭癌最为常见。尤其是舌癌，近年有上升的趋势，占口腔癌的41.8%。其次是颊癌，占口腔癌的30.2%。牙龈癌近年有下降的趋势，占口腔癌的22.5%。其他如腭癌和口底癌也占一定的比例。口腔癌的发生多因不良行为和不良习惯还有环境因素与生物因素所致。

口腔癌的发病率随年龄的增长而升高，如江苏扬州1981～1982年进行了一次口腔恶性肿瘤的普查，年龄从0～70岁以上，共80028人。其中30岁组恶性肿瘤的患病率为0.038%，60岁组上升至0.34%，增加近10倍。

四、牙颌异常 Dentofacial anomalies

牙颌异常指儿童在生长发育过程中，由于各种因素的影响，如不良习惯、疾病、替牙紊乱、发育异常、遗传等，导致牙列不齐、殆关系紊乱等。牙颌异常指儿童在生长发育过程中，由于各种因素的影响，如不良习惯、疾病、替牙紊乱、发育异常、遗传等，导致牙列不齐、殆关系紊乱等。

Estimates of the frequency of different traits of malocclusion are available from a number of countries, primarily in northern Europe and North America. For example, prevalence rates of dentofacial anomalies are reported at 10%, according to the Dental Aesthetic Index. Malocclusion is not a disease but rather a set of dental deviations which in some cases can influence quality of lift. There is insufficient evidence that orthodontic treatment enhances dental health and function. Treatment is often justified by the potential enhancement of social and psychological well-being through improvements in appearance.

2000年，中华口腔医学会口腔正畸专业委员会组织完成了第一次全国错㿻流行病学调查，共调查了12个省市的25392名儿童与青少年。结果表明，在我国儿童与青少年的错㿻患病率近40年来有明显上升，由20世纪60年代初的40%上升到2000年的67.82%。

五、口腔黏膜病 Oral mucosal diseases

It is noteworthy that at the global level few systematic epidemiological studies of oral mucosal diseases have been carried out. Prevalence rates of oral leukoplakia vary from 0.1% to 10.6% depending on region or geographical location. Erythroplakia seems less common with prevalence rates of 0.1% or less.

Qat is a leafy narcotic substance that is popular in several countries in East Africa and the Arabian Peninsula. Qat can be consumed as a liquid in form of tea or smoked like tobacco. However, the most common mode of ingestion is by chewing the fresh leaves. Consumption of Qat can lead to adverse oral effects including oral mucosal lesions, dryness of the mouth, discoloration of teeth, poor oral hygiene and periodontal disease.

In some developing countries, oral diseases are increasing and countries in Africa and Asia must urgently address a number of vary serious oral conditions including noma (cancrum oris), ANUG (acute necrotizing ulcerative gingivitis), oral precancer and cancer. Cases of noma are reported for young children aged 3 ~ 5 years in Africa, Latin America and Asia; with 90% of them dying without having received any care.

In addition, Africa and Asia have the highest prevalence of HIV/AIDS, oral manifestations of which are widespread. Analyses of HIV/AIDS cases show that oral manifestation such as candida infections, hairy leukoplakia, oral clcers and gingival bleeding, necrotizing periodontitis, leukoplakia and Laposi's sarcoma are frequent.

1978年许国祺等对上海地区不同职业人员进行口腔黏膜健康情况调查，受检人数共18769人，查出患白斑的病人1502人，患病率为8%。我国白斑的患病率为10.47%，这是1980年全国口腔黏膜白斑和扁平苔藓苔藓协作组对全国134个点、134492名人员的调查结果。

从白斑的流行病学分布来看，白斑好发的年龄为40岁以上中年人，并随年龄增加而增高。我国口腔黏膜白斑和扁平苔藓苔藓协作组在1980年的调查结果则显示，好发年龄为50 ~ 59岁。白斑患者以男性居多，1978年李辉奉等在武汉调查了15280人，男女比例是27：1。大量流行病学调查表明，白斑发生的部位多见于颊黏膜、上下唇等处。白斑是一种癌前病变，吸烟是引起白斑的主要危险因素，白斑有导致口腔癌的可能，据调查其癌变率为3%～6%，停止吸烟后白斑可以消除。

扁平苔藓（Lichen Planus）在流行病学调查时的评价指标主要为患病率。1980年我国口腔黏膜白斑和扁平苔藓协作组对134492人进行调查，我国口腔黏膜扁平苔藓患病率为0.51%。关于口腔扁平苔藓好发年龄的报道相差较大，1980年李辉菶报道最小年龄为12岁，最大年龄为68岁。但发病最多的年龄是中年人。口腔扁平苔藓女性比男性略为多发。发病原因尚不清楚。严重时亦有癌变的可能。

六、唇腭裂 Cleft lip and palate

Diagnosis and treatment of craniofacial anomalies such as cleft lip and palate resent a number of challenges to public health. Oro-facial clefts occur in around 1 per 500～700 births, the rate varying substantially across ethnic groups and geographical areas. Other conditions that may lead to special health care needs include Down syndrome, cerebral palsy, learning and developmental disabilities, and genetic and hereditary disorders with oro-facial clefts appear to have substantial environmental causes, higher risk first of all associated with maternal tobacco, alcohol and nutritional factors. There is no consistent evidence of time trends, nor is there consistent variation by socioeconomic status, but these aspects have not been adequately studied. In addition, there are many parts of the world in which there is little or no information available on the frequency of craniofacial anomalies, in particular parts of Africa, central Asia, eastern Europe, India and Middle East.

根据1986年中国出生缺陷检测协作组对我国29个省、市、自治区120多万人口的调查报告显示，我国的唇腭裂发生率较高，为1.8‰，其中唇裂合并腭裂者占61.4%，单纯唇裂占30.5%，腭裂占8.2%。青海、甘肃、贵州等省发生率最高，其中青海省为3.1‰，而湖南省发生率较低，为1.3‰。在我国，唇腭裂的发生在城乡之间有显著差别，城市唇腭裂的发生率为1.7‰，而农村的发生率为2.1‰。这种情况可能与农村近亲婚配，妇女文化教育程度低，缺乏孕期健康意识有关。据北京医科大学出生缺陷中心统计分析15万出生检测资料显示，唇腭裂缺陷率近亲婚配与非近亲婚配分别为6.7‰与1.7‰，相对危险度为3.9，即发生唇腭裂的机率高达4倍；不正当的人工流产和不科学的堕胎也可影响胎儿的发育；另外，营养缺乏也是唇腭裂发生率高的原因之一。在唇腭裂中，男性婴儿发生率比女性婴儿高，男婴唇腭裂发生率为2.0‰，女婴发生率为1.6‰。

七、颞下颌关节紊乱 Temporomonibular disorders

Disturbances of the temporomonibular joint, usually referred to as TMD or TMPDS (temporomonibular pain and dysfunction syndrome) , are a group of extremely painful and distressing conditions. There are 3 times as many women patients as men, although no one knows why. Diagnosis is not easy because TMD is often accompanied by generalized pain in the head and neck region. There is no agreement on what constitutes standard treatment procedures, and treatment outcomes are mixed. It is hardly surprising that the epidemiology of these conditions is poorly understood.

The difficulty in defining risk factors in TMD stems from the absence of a suitable case definition of TMD. To put the problem in perspective, disagreements on criteria for diagnosing caries exist only over a narrow range of clinical detection of an agreed-upon pathology. TMD conditions, however, go far beyond these relatively restricted definitional problems; they are more akin to the problems with measuring malocclusion. Where a condition cannot be defined, valid measurement is virtually impossible. Definitions of TMD exist, but they tend to be all-encompassing and nonspecific, and hence of not much operational value for research purposes.

Epidemiologic studies of TMD have measured various signs and symptoms in different population groups, so summation of the state of knowledge is difficult. Commonly measured signs and symptoms include pain in the joint or masseter muscles with joint movement, limitations in mandibular movement, mandibular deviations on opening, and joint clicking or crepitus. Studies have used both self-reported questionnaires and clinical examinations to obtain information. Many of what are referred to as epidemiologic studies in fact are clinical studies of patients receiving treatment, and so have to be interpreted cautiously.

There is agreement that the prevalence of the commonly measured conditions just listed is quite high, even among people who do not perceive that they have a problem that requires treatment. One study of a representative population in Toronto found that 49% of adults responded positively to one or more of 9 questions regarding symptoms, although need for treatment was found in only 3% to 10%, depending on the case definition used. It is far more difficult, however, to interpret what these data mean, for it is common to find prevalent symptoms having no clinical significance. Is a clicking joint, for example, a sign of impending trouble, or is it of no consequence? One longitudinal study found that a majority of patients with a painless click did develop joint pain in time, although it should be noted that the group studied were already TMD patients for other reasons. Other longitudinal studies, however, have shown that many of these measured signs and symptoms are unstable over time, meaning that they come and go. It has been noted that signs and symptoms are as common in children and adolescents as they are in adults, although again the interpretation of these findings is unclear. Clicking joint of adolescents have been related to growth stages that come and go in response to "natural longitudinal fluctuations." Cross-sectional studies therefore can yield misleading data with regard to prevalence and correlations. (Burt 1999)

小结 Summary

为适应长学制教学，口腔流行病学是在全国统编教材的基础上适当加以内容扩展和增加相关英文参考文献和教材段落编写的。理论课以主要概念、原则和方法为重点，扩展内容和相关英文参考文献和教材段落以自学阅读为主。

思考题 Review questions

1. 如何在临床实践中应用的口腔流行病学的原则和方法。
2. 如何开展社区口腔健康调查。
3. 国内外口腔常见疾病的流行趋势和特点是什么。

参考文献 References

1. Pine CM. Community oral health. Reed Educational & Professional Publishing Ltd, 1997
2. WHO. Oral health surveys basic methods 4th edition. World Health Organization Geneva, 1997
3. Burt BA, Eklund SA. Dentistry, Dental Practice, and the Community 5th edition W.B. Saunders Company, 1999
4. 全国牙防组. 第二次全国口腔健康流行病学抽样调查. 人民卫生出版社, 1998
5. Petersen PE. The world oral health report 2003. Community Dent Oral Epidemiol, 2003, 31 (Suppl. 1): 3-24
6. 卞金有. 预防口腔医学 (第 4 版). 人民卫生出版社, 2003
7. 傅民魁等. 中国25392名儿童与青少年错㿥畸形患病率的调查. 中华口腔医学杂志, 2002, 37: 371-373
8. 叶玮, 冯希平, 刘艳玲. 上海市幼儿猛性龋危险因素的流行病学研究. 上海口腔医学, 2001, 10 (2): 166-169
9. WHO. Fluorides and oral health. World Health Organization Geneva, 1994
10. Axelsson P. Diagnosis and risk prediction of dental caries. Quitessence Publishing Co, Inc, 2000

（王伟健）

第三章　口腔健康资料统计学基本方法
Chapter Ⅲ Statistical Methods for Oral Health Data

概述 Overview

本章介绍了口腔健康资料的类型、常用的统计指标以及统计方法，并简述了统计分析软件——SPSS的使用方法。通过对本章的学习，应掌握常用的口腔健康资料统计指标及计算方法。

This chapter introduces the types of measurement scale, the statistical indicators of oral health data, and simple application of SPSS software. Through this chapter, the main statistical indictors of oral health data and the calculation methods should be grasped.

要点 Key points

- 计量资料和计数资料的统计指标。
- 计量资料和计数资料的描述性统计分析方法。

第一节　口腔健康资料的统计指标
Section 1 Statistical Indicators in Oral Health Data

一、资料的种类 Types of measurement scale

资料收集过程中，研究者常常对每个观察单位的某项特征进行测量和观察，这种特征称为变量（Variable）。对变量的测得值称为变量值（Value of variable）或观察值（Observed value），亦称为资料（Data）。变量的观察结果可以是定量的，也可以是定性的。根据观察值的特点将资料分为三种类型。

（一）计量资料 Measurement data

是对每个观察单位用定量的方法测定某项指标所得的资料。这类资料大都是用测量工具或仪器测得的。带有度、量或其他单位，又称测量资料、定量资料（quantitative data）。如长度、身高、体重、龋失补牙数等。这类资料的统计分析指标常为均数、标准差等。

This scale involves measurements that indicate a continuous scale that begins at absolute zero. It includes all the usual measurements (or determinations) of length, height, money amount, weight, volume, area, pressure, sound intensity, brightness, velocity, and so on. For example, the number of decayed, missing and filled teeth.

（二）计数资料 Enumeration data

计数资料是按观察单位的某种特征（或属性）分类，再清点各种观察单位的个数所得到的资料。如男性和女性，有龋和无龋儿童等。计数资料一般是用定性的方法得到的资料故又称分类资料（categorical data）或定性资料（qualitative data）。这类资料可计算相对数，如率、构成比等。

This is the scale of equivalency, wherein objects or observations are fitted into classes or categories, such as male or female, normal or malocclusion, diabetes or no diabetes, etc. The characteristics on the enumeration data have no quantitative significance; they are qualitative. On this level, numbers may be assigned to the characteristic, but only for the purpose of identification or classification.

（三）等级资料 Ordinal data

等级资料是将观察单位按某种指标的等级顺序分组，再清点各组观察单位的个数所得的资料。这类资料具有计数资料的特点，又兼有半定量的性质，故称为半计数资料或半定量资料。如牙龈指数、牙菌斑指数、收入水平、学生成绩等。

This level of measurement classifies objects into mutually exclusive and exhaustive categories. However, unlike the enumeration data, the groups in an ordinal data have some hierarchical relation or ordering. Thus ordinal level of measurement is a rank order, such as on the basis of whether it is better, equal to, or worse than some criterion, or in the order of intensity. Such rankings of a characteristic as severity of periodontal disease, plaque index scores, income levels, or student rankings in a class are examples of the ordinal scale of measurement.

实际上，资料类型的划分是根据研究目的而确定的。根据需要，测量精确度高一级的资料可以转化成低一级的资料。如儿童的龋失补牙数是计量资料，若按照有龋与无龋划分则属于计数资料，若按照龋病患病程度划分重度患龋儿童、一般患龋儿童、无龋儿童则属于等级资料。

二、统计指标 Statistical indicators

在对口腔流行病学资料进行统计分析之前，必须首先确定所用的一些特定的统计指标，以便能定量地、简练地描述所收集到的数据。根据收集到的数据资料类型不同，选择不同的统计指标。计量资料通常描述资料的集中趋势与离散趋势，分类资料通常用相对数来描述。

To describe the data, it is necessary to represent a set of data by means of a single number which, in its way, is descriptive of the entire set. Exactly what sort of number we choose depends on the particular characteristic we want to describe. For measurement data, we normally describe the center of a set of data, i.e. the measure of central tendency, and the spread of a set of data, i.e. the measure of dispersion. For enumeration data and ordinal data, we normally describe the relative number.

（一）计量资料的统计指标 Statistical indicators for measurement data

1. 描述集中趋势的统计指标 Measures of central tendency

（1）均数和算术均数 Mean and arithmetic mean

分析计量资料常用均数，它是反映一组性质相同的观察值的平均水平或集中趋势的统计指标。均数包括算术均数、几何均数、中位数等，其中算术均数较为常用。

Mean is the average level of a set of data, it is used to measure the central tendency of a set of data. Mean includes arithmetic mean, geometric mean, and median etc. The arithmetic mean of a set of quantitative data is equal to the sum of the measurements divided by the number of measurements contained in the data set.

例 1　调查某校学生口腔健康状况，其中 12 岁男生共检查 120 人，检出 108 颗龋，从 120 个变量中得出一个平均数，即为每人平均患龋数。

均数有三种算法：直接法、加权法、和简捷法。当观察值的个数不多时，可用直接法计算，公式为：

$$\bar{X} = \frac{\sum X}{n} \tag{1}$$

当观察值较多时，可用加权法计算。公式为：

$$\bar{X} = \frac{f_1 x_1 + f_2 x_2 + ... + f_k x_k}{f_1 + f_2 + ... + f_k} = \frac{\sum fX}{\sum f} \tag{2}$$

$\bar{X}$ 代表平均数，式中的 Σ 为求和的符号，x 代表变量（观察值），f 代表频数，Σfx 代表各变量乘频数后相加的总和，n 代表受检人数。

本例：

$$\bar{X} = \frac{108}{120} = 0.9$$

120 名 12 岁男生，平均每人患 0.9 颗龋齿。

加权的含义是指各个不同的观察值在计算均数时，所起的作用不同。频数多，权数大，作用也大；频数少，权数小，作用也小。

（2）中位数 Median

是指将一组观察值从小到大或从大到小排序后居于中间位置的那个数值。全部观察值中，大于和小于中位数的观察值个数相等。任何分布的定量数据均可用中位数描述其分布的集中趋势，因而试用范围较广。

当观察值个数为偶数时，中位数为位于中间的两个观察值的均数；当观察值个数为奇数时，中位数为位于中间的那个观察值。

The median of a data set is the middle number when the measurements are arranged in ascending (or descending) order. If n is odd, the median is the middle observation. If n is even, the median is the mean of the middle two numbers.

（3）众数 Mode

众数是指一组观察值中出现次数最多的那个观察值。众数与中位数都不是通过全部观察值计算出的，而是将数据排序后从位置上直接得到的。

The mode is the measurement that occurs with greatest frequency in the data set. If all the numbers in the group are different, then we cannot have a modal value.

2. 描述离散趋势的统计指标 Measures of dispersion

集中趋势是数据分布的一个重要特征，但只有集中趋势指标还不能很好地描述数据的分布规律，还需要引入描述数据分布离散趋势的指标。表示数据分布离散趋势的指标有全距、方差、标准差以及变异系数等，最常用的指标是标准差。

Measures of central tendency describe one important aspect of a set of data-their "middle" or their "average" - but they tell us nothing about other characteristic. We also require ways of measuring the extent to which data are dispersed, or spread out about the average value, and the statistical measures which provide this information are called measures of dispersion.

（1）全距 Range

又称极差，是一组资料最大值与最小值之差。

The range of a set of data is the largest value minus the smallest.

（2）四分位间距 Interquartile range

四分位间距用 Q 表示，是上四分位数 Q_3（P_{75}）和下四分位数 Q_1（P_{25}）之差。其值越大，说明变异程度越大。

The interquartile range is defined as (Q_3 - Q_1). The bigger the value is, the more the dispersion of the data.

（3）标准差 Standard deviation

标准差是用来说明一组观察值之间的变异程度，即离散度。如检查2组儿童患龋病情况，每组检查8人，其龋数为24，龋均为3，但每组患龋情况的分布不尽相同：一组为3，4，2，2，5，3，4，1；另一组为0，1，1，9，8，1，2，2，前组分布比较集中，即每个人患龋的牙数变异较小，而后者比较分散，变异较大。标准差的计算方法可用标准差加权计算法。适用于有较多相同观察值的资料。

在例1中，120名12岁男生龋标准差计算方法见表3-1。

表3-1　标准差加权法计算表

分组 x	频数 f	fx	fx^2
0	70	0	0
1	15	15	15
2	18	36	72
3	11	33	99
4	6	24	96
合计	120	108	282

$\sum f=120 \quad \sum fx=108 \quad \sum fx^2=282$

公式：

$$S(\text{标准差})=\sqrt{\frac{\sum fx^2-(\sum fx)^2/\sum f}{\sum f-1}},\ \sum f=n \qquad (3)$$

$$S(\text{标准差})=\sqrt{\frac{282-(108)^2/120}{120-1}}=1.25$$

120 名男生龋的标准差为 1.25。

标准差可以用来反映一组观察值的离散程度，标准差越小，离散程度越小，均数的代表性越好。用于计算变异系数、标准误，结合均数与正态分布的规律估计参考值的范围。

（二）计数资料的统计指标 Statistical indicators for enumeration data

研究中清点分类资料得到的数据被称为绝对数。绝对数是研究客观事物或现象本质的基本信息，但不便于相互比较和寻找事物间的联系，因此，常根据研究目的计算相应的相对数指标，以便对资料进行统计学描述和深入的分析。相对数（relative number）是计数资料的统计指标。它是根据两种或两种以上的有关数据（绝对数）在同一基础上算出来的对比数值。相对数是两个有联系的指标之比。常用的相对数有率、构成比以及相对比。

1. 率 Rate

率又称频率指标，是用来说明某种现象发生的频率或强度。在评价口腔疾病的患病状况时，常用率来表示人群中疾病状况的高低。率常用 100 为基数，计算公式如下：

$$\text{率}=\frac{\text{某现象实际发生数}}{\text{可能发生某现象的总人数}}\times 100\% \tag{4}$$

如：

$$\text{患龋率}=\frac{\text{患龋人数}}{\text{受检人数}}\times 100\%$$

The prevalence of a disease is the probability of currently having that disease regardless of the duration of the time one has had the disease. It is obtained by dividing the number of people who currently have the disease by the number of people in the study population.

例 2　检查甲校 12 岁男生 400 人，患龋人数为 120 人。检查乙校同年龄男生 600 人，患龋人数为 150 人，不能认为乙校 12 岁男生的患龋情况比甲校严重，因为两校的受检人数不等，患龋率不同。两校学生的患龋率分别是：

甲校学生：$120/400 \times 100\% = 30.0\%$

乙校学生：$150/600 \times 100\% = 25.0\%$

结论应该是甲校 12 岁男生的患龋率高丁乙校。

2. 构成比 Proportion

是用来说明某事物内部各构成部分所占的比重。以龋病为例，龋、失、补的牙数各占龋总数的百分比即龋、失、补的构成比。计算公式如下：

$$\text{构成比}=\frac{\text{某一构成部分的个体数}}{\text{事物各构成部分个体数的总和}}\times 100\% \tag{5}$$

一组构成比之和应为 100%。

例 3　检查某校 12 岁学生 120 人，他们患龋病情况：未治龋共 80 颗，龋失牙为 10 颗，因龋已充填牙为 30 颗，其龋、失、补的构成比分别为：

$$\text{龋}= 80/120 \times 100\% = 66.67\%$$

$$\text{失}= 10/120 \times 100\% = 8.33\%$$

$$补 = 30/120 \times 100\% = 25.00\%$$

3. 相对比 Ratio

是用来说明两个同类指标或有关指标的比。通常以某种现象的数值为1或100作基数，另一个指标是它的几倍或百分之几。

（三）标准误 Standard error

在抽样调查中，使样本均数（或率）与总体均数（或率）之间出现差别的重要原因之一是存在抽样误差。标准误是用来表示抽样误差的大小。数理统计已经证明，标准误的大小与总体标准差成正比，随着样本含量的增多逐渐减小，如均数的标准误，当标准差不变时，与样本含量（n）的平方根成反比。由于总体标准差不易获得，故以样本标准差作为总体标准差的估计值。

The standard deviation of the sampling distribution is often called the standard error of the sample proportion or sample mean. It quantifies how good the sample proportion or sample mean is and how large an error might be made. Note that the standard error is not an estimate of any quantity in the population, but an indication of the variability among many sample proportions or sample means from the sample population, or alternatively, a measure of the uncertainty of a single sample proportion or sample mean as an estimate of the population proportion or population mean.

We can make two intuitive judgments about the standard error:

standard error will be smaller as the sample size n is getting bigger, i.e. big samples are more reliable than small samples.

standard error will depend on the variability of the observations. If the variability of the observations is small (i.e. if the variance and standard deviation is small), we would expect the standard error to be small. If it were large, the standard error may well be large too.

均数标准误计算公式为：

$$S_{\bar{X}}\,(\text{均数标准误}) = \frac{s}{\sqrt{n}} \tag{6}$$

如标准差为1.25，样本含量为120，则标准误的计算如下：

$s = 1.25$，$n = 120$，$S_{\bar{x}} = \dfrac{1.25}{\sqrt{120}} = 0.11$

率的标准误计算公式为：

$$S_p\,(\text{率的标准误}) = \sqrt{\frac{P(1-P)}{n}} \tag{7}$$

p 代表样本率，n 为样本量

如调查200名18岁青年患龋情况，其患龋率为60%，标准误的计算如下：

$$S_p\text{(率的标准误)}=\sqrt{\frac{60\%\times(1-60\%)}{200}}=3.46\%$$

（四）可信区间 Confidence interval

在抽样研究中，虽有抽样误差存在，但只要是随机样本，其样本均数（或率）围绕总体均数（或率）呈正态分布或近似正态分布，故可以样本均数（或率）和标准误对总体均数（或率）作出区间估计。区间估计有95%可信区间及99%可信区间。95%或99%可信区间即总体均数（或率）有95%或99%的概率（或可能性）在此区间范围内，即以上可信限为界，但不包括界值在内的一个范围。在实际工作中，95%的可信度更为常用。

A confidence interval is an interval calculated from the data in the sample in such a way that it contains the true value of the parameter to be estimated with a specified probability. This probability is referred to as the level of confidence. For instance, a 95% confidence interval for (population) mean is that, if samples were drawn repeatedly from the same population, 95% of confidence intervals calculated from these samples will contain the true value of mean.

样本观察例数在100例以上时，总体均数的95%可信区间为$X \pm 1.96S_{\bar{x}}$，总体均数的99%可信区间为$\bar{X} \pm 2.58S_{\bar{x}}$。

如：$\bar{X} = 0.9$　$S_{\bar{x}} = 0.11$　$n = 120$

95%可信区间的值为：$0.9 \pm 1.96 \times 0.11$　即0.68 ~ 1.12

99%可信区间的值为：$0.9 \pm 2.58 \times 0.11$　即0.62 ~ 1.18

当n足够大，且P不接近零时，

总体率的95%可信区间为：$P \pm 1.96Sp$

总体率的99%可信区间为：$P \pm 2.58Sp$

第二节　资料的整理

Section 2 Sorting Data

口腔流行病学的现场调查工作结束后，常会得到大量的数据资料，在这些资料中有许多数据需要进行统计学处理和分析，工作量极大。为了保证资料的完整性和准确性，就必须在统计分析前对收集到的资料进行认真细致的整理。整理工作一般分三步：

一、核对 Proof-reading

首先是对所有数据进行认真核对。资料收集以后，对调查表中的每一个项目都要仔细检查，一般项目中的性别、年龄、职业是否相符，口腔健康状况项目中是否有缺漏，有无不符合逻辑的错误，如在龋病检查中，明明在牙列状况一栏中某颗牙齿记录为“无龋”，但在牙周状况栏中却记录为“缺失牙”。这些差错在流行病学调查的资料中常会看到，一经发现，需要及时纠正，以保证分析的结果不致发生偏差。

二、分组 Sorting data

资料核对无误后，接下来的工作就是分组。分组是把调查资料按照一定的特性或程度进行归类。常按不同地区及不同人群的特征，如性别、年龄、城乡、种族等分组。也可按照某种疾病的患病严重程度进行分组，常见的如按患龋牙数或牙周袋深浅分组。分组是口腔流行病学调查中进行统计分析的关键一步，在“同质”条件下进行恰当的分组可以正确反映疾病的流行特征，提示各种影响流行的因素，并能建立病因假设，而不恰当的分组可能会掩盖许多有用的信息。例如：口腔疾病常与年龄有很密切的关系，随着增龄变化，患病率也会随之而改变，如果我们在对调查资料进行分组时没有按年龄分组，就难以看出年龄可能对疾病的影响。另外，在对连续性变量进行分组时还必须考虑到变量分界点的选择，应按照习惯的分界点或国际上普遍使用的分界点作为分组标志，这样可以对统计的数据进行相互比较。例如，当我们对某一调查资料按年龄分组时，如果国际上普遍以每 10 岁为一组，而我们却以每 5 岁为一组，结果相互之间就难以比较。

三、整理 Data set

资料分组后，就可以清点每组中的频数。人工整理时，可用计数法，将每一组中的频数相加。人工整理花时多，且误差大，尤其是在进行大规模的口腔流行病学调查时，变量多达几千万或更多，资料整理十分困难，因此，在有条件的地方可以使用计算机整理。计算机整理可以借助各种数据库软件，如 SPSS、FoxPro、dbase Ⅲ、Epi info 等。

In any study there is always the potential for errors to occur in a data set, either at the outset when taking measurements or when collecting, transcribing and entering the data onto a computer. It is hard to eliminate all of these errors. However, you can reduce the number of typing and transcribing errors by checking the data carefully once they have been entered. Simply scanning the data by eye will often identify values that are obviously wrong.

Typing mistakes are the most frequent source of errors when entering data. If the amount of data is small. Then you can check the typed data set against the original forms/questionnaires to see whether there are any typing mistakes. However, it is time-consuming if the amount of data is large. It is possible to type the data in twice and compare the two data sets using a computer program. Any differences between the two data sets will reveal typing mistakes. Although this approach does not rule out the possibility that the same error has been incorrectly entered on both occasions, or that the value on the form/questionnaire is incorrect, it does at least minimize the number of errors. The disadvantage of this method is that it takes twice as long to enter the data, which may have major cost or time implications.

第三节 资料的统计分析方法

Section 3 Statistical Methods in Oral Health Data

在抽样研究中，不可避免会产生抽样误差。当我们从同一总体中随机抽取若干例数相等的样本，计算他们的样本均数或样本率时，这些样本均数或率不可能都相等，也不可能都等于总体均数或率，这种误差为抽样误差。如调查某市小学生患龋病情况，随机抽取 6 ~ 11 岁学生 1200 人（每年龄组抽 200 人），龋均为 2.0；如再从该市随机抽取同年龄 1200 人，龋均就不一定仍为 2.0，也不一定恰好等于该市同年龄小学生的实际龋均。造成样本均数（或率）与总体均数（或率）差别的原因，可能是由于抽样误差所致，也可能两均数确实存在质的差别。对两种可能性进行判断的方法，就用假设检验，进行统计推断。

所以，假设检验的目的是以样本之间的差异，推断总体之间是否确有差异，是属于抽样误差所致的范围内的波动，还是有本质上的差别。若是由于抽样误差引起的可能性很小时，就可以推断它们之间确有本质差别。通常按下列标准作出统计学上的判断：

$p > 0.05$	统计学无显著意义 No statistically significant differences
$0.05 \geqslant p > 0.01$	统计学有显著意义 Statistically significant differences
$p \leqslant 0.01$	统计学有高度显著意义 High statistically significant differences

以 p 值表示概率大小，常用 5%（即 0.05）或 1%（即 0.01）作为判断统计学意义的标准。

数据统计分析可以使用公式计算，也可以借助计算机统计软件计算，常用的数据统计分析软件有SPSS（社会科学用统计软件包，Statistical Package for Social Science）、SAS（统计分析系统，Statistical Analysis System）等。下面介绍几种数据统计分析的方法。

一、计量资料的统计分析 Statistical analysis for measurement data

1. 两样本均数的比较 Two-sample t test

检验两个样本均数差异是否有统计学意义，若样本含量小，一般用 t 检验，样本含量大时一般用 u 检验。

例 4　1983 年抽样调查某市中、小学生龋病患病情况，检查 12 岁男、女学生各 300 人，结果男生龋均为0.99，女生龋均为1.90，男、女生龋均的标准差分别为1.62和2.00，问男、女生患龋情况是否有差异。

（1）检验假设：男生与女生龋均来自同一总体，其差异是由抽样误差所致。

（2）计算 u 值

公式：

$$u=\frac{|\bar{X}_1-\bar{X}_2|}{\sqrt{(S_{\bar{X}_1})^2+(S_{\bar{X}_2})^2}}=\frac{|\bar{X}_1-\bar{X}_2|}{\sqrt{\left(\frac{S_1}{n_1}\right)^2+\left(\frac{S_2}{n_2}\right)^2}} \tag{8}$$

本例　$\bar{X}_1 = 0.99$　　$\bar{X}_2 = 1.90$

　　　$S_1 = 1.62$　　$S_2 = 2.00$

$$S_{\bar{X}_1}=\frac{S_1}{\sqrt{n}}=\frac{1.62}{\sqrt{300}}=0.09$$

$$S_{\bar{X}_2}=\frac{S_2}{\sqrt{n}}=\frac{2.00}{\sqrt{300}}=0.12$$

代入公式 $$u=\frac{0.91}{\sqrt{0.008+0.014}}=6.14$$

（3）确定 p 值 当 $u=1.96$ 时，$p=0.05$，$u=2.58$ 时，$p=0.01$，本例 $u>2.58$ 故 $p<0.01$。

判断结果 本例男、女学生龋均的差别有统计学意义（$p<0.01$），故可以认为女生龋均明显高于男生。

2. 多个样本均数的比较 Analysis for variance，ANOVA

检验两组以上样本均数间的差别，通常用方差分析、秩和检验方法。以下为用方差分析检验的实例。

例 5 某医院于 1982 年对某市中、小学生患病情况进行抽样调查。根据学生来源不同，对城市、近郊城市、近郊农村及远郊农村的学生都进行了抽样。调查人数分别为826、630、630及 840 人；结果龋均分别为 1.40、1.67、1.27 及 1.31；其标准误分别为 0.07、0.07、0.07 及 0.06；问这 4 种来源的学生龋均的差别有无统计学意义。

（1）检验假设 4种来源学生的龋均来自同一总体，其差异是由抽样误差所致，见表3-2。

表 3-2 4 种来源学生患龋情况

	城市学生	近郊城市学生	近郊农村学生	远郊城市学生	合计
$\sum_{j=1}^{n_j} X_{ij}$	1153	1055	802	1104	4114 ($\sum X$)
n_i	826	630	630	840	2926 (n)
$\overline{X_i}$	1.40	1.67	1.27	1.31	1.41 ($\overline{X}$)
$\sum_{j=1}^{n_j} X_{ij}^2$	3869	3965	2872	3836	14542 ($\sum X^2$)

资料来源：杨是主编《口腔预防医学》（第二版）

（2）计算组间与组内变异的离均差平方和（SS 组间，SS 组内）及总变异的离均差平方和（SS 总）。

先按公式求校正数（C）

公式 $$C=\frac{(\sum X)^2}{n}$$

本例 $$C=\frac{(4114)^2}{2926}=5784.35$$

公式 $$SS_{组间}=\sum_{i=1}^{k}\frac{(\sum_{j=1}^{n_i} X_{ij})^2}{n_i}-C$$

$$SS_{组间}=\frac{(1153)^2}{826}+\frac{(1055)^2}{630}+\frac{(802)^2}{630}+\frac{(1104)^2}{840}-5784.5=63.74$$

公式 $SS_{总} = \sum X^2 - C$

本例 $SS_{总} = 14542 - 5784.35 = 8757.65$

公式 $SS_{组内} = SS_{总} - SS_{组间}$

本例 $SS_{组内} = 8757.65 - 63.74 = 8693.91$

（3）列方差分析表（表3-3）

表 3-3　方差分析表

变异来源	SS	n′	MS	F 值
总变异	8757.65	2925(n-1)		
组间变异	63.74	3(K-1)	$\frac{SS_{组间}}{k-1} = 21.25$	$\frac{SS_{组间}}{MS_{组内}} = 7.13$
组内变异	8693.91	2922(n-k)	$\frac{SS_{组内}}{n-k} = 2.98$	

资料来源：杨是主编《口腔预防医学》（第二版）

（4）确定 p 值　组间自由度 $n_1 = 3$，组内自由度 $n_2 = 2922$，查附表 F 值 $F_{0.01\,(3.00)} = 3.78$。本例 $F = 7.13 > 3.78$，故 $p < 0.01$。

（5）判断结果　4种来源的学生龋均差别有统计学意义（$p < 0.01$），即认为他们的龋均是有差别的。

（6）关于多组均数的两两比较，经方差分析各组均数之间差别有统计学意义时，就需进一步检验哪些均数间差别有统计学意义，哪些没有。上例经方差分析后，4种来源学生的龋均相互之间差别的统计学意义，按以下步骤计算。

① 检验假设　各组均数两两相等，见下表。

② 计算 q 值

公式：

$$q = \frac{\left|\bar{X}_A - \bar{X}_B\right|}{S_{(\bar{X}_A - \bar{X}_B)}}$$

式中 $S_{(\bar{X}_A - \bar{X}_B)}$ 为两均数 $\bar{X}_A$ 与 $\bar{X}_b$ 之差的标准误，按下式计算。

公式 $$S_{(\bar{X}_A - \bar{X}_B)} = \sqrt{\frac{误差的均方}{每组样本含量}}$$

本例每组样本含量不等，应先求出每组样本含量的均数 n_0。

公式 $$n_0 = \frac{1}{k-1}\left[\sum n_i - \frac{\sum n_i^2}{\sum n_i}\right]$$

代入公式 $n_0 = \frac{1}{4-1}\left(2926 - \frac{(826)^2 + (630)^2 + (630)^2 + (840)^2}{2926}\right) = 726.79$

本例 $k = 4 \quad \sum n_i = 2926$

均数组次

1	2	3	4
1.67	1.40	1.31	1.27
(近郊城市)	(城市)	(远郊)	(近郊农村)

$$S_{(\bar{X}_A - \bar{X}_B)} = \sqrt{\frac{2.98}{726.79}} = 0.06$$

1 与 4 比较，其 q 值为：

$$q = \frac{\bar{X}_1 - \bar{X}_2}{0.06} = \frac{1.67 - 1.27}{0.06} = 6.67$$

1 与 3，1 与 2，2 与 4，2 与 3，3 与 4 比较，其 q 值计算方法同上（表 3-4）。

表 3-4　各均数间两两比较

比较组 (A 与 B) (1)	差数 ($\bar{X}_A - \bar{X}_B$) (2)	a (3)	q (4)＝(2)/0.06	q 的界值 $p = 0.05$ (5)	$p = 0.01$ (6)	结论 (7)
1 与 4	0.40	4	6.67	3.63	4.40	**
1 与 3	0.36	3	6.00	3.31	4.12	**
1 与 2	0.27	2	4.50	2.77	3.64	**
2 与 4	0.13	3	2.17	3.31	4.12	
2 与 3	0.09	2	1.50	2.77	3.64	
3 与 4	0.04	2	0.67	2.77	3.64	

**n'=2922（为 q 值表中的∞项）

a = 4 时 $q_{0.05}$(∞，4)= 3.63　$q_{0.01}$(∞，4)= 4.40　资料来源：杨是主编《口腔预防医学》(第二版)

判断结果　近郊城市学生龋均与其他3种来源学生龋均的差异有统计学意义，即近郊城市学生的龋均分别高于近、远郊农村及城市学生的龋均。

二、计数资料的统计分析 Statistical analysis for enumeration data

1. 两个样本率差异的假设检验 u-test

检验两个样本率差异是否有统计学意义，一般用 u 检验，其步骤和方法如下：

例 6　某单位调查男、女学生各 300 人，男生患龋人数为 170，患龋率为 56.67%，女生患龋人数为 210，患龋率为 70%。男、女生患龋率差异的假设检验方法为：

检验假设　男生与女生患龋率的差异非本质差异。

计算 u 值

$$u=\frac{|p_1-p_2|}{\sqrt{(S_{P_1})^2+(S_{P_2})^2}}=\frac{|p_1-p_2|}{\sqrt{\frac{p_1q_1}{n_1}+\frac{p_2q_2}{n_2}}} \tag{9}$$

本例　$p_1=56.67\%$，$q_1=43.33\%$

$p_2=70\%$，$q_2=30\%$

$n_1=\ \ n_2=300$

$$u=\frac{|56.67-70|}{\sqrt{\frac{56.67\times 43.33}{300}+\frac{70\times 30}{300}}}=3.42$$

确定 P 值　据双侧检验，$u=1.96$，$p=0.05$；$u=2.58$，$p=0.01$

本例　$u>2.58$，故 $p<0.01$。

判断结果　本例两样本率的差别有统计学意义（$p<0.01$），可认为女生患龋率比男生高。

2. 卡方检验 Chi-square test

两个或两个以上样本率和构成比之间差别的假设检验常用卡方检验。

例 7　某医院在某市检查汉族小学生 1350 人，患龋率为 54.52%，检查相同年龄的维吾尔族小学生 600 人，患龋率为 45.33%。汉族与维吾尔族学生患龋率差别的假设检验如表 3-5：

表 3-5　汉族与维吾尔族学生患龋率比较

民族	患龋人数	未患龋人数	合计	患龋率 (%)
汉	736 (a)	614 (b)	1350 ($a+b$)	54.52
维吾尔	272 (c)	328 (d)	600 ($c+d$)	45.33
合计	1008 ($a+c$)	942 ($b+d$)	1950 (n)	51.69

资料来源：杨是主编《口腔预防医学》（第二版）

（1）检验假设　汉族与维吾尔族学生的患龋率相同，均等于两组学生合计的患龋率51.69%。

（2）计算 χ^2 值

$$\chi^2=\frac{(ad-bc)^2\times n}{(a+b)(c+d)(a+c)(b+d)} \tag{10}$$

本例

$$\chi^2=\frac{(736\times 328-614\times 272)^2\times 1950}{1350\times 600\times 1008\times 942}=14.03$$

(3) 确定 p 值：

计算自由度 (n')，n' = (行数 − 1) (列数 − 1)，

本例 $n' = (2-1)(2-1) = 1$。

查 χ^2 值表，$\chi^2_{0.01(1)} = 6.63$，本例 χ^2 值为 14.03 大于 6.63，故 $p < 0.01$。

(4) 判断结果　本例汉族与维吾尔族学生患龋率的差别有统计学意义 ($p<0.01$)。可认为汉族学生患龋率高于维吾尔族学生。

第四节　SPSS/PC 应用入门

Section 4 Access to SPSS/PC

SPSS (Statistical Package for the Social Science) 社会科学用统计软件包是世界上著名的统计分析软件之一。它和 SAS (Statistical Analysis System，统计分析系统)、BMDP (Biomedical Programs，生物医学程序) 并称为国际上最有影响的三大统计软件。

一、SPSS 的功能 Functions of SPSS

在开始 \ 程序菜单中双击"Spss for Windows"，就进入了 SPSS。SPSS 有两个窗口，一个是 SPSS 数据编辑窗口 (SPSS Data Editor)，另一个是 SPSS 输出窗口 (Output-SPSS Viewer)。

(一) SPSS 数据编辑窗口 Data edition

整个数据编辑窗口分为标题栏、菜单栏、工具栏、编辑栏、内容区和状态栏。SPSS 程序很大，命令和功能也很多，我们主要介绍菜单栏上的 10 个菜单命令。

1. File (文件) 菜单

文件菜单提供了对数据文件进行打开、保存、调用、打印、退出等16条命令。SPSS不仅能调用SPSS不同版本生成的数据文件，还能调用Excel、Lotus、Dbase、SYLK、Tab-delimited、Syntax 等生成的各类文件，也可以使用 ODBC 的文件数据源，能够调用 ABCII 的数据。当然，也可以直接在内容区中输入数据，但要注意先定义变量。

2. Edit (编辑) 菜单

编辑菜单提供了剪切、复制、粘贴、删除、查找、后悔、功能9条命令。其功能项类似于 Word 中的选项命令，可以对系统的各方面设置进行调节，如果不理解其中的一些命令，请尽量选择系统的默认值。

3. View (视图) 菜单

视图菜单提供了开关状态栏、工具栏、字体选择、内容区网格线、显示变量值标签、数据窗口与变量窗口转换等 6 条命令。

4. Data (数据) 菜单

数据菜单提供了定义变量、定义数据、模板、插入变量、插入个案、查找个案、个案排序、增加个案、增加变量等 15 条命令，其性质类似于数据库的编辑与管理。

5. Transform (转换) 菜单

转换菜单提供了计算、重新赋值、计数、随机测定、替换缺省值等 10 项实用功能。

6. Analyze (分析) 菜单

这是 SPSS 的精华，它提供了强大而完备的统计方法。

（1）Reports 报告　包括 Case Summaries 个案汇总；Report Summaries in Rows 行形式输出报告；Report Summaries in Columns 列形式输出报告。

（2）Descriptive Statistics 描述性统计分析　包括 Frequencies 频数分布表；Descriptives 描述统计量的过程；Explore 探索性分析；Crosstabs 列联表；Ratio 比率，这部分主要是对原始数据作整理和初步分析。

（3）Tables 表　包括 Custom Tables 定义表；Multiple Response Sets 多元反应项设定、Basic Tables 基本表、General Tables 总表、Multiple Response Table 多元反应项表、Tables of Frequencies 频数表。它们以表的形式将功能反映出来。

（4）Compare Means 比较均数　包括 Means 分组计算指定变量的描述统计量；One-Sample T Test 独立样本 T 检验；Independent-Samples T Test 非独立样本 T 检验；Paired-Samples T Test 配对样本 T 检验；One-Way ANOVA 单因素方差分析。这是对数据比较、求均数、标准差、做 T 检验以及单因素方差分析等。

（5）General Linear Model 一般线性模式　包括单因素、多因素、重复测量的 GLM 和 ANOVA，分类非常细，也可以作协方差分析（ANCOVA），这些统计方法是做实验经常用到的。

（6）Mixed Models 混合模型分析　包括 Linear 线性关系。

（7）Correlate 相关分析　包括 Bivariate 项计算两个变量间的相关系数并进行检验；Partial 项计算两个变量在控制了其他变量影响下的相关系数；Distance 项对变量或观测量进行相似性或不相似性测量。

（8）Regression 回归分析　包括 Lingear 线性回归、Curve Estimation 曲线回归、Binary Logistic 逻辑分析、Ordinal 序列分析、Probit 概率分析、Nonlinear 非线性回归、Weight Estimation 权重分析，Stage least Square 最小二乘法。

（9）Loglinear 逻辑线性分析　包括 General 项、Logist 项和 Model Selection 项。

（10）Clasify 聚类和判别分析　包括 Two Step Cluster 项执行两步快速聚类过程、Means Cluster 项执行快速聚类过程、Hierarchical Cluster 执行分层聚类过程、Discriminent 执行叛别分析过程。

（11）此外，统计菜单中还包括：Data Reduction -Factor 因子分析、Scale 比如、Nonparametric Test 非参数检验、Survival 生存分析、Multiple Response 多元反应项等。

7. Graphs（图形）菜单

用 SPSS 图形菜单制作图形可分为三步：建立数据文件，在数据窗口中录入数据或是从其他数据文件中调用数据；生成图形；修饰生成的图形。

Bar 选项可以生成简单条形图、分组条形图和分段条形图。

Line 选项可以生成单线图、多结图和垂线图。

Area 选项可以生成简单面积图和堆积面积图。

Pie 选项可以生成单圆图。

High-Low 选项可以生成高 - 低 - 收盘图、极差图和距限图。

Pareto 选项可以生成排列图或 Pareto 帕雷托图。

Control 选项可以生成最常见的工序控制图。

Eoxplot 选项可以生成探查数据的箱线图。

Error Bar 选项可以生成探查数据的误差条图。

Scatter 选项可以生成简单散点图、重叠散点图、矩阵散点图及三维散点图。

Histogram 选项可以生成直方图。

P-P 选项可以生成变量分布的百分位数对正态分布的百分位数的图形。

Q-Q 选项可以生成变量分布的分位数对正态分布的分位数的图形。

Sequence 选项可以生成变量分布分位数对正态分布分位数的图形。

Time Series 选项可以生成自相关图、偏相关图和互相关图。

8. Utility（实用程序）菜单

实用程序菜单提供了变量信息、文件信息、定义设置、用户设置和自动增加新个案等7个命令。

9. Windows（窗口）菜单

窗口菜单提供了 SPSS 最小化、SPSS 数据编辑窗口和 SPSS 输出窗口的切换之功能。

10. Help（帮助）菜单

帮助菜单提供了帮助主题、SPSS 教程、SPSS 语句指南、SPSS 漫游、关于 SPSS 等 8 个功能。

（二）SPSS 输出窗口 Output windows

SPSS输出窗口是用于展示SPSS的统计分析结果。其菜单命令与数据编辑窗口相似，只是减少了几个菜单项，而增加了一个INSERT菜单项，提供了插入新标题、插入新文本、插入图表、插入文本文件、插入对象等，所以需要用这些菜单命令进行调整修饰，在图形编辑窗口中，可以作图形转换，加入图形要素，展示图列和作图属性的修改（包括对图形颜色、标记符号、图线样式、标签、字体字号的选择和立方体图形旋转、分离圆图等）。

切记SPSS只是提供了强大的统计分析程序，至于选取哪种统计方法处理数据，还需要从统计学原理出发加以选择。

二、数据文件的管理 Data handling

一切统计分析都是以数据为基础的，因此统计软件的数据管理能力非常重要。SPSS 为用户提供了便捷的数据管理功能。

1. 建立与保存数据文件 Set up and save a data file

SPSS中数据文件的管理功能基本上都集中在File菜单上。SPSS 12.0有三个主要窗口界面：数据管理窗口、程序编辑窗口及结果浏览窗口，另有两个不常用的窗口：结果草稿浏览窗口和VBs脚本语言编辑窗口。他们共享许多菜单项，如File菜单就大部分相同，这里介绍的许多内容在五个窗口中都是通用的。

（1）新建数据文件

课题数据收集上来后要进行统计分析，首先要新建一个数据库，然后将所有的数据从纸上录入到计算机里。在SPSS中，新建一个数据库非常容易。当进入SPSS系统时，系统就已经生成了一个空数据文件，即打开后看到的空白的数据管理界面。只要按自己的需要定义变量，输入数据就可以了。

（2）打开其他格式的数据文件

SPSS 提供了以下几种方法来打开其他格式的数据文件。

1）直接打开　SPSS 可以直接读入许多格式的数据文件，其中就包括 Excel 各个版本的数据文件。选择菜单File==>Open==>Data或直接单击快捷工具栏上的“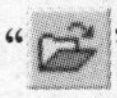”按钮，系统就会弹出 Open File 对话框，单击“文件类型”列表框，在里面能看到直接打开的数据文件格式见表 3-6。

表 3-6　SPSS 直接打开的数据文件格式

SPSS (*.sav)	SPSS 数据文件 (6.0 ~ 12.0 版)
SPSS/PC+ (*.sys)	SPSS 4.0 版数据文件
Systat (*.syd)	*.syd 格式的 Systat 数据文件
Systat (*.sys)	*.sys 格式的 Systat 数据文件
SPSS portable (*.por)	SPSS 便携格式的数据文件
EXCEL (*.xls)	EXCEL 数据文件 (从 5.0 版～ 2000 版)
Lotus (*.w*)	Lotus 数据文件
SYLK (*.slk)	SYLK 数据文件
dBase (*.dbf)	dBase系列数据文件，（从 dBase Ⅱ ~ Ⅳ）
Text (*.txt)	纯文本格式的数据文件
data (*.dat)	纯文本格式的数据文件

选择所需的文件类型，然后选中需要打开的文件，SPSS 就会按你的要求打开你要使用的数据文件，并自动转换为数据 SPSS 格式。

2）使用数据库查询打开　SPSS可以直接打开许多类型的数据文件，但并不是所有类型的数据文件都可以直接打开，比如FoxPro 3.0以上版本的*.dbf文件就不能直接打开。为此，SPSS 还提供了另一个适用范围更广、但较为专业的数据接口——数据库查询。

选择菜单File==>Open Database==>New Query，系统会弹出数据库向导的第一个窗口，其中会列出所使用的机器上已安装的所有数据库驱动程序，选中所需的数据源，然后单击下一步，向导会一步一步的提示如何做，直至将数据读入 SPSS。

3）使用文本导入向导读入文本文件　选择菜单File==>Read Text Data，系统就会弹出Open File 对话框，只是文件类型自动跳到了 Text（*.txt）。实际上，该功能在 SPSS 中已被整合到了 Open File 对话框中，之所以在菜单上保留该条目的原因是为了和 SPSS 老版本的使用上保持兼容，而且读入纯文本的情况非常普遍，放在这里更加醒目。

（3）保存数据文件

在对数据做了修改后，保存数据文件是必不可少的工作之一。选择菜单File==>Save，如果数据文件曾经存储过，则系统会自动按原文件名保存数据；否则，就会弹出和选择 Save as 菜单时相同的 Save as 对话框。里面可以保存的数据类型和可以打开的几乎一样多，选择合适的类型确定。

(4) File 菜单中的其他条目

【Display Data Information】

该菜单项用于显示数据的基本信息，选择它后会弹出类似于打开文件的一个对话框用于选择数据文件，选择好后按OK，系统就会在结果窗口中列出所选数据的基本情况，如建立时间、标签设置、记录数、变量设置等。

【Mark File Read Only】

将数据文件标记为只读文件以防无意中的数据修改。

【Cache Data】

建立数据缓冲区。以前SPSS每执行一条命令都会重新读取所需的数据，如果是从远程用SQL调用数据库，非常费时。现在使用Cache Data，可以将数据全部读入暂存盘，建立活动数据的缓冲区，加快处理速度。

【Print 和 Print Preview】

这两个菜单项用于将数据管理窗口中的数据以表格的形式打印出来，其中 Print Preview 是打印预览，不过和 SPSS 结果的打印程序一样，用 SPSS 直接打印数据非常浪费纸张。

【Stop Processor】

用于停止执行当前的 SPSS 命令。

2. 编辑数据文件 Edit a data file and data transformation

在 SPSS 中，数据文件的编辑、整理等功能被集中在 Data 和 Transform 两个菜单项中。

(1) 定义新变量

1) 直接定义新变量　大多数情况下，我们需要从头定义变量，在 SPSS 12.0 中，定义变量的操作界面只需单击左下方的 Variable View 标签就可以切换到变量定义界面开始定义新变量。

例 8　对某幼儿园小班儿童的口腔健康状况进行调查，共检查126名儿童，其中男孩68名，女孩58名。龋齿的检查标准按照WHO（1997）口腔健康调查基本方法记录每颗乳牙的牙冠龋齿状况。变量定义如下所示：

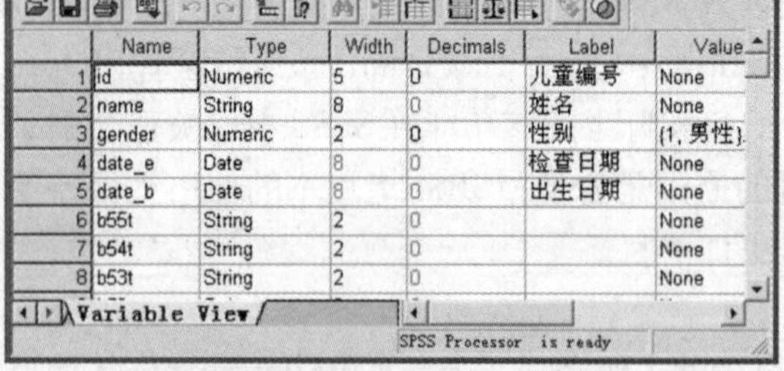

以变量“id”为例：变量名为“id”，类型为 Numeric，宽度为 5，小数位数 0 位，变量标签位为“儿童编号”。右侧在图中未能看到的依次为 Values，用于定义具体变量值的标签；Missing，用于定义变量缺失值；Colomns，定义显示列宽；Align，定义显示对齐方式；Measure，定义变量类型是连续、有序分类还是无序分类。

使用该窗口，我们可以一次定义许多新变量。

变量标签（Label）和变量值标签（Values）的定义：

变量标签和变量值标签被分开设置，变量标签就在Label框中直接输入，变量值标签则在它右侧的 Value 框定义。以性别“gender”为例，单击 Value 框右半部的省略号，会弹出变量值标签对话框如下：

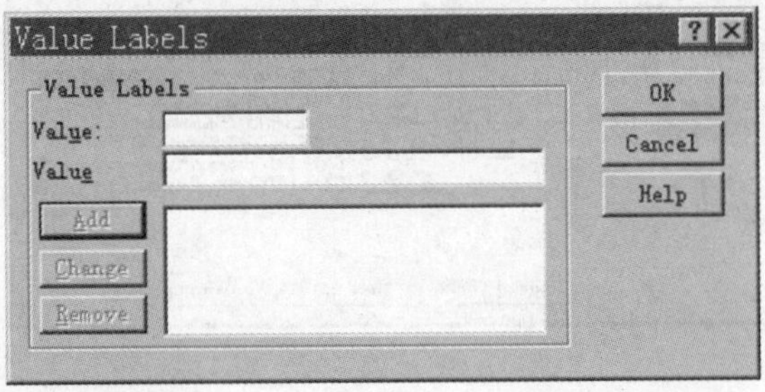

上部的两个文本框分别为变量值输入框和变量值标签输入框，分别在其中输入“1”和“男性”，此时下方的Add钮变黑，单击它，该变量值标签就会被加入下方的标签框内。与此类似定义变量值“2”和“女性”，最后按OK，变量值标签就设置完成。此时做任何分析，在结果中都有相应的标签出现。

缺失值的定义　单击 missing 框右侧的省略号，会弹出缺失值对话框如下：

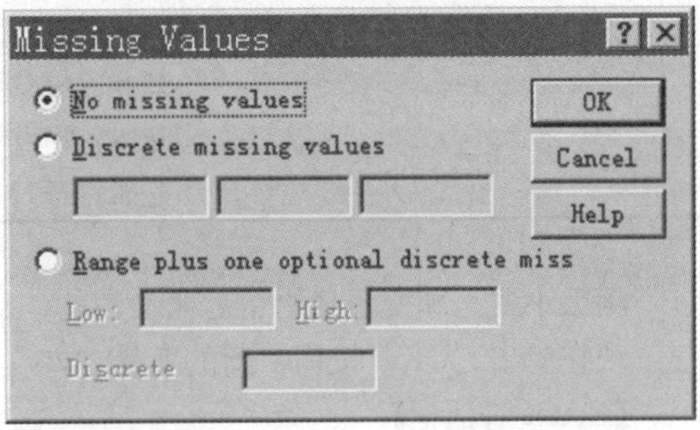

界面上有一列三个单选钮，默认值为最上方的“无缺失值”；第二项为“不连续缺失值”，最多可以定义3个值；最后一项为“缺失值范围加可选的一个缺失值”。

2）从原有变量计算新变量　从定义变量开始的情况多数在建立数据库时出现。但是，当数据库已经建立，需要整理、转换变量时，就需要根据某种条件从原有变量计算新变量。下面我们将按菜单条目的顺序依次讲解他们的功能。

【Compute 对话框】

例 9　在例 8.sav 中建立新变量 yrs，用来计算儿童的年龄，儿童年龄的计算是用检查日期（date_e）减去儿童出生日期（date_b），再除以 365 天即可。

计算公式为：yrs ＝(date_e - date_b)/365。

这里需要用到 Compute 对话框。选择菜单 Transform==>Compute，弹出 Compute Variable 对话框如下：

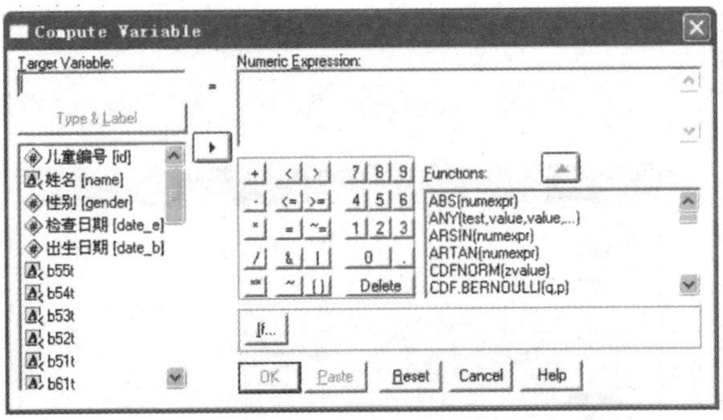

左上角为需要计算的变量名，在其中键入“yrs”，此时“Type & Lable”按钮就会变黑，用来对 yrs 进行详细的定义；软键盘右侧为函数窗口，可以在这里找到并使用所需的 SPSS 函数，计算儿童年龄需要应用函数CTIME.DAYS，选择进入右上方的数值表达式窗口；从左下方为候选变量列表中选择检查日期变量 date_e 进入 CTIME.DAYS（）中；从中部的类似计算器的软键盘，用鼠标按键输入符号减号“-”进入CTIME.DAYS（date_e -）；再从左下方候选变量列表中选择儿童出生日期变量 date_b

进入CTIME.DAYS（date_e-date_b）中；最后从中部的软键盘用鼠标按键输入“/365”，完成儿童年龄的计算公式输入，对话框如下：

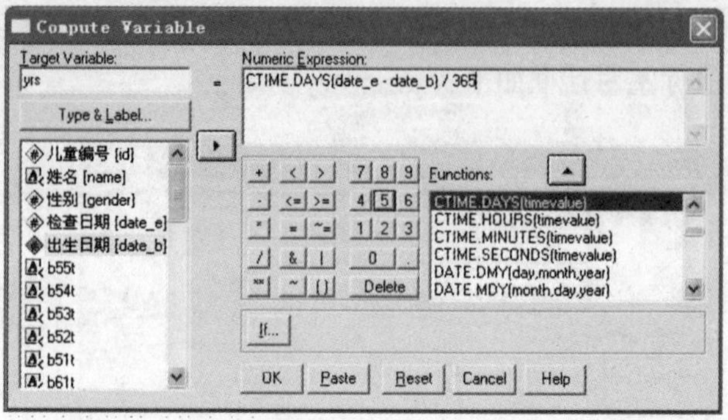

软键盘上的符号的含义如下：

~ =	不等号，等价于<>
&	逻辑符号 AND
|	逻辑符号 OR
**	乘方，相当于函数 EXP（）
~	逻辑符号 NOT

函数主要是和变量名组合起来使用的，比如说 ABS（x）就是取变量 x 的绝对值。

现在单击“OK”按钮，新的变量“yrs”就出现在数据库中。

【Count 对话框】

Count对话框用于计算某个值或某些值在某个变量的取值中是否出现，比如想看看每名儿童有几颗完好的乳牙。选择菜单 Transform==>Count，系统弹出 Count 对话框如下：

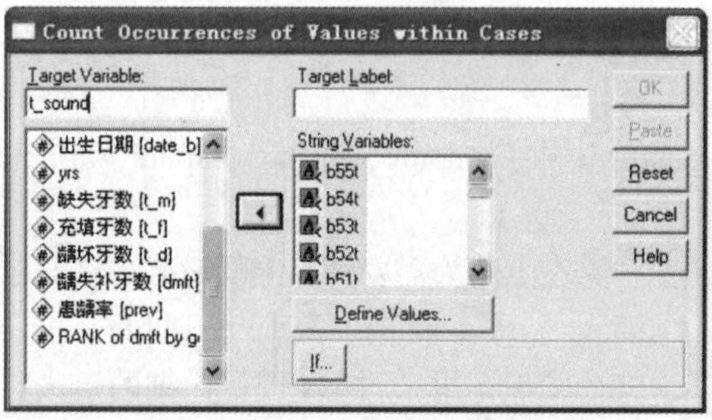

Target Variable 框中用于指定记录变量值是否出现的变量名，在这里输入t_sound；从候选变量列表中选中口内 20 颗乳牙相应的变量“b55t， b54t...b85t”，将其选入Variables窗口，此时“Define Values”按钮变黑，单击它，系统弹出变量值定义窗口如下：

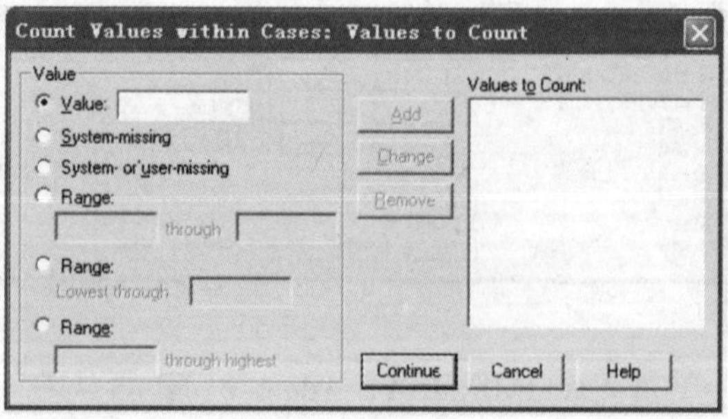

左半部为变量值定义窗口，可以定义某个值、系统缺失值、系统或用户定义缺失值、变量值范围、小于某值或大于某值。我们这里是第一种情况：选择 Value，键入 A，然后单击已变黑的“Add”按钮，“A”就会被加入“Values to Count”框内。然后单击“Continue”，再单击Count对话框的“OK”，可以看到系统自动生成变量 t_sound。

【Recode 对话框】

Recode对话框用于从原变量值按照某种一一对应的关系生成新变量值，可以将新值赋给原变量，也可以生成一个新变量。

例 10　在例 8.sav 中生成新变量——患龋情况（prev），当龋失补（dmft）等于 0 时取值为 0，大于 0 时取值为 1。

选择菜单 Transform==>Record==>Into Different Variables，Recode 对话框如下：

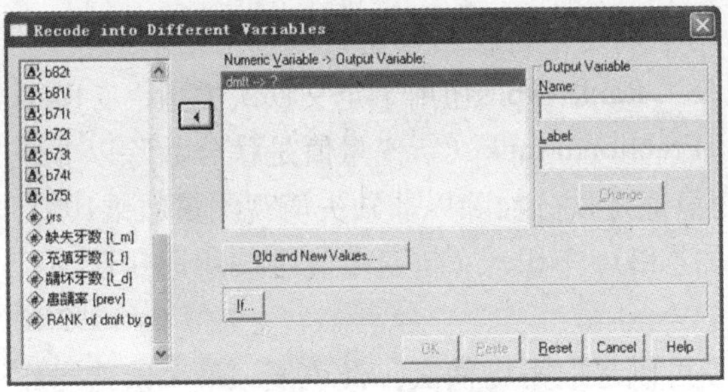

将龋失补牙数（dmft）选入 Input Variable->Output Variable 框，此时 Output Variable 框变黑，在其中键入新变量名 prev 并单击 Change，可见原来的 dmft->?变成了 dmft->prev。现在单击“Old and New Values”，系统弹出变量值定义对话框如下：

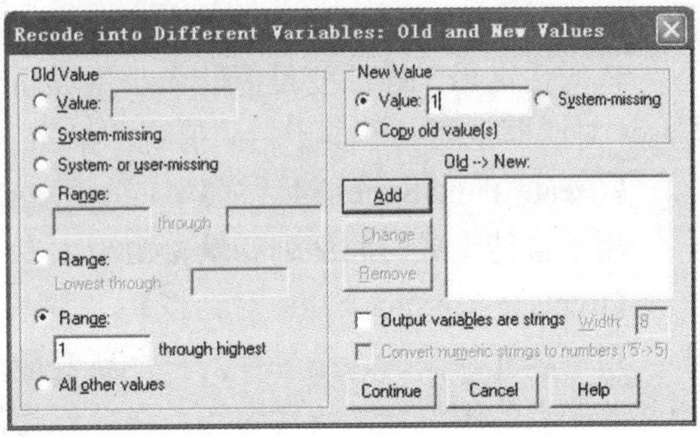

按照题目的要求，选择 Range: through highest，在左侧框中键入 1，然后在右上方的 Value右侧框中键入对应的新变量值1，此时下方 Add 键变黑，单击它，Old->New 框中就会加入1 thru Highest->1；选择Value，在右侧框中键入 0，然后在右上方的 Value 右侧框中键入对应的新变量值 0，此时下方 Add 键变黑，单击它，Old->New 框中就会加入 0->0；最终 Old->New 框中共有0->0，1 thru Highest->1 两条，现在单击 Continue，再单击 OK，系统就会按要求生成新变量 prev。

简单叙述操作步骤如下：

Input Variable->Output Variable 框中选入 dmft

Output Variable 框：选入 prev

Output Variable Name 框：键入患龋率：单击 Change 钮

选中 dmft->prev：单击 Old and New Values 钮：

Range: through highest 单选钮：键入 1：New Value Value 单选钮：键入 1：单击 Add 钮

Value 单选钮：右侧键入 0，New Value Value 单选钮：键入 0，单击 Add 钮

单击 Continue

单击 OK

【Rank Cases 对话框】

例 11　例 8.sav 中将男女分组，计算龋失补牙数（dmft）的秩和。

解：选择菜单 Transform==>Rank Cases，弹出 Rank Cases 对话框如下：

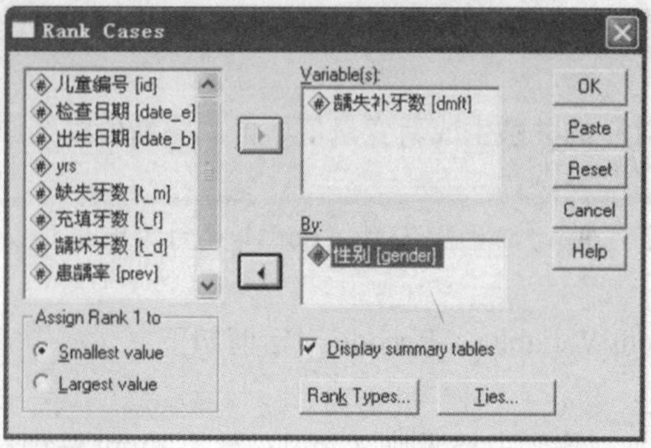

将龋失补牙数dmft选入Variable框，分组变量 gender 选入 By 框，单击 OK 即可。系统会建立一个新变量 Rdmft（即原变量名前加 R 表示 Rank 之意），其取值为 dmft 分组的秩次。

Rank Cases 对话框的其他几个选项：

左下角的 Assign Rank 1 to 框架用于选择将秩次 1 赋给最小值还是最大值；

中下部的 Display summary tables 复选框用于确定是否在结果窗口内输出结果报表；

Rank Types钮用于定义秩次类型，有Rank（秩分数）、Savage评分（新变量值按指数分布）、Fractional rank（新变量值是秩分数除以非缺失值观测量的权重之和）、Fractional rank %（新变量值是秩分数除以非缺失值观测量数乘100）、Sum of case weights（新变量值是各观测量的权重之和）、Ntiles（新变量值是按所选变量的百分位数分组的组序号），默认值为 Rank。

Ties钮用于定义对相同值观测量的处理方式，可以是取平均秩次、最小值、最大值或当作一个记录处理，默认值为取平均秩次。

【Automatic Record 对话框】

该对话框用于按原变量值的大小生成新变量，变量值就是原值的大小次序，功能和 Rank Cases 对话框重复（等价于相同值观测量当作一个记录处理的情况）。

【Create Time Series 对话框】

用于自动生成时间序列变量，由于太专业，这里不做过多解释。

【Replace Missing Value 对话框】

用于填充缺失值，结果存入一个新变量。填充方法有：序列的均数、相邻若干点的均数、相邻若干点的中位数、线性内插、线性外延，默认值为序列的均数。

（2）数据的录入

1）直接录入　直接录入就是直接将数据输入数据库中。

2）数据录入技巧　和其他常用统计软件相比，SPSS数据界面最大的优势就是支持鼠标的拖放操作，以及拷贝粘贴等命令，下面的数据录入技巧就是对这些功能的利用。

【连续多个相同值的输入】

如前面gender变量有连续多个1，如果直接输入，可以在第一格内输入1并回车，然后回到刚才的单元格并单击右键，选择copy，最后用拖放方式选中所有应输入1的单元格，单击右键并选择 paste，所有选中的单元格就会都被刚才拷贝的 1 填充。

【将 EXCEL 数据直接引入 SPSS】

Excel 已经打开原数据，并且数据量较少的时候，可以直接用拷贝粘贴的方法将数据引入SPSS：先在EXCEL中选中所有的数据（不包括变量名），然后选择拷贝命令；然后切换到SPSS，最好使行1列1单元格成为当前单元格，然后执行粘贴命令，数据就会全部转入SPSS，再定义相应的变量即可。

3. 进一步整理数据文件 Further editing a data file

在许多情况下，我们需要先对数据进行一些整理（如分组、合并、加权等）才能将其用于最终的统计分析。这些功能基本上都集中在Data菜单项中，下面我们就对这些对话框做逐一介绍。

【Sort Cases 对话框】

例 12　对数据库例 8.sav 按 id 升序，dmft 降序的次序排列。

选择菜单Data==>Sort Cases，系统弹出Sort Cases对话框，该对话框比较特殊的是下方的Sort Order 单选钮，有升序和降序两种选择。该单选钮是和上方的 Sort By 框一起使用的，具体方法如下：

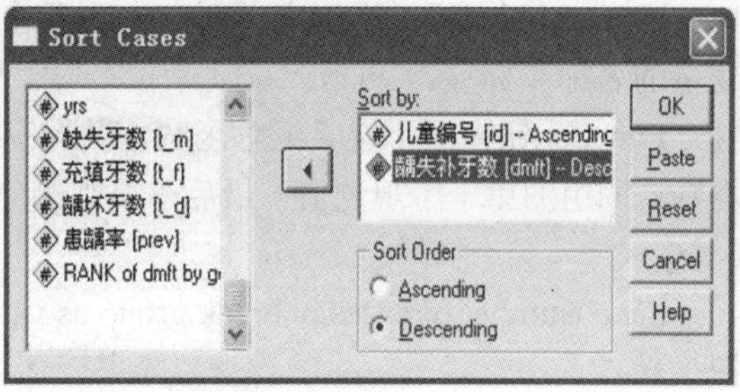

确认升序单选钮被选择，将id选入Sort By框；

选择降序单选钮，将dmft选入Sort By框。id 和 dmft 后面分别跟着 Ascending 和 Descending，表明前者是按升序、后者按降序排列；由于 id 在前，因此排序时以 id 优先。

【Transepose 对话框】

该对话框用于对数据进行行列转置，可以在原数据文件中指定一个变量记录转置后的变量名。原变量名则自动保存在系统产生的名为 case_lbl 的字符变量中。

该对话框左侧为候选变量框；右上方为Variable框，用于选入需要转置的变量，一般应选入除名称变量外的所有其他变量，如果有变量未选入，则转置时会被自动丢弃；右下方为Name Variable框，用于指定原数据文件中记录转置后变量名的字符变量，但不是必需的，此时系统会将新变量自动按 var001、var002...的顺序命名。

【Merge Files 对话框】

用于合并数据文件，实际上包括了两个对话框，分别对应了两种合并方式：

（1）从外部数据文件中增加记录到当前数据文件中，称为纵向合并，用Add Cases对话框完成，相互合并的数据文件中应该有相同的变量。选择菜单Data==>Merge Files==>Add Cases，系统首先弹出打开数据文件对话框，选中需要添加的数据文件并按OK，系统才弹出Add Cases对话框，左侧显示的是新、老数据文件中不匹配的变量名，右侧显示的是已经匹配的变量名。可以用 Rename 按钮对不匹配变量改名（先选中）或用鼠标强行匹配（即先按 Ctrl 键选中匹配的两个变量再单击 Pair 钮）。右下方的 Indicate case source as variable 复选框用于定义一个新变量以区分哪些记录是后来添加的。选择完成后单击 OK。

注意：用于合并的两个数据库文件必须事先按照匹配变量升序排列。

（2）从外部数据文件增加变量到当前数据文件，称为横向合并，用Add Variable对话框完成，相互合并的数据文件中应包含同样的记录。选择菜单Data==>Merge Files==>Add Variable对话框，系统同样先弹出打开数据文件对话框，单击OK 后弹出和前面相似的 Add Variable 对话框。按需选择即可。

【Aggregate 对话框】

用于对数据进行分类汇总，所谓分类汇总就是按指定的分类变量对观测值进行分组，对每组记录的各变量值求指定的描述统计量，结果可以存入新数据文件，也可以替换当前数据文件。

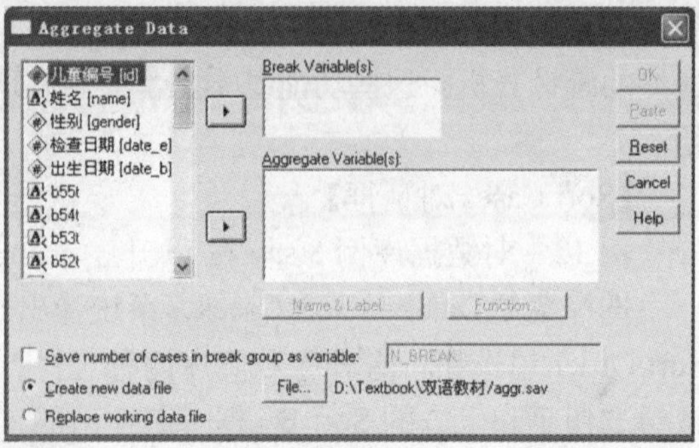

上图中各个选项的含义如下：

Break Variables 框：用于选择分组变量；

Aggregate Variables 框：用于选择被汇总的变量；

Name&Label钮：用于定义新产生的汇总变量的名称和标签；

Function钮：用于定义汇总函数，共有三组函数，以最常用的第一组为例，可选的函数有均数、同组的第一个观测值、最后一个观测值、同组记录数、标准差、最小值、和、最大值共 8 个；

Save Number of cases in break group as variable复选框：用于定义一个新变量以存储同组的记录数；

Create new data file 单选钮：定义一个新文件以存储汇总的结果，右侧的 File 钮用于具体文件名的定义，默认文件名为 aggr.sav；

Replace working data file 单选钮：用汇总的结果替换原来的数据。

例 13　计算例 8.sav 中男女儿童的龋失补牙数 dmft 的标准差。

通常用更简单的方法完成，这里只是演示一下汇总对话框的用法。

Break Variables 框：gender

Aggregate Variables 框：dmft

Function 钮：（Standard deviation 单选钮：Continue 钮）

Replace working data file 单选钮：选中

OK

【Split File 对话框】

用于将数据文件分组进行处理，各对话框选项的用途：

Analyze all cases 单选框：和下面的两个单选框为一组，选中本框不拆分文件；

Compare groups单选框：按所选变量拆分文件，各组分析结果紧挨在一起便于相互比较；

Organize output by groups 单选框：按所选变量拆分文件，各组分析结果单独放置；

Groups based on 框：用于选择拆分数据文件的变量；

Sort the file by grouping variables 单选框：将数据按所定的拆分变量排序；

File is already sorted 单选框：数据保持原状，不按所定的拆分变量排序。

【Select Cases 对话框】

很多时候不需要分析全部的数据，而是按某种要求分析其中的一部分（比如只分析男性的龋失补牙数、只对前200个数据进行分析以了解大概情况），这时使用Select Cases对话框可以简化工作。该对话框界面如下所示：

其中主要的对话框选项为：

All cases 单选钮：和下面的 4 个单选钮为一组，选中它则分析所有的记录；

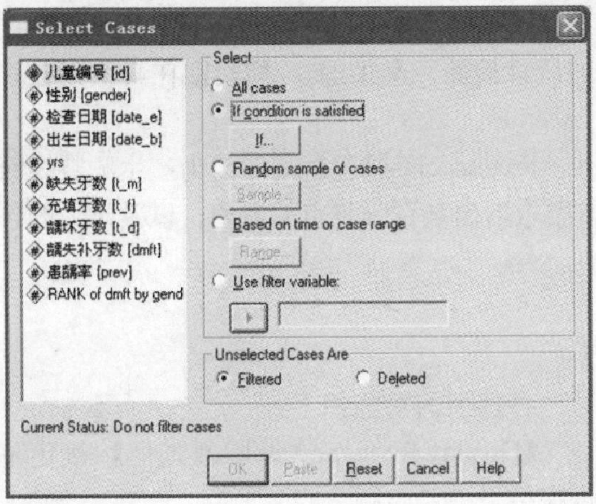

If condition is satisfied 单选钮：只分析满足条件的记录；

If按钮：和If单选钮一起使用，单击后弹出 If 对话框；

Random sample of cases 单选钮：从原数据中按某种条件抽样；

Sample 按钮：和 Random 单选钮一起使用，可以设定按百分比抽取记录，或者精确设定从前若干个记录中抽取多少个记录；

Based on time or case range 单选钮：基于记录序号来选择记录；

Range 按钮：和 Based 单选钮一起使用，用于输入记录序号范围；

Use filter variable 单选钮：使用筛选指示变量来选择记录，必须在下面选入一个筛选指示变量，该变量取值为非 0 的记录将被选中，进入以后的分析；

Filtered单选钮：和下面的Deleted单选钮为一组，表示未被选中的记录只是被隔离，这些记录的记录号会被加上斜杠以示区别；

Deleted 单选钮：未被选中的记录将被删除，一般不要使用。

当对数据库作出筛选后，所作的筛选将在以后的分析中一直有效，直到再次改变选择条件为止。同时在多数情况下，系统会自动产生一个名为filter_$的筛选指示变量，被选中的记录该变量取值为 1，反之则为 0。

【Weight Cases 对话框】

在默认情况下，每一行就是一条记录，这在多数情况下没有什么问题，但有时却非常麻烦，如果需要计算一个四格表卡方，有100例，如果每一行就是一条记录，就需要输入100条记录。如果希望在计算过程中利用不同的变量对数据进行加权处理，就需要用到Weight Cases 对话框。该对话框的界面上有两个单选钮，分别是不权重记录和用某变量权重记录，如果选择后者，则需要选中一个权重变量。

【Data 菜单中的其余对话框】

Define dates 对话框：可以自动生成时间变量。

Insert Variable 命令：在当前列插入新变量。

Insert cases 命令：在当前行插入新记录。

Goto cases对话框：到达指定记录号的记录，该命令在记录数极多时（1000条以上）非常有用。

三、描述性统计分析 Descriptive statistics

描述性统计分析是统计分析的第一步，做好这一步是下面进行正确统计推断的先决条件。SPSS的许多模块均可完成描述性分析，但专门为此设计的几个模块则集中在Descriptive Statistics 菜单中，最常用的是列在最前面的四个过程：Frequencies过程是产生频数表；Descriptives

过程则进行一般性的统计描述；Explore过程用于对数据概况不清时的探索性分析；Crosstabs过程则完成计数资料和等级资料的统计描述和一般的统计检验，常用的 χ^2 检验则在其中完成。

1. Frequencies 过程

频数分布表是描述性统计中最常用的方法之一，Frequencies过程就是专门为产生频数表而设计的。它不仅可以产生详细的频数表，还可以按要求给出某百分位点的数值，以及常用的条图，圆图等统计图。

（1）界面说明

Frequencies 对话框的界面如下所示：

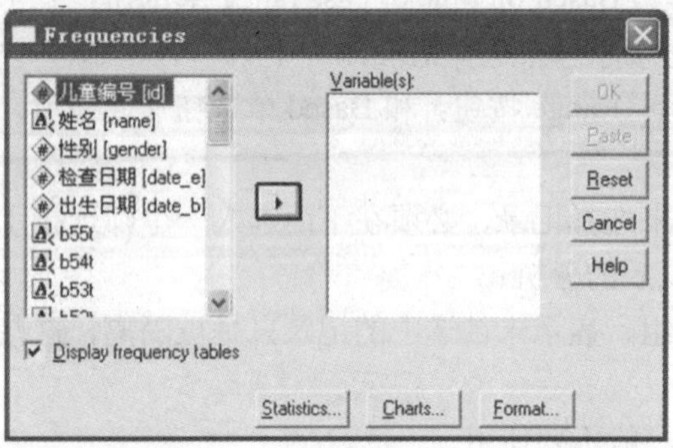

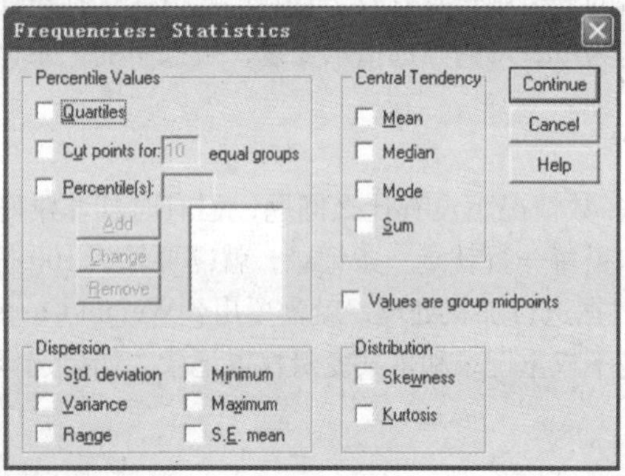

各选项的功能如下：

【Display frequency tables复选框】 确定是否在结果中输出频数表。

【Statistics钮】 单击后弹出Statistics对话框如下，用于定义需要计算的其他描述统计量。

其中：

Percentile Values 复选框组　定义需要输出的百分位数，可计算四分位数（Quartiles）、每隔指定百分位输出当前百分位数（Cut points for equal groups）、或直接指定某个百分位数（Percentiles），如直接指定输出 P2.5 和 P97.5。

Central tendency复选框组　用于定义描述集中趋势的一组指标：均数（Mean）、中位数（Median）、众数（Mode）、总和（Sum）。

Dispersion 复选框组　用于定义描述离散趋势的一组指标：标准差（Std.deviation）、方差（Variance）、全距（Range）、最小值（Minimum）、最大值（Maximum）、标准误（S.E.mean）。

Distribution 复选框组　用于定义描述分布特征的两个指标：偏度系数（Skewness）和峰度系数（Kurtosis）。

Values are group midpoints 复选框　当输出的数据是分组频数数据，并且具体数值是组中值时，选中该复选框以通知 SPSS。

【Charts 钮】

弹出 Charts 对话框，用于设定所做的统计图。

Chart type 单选钮组　定义统计图类型，有四种选择：无、条图（Bar chart）、饼图（Pie chart）、直方图（Histogram），其中直方图还可以选择是否加上正态曲线（With normal curve）。

Chart Values单选钮组　定义是按照频数（frequencie）还是按百分比（percentage）作图（即影响纵坐标刻度）。

【Format 钮】

弹出 Format 对话框，用于定义输出频数表的格式。

Order by 单选钮组　定义频数表的排列次序，有四个选项：Ascending values 为根据数值大小按升序从小到大作频数分布；Descending values为根据数值大小按降序从大到小作频数分布；Ascending counts 为根据频数多少按升序从少到多作频数分布；Descending counts 为根据频数多少按降序从多到少作频数分布。

Multiple Variables 单选钮组　如果选择了两个以上变量做频数表，则 Compare variables 可以将他们的结果在同一个频数表过程输出结果中显示，便于互相比较，Organize output by variables 则将结果在不同的频数表过程输出结果中显示。

Suppress Tables more than...复选框　当频数表的分组数大于下面设定数值时禁止它在结果中输出，这样可以避免产生巨型表格。

(2) 分析实例

例 14　例 8.sav 中将儿童的龋失补牙数 dmft 结果绘制频数表、直方图，计算均数、标准差、变异系数 CV、中位数 M、P2.5 和 P97.5。

频数表的操作步骤如下：

Analyze==>Descriptive Statistics==>Frequencies

Variables 框：选入 dmft

单击 Statistics 钮：

选中 Mean、Std.deviation、Median 复选框

单击 Percentiles：输入 2.5：单击 Add：输入 97.5：单击 Add：

单击 Continue 钮

单击 Charts 钮：

选中 Bar charts

单击 Continue 钮

单击 OK

得出结果后手工计算出 CV。

(2) 结果解释

输出结果的界面如下：

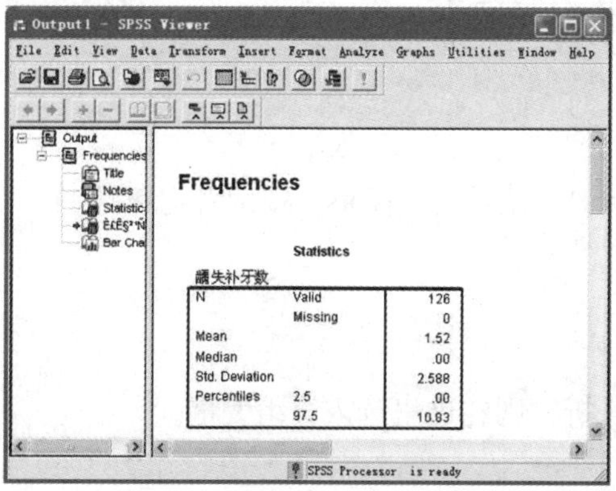

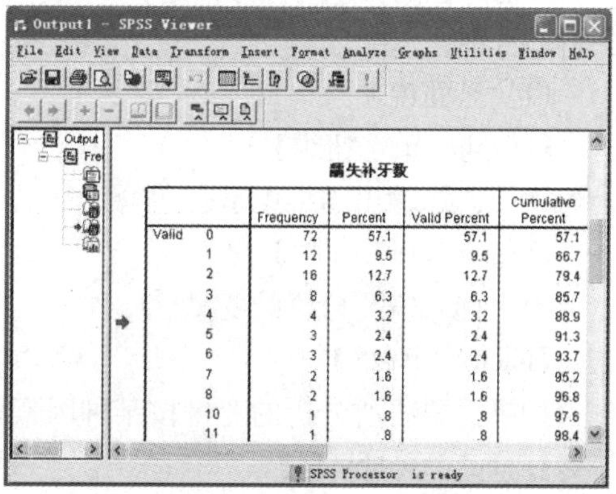

最上方为表格名称，左上方为分析变量名，可见样本量N为126例，缺失值0例，均数Mean = 1.52，中位数 Median = 0，标准差 Std. = 2.588，P2.5 = 0，P97.5 = 10.83。

系统对变量dmft作频数分布表（此处只列出了开头部分），Valid右侧为原始值，Frequency为频数，Percent 为各组频数占总例数的百分比（包括缺失记录在内），Valid percent 为各组频数占总例数的有效百分比，Cummulative Percent 为各组频数占总例数的累积百分比。

2. Descriptives 过程

Descriptives过程是连续性资料统计描述应用最多的一个过程，可对变量进行描述性统计分析，计算并列出一系列相应的统计指标。该过程的特殊功能在于可将原始数据转换成标准正态评分值并以变量的形式存入数据库供以后分析用。

（1）界面说明

【Save standardized values as variables 复选框】

确定是否将原始数据的标准正态评分存为新变量。

【Options 钮】

弹出 Options 对话框，大部分内容均在前面 Frequences 过程的 Statistics 对话框中见过，只有最下方的Display Order单选钮组是新的，可以选择为变量列表顺序、字母顺序、均数升序或均数降序。

（2）结果解释

下面是一个典型的 Descriptives 过程结果统计表表 3-7（例 1 中儿童龋失补牙数 dmft 的描述性统计结果）：

表 3-7 Descriptive Statistics

	N	Minimum	Maximum	Mean	Std. Deviation
dmft 126		0	12	1.52	2.588
Valid N (listwise)	126				

3. Explore 过程

Explore过程可对变量进行更为深入详尽的描述性统计分析，主要用于对资料的性质、分布特点等完全不清楚时，故又称之为探索性分析。它在一般描述性统计指标的基础上，增加有关数据其他特征的文字与图形描述，如枝叶图、箱图等，显得更加详细、全面，有助于制定继续分析的方案。

（1）界面说明

【Display 单选钮组】

用于选择输出结果中是否包含统计描述（statistics）、统计图（plots）或两者均包括。

【Dependent List 框】

用于选入需要分析的变量。

【Factor List 框】

如果需要将所分析的变量按某种因素取值分组分析，则在这里选入分组变量。

【Label cases by 框】

选择一个变量，他的取值将作为每条记录的标签。最典型的情况是使用记录ID号的变量。

【Statistics 钮】

弹出 Statistics 对话框，用于选择所需要的描述统计量。有如下选项：

Descriptives 复选框：输出均数、中位数、众数、5% 修正均数、标准误、方差、标准差、最小值、最大值、全距、四分位全距、峰度系数、峰度系数的标准误、偏度系数、偏度系数的标准误及指定的均数可信区间。

M-estimators 复选框：作中心趋势的粗略最大似然确定，输出四个不同权重的最大似然确定数。

Outliers 复选框：输出五个最大值与五个最小值。

Percentiles 复选框：输出第 5%、10%、25%、50%、75%、90%、95% 位数。

【Plot 钮】

弹出 Plot 对话框，用于选择所需要的统计图。选项如下：

Boxplots 单选框组：确定箱式图的绘制方式，可以是按组别分组绘制（Factor levels together），也可以不分组一起绘制（Depentends together），或者不绘制（None）。

Descriptive 复选框组：可以选择绘制茎叶图（Stem-and-leaf）和直方图（Histogram）。

Normality plots with test 复选框：绘制正态分布图并进行变量是否符合正态分布的检验。

Spread vs. Level with Levene Test单选框组：当选择了分组变量时，绘制spread-versus-level 图，设置绘图时变量的转换方式，并进行组间方差齐性检验。

【Options 钮】

用于选择对缺失值的处理方式，可以是不分析有任一缺失值的记录、不分析计算某统计量时有缺失值的记录，或报告缺失值。

（2）结果解释

例 15　一项评价口腔维护对糖尿病患者血糖控制效果的研究，83 名糖尿病患者接受口腔治疗，进入口腔维护期的基线糖化血红蛋白（HbA1c）水平和口腔维护一年后的评价糖化血红蛋白水平已经输入数据库中（变量分别为hba1c_b，hba1c_e）。请对评价时的糖化血红蛋白水平进行 Explore 描述。

数据库界面如下：

按默认方式下的选择，Explore 过程的输出界面如下：

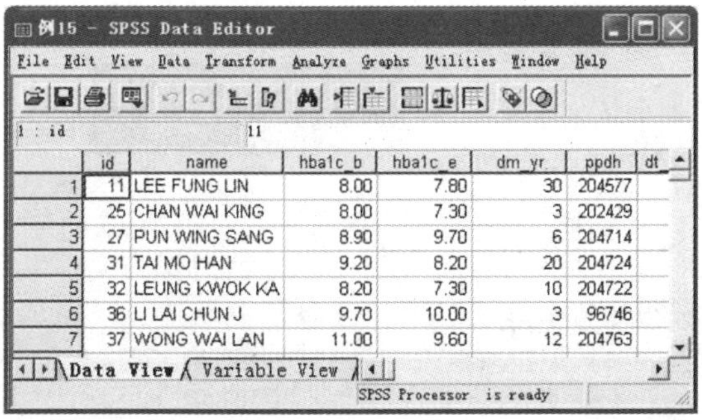

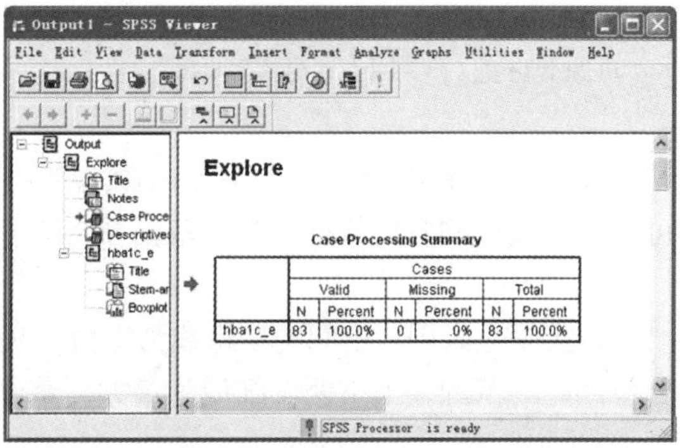

上图未显示的输出结果如下：

表 3-8 Descriptives

			Statistic	Std. Error
hba1c_e		Mean	8.0964	0.10696
	95%Confidence Interval for Mean	Lower Bound	7.8836	
		Upper Bound	8.3092	
	5% Trimmed Mean		8.0718	
	Median		7.9000	
	Variance		0.950	
	Std. Deviation		0.97448	
	Minimum		5.90	
	Maximum		10.80	
	Range		4.90	
	Interquartile Range		1.20	
	Skewness		0.575	0.264
	Kurtosis		0.184	0.523

hba1c_e

hba1c_e Stem-and-Leaf Plot

```
Frequency    Stem &  Leaf

 1.00        5 .     9
 4.00        6 .     2669
37.00        7 .     0000111233333344455555677788888889999
27.00        8 .     000000111223344555666789999
 9.00        9 .     002267799
 4.00       10 .     0022
 1.00 Extremes (>= 10.8)

Stem width:     1.00
Each leaf:      1 case (s)
```

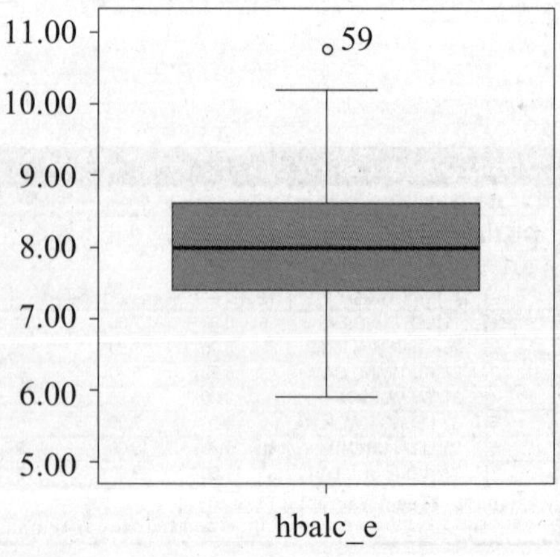

以上是茎叶图，整数位为茎，小数位为叶。这样可以非常直观的看出数据的分布范围及形态。

以上是箱式图，中间的黑粗线为均数，灰框为四分位间距的范围，上下两个细线为最大、最小值。

4. Crosstabs 过程

Crosstabs过程用于对计数资料和等级资料进行统计描述和简单的统计推断。在分析时可以产生二维至n维列联表，并计算相应的百分数指标。统计推断则包括了常用的χ^2检验、Kappa值，分层χ^2（$\chi^2_{M\text{-}H}$）。如果安装了相应模块，还可计算χn维列联表的确切概率（Fisher's Exact Test）值。

（1）界面说明

【Rows 框】

用于选择行 * 列表中的行变量。

【Columns 框】

用于选择行 * 列表中的列变量。

【Layer 框】

Layer 指的是层，对话框中的许多设置都可以分层设定，在同一层中的变量使用相同的设置，而不同层中的变量分别使用各自层的设置。如果要让不同的变量做不同的分析，则将其选入 Layer 框，并用 Previous 和 Next 钮设为不同层。Layer 在这里用的比较少，在多元回归中应用较多。

【Display clustered bar charts 复选框】

显示重叠条图。

【Suppress table 复选框】

禁止在结果中输出行 * 列表。

【Exact 钮】

如果你在安装 SPSS 时没有安装 EXACT 模块，则此处对话框中不会出现 Exact 钮。针对2*2以上的行*列表设定计算确切概率的方法，可以是不计算（Asymptotic only)、蒙特卡罗模拟（Monte Carlo）或确切计算（Exact)。蒙特卡罗模拟默认进行10000次模拟，给出99%可信区间；确切计算默认计算时间限制在 5 分钟内。这些默认值均可更改。

【Statistics 钮】

弹出 Statistics 对话框，用于定义所需计算的统计量。

Chi-square 复选框：计算χ^2值。

Correlations 复选框：计算行、列两变量的 Pearson 相关系数和 Spearman 等级相关系数。

Norminal 复选框组：选择是否输出反映分类资料相关性的指标。

Contingency coefficient 复选框：即列联系数，其值界于 0 ~ 1 之间。

Phi and Cramer's V 复选框：这两者也是基于χ^2值的，Phi 在四格表χ^2检验中界于 −1 ~ 1 之间，在 R*C 表χ^2检验中界于 0 ~ 1 之间；Cramer's V 则界于 0 ~ 1 之间。

Lambda 复选框：在自变量预测中用于反映比例缩减误差，其值为 1 时表明自变量预测应变量好，为 0 时表明自变量预测应变量差。

Uncertainty coefficient复选框：不确定系数，以熵为标准的比例缩减误差，其值接近1时表明后一变量的信息很大程度来自前一变量，其值接近0时表明后一变量的信息与前一变量无关。

Ordinal 复选框组：选择是否输出反映有序分类资料相关性的指标。

Gamma 复选框：界于 0 ~ 1 之间，所有观察实际数集中于左上角和右下角时，其值为 1。

Somers'd 复选框：为独立变量上不存在同分的偶对中，同序对子数超过异序对子数的比例。

Kendall's tau-b 复选框：界于 −1 ~ 1 之间。

Kendall's tau-c 复选框：界于 −1 ~ 1 之间。

Eta 复选框：计算 Eta 值，其平方值可认为是应变量受不同因素影响所致方差的比例。

Kappa 复选框：计算 Kappa 值，即内部一致性系数。

Risk 复选框：计算比数比 OR 值。

McNemar 复选框：进行 McNemar 检验（一种非参检验）。

Cochran's and Mantel-Haenszel statistics复选框：计算$\chi^2_{M\text{-}H}$统计量（分层χ^2，也有写为χ^2_{CMH}的），可在下方输出 H_0 假设的 OR 值，默认为 1。

【Cells 钮】

弹出 Cells 对话框，用于定义列联表单元格中需要计算的指标：

Counts 复选框组：是否输出实际观察数（Observed）和理论数（Expected）；

Percentages复选框组：是否输出行百分数（Row）、列百分数（Column）以及合计百分数（Total）；

Residuals 复选框组：选择残差的显示方式，可以是实际数与理论数的差值（Unstandardized）、标化后的差值（Standardized，实际数与理论数的差值除理论数），或者由标准误确立的单元格残差（Adj. Standardized）；

【Format 钮】

用于选择行变量是升序还是降序排列。

（2）分析实例

例 16　在例 8.sav 中，比较男女儿童龋病的患病率是否有差别。

如果 126 名儿童按照性别列出患龋状况的频数表如下：

	无龋	有龋	合计
男性	40	28	68
女性	32	26	58
合 计	72	54	126

在建立数据库时可以直接输入三个变量——行变量、列变量以及指示每个格子中频数的变量，然后用 Weight Cases 对话框指定频数变量，最后调用 Crosstabs 过程进行 χ^2 检验。假设三个变量分别名为 R、C 和 W，则数据集结构和命令如下：

R	C	W
1.00	1.00	40
1.00	2.00	28
2.00	1.00	32
2.00	2.00	26

Data==>Weight Cases
Weight Cases by 单选框：选中
Freqency Variable：选入 W
单击 OK 钮
Analyze==>Descriptive Statistics==>Crosstabs
Rows 框：选入 R
Columns 框：C
Statistics 钮：Chi-square 复选框：选中：单击 Continue 钮
单击 OK 钮
（3）结果解释
上例的结果如下：
Crosstabs

表 3-9　Case processing summary

	Cases					
	Valid		Missing		Total	
	N	Percent	N	Percent	N	Percent
R * C	126	100.0%	0	0.0%	126	100.0%

首先是处理记录缺失值情况报告，可见 126 例均为有效值。
R * C Crosstabulation

表 3-10　Count

		C		Total
		1.00	2.00	
R	1.00	40	28	68
	2.00	32	26	58
	Total	72	54	126

上面为列出的四格表，实际使用时可以在其中加入变量值标签，使看起来更清楚。

表 3-11　Chi-Square tests

	Value	df	Asymp. Sig. (2-sided)	Exact Sig. (2-sided)	Exact Sig. (1-sided)
Pearson Chi-Square	0.170 (b)	1	0.680		
Continuity Correction (a)	0.054	1	0.816		
Likelihood Ratio	0.170	1	0.680		
Fisher's Exact Test				0.720	0.408
Linear-by-Linear Association	0.169	1	0.681		
N of Valid Cases	126				

a. Computed only for a 2 × 2 table
b. 0 cells (.0%) have expected count less than 5. The minimum expected count is 24.86

上表给出了一堆检验结果，从左到右为：检验统计量值（Value）、自由度（df）、双侧近似概率（Asymp.Sig.2-sided）、双侧精确概率（Exact Sig.2-sided）、单侧精确概率（Exact Sig.1-sided）；从上到下为：Pearson 卡方（Pearson Chi-Square 即常用的卡方检验）、连续性校正的卡方值（Continuity Correction）、对数似然比方法计算的卡方（Likelihood Ratio）、Fisher's 确切概率法（Fisher's Exact Test）、线性相关的卡方值（Linear by Linear Association）、有效记录数（N of Valid Cases）。另外，Continuity Correction 和 Pearson 卡方值处分别标注有 a 和 b，表格下方为相应的注解：a.只为 2 × 2 表计算。b.0% 个格子的期望频数小于 5，最小的期望频数为 24.86。因此，这里无须校正，直接采用第一行的检验结果，即 $\chi^2 = 0.170$，$p = 0.680 > 0.05$。拒绝 H_0，接受 H_1，不能认为男女儿童龋病的患病率有显著性差异。

四、均数间的比较 Compare means

该菜单集中了几个用于计量资料均数间比较的过程。具体有：

Means 过程对准备比较的各组计算描述指标进行预分析，也可直接比较。

One-Samples T Test 过程进行样本均数与已知总体均数的比较。

Independent-Samples T Test 过程进行两样本均数差别的比较，即通常所说的两组资料的 *t* 检验。

Paired-Samples T Test 过程进行配对资料的显著性检验，即配对 *t* 检验。

One-Way ANOVA过程进行两组及多组样本均数的比较，即成组设计的方差分析，还可进行随后的两两比较。

1. Means 过程

Means过程的优势在于各组的描述指标被放在一起便于相互比较，并且如果需要，可以直接输出比较结果，无须再次调用其他过程。

（1）界面说明

【Dependent List 框】用于选入需要分析的变量。

【Independent List 框】用于选入分组变量。

【Options 钮】弹出 Options 对话框，选择需要计算的描述统计量和统计分析：

【Statistics 框】可选的描述统计量。它们是：

sum，number of cases 总和，记录数

mean，geometric mean，harmonic mean 均数，几何均数，修正均数

standard deviation，variance，standard error of the mean 标准差，均数的标准误，方差

median，grouped median 中位数，频数表资料中位数（比如 30 岁组有 5 人，40 岁组有 6 人，则在计算 grouped median 时均按组中值 35 和 45 进行计算）

minimum，maximum，range 最小值，最大值，全距

kurtosis，standard error of kurtosis 峰度系数，峰度系数的标准误

skewness，standard error of skewness 偏度系数，偏度系数的标准误

percentage of total sum，percentage of total N 总和的百分比，样本例数的百分比

【Cell Statistics 框】选入的描述统计量

Statistics for First layer 复选框组

Anova table and eta 对分组变量进行单因素方差分析，并计算用于度量变量相关程度的eta值。

Test for linearity 检验线性相关性，实际上就是上面的单因素方差分析

（2）结果解释

例 17　以例 8 的数据为例，计算男女儿童平均龋失补牙数（dmft），输出如下：

Means

表 3-12　Case processing summary

	Cases					
	Included		Excluded		Total	
	N	Percent	N	Percent	N	Percent
dmft * gender	126	100.0%	0	0.0%	126	100.0%

上表是缺失值报告。

Report

表 3-13　dmft

性别	Mean	N	Std. Deviation
男性	1.40	68	2.462
女性	1.67	58	2.743
Total	1.52	126	2.588

常用统计描述量报表。这里按默认情况输出均数，样本量和标准差。由于选择了分组变量，因此三项指标均给出分组及合计值，可见以这种方式列出统计量可以非常直观的进行各组间的比较。

表 3-14　ANOVA table

		Sum of Squares	df	Mean Square	F	Sig.
dmft * 性别	Between Groups (Combined)	2.373	1	2.373	0.352	0.554
	Within Groups	835.055	124	6.734		
	Total	837.429	125			

上表为单因素方差分析表。在选择了 Anova table and eta 或 Test for linearity 复选框时出现。实际上就是在检验各组间均数有无差异。上面各项的具体含义将在单因素方差分析一节中解释。

表 3-15　Measures of association

	Eta	Eta Squared
dmft * 性别	0.053	0.003

相关性度量指标，给出 Eta 值以及 Eta 值的平方根。

2. One-Samples T Test 过程

One-Samples T Test 过程用于进行样本所在总体均数与已知总体均数的比较，可以自行定义已知总体均数为任意值，该对话框的界面非常简单。

（1）界面说明

【Test Variables 框】用于选入需要分析的变量

【Test Value 框】在此处输入已知的总体均数，默认值为 0

【Options 钮】弹出 Options 对话框，用于定义相关的选项，有：

Confidence Interval 框　输入需要计算的均数差值可信区间范围，默认为 95%。如果是和总体均数为 0 相比，则此处计算的就是样本所在总体均数的可信区间。

Missing Values 单选框组　定义分析中对缺失值的处理方法，可以是具体分析用到的变量有缺失值才去除该记录（Excludes cases analysis by analysis），或只要相关变量有缺失值，则在所有分析中均将该记录去除（Excludes cases listwise）。默认为前者，以充分利用数据。

（2）结果解释

One-Samples T Test 过程的输出也是比较简单的，由描述统计表和 *t* 检验表组成。

例 18　检验数据例 8.sav 中 dmft 的总体均数是否等于 3，结果输出如下：

T-Test

表 3-16　One-sample statistics

	N	Mean	Std. Deviation	Std. Error Mean
dmft	126	1.52	2.588	0.231

所分析变量的基本情况描述，有样本量、均数、标准差和标准误。

表 3-17　One-sample test

	Test Value = 3					
	t	df	Sig.(2-tailed)	Mean Difference	95% Confidence Interval of the Difference	
					Lower	Upper
dmft	-6.402	125	0.000	-1.476	-1.93	-1.02

上表为单样本 *t* 检验表，第一行注明了用于比较的已知总体均数为 3，下面从左到右依次为*t*值（*t*）、自由度（*df*）、*P*值（Sig.2-tailed）、两均数的差值（Mean Difference）、差值的95%可信区间。由上表可知：$t = -6.402$，$P < 0.001$。因此可以认为 dmft 的总体均数不等于 3。

3. Independent-Samples T Test 过程

Independent-Samples T Test 过程用于进行两样本均数的比较，即常用的两样本 *t* 检验。该对话框的界面和上面的 One-Samples T Test 对话框非常相似。

（1）界面说明

【Test Variables 框】用于选入需要分析的变量

【Grouping Variable 框】用于选入分组变量。注意选入变量后还要定义需比较的组别

【Define Groups 框】用于定义需要相互比较的两组的分组变量值

【Options 钮】和 One-Samples T Test 对话框的 Options 钮完全相同

(2) 结果解释

例 19　检验数据例 8.sav 中男性与女性的 dmft 是否相同，用 Independent-Samples T Test 过程的结果输出如下：

T-Test

表 3-18　Group statistics

	性别	N	Mean	Std. Deviation	Std. Error Mean
dmft	男性	68	1.40	2.462	0.299
	女性	58	1.67	2.743	0.360

两组需检验变量的基本情况描述。

表 3-19　Independent samples test

		Levene's Test for Equality of Variances		*t*-test for Equality of Means						
		F	Sig	*t*	*df*	Sig.(2-tailed)	Mean Difference	Std. Error Difference	95% Confidence Interval of the Difference	
									Lower	Upper
dmft	Equal variances assumed	0.700	0.404	-.594	124	0.554	-.275	0.464	-1.193	0.643
	Equal variances not assumed			-.589	115.768	0.557	-.275	0.468	-1.202	0.651

可见该结果分为两大部分：第一部分为Levene's方差齐性检验，用于判断两总体方差是否齐，这里的检验结果为 $F = 0.700$，$p = 0.404 > 0.05$，可见在本例中方差是齐的；第二部分则分别给出两组所在总体方差齐和方差不齐时的 t 检验结果，由于前面的方差齐性检验结果为方差齐，第二部分就应选用方差齐时的 t 检验结果，即上面一行列出的 $t = 0.594$，$df = 124$，$p = 0.554 > 0.05$。从而最终的统计结论为按 $\alpha = 0.05$ 水准，拒绝 H_0，接受 H_1，不能认为男性和女性儿童龋病的患病状况有显著性差异。最后面还附有一些其他指标，如两组均数的可信区间等，以对差异情况有更直观的了解。

4. Paired-Samples T Test 过程

该过程用于进行配对设计的差值均数与总体均数0比较的*t*检验，此功能实际上是和One-Samples T Test 过程相重复的（等价于已知总体均数为0的情况），但Paired-Samples T Test 过程使用的数据输入格式和前者不同，即统计表格格式，因此仍然有存在的价值。

（1）界面说明

Paired Variable 框用于选入需要进行比较的一对或几对变量——注意这里的量词是对而不是个。选入变量需要成对成对的选入，即按住Ctrl键，选中两个成对变量，再单击 ▸ 将其选入。如果只选中一个变量，则 ▸ 按钮为灰色，不可用。

（2）分析实例

例20　以例15的数据为例，问接受口腔治疗后，糖尿病患者的血糖水平与基线比较有无差别?

Analyze==>Compare Means==>Paired Samples T test

同时选中 hba1c_b、hba1c_e：选入 Paired Variables 框

单击 OK 钮

（3）结果解释

上述输出结果如下：

T-Test

表 3-20　Paired samples statistics

		Mean	N	Std. Deviation	Std. Error Mean
Pair 1	hba1c_b	8.9554	83	0.93967	0.10314
	hba1c_e	8.0964	83	0.97448	0.10696

配对变量各自的统计描述，此处只有1对，故只有 Pair 1。

表 3-21　Paired samples correlations

		N	Correlation	Sig.
Pair 1	hba1c_b & hba1c_e	83	0.284	0.009

此处进行配对变量间的相关性分析。等价于 Analyze==>Correlate==>Bivariate。

Paired Samples Test

		Paired differences					*t*	*df*	Sig. (2-tailed)
		Mean	Std. Deviation	Std. Error Mean	95% confidence interval of the difference				
					Lower	Upper			
Pair 1	hba1c_b-hba1c_e	.85904	1.14551	0.12574	0.60891	1.10917	6.832	82	.000

配对t检验表，给出最终的检验结果，可见$p < 0.001$，故可认为接受口腔维护后糖尿病患者血糖水平与基线比较有差异，即口腔维护对糖尿病患者血糖的控制有显著影响，口腔维护有利于糖尿病患者的血糖控制。

5. One-Way ANOVA 过程

One-Way ANOVA过程用于进行两组及多组样本均数的比较，即成组设计的方差分析，如果做了相应选择，还可进行随后的两两比较，甚至于在各组间精确设定哪几组和哪几组进行比较。

（1）界面说明

【Dependent List 框】选入需要分析的变量，可选入多个结果变量（应变量）

【Factor 框】选入需要比较的分组因素，只能选入一个

【Contrast钮】弹出Contrast对话框，用于对精细趋势检验和精确两两比较的选项进行定义

Polynomial 复选框　定义是否在方差分析中进行趋势检验

Degree下拉列表和Polynomial复选框配合使用，可选择从线性趋势一直到最高五次方曲线来进行检验

Coefficients框　定义精确两两比较的选项。这里按照分组变量升序给每组一个系数值，注意最终所有系数值相加应为 0。如果不为 0 仍可检验，只不过结果是错的。

【Post Hoc 钮】弹出 Post Hoc Multiple Comparisons 对话框，用于选择进行各组间两两比较的方法，有：

Equal Variances Assumed 复选框组　一组当各组方差齐时可用的两两比较方法，共有 14 中种，最常用的为 Bonferroni 和 S-N-K 法。

Equal Variances Not Assumed 复选框组　一组当各组方差不齐时可用的两两比较方法，共有 4 种，其中以 Dunnetts's C 法较常用。

Significance Level 框　定义两两比较时的显著性水平，默认为 0.05。

【Options 钮】弹出 Options 对话框，用于定义相关的选项，有：

Statistics 复选框组　选择一些附加的统计分析项目，有统计描述（Descriptive）和方差齐性检验（Homogeneity-of-variance）

Means plot 复选框　用各组均数作图，以直观的了解它们的差异。

Missing Values 单选框组　定义分析中对缺失值的处理方法，可以是具体分析用到的变量有缺失值才去除该记录（Excludes cases analysis by analysis），或只要相关变量有缺失值，则在所有分析中均将该记录去除（Excludes cases listwise）。默认为前者，以充分利用数据。

（2）分析实例

例 21　某幼儿园对 3、4、5 岁的儿童进行了口腔健康状况检查，计算乳牙龋失补牙数（dmft）。问三个年龄组儿童龋病的患病状况有无差别?

假设数据已经输好，数据库界面如下：

分组变量为 age，取值分别为 3、4、5，龋失补牙数变量为 dmft。此处先进行单因素方差分析，然后进行两两比较，这里选择 Bonferroni 法进行两两比较。操作如下：

Dependent List 框：选入 dmft

Factor 框：选入 age

Post Hoc 钮：选中 Bonferroni 复选框：单击 Continue 钮

单击 OK 钮

（3）结果解释

上题的输出结果如下：

Oneway ANOVA

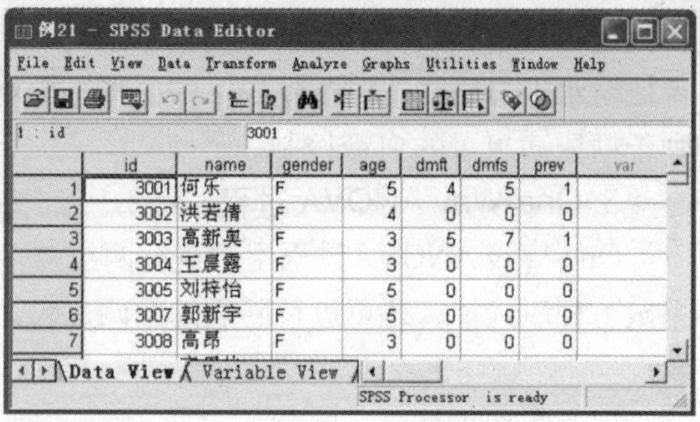

表 3-22 dmft

	Sum of Squares	*df*	Mean Square	F	Sig.
Between Groups	80.010	2	40.005	4.374	0.014
Within Groups	2003.107	219	9.147		
Total	2083.117	221			

上面实际上是一个典型的方差分析表。给出了单因素方差分析的结果，可见 $F = 4.374$，$P = 0.014 < 0.05$。因此可认为三个年龄组儿童乳牙龋病的患病程度不同。

Post Hoc Tests

Multiple Comparisons

表 3-23 Dependent variable: dmft

	(I) age	(J) age	Mean Difference (I-J)	Std. Error	Sig.	95% Confidence Interval Lower Bound	95% Confidence Interval Upper Bound
Bonferroni	3	4	-.458	0.509	1.000	-1.69	0.77
		5	-1.404 (*)	0.484	0.012	-2.57	-.24
	4	3	0.458	0.509	1.000	-.77	1.69
		5	-.946	0.503	0.184	-2.16	0.27
	5	3	1.404 (*)	0.484	0.012	0.24	2.57
		4	0.946	0.503	0.184	-.27	2.16

* The mean difference is significant at the. 05 level.

上表是用 Bonferroni 法进行两两比较的结果，3 岁儿童和 5 岁儿童龋病的患病程度在统计学上有显著性差异（$p = 0.12 < 0.05$）；而 3 岁儿童和 4 岁儿童或 4 岁儿童和 5 岁儿童龋病的患病程度间在统计学上没有显著性差异。

表 3-24 Student-Newman-Keuls

age	N	Subset for alpha = .05	
		1	2
3	76	1.42	
4	66	1.88	1.88
5	80		2.83
Sig.		0.360	0.059

Means for groups in homogeneous subsets are displayed

a Uses Harmonic Mean Sample Size = 73.512

b The group sizes are unequal. The harmonic mean of the group sizes is used. Type I error levels are not guaranteed

上表进一步说明组间两两比较的结果，在表格的纵向上各组均数按大小排序，然后在表格的横向上被分成了两个亚组，两个亚组间的p值小于0.05，而同一亚组内的各组均数比较的p值则大于0.05。从上表可见，3岁儿童和4岁儿童分在一个亚组中，而4岁儿童和5岁儿童又分在一个亚组中，说明只有3岁儿童和5岁儿童龋病的患病程度间有显著性差异。最下方是组内两两比较p值均分别为0.360和0.059，都大于0.05。

思考题 Review questions

1. 掌握算术均数、标准差、标准误的计算方法。
2. 掌握计量资料和计数资料的描述性统计分析方法。

参考文献 References

1. Richard F. Morton J. Richard Hebel, Robert J. McCarter ed, A study guide to epidemiology and biostatistics. 4th ed, Gaithersburg, MD. Aspen Publishers, 1996
2. Aviva Petrie, Caroline Sabin. Medical statistics at a glance. Oxford ; Malden, MA: Blackwell Science, 2000
3. 杨是, 石四箴主编. 口腔预防医学及儿童口腔医学. 第二版, 人民卫生出版社, 1995

（王伟健　荣文笙）

第四章　龋病预防与控制

Chapter Ⅳ Prevention and Control of Dental Caries

概述 Overview

本章叙述龋病的主要内容，包括：1. 龋病病因及其致病因素；2. 龋病危险因素及其预测方法；3. 龋病预防的科学基础与主要策略；4. 窝沟封闭与预防性修复；5. 非创伤修复治疗（ART）

This chapter describes major contents of Dental Caries. Including:

- *Aetiology of dental caries and its cariogenic factors.*
- *Caries risk factors and its predicting methods.*
- *The scientific basis and main strategies for caries prevention.*
- *The pit and fissure sealants and preventive restoration.*
- *Atraumatic restorative treatment (ART) .*

要点 Key points

- 致龋因素 cariogenic factors
- 细菌病因学说 etiological theory of bacteria
- 抗酸作用 anti-acid effect
- 脱矿化与再矿化 demineralization and remineralization
- 龋危险因素 caries risk factors
- 菌斑控制 plaque control
- 糖替代品 sugar substitutes
- 窝沟封闭 pit and fissure sealants
- 预防性树脂充填 preventive resin restoration
- 非创伤性修复治疗 atraumatic restorative treatment, ART

第一节　龋病病因及其致病因素

Section 1 Etiology of Dental Caries and its Cariogenic Factors

在人类发展的历史中，龋病的最早发现是440～150万年前的非洲南部“南方古猿”磨牙龋的化石。在我国旧石器时代，距今10万年，发现了广西“智人”化石的龋病痕迹。5000～6000年前，新石器时期，从中国北方大量出土的人体骨骸中证实了龋发病情况与现代人相近。公元前1300年殷商时代就已有甲骨文对龋的记载。公元前180年到汉代淳于意提出“食而不漱”的朴实主张。确切的病因学探讨是从19世纪初开始，如Parmly（1918）、Roberson（1835）、

Regnart（1938）的化学学说（The chemical theory）及Erall（1843）的细菌学说（The bacterial theory）。有影响的研究是 W.D.Miller（1890）的化学细菌学说（The chemoparasitic theory），此后又出现了 Cottlieb（1944）蛋白溶解学说（The proteolytic theory），Schalation（1945）蛋白溶解螯合学说（The Proteolysis-chelation theory）。20世纪中Oraland（1955）和Keys（1960）提出：细菌、食物、宿主相互作用的龋病三因素理论（The theory of three factors），在此基础上Newhrum（1978）增加了“时间因素”，形成了四因素理论（The theory of four factors）（Table4-1）。这个理论至今仍被多数人接受，并列入教学课程中。近年来 Philip Marsha（1999）等人，将微生态学观点融入到龋病理论中，提出：关键的口腔微生物、敏感的宿主、环境的刺激之间的复杂作用及这些因素对微生态的影响，这种提法已被越来越多的关注。随着近代科学的发展，对龋病发病机理研究，结合了分子生物学、分子遗传学内容及社会经济及文明发展的相关性探讨，从而加深了认识，促使多种综合防治龋病措施的产生，使一些国家的龋发病率明显下降。近些年来由于我们国家的重视，及防治工作的开展，则在龋病防治上看到了明显的成效。

表 4-1 Historical progress of caries research in the modern time

Time	Scholar	Theory	Content
1918~1867	Parunly	The chemical theory	Food stagnated on the surfaces of enamel, The lesion was involved by a chemical agent
1843	Erdl	The bacterial theory	The bacterial destruction of teeth
1890	Miller	The chemoparasitic theory	Dental decay have two stages-dissolution of the tissues and dissolution of the softened residue The process of destruction could be mediated by any microorganism capable of acid production and protein digestion
1944	Gottlieh	The proteolytic theory	The proteolytic enzymes of bacteria first attack organic components , Acid dissolution of the mineral phase was a secondary phenomenon
1945	Schalation	The proteolysis chelation Theory	The proteolytic enzymes initially breakdown organic components of enamel, then organic phase have chelating, that lead to dissolution of enamel minerals
1955~1960	Oraland, Keys	The theory of three factors	Caries result from a complex interaction of microbial, diet, and host factors, three factors must exist simultaneously
1978	Newbrum	The theory of four factors	The dental lesion was involved by microbial, diet ,host and time factors

一、龋病病因学 Etiology of dental caries

龋病是慢性细菌感染性疾病，是以细菌、宿主、食物及时间多因素引起的牙硬组织慢性腐蚀性疾病。

（一）细菌因素 Bacterial factor

1. 细菌病因学说 Etiological theory of bacteria

龋病病原学说有三种主张

特异性菌斑学说（The specific plaque hypothesis）：认为龋病是菌斑内个别菌的活性作用。

非特异性菌斑学说（The non-specific plaque hypothesis）：龋病是菌斑内微生物的共同作用所致。

菌斑生态学说（The ecological plaque hypothesis）：认为龋病发生是菌斑内常在菌（Residents）所生存环境的改变使平衡失调而致（Table 4-2）。

2. 病原菌确定（Pathogenic determination）

经多年龋病致病菌的探讨，公认确定致病菌应有如下条件：

局部的细菌与龋病的发生呈正相关。

相关的细菌应在龋病初期病变有足够数量。

在患龋者体内有相应高水平的特异性抗体。

能产生相关的毒性作用。

排除有关菌而使龋病减少。

相关菌能在动物口腔内造成龋病模型

The follows is recognized requirement of cariogenic bacteria：

Local bacteria is positive correlation with caries lesions.

A microbe should be present in sufficient numbers to initiate disease.

The microbe should generate high levels of specific antibodies.

The microbe should produce relevant virulence factors.

Elimination of the microbe should result in clinical improvement.

The microbe should cause disease in an appropriate animal model .

表 4-2 Pathogens hypothesis of caries

Hypothesis	Proposed
The specific plaque hypothesis	Only a few species are actively involved
The non-specific plaque hypothesis	The outcome of the overall activity of the total plaque microflora.
The ecological plaque hypothesis	Caries is a result of shift in the balance of the resident microflora due to a change in local environmental conditions.

3. 致病菌（Pathogens）

经历了一个世纪的探讨，目前公认：变形链球菌群、乳酸杆菌及放线菌属内几个菌种为人类的致病菌。

（1）变形链球菌群（*Streptococcus mutans group*）

变形链球菌群是链球菌属内口腔固有链球菌内的一个菌群。这个菌群有7个菌种，含8个血清型（Table4-3）其中5个菌种由人口腔内分离，其中变形链球菌（*S.mutans*）检出为74%～100%，其次为远缘链球菌（*S.sobrinus*）约为20%，而仓鼠链球菌（*S.cricetus*）、鼠链球菌（*S. rattus*）及道恩链球菌（*S.downei*）检出较少。也可从人口腔内同时检出2个以上菌种。野生鼠链球菌（*S.ferus*）及猕猴链球菌（*S.macacal*）从动物体检出。

表 4-3　Species and serotypes of *S.mutans* group

Species	Serotypes	Isolation	
		Humans	Animal
S.mutans	c、e、f	+	–
S.sobrinus	d、g	+	–
S.cricetus	a	+	–
S.rattus	b	+	–
S.downei	h	+	–
S.ferus	c	–	+
S.macacae	c	–	+

流行病学研究证实，变形链球菌群主要从早期龋损处检出数量明显增加，唾液中变形链球菌数量，在龋活性的儿童中明显高于非活性儿童。体外实验室及动物模型的研究也证实了这个菌群的致龋性，并且可致牙各个面龋。

变形链球菌群在口腔内定植，最早在出生后19～31个月（平均26个月），这个定植时间称窗口感染（Windows of infectivity）。了解了这个规律，可以用替代菌定植，阻止或减少致病变形链球菌定植，达到减少龋病的发生。

菌群特征：革兰阳性球菌，也可是球杆菌，呈长链或短链。在轻唾培养基生长的典型菌落多为坚韧，有多糖株。发酵甘露醇、山梨醇、乳糖、葡萄糖，产生乳酸、乙酸、丙酸等。蔗糖促进生长，能合成葡聚糖及果聚糖。在微需氧及厌氧环境中生长。

Streptococcus mutans group are oral indigenous microflora in the genus streptococcus. Eight serotypes and seven species were recognized. Five species is isolated from human (Table4- 3). Epidemiological studies with showed that S. mutan accoumted for 74%～100% of S.mutans group, S. sobrinus is the second most mommun (20%).

Window of infectivity: The acquisition of some bacteria may occur optimally only certain ages. Transmission of mutans streptococci to children have a specific window of infectivity between 19 and 81 months (median age=26 months).

（2）乳酸杆菌（*Bactobacillus*）

口腔正常菌群，革兰阳性无芽胞杆菌，菌落光滑型，为圆形凸起，表面光滑，半透明。粗糙型表面干燥，边缘不齐。有两种发酵碳水化合物产酸类型：同质发酵仅产生乳酸；异质发酵产生乳酸、乙酸、甲酸、琥珀酸、丁酸、延胡索酸。产酸力强，耐受pH3.8环境，在CO_2及微需氧环境生长。

龋病相关的菌种主要有：干酪乳杆菌（*L.casei*）、嗜酸性乳杆菌（*L.acidphilus*）、发酵乳杆菌（*L.fermentum*）。

致龋作用：促进龋的发展，也可在一定条件下单独致龋，也可与变形链球菌、放线菌协同致龋。

Lactobacillus is the normal microflora. Cell are usually long rod. Faculalative anaerobes, Growth is generally enhanced by 5% CO_2. They can be divided into two groups: the homo-fermentative species with produce mainly lactic acid, and hetero-fermentative species with produce lactic acid acefate.

The most commonly isolated to be L.acidophilus, L.casei and L.fermentum. The lactobacillus is involved more in the progression of caries lesion deep of enamel and dentine.

（3）放线菌属（*Actinomyces*）

属口腔正常菌群，革兰阳性无芽胞杆菌，可有分枝或丝状，也可为多形性。菌落形态各异，多从牙邻面及龈缘菌斑分离，发酵碳水化合物产生乳酸、乙酸、甲酸、琥珀酸，能利用蔗糖产生细胞外多糖。在微需氧及厌氧环境生长。主要与邻面及根面龋有关。

与致龋相关的菌有：内氏放线菌基因Ⅰ型（A.naeslundii genspecies Ⅰ）、内氏放线菌基因Ⅱ型（原粘性放线菌）（A.naoslundii genspeciesⅡ）、溶牙放线菌（A.odontolyticus）（Table4-4）。

Actionmyces belong to oral normal microflora. Cell is irregular, nonsparing gram-positive rods, filaments and branching. Facultative anaerobes. Requiring added CO_2 for good growth. fermentative carbohydrates producing formic, acetic, lactic and succiuic acids, and produce extracelluar polysaccharides.

Acitinomyes is isolated from approximal site and the gingival crevicl of dental plaque, that has been associated with root caries and approxinmal surface caries.

（4）其他致龋菌（Other Cariogenic Bacteria）

近些年来对致龋菌探讨中，已发现在一些龋病发生的部位常检不到上述三种致病菌，而非变形链球菌（Non-Streptococcus mutans）的致龋作用引起人们的关注，这些菌多指非变形链球菌的产酸菌。另外在根面龋的致龋菌研究发现：一些根面龋发生的部位，检查不到变形链球菌、乳酸杆菌、放线菌，而有关牙周相关菌种增加，如中间普氏菌（P.intermedia）、嗜二氧化碳噬纤维菌（Capnocytophaga）。

表 4-4 Major cariogenic bacteria

Genus	Species	Caries
Stretococcus mutans group	S.mutans	White spot and advanced caries at crown
	S.sobrinus	fissure, approximal and root surface
,Lactobacillus	L.casei	
	L.acidphilus	Progression of Lesions
	L.fermentum	
Actinomyes	Viscosus A.naeslundii	
	genspeclesi Ⅰ and Ⅱ	Lesions at approximal, root surface
	A.odontolyticus	

4. 致病菌毒性作用 The virulence effect of the cariogenic bacteria

龋病是多菌、多毒性疾病，归纳为三类毒性作用：粘附（Adhesion）、产酸（acidgenic）、耐酸（aciduric）。

（1）粘附（Adhesion）

粘附是致龋菌在牙表面定居的首要功能，致龋菌除自身附着在牙表面，同时能凝集其他细菌，促进菌斑形成。主要附着机理是细菌表面粘附素（Adhesins）和牙表面获得膜表面受体（Receptors）的生物化学的分子结合。

变形链球菌（*Mumans Streptococci*） 变形链球菌群附着功能有：①变形链球菌表面抗原家族（Antigen Ⅰ/Ⅱ family），多为肽粘附蛋白，可与获得膜（the acquired pellicle）上糖蛋白凝集素（Salivary agglutinin glycoprotein-SAG）结合。这种功能是变形链球菌向牙表面附着定植起主要作用。目前已有Ⅰ/Ⅱ基因疫苗的研究。②变形链球菌细胞壁的脂磷壁酸（lipoteichoic acid-LTA）与获得膜血族反应的糖蛋白（Blood group reactive glycoprotein）结合附着在牙表面。③葡聚糖连接蛋白（Gluean binding protein-GBPs）这个蛋白包含在葡糖基转移酶（Glucosyltrsferase-GTF）基因序列的C末端片段，大约有500个氨基酸。GBPs与葡聚糖（Glucan）结合，使变形链球菌在牙面上定植，并促进菌斑形成。GTFs有三种：①受gtfB基因支配的GTF-I，主要在蔗糖存在下催化合成不溶性葡聚糖（Insoluble glucan）②受gtfC调控的GTF-I ③受gtfD调控的GTF-S主要产生水溶性葡聚糖（Soluble glucan）。

另外变形链球菌还有果糖基转移酶（fructosyltransferase-FTF）与GTFs利用蔗糖合成葡聚糖和果聚糖，作为细胞外多糖构成菌斑基质，也可为产酸菌细胞外能源贮备。GTF-I产生不溶性葡聚糖对菌斑起到抗唾液溶解的保护作用。是主要致龋因素之一。

由此看出，GTFs、FTF、GBPs参与了致龋菌定植及致龋作用。

放线菌属中内氏放线菌（Actimomyces naeslundii）有Ⅰ型和Ⅱ型菌毛，其中Ⅰ型菌毛（肽蛋白）与获得膜的富脯蛋白（Prolime-rich protein）结合而附着在牙表面上（表4-5）。

除了致龋菌以附着素直接附着在牙表面获得膜上，它们自身还具有接受其他菌附着素的相应受体而产生共聚（Coadhesion）而促使菌斑形成多菌种的群体。

表4-5 Adhesin and receptor of cariogenic bacteria

Bacteria	Adhesin	Receptor
S.mutans	LTA	Blood group reactive glycoprotein
	Antigen Ⅰ/Ⅱ	Salivary agglutinin
	Glucan binding protein	Glucan
A.naesludii	Type Ⅰ fimbriae	Proline-rich protein

Adhesion is living function of carigenic bacteria on teeth surface. Some adhesion mechanisms involve specific molecular interaction between components on the microbial cell surface adhesion and receptors in the acquired pellicle. For example:

Interaction surface glucan binding protein PRPS of S.mutans with glucan in acquired pellicle.

Antigen I/II protein from S.mutans interacts with salivary agglutinins.

Lipoteichoic acid (LTA) of S.mutans combines with blood group reactive substances.

Type 1 fimbrial adherene to PRSs on the acquired pellicle.

（2）产酸（Acidogenicity）

致龋菌利用口腔内碳水化合物代谢产生乳酸（Lactic acid）、乙酸（Acetic acid）、甲酸（Formic acid）、丙酸（Propionic acid）等酸性产物，乳酸是主要酸性产物。酸性产物在菌斑内滞留，使牙表面脱钙，形成龋洞，因此致龋菌的代谢产酸功能是致龋菌的重要毒性因素，其特点是：

产酸能力强：表现代谢碳水化合物产酸快，DisHer（1983）及Margolis（1992）证实变形链球菌在蔗糖存在下菌斑内乳酸产物在5～7分钟达到最高峰，而使pH下降至临界pH以下。

有细胞外糖原储备能力：变形链球菌具有葡糖基转移酶（Glucosyltransferase-GTF）和果糖基转移酶（Fructosyltranferase-FTF），两个酶利用蔗糖合成-葡聚糖（glucans）及果聚糖（fructans）构成牙菌斑的主要基质成分，作为菌斑内细菌细胞外能源的储备，另外粘性放线菌也具有合成葡聚糖的能力。

细胞内多糖：变形链球菌有完善的糖磷酸转移酶系统（Phosphotransferase sugar transport system-PTS）可以迅速将细胞外碳水化合物转入细胞内，一部分代谢产酸，一部分形成细胞内多糖（Intracellular golysaccharide-IPS）作为细胞内糖源储备。当细胞外能源缺乏时，能继续代谢产酸，因此细胞内多糖也是致病因子之一。

The virulence characteristics of Acidogenicity include:

① High acidogenicity with the ability to rapidly metabolize carbohydrates to lactic, acetic and formic acid.

② Intracellular glycogen synthesis in the presence of high sugar concentration in order to sustain the cell in periods of low exogenous carbohydrates.

③ Synthesis of extracellular glucan and fructan from sucrose that aid in colonization of the organism in the plaque.

（3）耐酸（acid tolerance）

Hamilton (1987) 及 Svensater (1997) 证实 S.m 在 pH4.8，*A.naeslandii* pH4.86，*L.casei* pH3.81 环境中仍能生存（Table 4-6）。其原理是致龋菌有质子转移酶（Protor translocating ATPase-H+/ATPase），使酸中 H+ 从胞膜排出，使胞内保持稳定的 pH (Margais 1995 and Bowden 1998)。因此在低pH状态菌斑内部一些菌不能存活，则耐酸菌能持续产酸，以致发挥脱钙作用。

表 4-6 The pH tolerance of cariogenic bacteria

Organism	Acid formed from glucose	Terminal pH during growth	Killing pH
S.mutans	Lactate, Acetate formate	4.28	3.0
A.naeslundii	Lactate, Acetate formate, Succinate	4.64	3.2
L.casei	Lactate, Acetate formate, Fumarote	3.81	2.3

The mechanisms of acid tolerance

Acid tolerant mechanisms of carieogenic bacteria is proton extrusion via membrane-associated , proton-translocating ATP (Adrenosine triphosphate) synthase (H+/ATPase) (adrenosine triphosphatase) and acid endproduct efflux. S.mutans and Lactobacill have higher levels of ATP-synthase acitity.

（二）宿主因素 Host factor

1. 牙齿 Teeth

牙齿可以由于全身及局部的先天及后天的原因，使牙及牙列出现多种龋易感的弱点。

（1）正常发育的缺陷 Normal developmental defect

人的咀嚼器官在人类进化过程中属于退化器官，因此在近代人类的牙及牙列的发育及萌出形成自然的发育性缺陷。

解剖结构异常：牙冠的窝沟及异常发育沟是不易驱除菌斑的滞留区。窝沟深而细，沟内壁釉质层较薄，钙磷含量低，蛋白成分多，易受酸蚀。

牙弓排列异常：牙列不齐增加了菌斑滞留区，即是龋易感区，如前倾及水平等阻生齿，使第二磨牙远中易出现邻面龋。

发育中的易感：年青恒牙釉质表面多微孔，釉柱间质宽，矿化程度低，抗酸蚀能力弱。

（2）异常发育缺陷 Abnormal developmental defect

在恒牙发育时期，儿童患有全身疾病及营养不良，而使牙釉质形成障碍，常出现釉质发育不全及钙化不全，形成龋病易感条件。

（3）局部炎症（local inflammation）

由于乳牙根尖化脓性炎症使将萌出的恒牙冠出现釉质缺损的特奈氏牙齿，出现龋易感区。慢性牙周炎发展使牙周组织退缩，牙根暴露，根面牙骨质矿化程度差，有机物成分含量多，容易受菌斑有关细菌水解有机物及脱矿。

（4）医源性原因（Medical reason）

正畸矫正器托槽周围，固定修复体颈部边缘，邻面洞充填体悬突等都可以造成人为的菌斑堆积的死角，而形成龋易感区。

环境原因（Environmental reason）

在酸性环境中作业的工作人员，牙齿易受到酸蚀性脱钙而后发展成为龋。高氟区人群，牙齿长期受到水氟的侵蚀，出现严重的氟牙症患者的口腔内，在氟斑的基础上发展的龋，常常是一个牙存有 2 个以上的多个龋洞。

2. 唾液（Saliva）

唾液主要指混合唾液（whole saliva），唾液内有多种成分，在维持口腔微环境平衡起到重要作用。

（1）清洁口腔（cleansing mouth） 唾液的静态流量是0.33ml/min，动态流量是1.89ml/min，正常的流量起到机械清除口腔微生物的作用，流量减少则易发生龋病，例如患头颈部癌的病人，作放射线治疗后造成涎腺损伤引起干燥综合征（Xerostomia），在口腔内唾液变形链球菌比例由 0.6% 增加到 44%，乳酸杆菌比正常增加 1000 倍，常易患猖獗龋（Rampant caries）。

唾液清除口腔内微生物不是单独机械清除，是和唾液内的凝集作用协同完成，如唾液内粘蛋白（Mucin）和凝集素（Agglutinins）对悬浮的微生物凝集后，再通过唾液被吞咽及吐出清除细菌。

（2）抑制微生物（Inhibiting microorganism） 唾液里有多种抑制微生物的特异性及非特异性的物质，控制着口腔内微生态的平衡环境。非特异性抑菌物质有：唾液的流动、粘蛋白、凝集素、乳铁蛋白、溶菌酶、唾液过氧化酶系统、富组蛋白、富酪蛋白及抗菌肽等。特异性的有：淋巴、郎氏细胞、SigA、IgG、IgA、IgM、补体、嗜中性白血球及巨噬细胞等（表 4-7）。

表 4-7 Specific and non-specific host defence factor of the mouth

Defence factors	Function
Specific	
Epithelial lymphocytes and Langerhans cell	Cellular barriers to penetrating bacteria
SIgA	Prevents microbial adhesion
IgG，IgA，IgM	Prevents microbial adhesion
Neutrophils macrophaga	Phagocytesis
Complement	Activates neutrophils
Non-specific	
Saliva flow, Mucin, afflutinins	Physical removal of bacteria
Lysozyme	Cell lysis
Lactoferrin	Cell killing
Sialoperoxidase system	Hypothiocyanite production Hypocyanous acid production
Histidine-rich peptides	Antibacterial activity

（3）抗酸作用（Anti-acid effect） 口腔恒定的中性环境（pH6.0 ～ 7.0）主要是有碳酸盐缓冲系统及磷酸盐缓冲系统维持中和口腔内酸性产物，其次还有尿素分解和蛋白分解的氨基酸产物也起到升高口腔 pH 作用。

（4）再矿化作用（Effect of remineralization） 牙釉质表面滞留的菌斑内产酸菌（The acidogenic bacteria）代谢碳水化合物产酸（乳酸、乙酸等），使菌斑内菌斑液pH下降，当pH维持在临界pH5.0～5.5（Critical pH5.0～5.5）以下时，釉质表面羟基磷灰石（Hydoxypatite-HA）被降解，钙及磷酸盐溶出，出现牙脱矿（Demineralization），脱矿继续则出现龋洞（图 4-1）。

唾液内缓冲系统及钙、磷、氟可使唾液及菌斑内 pH 上升及促使钙磷再沉积，这个过程为再矿化（Remineralization）。脱矿和再矿化是伴随发生的过程，是口腔内菌斑与宿主在微环境内平衡内容之一。菌斑酸性产物持续及滞留则平衡失调而牙脱矿发生，当菌斑代谢得到控制，则唾液起到了再矿化作用，因此控制菌斑，增加唾液的再矿化作用，则是防治龋病发生重要环节。

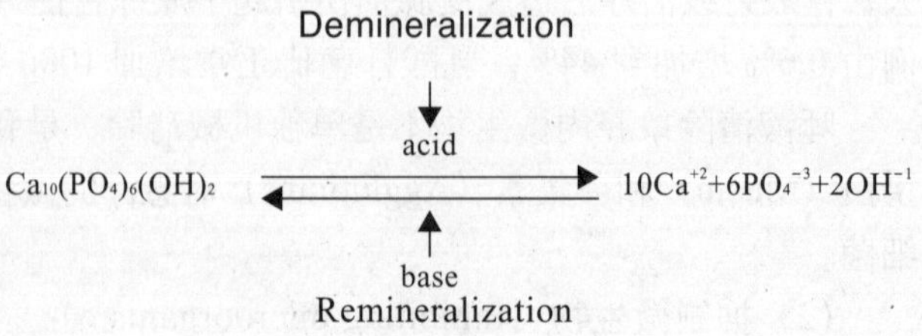

图 4-1 脱矿与再矿化

3. 人的行为和生活方式 Human behaviour and lifestyle

人的行为首先是对疾病的认识，在此基础上不仅是个人的防病能力的提高，而是变为社会行为，使之有目的有计划的采取有效的社会性的防治措施。从发达国家半个世纪的社会防治及我国近些年牙病防治工作发展经验，证实了人对疾病认识的重要作用。

生活方式指，与龋病相关的生活习惯和饮食结构。人们渐渐认识到，如果没有良好的口腔卫生习惯，嗜烟，饮食含糖量多、纤维食物少的不合理膳食，婴幼儿牙胚发育时期的全身疾病及营养障碍等造成的龋病易发的危险因素，改变龋病易发的生活方式也是防治龋病发生的重要内容。

（三）食物因素 Dietary factor

1. 营养的种类与龋病关系 Relationship between nutrient type and caries

食物是人的主要营养来源，而口腔内微生物的能源包括有：内源性营养（Endogenous Nutrients）和外源性营养（Exogenous Nutrients）。内源性营养由各涎腺分泌及龈沟液构成的各种氨基酸、肽、蛋白、糖蛋白及微量元素。这些成分是口腔内微生物定居初期的基本营养来源。这部分营养，限定了微生物在口腔内种类及数量，维持着口腔微环境的平衡。外源性营养指食物。食物种类不同则对龋病发生的作用不同。碳水化合物食物是口腔内产酸菌代谢的能源，口腔内碳水化合物过多则有利致龋菌及产酸菌生长，使菌斑内菌群比例失调，有利龋发生。蛋白类食物如奶类食品，在口腔内分解氨基酸等产物，可以升高口腔内pH，有利于磷酸钙再矿化。蛋白本身可以结合钙，也可作为钙的储备。食物中蛋白可以附着在获得膜上，阻止变形链球菌吸附。

脂类食物到目前为止还没有证实与龋的关系。食物中的微量元素：钙磷是牙矿化原料，氟可以促进矿化，抗酸蚀及抑制致龋菌，锌可以抑制致龋菌在牙表面附着，镉、钼也可以提高牙的抗酸能力。

Endogenous nutrients is whole saliva (salivary secretion and gingival crevicular fluid), which contain amino acid, peptide, protein glycoprotein and elements, that primarily nutrients of resident oral microflara. Endogenous nutrients maintaiming balance of micro-enviroument.

Exogenous nutrients is diet. Fermentable carbohydrates makes S.mutans and Lactobacill increase. The milk products can protect the teeth, reduce adhesion of S.mutans and elevate plaque pH.

2. 碳水化合物食物与龋的关系 Relationship between carbohydrate food and caries

碳水化合物是产酸菌的代谢能源，但碳水化合物种类、用量及食用频率影响着致龋作用。

（1）种类与龋 Type of sugar and caries 蔗糖（Sucrose）致龋作用是：①致龋菌利用蔗糖代谢产酸较快，Margrlis 利用10%蔗糖给受试者漱口，龋活性菌斑内7分钟pH下降到临界pH以下。②致龋菌可以转运蔗糖到细胞内，合成细胞内多糖，作为持续产酸的糖原储备。③致龋菌细胞外葡糖基转移酶可合成细胞外多糖（葡聚糖），而促进菌斑形成。④可以合成多种细胞外多糖（葡聚糖、果聚糖、杂多糖等）作为菌斑基质及细胞外能源储备。

（2）其他糖类如葡萄糖、淀粉、乳糖、果糖及麦芽糖等都可被致龋菌代谢产酸，但致龋作用相对比蔗糖弱。木糖醇、山梨醇、甘露醇及甜叶菊糖等一般不能被致龋菌利用。常作为糖代用品，阻止致龋菌产酸脱钙。

Many sweet foods are composed of mono or disaccharide (glucose or sucrose) which are easily

metabolized by plaque bacteria and predispose enamel to dental caries.

Sugar substitutes (mannital, sorbitol and xylitol) cannot be metabolized by plaque bacteria and can reduce caries.

3. 糖的食用频率与龋病关系 Relationship between frequency of eating sugar and caries

Gustafsson研究对受试者每天三餐加蔗糖330g，连续观察2年，无明显龋发生。另一组受试者除每日三次外，在三餐间隔加餐含糖类食物，每次2～3g蔗糖，则2年观察龋发生明显，Gustafsson用Stephan观察了受试者每餐的牙菌斑pH变化发现：一日三餐大量食糖，pH下降在临界pH（The critical pH）以下一次持续时间为为40～60分钟，占全天时间的8%～10%时间，而三餐间加餐甜食，则使pH在临界pH以下持续时间增加到280～420分钟，占全天19%～29%的时间，则增加致龋菌在菌斑酸性产物停留的时间及脱钙的危险性（图4-2）。

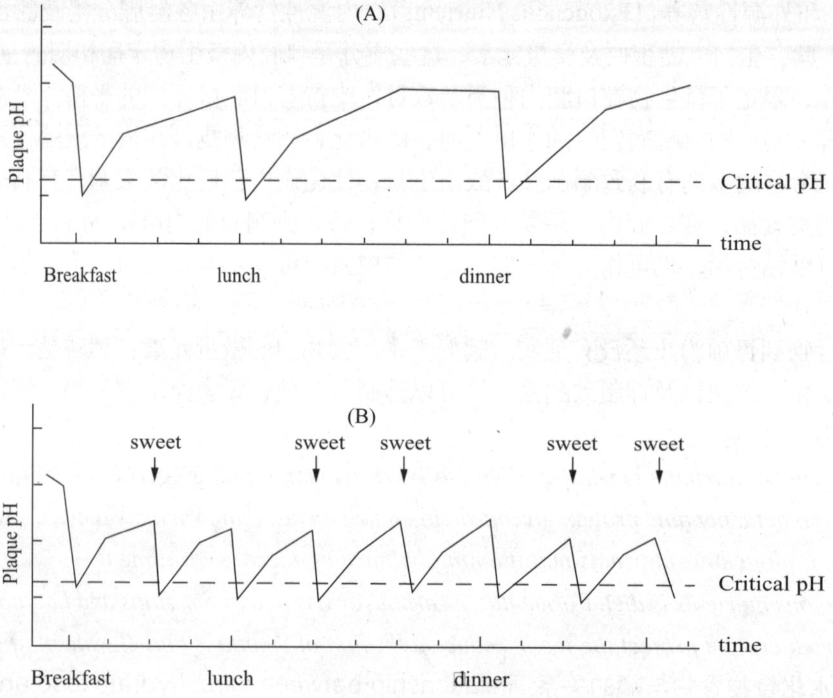

图4-2 (A) limits their carbogydrate intake to main meals only, (B) Has freqent intake fermentable carbohydrate during the day.

4. 牙发育期营养与龋的关系 Relationship between nutrient and caries during teeth development

乳牙在胚胎期形成，此时母亲的营养状况直接影响乳牙的发育。恒牙冠在出生后约在3岁以前发育形成时期，儿童机体出现营养障碍或全身疾病，使恒牙发育必要成分钙、磷及维生素A、D等微量元素摄取不足，使恒牙发育易出现釉质发育不全及钙化不全。

（四）时间因素 Time factor

龋病是以牙硬组织破坏的慢性感染性疾病和一般慢性疾病一样，有一定时间的病理发展进程。龋病的发生因素的具体时间含义应是：致龋菌斑内酸性产物滞留在牙表面的时间及菌斑内低的临界 pH 所持续时间。时间越长，脱钙的危险性越大。

The carious process consists of alternating periods of destruction and repair and the saliva has the ability to delay progression of lesions. Thus, when saliva is present, caries does not destroy the tooth in days or weeks but rather in months or years, or not at all. There is a great deal of scope to modify the carious progress.

二、龋病分类 Classification of dental caries

龋病有多种分类方法，常根据牙体破坏的组织病理、病程、损害部位进行分类。

（一）病理分类 Pathalogical classification

釉质龋（Enamel Caries）龋损限于牙釉质内。

牙本质龋（Dentinal caries）损害达牙本质层。

牙骨质龋（Cementum caries）损害牙根表牙骨质层。

（二）病程分类 Classification of carious process

急性龋（Acute caries）病程破坏快，腐质软而湿润，色浅，也称湿润龋，多发生儿童及青年。如多数牙同时出现龋损称猖獗龋或称猛性龋（Rampant Caries）。干燥综合征（Xerostomia）、舍古林综合征（Sjogren's syndroml）、奶瓶龋（Nursing bottle caries）易患猖獗性龋。（表 4-8）

表 4-8 The particular group of Rampant caries

Group of people	Reason	Mechanism
Xerostomic patients	Radiation treatment for head and neck cancer	Reduced rate of salivary flow
Patients with sjogren syndrome	Disease of the body or medication	Reduced rate of salivary flow
Young infants with Nursing bottle caries	Frequent feeding with bottle	High concentration of fermentable carbodydrate

慢性龋（chronic caries）常见的龋损类型，龋损破坏速度慢，腐质色黑，质地干，又称干性龋。病损局部环境的改变，则破坏可停止进行，则此状态称静止龋。

继发龋（Secondary Caries）龋洞经治疗充填后，龋坏再发生。主要由于充填物与洞壁不密合出现细菌的滞留的间隙，如邻面充填物悬突，充填物表面处理不够光滑，则易再发生龋。

（三）根据解剖部位分类 Classification of carious lesion by anatomical site

窝沟龋（Fiffure caries）多见的龋损类型。常见的是磨牙[殆]面窝沟及后牙颊侧沟。窝沟内细深，沟内釉质壁薄，滞留的菌斑不易清除。是龋发生率最高的部位。

邻面龋（Appoximal surface caries）多发于后牙（前磨牙、磨牙）之间接触点下，菌斑滞留处，早期不易被发现。

根面龋（Root surface caries）好发于牙根外露的牙骨质表面的成年及老年人。

光滑面龋（Smooth surface caries）由于牙光滑面（颊舌侧）菌斑易清洁，龋发生较少，如配带的固定矫正器患者托槽周围易堆积菌斑，则常出现光滑面的早期龋损。

线形釉质龋（Linear ename caries）好发乳牙前牙唇面。

（四）根据龋损深度分类 Classification of carious lesion by depth

浅龋（shallow caries）损害限于牙釉质及牙骨质浅层，一般无症状。

中龋（Middle caries）损害限于牙本质，常对冷热、酸有反应，除去刺激则症状消失。

深龋（Deep Caries）损害达牙本质深层，常有牙髓症状出现。

三、龋病的进展 The progress of dental caries

（一）初期龋局部菌斑的变化 Local change of dental plaque in initial caries

龋病发生早期牙釉质（骨质）表面滞留的菌斑菌群与健康部位有明显的不同。

菌群变化 龋发生的早期局部菌斑内致龋菌及耐酸菌比例增加，变形链球菌数量可增加 10 ~ 100 倍，乳酸杆菌及耐酸菌也相应增加。

菌斑对糖的反应 Fejerskov（1992）观察。龋活性及非活性菌斑儿童，用蔗糖漱口，并连续观察菌斑变化，发现与健康部位比较菌斑pH漱口后，菌斑pH下降至临界pH以下，持续时间长，回升慢（图 4-3）。

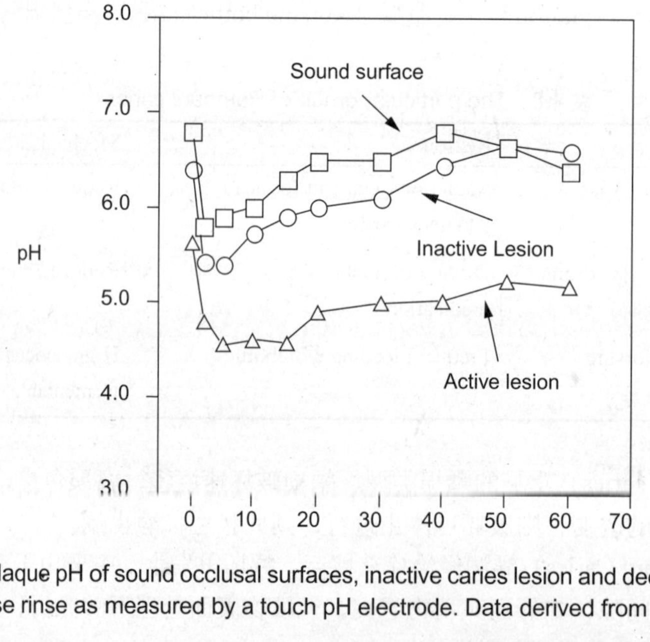

图4-3 The in situ plaque pH of sound occlusal surfaces, inactive caries lesion and deep, active occlusal caries lesion after a sucrose rinse as measured by a touch pH electrode. Data derived from Fejerskov et al., (1992)

酸性产物 Margolis（1992）用蔗糖液给龋活性及非活性受试者漱口，发现活性菌斑乳酸产物比非活性菌斑产生快。乳酸产物在 30 分钟达到高峰，其他酸性产物也相应增加。

（二）釉质表面下脱钙 Demineralization underlying enamel surface

牙表面滞留的菌斑内，酸性产物侵蚀釉质表面，使釉质多孔结构被侵蚀，透过抗酸强的表层，通过多孔结构进入釉质表面下，引起脱钙，形成脱矿带，继续脱矿则在X线片上出现釉质表面下透影区，临床表现为白垩色斑（white spot）。如果局部酸蚀终止，唾液及菌斑内饱和钙、磷可以在脱矿部位沉积再矿化，此阶段为可逆时期。

这个再矿化过程受到菌斑滞留时间、致龋及产酸菌的数量，碳水化合物的提供量，局部钙、磷、氟的浓度及唾液流量等因素的影响。

（三）龋洞形成 Cavitation

釉质表面下脱钙继续扩大，釉质表面下组织崩解到一定程度，釉表面层塌陷形成釉质龋洞。这个时期则成为不可逆的过程。釉质龋损继续发现到深层沿牙本质小管方向破坏，因牙本质钙、磷含量相对少，有机物质多，则龋损坏更容易，此时期继续则可能出现牙髓及根尖炎症并发症的危险。

Dental caries is a multifactorial ubiquitous, plaque-related chronic infection disease.

Interaction of the factors involved in dental caries are the tooth, saliva, bacterial of plque, the diet (sucrose) and time. Interaction of the factors result from imbalance of ecological plaque.

The major form of tooth destruction is demineralization of enamel, dentine, cementum by acids generated during carbohydrate matabolism by the acidogenic oral microflora.

第二节　龋病危险因素及其预测方法

Section 2 Caries Risk Factors and its Predicting Methods

龋病危险因素是可能发生龋的潜在因素，它包含关键微生物、敏感宿主、含碳水化合物食物等因素。危险因素的预测是防治工作的重要内容。

Caries risk factors are potential factors that can occur dental carie. These include the key oral microorganisms, susceptible host and dietary carbohydrate. The predication of caries risk factors is impordont content in caries prevention.

一、确定龋病危险因素的方法 The methods for determining caries risk factors

（一）流行病学研究 The epidemiological study

根据人群口腔内龋病现状的预测

儿童及青少年人群：研究证明患乳牙龋的多少与第一恒磨牙新生龋有相关性。第一恒磨牙窝沟新生龋与恒牙龋发生有相关性，因此乳牙及第一恒磨牙龋发病情况可以作为危险因素预测信号。

成年及老年人：患根面龋的发病率较高，因此牙根外露是根面龋发生的危险因素。

患相关全身疾病人群：儿童营养不良、早产儿、影响儿童恒牙胚发育的全身感染性疾病等是儿童恒牙出现钙化不全、釉质发育不全等是龋的易感因素。接受放射治疗的头颈癌患者，涎腺受损唾液分泌障碍是易患猖獗龋（Rampant Caries）的危险因素。

（二）牙菌斑微环境改变的研究 The study on microenvironmental change in dental plaque

1. 致龋菌数量增加 Increasing the amount of cariogenic bacterias

Loesche W等研究证明：釉质表面早期龋患部位菌斑与周围健康部位比较，变形链球菌（S. mutans）数量增加10～100倍，在窝沟及邻面早期龋，变形链球菌、乳酸杆菌（Lactobacillus）及放线菌（Actinomyes）有明显增加。Matsukubo.T等人的追踪观察，变形链球菌在牙菌斑及唾液内菌数＞10^5CFU/ml，乳杆菌＞10^4 CFU/ml 为龋活性。杨圣辉（1999）对 2000 名幼儿园儿童观察证实，唾液中变形链球菌数＞10^5CFU/ml，两年后 60% 儿童有新生龋。

2. 耐酸菌数增加 Increasing the number of aciduric bacterias

有部分研究对变形链球菌及乳酸杆菌的危险预测提出相反看法，Brail Stord提出了非变形链球菌的耐酸菌可作为龋危险因素预测，但目前为止，还没有确定预测界线，但比较公认的研究是牙表面菌斑 pH5.0 ～ 5.5 以下为釉质表面脱钙危险因素的临界 pH（The critical pH）。

What is critical pH?

The critical pH is the pH below which demineralization of enamel is favoured.

（三）糖与危险因素的研究 The study on risk factor and sugar

有利于致龋菌及耐酸菌产酸的营养物质，主要是蔗糖（Sucrose），其他为葡萄糖、淀粉、乳糖等碳水化合物类食物。对产酸关系密切的主要是糖在口腔内停留的时间，因此吃含糖食物及糖的频率比量更重要（图 4-2）。

二、龋病的危险因素 The risk factor of dental caries

1）致病菌在口腔唾液内及牙菌斑里菌数增加，变形链球菌＞10^5CFU/ml，乳酸杆菌＞10^4 CFU/ml，为危险因素预测指标，也可称高龋活性（the High Caries Activity）。

2）牙菌斑内耐酸菌比例增加。

3）牙菌斑内 pH 持续在 5.0 ～ 5.5 以下（below the Critical pH）

4）乳牙及第一恒磨牙龋，特别是新生龋存在，可作为以后恒牙龋的危险因素。

5）牙根外露的成年及老年人。

6）发育缺陷的牙如钙化不全、釉质发育不全、 殆面窝沟及颊面沟。

7）口干症患者（Xerostomic Patients）易发生猖獗龋。

8）长时间频繁食用含糖食物及饮料的人群

9）长期菌斑滞留的部位。

10）影响牙胚发育的相关疾病，如早产儿、营养不良等（表 4-9）。

表 4-9　Risk factors of dental caries

Cariogenic Factors	Risk factors
Micro flora	Increase proportion of cariogenic bacteria in plaque The plaque pH is below the critical pH Increased proportion of aciduric bacteria
Host	Exposed cementum surface of the root Growth defect of teeth Incipient young permanent Xerostomic patients
Food	Frequent intake of carbohydrate food
Time	Plaque Accumulate no the enamel surface for long time

三、龋病危险因素预测及早期诊断 The predication of caries risk factor and diagnosis in its early stage

（一）龋病预测方法 The method of predicative caries

The caries activity test is a testing method to detect caries risk factor by using microbiological theory. The method include Dentocult SM test, Dontocule LB test, Cariostat test and Dentobuff strip.

1. 实验方法 Experimental methods

实验室龋危险因素的检测又称龋活性试验（The Caries Activity Test），目前已成为产品的常用几种简易的方法：

（1）Dentocult SM 试验

目的：观察变形链球菌群各菌种再唾液中每毫升菌落的数量，确定龋活性。

试剂盒：包括又含 MSB 培养液的螺帽培养瓶，杆菌肽纸片，附着板及石蜡丸。

使用方法：检测时受试者先咀嚼一粒石蜡丸1分钟，然后持附着板在受试者舌背面反转涂抹10次，然后将附着板放置培养瓶内，37℃，48小时培养后，记录变形链球菌附着生长板上的蓝色菌落密度。

结果判断：分四级 “0 和 1”$<10^5$，“2” $10^5\sim10^6$，“3” $>10^6$，“3” 为高龋活性。

（2）Dentocule LB 试验

目的：主要观察乳酸杆菌在唾液及菌斑内每毫升菌落的数量，判断龋危险因素。

试剂盒：螺帽培养瓶，含有 Rogosa agar 固体培养的试板。

检测方法：受试者先咀嚼石蜡丸1分钟后，收集唾液于容器内，再将唾液均匀浇在培养板的琼脂培养基表面，多余唾液倾去，放置35℃，4天培养后，记录培养板上生长的乳酸杆菌菌落密度。

判断标准：1000/ml (10^3/ml)、10000 (10^4/ml)、100000 (10^5/ml)、1000000 (10^6/ml)，> 10000/ml (> 10^4/ml) 为高龋活性。

以上两种为常用的龋危险因素预测细菌学方法。

（3）Cariostat 试验

目的：检测牙表面菌斑内产酸菌产酸能力。

试剂盒：含有溴甲酚紫及溴甲酚绿的液体培养管，标准的棉签。

检测方法：用棉签涂擦一侧后牙颊面4～5次，将棉签放置培养管内，37℃，48小时培养后，观察培养液的颜色变化。

结果判断：蓝紫色（－），绿色（+），黄绿色（++），黄色（+++），黄绿色（++）培养管 pH5.0 ～ 5.5 为龋危险龋活性，黄色（+++）为明显龋活性。

（4）Dentobuff Strip 试验

原理：标准化的黄色试条，为酸性状态的指示条，接触唾液后试条受到唾液缓冲作用的影响，试条 pH 升高则指示剂发生变色，变色则说明唾液缓冲能力。

产品：黄色试条

方法及结果判断：用试条浸受试者唾液后，试条变为蓝色，表示pH＞6.0，说明唾液有缓冲能力，否则缓冲能力异常。

表 4-10 Dentocult S.M. and L.B. caries activity test

Methods	Instructions for use	High caries activity
Dentocult SM	Estimate mutans streptococcus count in Saliva and plaque	$>10^6$ CFU/ml
Dentocult LB	Estimating the Salivary Lactobacillus Count	$>10^4$ CFU/ml

除上已产品化的龋活性试验方法外，还有一些方法如刃天青纸片法（Resazarin disc test）Sngder test 等方法。

2. 口腔现状检查 Examination of dental status

进食碳水化合物情况：特别是含蔗糖食物及饮料，了解进食量、频率及种类，时间多。

口腔现状：乳牙多龋及新萌出恒牙（第一恒磨牙）新生龋，是预示以后恒牙龋发生的危险信号。

牙根外露的老年人，牙发育异常，牙列不齐有菌斑滞留易发生龋。

口腔内固定矫正器，固体修复体是否有菌斑滞留存在的危险因素。

（二）龋病的早期诊断 Early diagnosis of dental caries

早期龋诊断的内容应重视早期釉质浅龋。

釉质光滑面及窝沟表面下脱钙诊断：检查可见到白垩色斑及变色（黑色）现象，龋进一步发展可探到釉质表面粗糙感，近来也有用DIANO dent龋病检测仪（为半导体激光检测仪），可以早期提高㓖面龋诊断率。

邻面早期龋诊断：用探针检测表面粗糙感，确定釉质表面的早期龋。表面下脱钙有效方法：临床多用X线合翼片（Bitiwing Rodography）观察早期表面下脱钙透影区。也有用DIANO dent检测仪检测邻面龋。

根面牙骨质龋诊断，临床主要用探针检查粗糙面，也存在试用重氮盐染料类物质的显色观察根面早期龋。

Caries risk factors are among the key oral microorganisms, susceptible host, dietary carbohydrate. Patients with extensive or recurrence caries should be evaluated to identify relevant risk factors. High Salivary or plaque count of lactobacillus and mutans streptococcus are related in many caries to a high risk factors.

第三节 龋病预防的科学基础与基本对策

Section 3 The Scientific Basis and Main Strategies for Caries Prevention

龋病是多因素、慢性感染性疾病，因此在防治上应是综合性防治。

Dental Caries is a multifactorial ,chronic infections disease. Therefore strategies of caries prevention should be comprehensive measure.

一、菌斑控制 Plaque control

（一）机械方法 Mechanical methods

机械清除菌斑是简易的自我保健方法。包括有牙刷、牙膏、牙线、牙签、牙间刷及牙间充洁器。目前牙刷的刷头种类繁多，但基本的原则是：最大限度清除牙表面菌斑、减少对牙表面的磨损及牙龈损伤。

（二）抗菌剂 Antimicrobial agents

1. 杀菌剂 Bactericidal agents

氯已定（chlorhexidine）有叫洗必太，为双胍类，为广谱杀菌剂。对革兰氏阳性、阴性菌、真菌有效。变形链球菌对它敏感。作用原理：

阻止细菌代谢中磷酸转移酶系统（PTS）的糖转移功能。

影响细菌胞膜三磷酸腺苷酶合成（ATP-synthanl）和膜离子的渗透性。

抑制牙龈卟啉单胞菌蛋白酶的活性。

氯已定与牙表面获得结合，沉积在牙表面起到药物缓慢释放作用。

副作用：使牙表面积舌背部着色，对口腔黏膜有刺激作用。

氯已定使用日趋势小，因为它是广谱杀菌剂，不宜长期使用。但对危险人群中如因头颈部痛作放射治疗的患者防止猖獗龋的发生受到一定的效果。

剂型，含漱剂（0.12% ~ 0.2%），凝胶（1%）。

Effected theory of chlorhexidine

- *abolish the acitivity of the PTS sugar transport system and thereby markedly inhibit acid production in streptococci.*
- *inhibit a major protease of P.gingivalis.*
- *affect varion membrane functions including the ATP-synthase.*

2. 植物提取物 Plant extracts

这类提取物包括有黄芩、厚朴、五倍子、金银花、三颗针、二面针等功能是抑制细菌作用，副作用少。剂型多为漱口剂及牙膏。

（三）酶类 Enzymes

酶类有特异性及非特异性酶。非特异性蛋白酶类破坏细菌细胞膜。特异性的有葡聚糖酶（变聚糖酶 mutanase 及葡聚糖酶 glucanase），用于溶解葡聚糖，减少菌斑在牙表面堆积。

（四）抗菌斑附着剂 Aati-adherence agants

包括有茶多酚、甲壳胺等，这些物质除有弱的抑菌作用外，主要作用是阻止菌斑在牙表面附着，阻止葡聚糖合成。甲壳胺是氨基多糖类物质，有表面阳离子活性，可以吸附凝集口腔内细菌，阻止菌斑堆积，同时也有解吸附功能，使已附着牙面的菌斑脱落。

茶多酚可以放在含漱剂中。甲壳胺可以放在牙膏、含漱剂内。

（五）氟化物 Fluorides

氟化物防龋核心是氟离子，其作用有多方面，具体包括有：

1. 对牙体的作用

氟在口腔内唾液内适当浓度下，与牙表面羟基磷灰石（hydrooxyapatite）结合形成氟羟基磷灰石（fluoroapatite），增加釉质的硬度及抗酸蚀作用，在脱钙与在矿化过程中，有氟存在则可以促进在矿化。

2. 对致龋变形链球菌作用

氟化物抑制变形链球菌体内烯醇化酶（Enolase），减少糖分解作用。

阻止了磷酸转移酶系统中磷酸烯醇丙酮盐（phosphoenolprrurate 简称 PEP）的产生，间接抑制了糖向细胞内转运 。

干扰了细胞膜的离子渗透。

氟离子进入细胞内结合 H+ 为 HF 使细胞酸化而使关键子代谢酶失活

抑制了细胞内多糖（Intracellular polysaccharide IPS）合成（图 4-4）。

Effects of the fluoride

① reducing glycolysis by inhibition of enolase

② indirectly inhibiting sugar trauspout by blocking the production of PEP for the PTS system;

③ interfering with bacterial membrane permeabilrty to ionic transfer;

④ acidifying the interiou of cell, and hence inactivating key metabolic enzymes;

⑤ inhibiting the synthesis of intracellular storage. (IPS) (图 4-4)

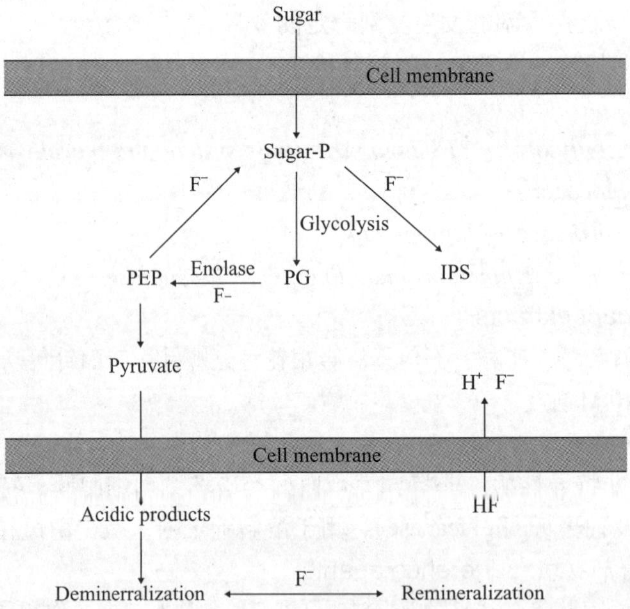

图 4-4　Effect of fluoride F Fluoride IPS intracellular polysaccharide PG phosphoglycerate PEP phosphoenolpyruvate

临床研究证明：连续使用含1ppm氟水含漱，则牙菌斑内氟含量增加到190ppm，一般与菌斑内有机物结合，当菌斑内 pH 下降时，则可以在释放，达到限制菌斑内产酸作用。

关于致龋菌耐氟问题，在实验室研究中显示变形链球菌、乳酸杆菌对高氟的耐受性。但临床观察还没有证据说明对产酸及致龋作用有影响，有待进一步深入研究中。

（六）替代疗法 Replacement therapy

是用于致龋菌毒性因子缺陷株替代野生株定植口腔的方法，以达到减少龋齿发生的作用。替换毒性缺陷株必须有附着及生存代谢的能力。较早的研究有，Johuson and Hillman（1982）用化学方法诱变了变形链球菌乳酸脱该酶（Lactec dehydroyenase 称 LDH）缺陷株，定植在牙面，证实了在碳水化合物存在下，不能代谢产生乳酸。但它存在多基因损伤问题。Hillman（1996 ~ 1999）先后用基因重组构建成变形链球菌 LDH 缺陷株 CHTS 及 BCS3-L1 株，经实验鼠证明有稳定的附着功能。

Clancy andBurne（1997）构建成含有唾液链球菌尿素酶基因（UreA-G）变形链球菌 GS-5 株，经实验鼠证明 GS-5 株具有尿素酶活性，具有分解菌斑及唾液中尿素产生氨基酸，阻止菌斑内碳水化合物分解产酸后 pH 下降的能力。

Replacement therapy would replaced the pathogen native to dental plaque with an altered strain that would be less virulent. for example, More recently a mutans strains of S.mutans BCS3-L1 was derived entirely deficient in LDH activity replacement wild-type strain in gnotobiotic rats producing from sugar substrates less lactic acid.

（七）疫苗 Vaccine

防龋疫苗为主动免疫，以致病的特异性抗原，使机体产生特异性抗体，而中和致龋菌的毒性因子，能使机体保持较长时间防治作用，这个方法比较适合危险人群的防治。由于当前分子生物学发展，用基因工程的方法能研制出纯的抗原，而避免了多克隆抗原造成与心内膜交叉反应的副作用。目前针对变形链球菌致龋毒性的疫苗研制主要有两种毒性抗原研制途径：

含葡聚糖转移酶（glucosyl trensferases GTF）基因疫苗研究 GTF 是蛋白结构基因包括催化（catalytic damain）段和结合葡聚糖连接蛋白（glucona-binding protein 称 GBPs）部分。催化段在酶结构的 N 末端 Gtf，作用是催化蔗糖（sucrose）合成细胞外葡聚糖，组成菌斑基质，促进菌斑堆积。 GBPs 在 C 末端使葡聚糖与牙表面获得结合，促使变链附着在牙面。Smith 和 Tanbman 研制出纯的 59KD（ GBP59）肽蛋白。Smith1999 研究 S.mGTFb5、b7 纯的催化段肽蛋白，免疫鼠模型证实了抗龋活性的作用。

变形链球菌表面附着蛋白疫苗研究　疫苗是变形链球菌表面Ⅰ/Ⅱ蛋白，是菌毛蛋白黏附素与牙表面获得膜内糖蛋白受体（Receptor）结合，附着在牙表面。这个基因疫苗已证实了主要是阻止变形链球菌定植，特别是儿童窗口感染期（Window of infection）起到阻止定植作用。

疫苗的研究还处在研制阶段，研究技术已趋成熟，但在龋齿防治研究历程中，它是迟到的研究。当前在发达国家，氟防龋及其他方法，使龋发病率下降了50%，可疫苗还需等待一个时期。不过被动免疫方式的变链菌的特异性抗体产品已上市，如含致病因子的变链免疫的蛋白（IgY）抗体的局部口腔喷雾剂开始应用。

Vaccine of preventing caries is active immunization. The specific antigen immunize to obtain specific antibody. That would protect against dental caries. For example, the N-termina region of Gtf and C-tormind third of protein of S. mutans have been used to immunize rats to induce specific antibody, that shown to inhibit dental caries.

二、糖替代品 Sugar substitutes

糖类是人类的主要营养素之一，日常生活中人食用的糖类有：蔗糖、淀粉、乳糖等，特别是蔗糖是公认的致龋食物。蔗糖在口腔内停留，打破口腔菌群平衡，激活致龋变形链球菌过度生长，产生细胞外多糖（Extracellular polymers）促进菌斑形成，同时促进细胞内多糖（Intracellular polymers）储存，增加代谢产酸能力而使牙表面脱钙形成龋洞。

蔗糖代用品有两种：一种为高甜度的代用品，如糖精（Sweeteners），天冬苯西二肽脂（Aspartame），甜叶菊糖，这些糖比蔗糖甜若干倍，同时有弱抑菌作用。另一类低甜度代用品，如木糖醇（Xylitol），山梨醇（Sorbitol），甘露醇（Mannitol）等。

目前在防龋上使用的代用品最多的是木糖醇（Xylitol）代用品。经研究证明：①木糖醇刺激唾液分泌，增加对pH下降的缓冲调节及促进再矿化作用。②木糖醇由变形链球菌的果糖转移酶转移系统（Fructose-PTS）带入菌体内，进入无效磷酸化循环（Fatile cycleofphosphorylation），消耗了糖代谢中磷酸烯醇丙酮酸盐（Phosphoenolpyravate-PEP），干扰了变形链球菌的糖代谢，抑制了糖分解产酸能力，而达到阻止酸蚀作用。

在实际生活中，糖代用品还不能完全代替蔗糖，因此控制进糖频率及吃糖后及时清洁口腔，减少糖在口腔内滞留时间尤为重要。

Sugar substitutes are of two types: the intense type . more sweeter than sucrose, including saccharin, Aspartame. These agents use for drinks. That have some weak antimicrobial effects. The bulk type, which are usually not as sweet including mannitol and soubital and xylital. xylital have been widely used.

三、增强宿主的抵抗力 Strengthening host ability to anti-caries

（一）加强孕期及婴幼儿保健 Strengthening oral care for pregnant women，infant & toddler

孕期注意口腔保健：①对患有龈炎、牙周炎孕妇应及时治疗，并加强口腔卫生，减少经口腔途径感染胎儿，防止早产儿。②注意孕期母亲的营养及全身健康，保证胎儿正常发育。

婴幼儿时期 在乳牙未萌出到恒牙胚发育期（3岁以内）应重视正确喂养及补钙，促使乳牙正常萌出及恒牙正常发育，减少牙冠钙化不全及釉质发育不全的出现。

（二）加强儿童及青少年口腔保健 Strengthening oral care for children & adolescent

在乳牙替换及恒牙萌生时期（5～12岁）应合理使用氟化物，促使年青恒牙钙化完全，增强抗腐蚀能力。

进行颊、猞面窝沟封闭，阻止菌斑滞留及龋病发生率。

建立合理饮食习惯，增强儿童咀嚼功能，促进颌骨发育，保证牙齿正常替换，减少因替换异常造成的牙列不齐。

加强儿童及青少年健康教育及建立良好自我保健习惯及意识（Table11）。

（三）建立口腔卫生保健网 Establishing oral heath care network

口腔卫生保健网的建立是口腔病防治的组织的保障。保健网应包括信息网。在我国保健网应有城市及农村两个系统。

农村口腔卫生保健网

一级：在省防治机构领导指导下的县级防治中心（或县医院口腔专科）专业口腔医师承

担。任务是：贯彻防治策略，进行技术指导及培训初级保健人员，能承担口腔常见病的诊断及治疗，并定期收集及反馈信息。

二级：指地区防治机构（或地区医院口腔科），有牙科助理医师组成的技术队伍。任务是贯彻防治措施，宣传口腔卫生知识，进行口腔防治：如窝沟封闭、氟保护期、早期充填等。

三级：村镇口腔保健站，由初期口腔卫生保健人员承担，任务是：宣传及指导人群自我保健，具有检查发现常见口腔病的能力，建立村镇人群口腔情况档案，定期向上级反馈信息。

城市口腔卫生保健网

一级：由市中心医院或牙病防治中心（所）承担，有中高级口腔防治人员组成的防治队伍。任务是负责落实组织防治工作的实施，指导及培养下级保健人员，解决口腔疑难病的诊断及治疗，制定每年的防治计划及建立完善的信息网络。

二级：主要指市区医院及防治组织，由地区防治机构及地区医院的中高级专业防治人员承担。任务是贯彻落实上级防治措施，培养指导初期保健人员，承担口腔常见病的诊断治疗，定期反馈口腔病发生及防治效果的信息。

三级：指社区医院及防治组织，由中高级口腔卫生保健人员承担的社区保健站，任务是落实防治措施，进行口腔健康教育，进行社区人群口腔健康监控，建立人群口腔健康档案，指导自我口腔保健知识及使用方法，能实行常见口腔保健措施如窝沟封闭，氟凝胶，预防性充填等措施，并定期反馈人群口腔防治信息。

表 4-11　Method of control caries

Caries factors	Method
Host	The resistant to demineralization (e.g fluoride)
	The use of sealants
	The use of plaque inhibitory varnishes
Euvironment	Reduce the consumption of sugar-containing food
	Reduce of eat carbohydrate containing food
	use sugar substitutes
Microflara	Oral hygiene
	Apply anti-microbial agents
	The use of replacemene therapy
	The use of vaccines

Strategies to control or prevent dental caries are based on ①Reducing levels of plaque, use to anti-plaque or antimicrobial agents ②using fluoride to encourage remineralization and to strengthen the resistance of enamel to acid attack ③reducing bacterial acid production by avoiding the frequent intake of fermentable carbohydrates in the diet, by replaceing such carbohydrates with sugar substitutes or by interfering with bacterial metabolism with fluoride of antimicrobial agents ④Enhancing the colonization resistance of plaque by replacecement therapy ⑤ using viccination or passive immunization against mutans streptococci.

第四节 窝沟封闭及预防性修复

Section 4 The Pit & Fissure Sealants and Preventive Restorations

Fluorides are highly effective in reducing the number of carious lesions occurring on the smooth surfaces of enamel and cementum. Unfortunately, fluorides are not equally effective in protecting the occlusal pits and fissures, where the majority of carious lesions occur. Considering the fact that occlusal surfaces constitute only 12% of the total number of tooth surfaces, it means that the pits and fissures are approximately eight times as vulnerable as the smooth surfaces. The placement of sealant is a highly effective means of preventing there.

窝沟封闭又称点隙裂沟封闭（Pit and Fissure sealant），是指不损伤牙组织，用一种树脂粘结材料涂布牙冠𬌗面、颊舌面点隙裂沟，目的是阻止致龋菌、产酸菌及酸性产物对牙体的侵蚀，以达到早期有效地防止龋病发生的有效方法。

Pit and Fissure is sealant applied to occlusal surfaces of the tooth, and the most effective means known to date for preventing and controlling occlusal caries sealing a suspected carious pit and fissure area of the teeth with a resinour sealant. It can prevent bacteria invasion and acid production for corroded tooth and to achieve effect iveness of preventing dental decay.

一、窝沟龋流行病学 Epidemiological status of fissure caries

国内外流行病学调查证实：乳牙龋病好发牙位首先是下颌第二乳磨牙，其次是上颌第二乳磨牙，依次第一乳磨牙及上乳前牙、下乳前牙。恒牙下第一磨牙最高，依次为下第二磨牙、上第一、第二磨牙、前磨牙、第三磨牙及上下前牙。总计磨牙在龋患比例最多。1980年岳松龄调查证实了恒牙咬𬌗区发生率最高。1978 ~ 1980 年美国的调查证实 5 ~ 17 岁 83% 与点隙窝沟有关，1982 ~ 1983 年调查显示 94% 的儿童为点隙窝沟。

1995年我国第二次口腔健康流行病调查显示，12岁人群窝沟龋占总龋的90.32%，光滑面龋为9.68%（表4-12）。

表 4-12 Comparison between fissure and smooth surface caries in 12 years group

	Number	Fissure caries	Smooth surface caries
DMFT	23 452	0.8	0.09
%	23 452	90.32	9.68

Epidemiological studies from the united states indicated that the molar pits and fissures are those most lihely to become carious.occlusal caries has been shonw to account for 83% of the total caries burdem in children between 5 and 17 years of age. There is good evidence from these data on both children and adults to indicate that the predilection for caries to develop on these specific sites continues through from time of eruption into early adult life. The second national epidemiological data in 1995 also indicate that occlusal caries rate at 12 years old is 90.32%.

总之，无论是乳牙还是恒牙，龋好发部位是磨牙，好发牙面是咬䅁面，好发点是点隙窝沟，则说明点隙窝沟是现代人类牙列中龋病特异性的易感部位。

二、牙䅁面点隙裂沟的解剖形态和龋损 Anatomic morphology of pit and fissure of the molar occlusal surface and carious lesion

点隙裂沟主要存在于磨牙咬䅁面，部分在下颌磨牙的颊侧面。磨牙咬䅁面裂沟有单个或多个点隙，前磨牙少，后磨牙多。根据解剖学形态分为 I、V、U、P、I、K 及 C 6 种类型。

但实际上可将其分为两个类型；V 型沟浅，口宽底尖；I型沟深沟窄底部膨大，龋易感的是 I 型，沟直径比牙刷毛还细，深沟底端呈膨大状，窝沟内壁釉质薄，钙磷含量相对少，而有机成分多（图 4-7）。

由于窝沟的解剖形态，容易滞留牙菌斑、唾液成分及精细的食物，无法清除，为菌斑内致龋菌的生长繁殖建立一个良好环境，则形成了龋好发的易感区域。

在沟内，早期发生的表面下脱钙，首先是沟壁部分，随着龋损发生则扩展到沟底部，在底部沿釉柱方向破坏病变已形成，继续较快的达到牙本质（图 4-6）。

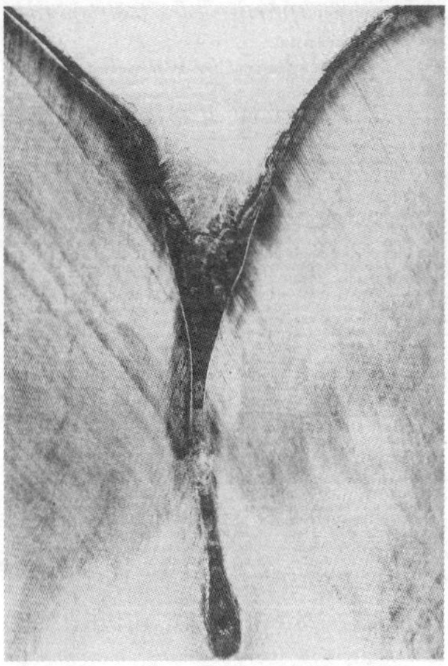

图 4-5 Dental plaque in a fissure on the occlusal surface of a molar.(Original magnification approx. × 100; courtesy K.U. Pang)

The susceptibility of the occlusal surface to carious attack results from the saclike morphology of the pit and fissures (图4-6). Occlusal fissures consist of deep narrow faults extending into the enamel

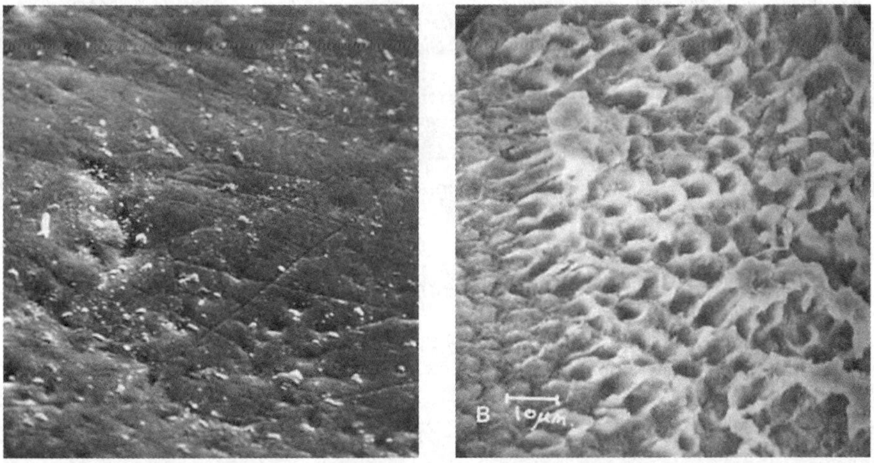

图 4-6 Scanning electron photomicrographs of human enamel surface. A. Unetched enamel. B. Etched enamel (× 1000)

and provide ideal sites for the entrapment of bacteria, food debris,and nutrients. Since the fissure widths usually measure only a fracton of the diameter of a toothbrush bistle, cleansing by conventional methods becomes almost impossible. Therefore, decay can readily occur.

Although pits and fissure are found predominatly in the occlusal surface of molars and premolars, pits are occasionally found at the cingulum of anterior teeth, particularly in the cingulum is pronounced, it is usually accomparnied by a deep pits.

Analysis of fissure contents indicates that the fissure are filled with food debris and plaque, which is made up of a variety of microorganisms. Studies by Theilade and coworkers in which surgicslly removed impacted molar crowns were placed in the mouths of volunteers, show that microorganisms invade the fissure areas within 24 hours following exposure to the oral environment vary with time and from patient to patient.

The carious process in occlusal surfaces beging with the accumulation of microorganisms and nutrients within the pits and fissure. Fissures with steep walls and narrow openings are particuiarly susceptible. The thin enamel at the base of the fissure udually leads to early dentinal involvement.

Enamel rods fan out in a radial fashion at the base of a pit or fissure. Enamel decalcification during caries attack proceeds along the enamel rods. As a result fissure caries are characterized by a cone or triangular shaped lesion having the apex at the enamel surface and its base at the dentioenamel junction (图4-7). This carious process spreads the area of attack across a large area of the dentin involving large numbers of dentinal tubules. This process can lead to considerable cavitation ans undemmining with little evidence of changes at the enamel surface.

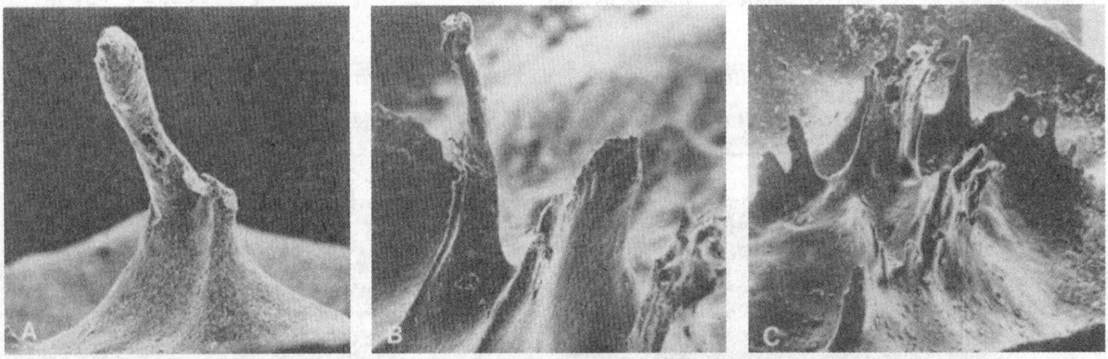

图 4-7 Replicas of fissures. (Galil, K. A. Gwinnet.A.J, Arch Oral Biol 20; 493, 1963) (× 100)

三、封闭剂的粘附机理 Adhesive mechanism of sealants

封闭剂与牙釉质表面粘附包括有：化学及机械的两种粘附作用。

1. 化学粘附（Chemical adhesion）

初期结合是封闭剂的离子和釉质表面羟基磷灰石的结合。第二种是两者氢键的分子结合。

2. 机械粘附（Mechanical adhesion）

是主要的结合。封闭剂与釉质表面的机械粘附基础必须先对釉质表面进行酸蚀（Acid

etching)。酸蚀首先是清除釉质表面菌斑及有机物质，之后使釉质表面粗糙，增加树脂的粘附面积。酸蚀后的釉质表面在偏光显微镜下可观察到三层组织学变化：第一层为酸蚀层，深达10μm，第二层叫丰富微孔层，深约20μm，第三层是定量微孔层，深约20μm。当釉质表面涂布封闭剂时，在封闭剂未固化时，可深入釉质微孔内25～50μm，形成树脂突与釉质形成牢固的机械结合。

Problems with Adhesion to tooth enamel

Successful adhesive bonding to enamel. Whether chemical or mechanical ,relies on tailoring the characteristics of the adhesive to those of the enamel surface. Bonding to enamel presents some difficult problems owing to surface contamination, the ever-present moist environment, and the nature of the enamel surface.

A considerable effort has been expended during the last two decades in search of materials that will form durable bonds weth the rather complex enamel surface. In general, effective adhesive bonding to a given surface can be achieved through a chemical and /or mechanical bonding. Chemical adhesion can occur by two mechanisms, primary chemical bonding (ionic, metallic, or covalent) and secondary chemical bonding (intermolecular forces such as hydrogen bonding or Van der Waal' forces).

Most adhesives do not rely on primary chemical bonding. In the case of pit and fissure sealants primary chemical bonding would require either direct covalent bonding between the tooth enamel and the sealant or incorporation of the sealant with the hydroxy-apitite crystal lattice through ionic bonding.

Acid etching of tooth enamel effectively removes the surface layer of enamel. The depth of the etch depends on the acid and its concentration.

Silverstone, investigating the etching process, has measured the loss of surface contour and the depth of histologic change obtained with various phosphoric acid concentration, including zinc oxide-buffered acid (表4-13). His results show that the greatest loss of contour and greatest histologic changes occur with acid concentrations in the 20 percent-30 percent range.

With 30 percent phosphoric acid there is a loss of controur some 10um in depth. In addition the histologic change (micropores) reaches an additional 20mm. The resin flows into the micropores leading to the sealant "tags", which provide micromechanical retention.

Etched enamel not covered by sealant soon returns to a normal appearance.

表 4-13　Depth of etch wnd histologic change in enamel（to nearest mm）after a 1-min exposure to various concentrations of phosphoric acid

	Concentration of phosphoric aicd（%）						
	20	30	40	50	50 ZnO	60	70
Depth of etch	14	10	9	7	6	2	2
Depth of histologic	20	20	15	12	10	4	2
Total depth of enamel afftected	34	30	24	19	16	6	4

（Siverstone LM: caries Reg8:2, 1974, Basel. S karger A6）

Chemically cures sealant are usually supplied as two liquids commonly called a catalyst and a universal or base. The catalyst contains sealant monomers and a peroxide, usually benzoyl peroxide, which is capable of producing polymerization-inducing free radicals.

Light-polymerized sealants are usually supplied a single sealant liquid that is painted onto the tooth surface and cured by exposure to an intense light of the proper wavelength. To ensure adequate shelf life, the photoinitiator may be supplied as a separate component that is mixed with the sealant before use.

Relationship between sealant physical properties and bonding

As discussed earlier, effective sealant bonding depends on microscopic mechanical interlocking and eletrostatic attraction between the sealant and etched enamel. Factors contributing to good bond strengths include the tensile strength of the sealant and the ability of the sealant to wet the enamel and to penetrate into the rough etched surface. Sealants that exhibit the greatest penetration into tooth enamel have low contact angles and low viscosities.

四、窝沟封闭的防龋作用 Caries preventive effectiveness of fissure sealants

1. 消除了人磨牙冠颊部窝沟滞留菌斑的发育缺陷。
2. 阻止了致龋菌、产酸菌在沟内定居。
3. 阻断了沟内细菌营养来源，特别是碳水化合物及菌斑的酸性产物在沟内停留，从而影响了细菌在沟内生存。
4. 封闭釉质表面多孔结构，阻止酸性产物渗入。
5. 如果封闭剂内有一定氟离子存在，则有利于釉质，特别是年青恒牙的矿化作用。

Efficiency and effectiveness of fissure sealants

Whether a method is efficient or effective, that is, does it do the job for least cost and does it achieve the stated objective, is a matter of real concern to clinicians.

Similarly, clincians need to be confident that sealants will be retained and that caries of the partial or non-sealed surface, which may go undetected, will not result.

The first longitudinal study to report on the use of fissure sealants employed a self-curing resin that was applied only once and not topped-up at any time subsequently. After 15 years, 28% of the Sealants were totally retaines and 35% were partially retained significantly nificantly, more of the sealed teeth remained caries free:68% as compared with 17% in the non-sealant group. A similar trial in Sweden took the opportunity to repair the sealants on first molars when the second molars were sealed. Data from this trial indicated that after 20 years, 87% of the surfaces were either fully or partially sealed and only 13% had active caries or had been restored.

五、殆面龋预防方法的研究进展 Study progress of preventative method of the occlusal caries

殆面部点隙裂沟龋的防治研究，早在20世纪20年代末用预防性银汞充填及窝沟磨除法，但都没有得到满意的效果。60 年代 Buouocore 在对牙釉质酸蚀研究基础上，开始了窝沟封闭剂的作用，当时所用的材料是氰基丙烯醇脂和聚氨基甲酸乙酯，但材料性能有限，未达到预期效果。

60年代以后，Reydhouse（1968）使用Bis-GMA进行了三年观察，显示了防龋的效果。Bis-GMA 为双酚 A 和甲基丙烯酸缩水甘油酯或双酚 A 二缩水甘油醚环氧与甲基丙烯酸混合反应。材料的聚合与釉质有较强的结合力。则 Bis-GMA 被广泛用于窝沟防治。但此时期为 365nm 紫外光固化封闭剂，但材料表面吸附紫外光多，影响深层固化完全、能量低、固化需要时间长、效果不理想。此后出现Bis-GMA自凝固化材料（化学固化），70年代后又研制出可见光固化机和固化剂，高强度光源使固化时间缩短在 10 ~ 20 秒内，操作比以前更方便，产品有 Consise（美国）。

近年进入封闭剂与氟结合研制时期，目前有两种形式含氟产品：一种是封闭剂内含氟盐。作用是封闭后释放氟离子，另一种是有机氟加入封闭材料内，以变换形式释放氟离子，这类材料有Teethmate（日本）、pulpdent（美国）两种。目前也有以含氟玻璃粒子材料作为封闭剂已达到封闭后释放氟的作用。最新的研制是激光固化，目的是增加釉质抗龋的强度最小限度地缩小凝固时间。

窝沟封闭剂自 60 年代研制以来，不断提高及完善封闭的效果，简化操作，使之更有利于广泛开展人群的早期有效地龋病防治。

Historically several agents have been tried to protect deep pits and fissures on occlusal surfaces.

In 1895, Wilson reported the placement of dental cement in pits and fissures to prevent caries. In 1929, B ǒ decker suggested that deep fissures could be broadened with a large round bur to make the occlusal areas more self-cleansing, a procedure that is called enameloplasty.

In 1923 and again in 1936 Hyatt advocated the early insertion of small restorations in deep pits and fissure before carious lesions had the opportunity to develop.

In the late 1960s and early 1970s, another option became available-the use of pit-and-fissure sealants. With this opton, a liquid resin is flowed over the occlusal surface of the tooth where it penetrates the deep fissures to fill areas that cannot be cleaned with the toothbrush. The hardened sealant presents a barrier between the tooth and the hostile oral environment. Concurrently, there is a signifi-cant reauction of Streptococcus mutans on the treated tooth surface. Pits and fissures serve as reservoirs for mutans streptococci, sealing the niche thereby reduces the oral count.

六、封闭剂的组成和种类 Component and type of sealants

1. 组成（Component）

窝沟封闭剂一般由三部分组成：

（1）基质　目前多用双酚 A- 甲基丙烯酸缩水甘油酯（Bis-GMA）。

（2）稀释剂　多为基质的单体成分，为增加流动性。常用的有甲基丙烯酸甲酯（牙托水）、三缩三乙醇双甲基丙烯酸酯和甲基丙烯酸缩水甘油酯。

（3）催化剂　也称促凝剂，包括两种：自凝引发剂有过氧化苯甲酰和芳香胺；光固引发剂；紫外光固引发剂为安息香醚类，可见光引发剂为 a- 二酮类光敏剂。

2. 种类（Type）

分为自凝及光固化两种：

（1）自凝固化封闭剂　基质加催化剂。使用时两种混合调拌，约2分钟固化，调后及时涂于窝沟处，注意防湿。此封闭剂使用简单、经济，不需要光照设备，不足之处容易产生气泡。

（2）光固化封闭剂　涂后需要照射可见光（430～490nm）或用紫外光源照射，此法固化快（10 ~ 20 秒）抗压强大，表面光滑、耐磨，操作容易，不用调拌，但要注意保护操作者眼睛。

The most successful materials as fissure sealants, in terms of retention and thus caries prevention, are the bis-GMA resins, These have been in use since the 1970s and have not been superseded, although newer materials enjoy a vogue until longevity studies indicate that they do not compare well with the conventional resins. There has been concern in recent years over the potential oestrogenicity of resin-based sealant materials. Bis-GMA is synthesized from Bisphenol A (BPA) and, theoretically, residual BPA could mimic the role of natural steroid hormones. This risk is negligible and should not dettact from the very positive health gain for a targeted sealant programme.

Materials used as fissure sealants: Early materials (1904 ~ 1950)

Silver nitrate

Zinc phosphate/amalgam (Prophylactic odontotomy)

Black copper cement.

Newer materials (1966-present day)

Cyanoacrylate resins

Urethane resins

Bis-GMA resins

Glass ionomer cements

Resin-modifired glass ionomer cements

The conventional resin-based materials may be either filled or unfilled, and light -or self-polymerizing.

The choice of material and thus the mode of polymerization is more a matter for personal choice, since there is no significant difference in retention rates between the different modalities. Visible light curing of resins or modified GICs for that matter, gives the clinician more control over the setting of the matter.

Variations in the type of materials that may be used as sealants

Filled or unfilled resins

Chemical or light-cured resins

Tinted clear or opaque resins

Resins, GICs or resin-modified GICs

Fluoride-releasing or fluoride-free

The primary difference between sealants is their method of polymerization. First-generation sealants were initiated by ultraviolet light, second-generation sealants are autopolymerized, and third-generation sealants use visible light.

Polymerization of the sealants

Two methods have been employed to catalyze polymerization: (1) light curing by use of a visible blue light (synonyms:photocure, photoactivation, light activation). And (2) self-curing, in which a menomer and a catalyst are mixed together (synonys: cold cure autopolymerization, and chemical activation).

Light-cured versus self-cured sealants

The main advantage of the light-cured sealant is that the operator can initiate polymerization at any suitable time. Polymerization time is shorter with the light-cured products than with the self-curing sealants.

Conversely, the self-curing resins do not require an expensive light source. They do, however, have the great disadvantage that once mixing has commenced, if some minor problem is experienced in the operating field, the operator must either continue mixing or stop and make a new mix.

The light-cured sealants have a higher compressive strength and a smoother surface; which is probably caused by air being introduced into the self-cure resins during mixing. Despite these differences, both the photocured and the autopolymerizing products appear to be equal in retention.

七、适应证、禁忌证 Indication、Contraindication

（一）适应证 Indication

1. 牙冠萌出，未发生龋损的乳牙及年青恒磨牙。乳牙在3～4岁，第一恒磨牙在6～7岁，第二恒磨牙在11～13岁为最适宜的封闭年龄。

2. 牙冠发育异常，如釉质发育不全。

3. 有充填物的牙，相邻牙无龋的窝沟。

Indications for sealants

Sealant placement needs to be considered in the context of risk factors, both for the individual patient and for individual teeth. It is vital that sealants are placed where there are sound clinical indications for doing so, supported by appropriate radiographs, in this case bitewings, and with consideration for the medical, dental, and social history of the patient.

As far as patient selection is concerned, the essential elements of those guidelines are that sealants are advised where a child or a young person is compromised in some way, and in whom the development of caries and /or its treatment is a risk. This is the main category of patients in whom sealants for the primary dentition may be advisable. The other categories of patients for whom sealants are advised are those who have experience of patients of caries in primary teeth.

If the risk factors outlined above are identified in a patient, then it is prudent to seal all susceptible sites on permanent teeth, as soon after eruption as is practicable.Where caries has affected one or more permanent molar teeth, the remaining sound pits and fissure should be sealed.

Criteria for selecting teeth for sealant placement

Following are the criteria for selecting teeth for sealing. Because no harm can occur from sealing, when in doubt, seal and monitor.

A deep occlusal fissure, fossa, or incisal lingual pit is present.

A sealant is contraindicated if:

Patient behavior does not permit use of adequate dry-field techniques throughout the procedure.

An open carious lesion exists.

Caries exist on other surfaces of the same tooth in which restoring will disrupt an intact sealant.

A large occlusal restoration is already present.

A sealant is probably indicated if:

The fossa selected for sealant placement is well isolated from another fossa with a restoration.

The area selected is confined to a fully erupted fossa, even though the distal fossa is impossible to seal due to inadequate eruption.

An intact occlusal surface is present where the contralateral tooth surface is carious or restored; this is because teeth on opposite sides of the mouth are usually equally prone to caries.

An incipient lesion exists in the pit-and fissure.

Sealant material can be flowed over a conservative class 1 composite or amalgam to improve the marginal integrity, and into the remaining pits and fissures to achieve a de facto extension for prevention.

（二）禁忌证 Contraindication

1. 窝沟龋进入牙本质深层，不易做封闭。
2. 窝沟处有龋损，同时出现牙髓炎症状 。

Other considerations in tooth selection

All teeth meeting the previous criteria should be sealed and resealed as needed. Where the cost-benefit is critical and priorities must be established, such as occurs in many public health programs , ages 3 and 4 years are the most important times for sealing the eligible deciduous teeth; ages 6 to 7 years for the first permanent molars; and ages 11 to 13 years for the second permanent molars and premolars.

The disease susceptibility of the tooth should be considered when selecting teeth for sealants, not be age of the individual . Sealants appear to be equally retained on occlusal surfaces in primary, as well as permanent teeth .Sealants should be placed on the teeth of adults if there is evidence of existing or impending caries susceptibility, as would occur following excessive intake of sugar or as a result of a drug-or radiation-induced xerostomia. They should also be used in areas where fluoride levels in community water is optimized, as well as in non-fluoridated areas.

八、临床效果及评价 Clinical effect and evaluation

（一）评价方法 Method of evaluation

窝沟封闭的临床效果评价包括：使用封闭剂的保留率和龋降低率，具体计算指标有：

保留率 计算是以单个牙为单位，可在一定时间内封闭后，殆面封闭剂的完整保留、部分及全部脱落三种占总封闭牙的百分比。

龋降低率　公式

$$\text{龋降低率} = \frac{\text{对照组总龋牙数} - \text{实验组患龋牙数}}{\text{对照组患龋牙数}} \times 100\%$$

（二）设计方法 Design methods

可采用自身半口对照，选择受试者口内同名对称磨牙，随机选一个牙作封闭，对侧牙为对照，进行观察分析。也有研究选择一种认可的封闭剂作阳性对照，不作处理的牙为阴性对照，作封闭剂为试验组，这样可以做到双盲。

（三）临床效果 Clinical effectiveness

Lewis Menaker 总结前人的临床窝沟封闭工作发现光固化封闭剂（Light-cured sealant）三年保留率为 58.3%，自凝封闭剂（Chemically cured sealant）为 84.2%（表 4-14）

表 4-14 Results from 3-year comparative study

	Light			Chemically cured sealant		
	1yr	2yrs	3yrs	1yr	2yrs	3yrs
Number of sealant-control pairs examination Retention (%)		258			233	
Complete	86.5	58.9	58.3	96.4	86.1	84.2
Partial	8.3	25.0	20.8	1.2	10.3	9.7
None	5.4	16.1	20.8	2.4	3.6	6.1

A quototion from J.D.Brook et a JADA 1979，99: 42 ～ 46

Weintraub 对以往窝沟封闭临床工作总结证明：7 年的完整保留率为 66%、10 年为 57%。观察到已有部分及全部脱落仍有防龋作用。研究公认，封闭剂保留率上颌较下颌高，前磨牙比磨牙高，其中原因归于牙位及操作难易（表 4-15）。

表 4-15 Effectiveness and evaluation of sealant

Years	Retentong (%)	Caries incidence (%)	Caries drop (%)
1	92	4	83
2	85	7	81
3	71	14	69
4	71	23	62
5	67	26	55
6	67	27	56
7	66	31	55
10	57	22	68

A quototion from Brunelle JA. Public Health Dent 1989, 49:317

Llodra 等（1993）对窝沟封闭临床效果进行了Mete分析，得出：①窝沟封闭剂是有效方法；②自凝封闭剂在保存率和龋降率上比光敏剂效果好；③封闭效果随时间延长而下降；④封闭剂与氟化物有相关作用；⑤1976年封闭效果龋下降不如 1976 年以前。

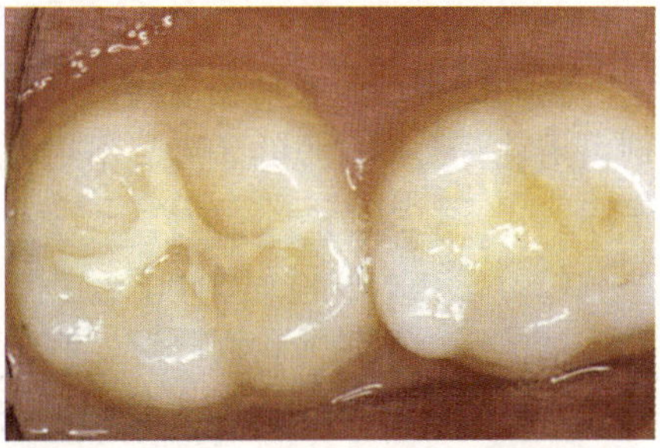
图 4-8 窝沟封闭临床效果

操作者对效果影响有待进一步观察。

从上述资料说明，窝沟封闭剂对龋的主要易感区—窝沟龋防治是有效的措施，应在社区人群特别是儿童及青少年人群中推广。

Evaluating retention of sealants

Resin sealants are retained better on recently erupted teeth than in teeth with a more mature surface; they are retained better on first molars than on second molars. They are better retained on mandibular than on maxillary teeth. This latter finding is possibly caused by the lower teeth being more accessible, direct sight is also possible; also, gravity aids the flow of the sealant into the fissure.

Teeth that have been sealed and then have lost the sealant have had fewer lesions than control teeth.

The number of retained sealants decreases at a curvilinear rate. Over the first 3 months, the rapid loss of sealants is probably caused by faulty technique in placement. The fallout rate then begins to plateau, with the ensuing sealant losses probably being due to abnormal masticatory stresses. After a year or so, the sealants become very difficult to see or to discern tactilely, especially if they are abraded to the point that they fill only the fissures. In research studies this lack of visibility often leads to underestimating the effectiveness of the sealants that remain but cannot be identified. Because the most rapid falloff of sealants occurs in the early stages, an initial 3-month recall following placement should be routine for determining if sealants have been lost. If so the teeth should be resealed. Teeth successfully sealed for 6 to 7 years are likely to remain sealed.

In a review of the literature, longest-term study reported that at the follow-up examination of the first molars, 20-years after sealant had been applied, 65% showed complete retention and 27% partial retention without caries. At a 15-year follow-up of the same sealants the second molars demonstrated the corresponding figures 65% and 30%, respectively. This study showed that pit-and-fissure sealants applied during childhood have a long-lasting, caries preventive effect. Mertz-Fairhurst cited studies in which 90 to 100% of the original sealants were retained over a 1-year period . One 10-year study using 3M Concise Sealant had a 57% complete retention and a 21% partial retention of sealant, all with no caries. Another study, using Dilton, registered 68% retention after 6 years. These are studies in which the sealant was paced and then observed at periodic intervals; there was no resealing when a sealant was lost. Where reseading is accomplished as needed at recall appointments, a higher and more continuous leves of protection is achieved. More recent studies report 82% of the sealants placed are retained for 5 years.

九、窝沟封闭的操作方法 Operating method of pit and fissure sealants

窝沟封闭的操作分为牙面清洁、酸蚀、冲洗、干燥、涂布、固化及检查 6 个步骤：

（一）牙面清洁 Cleansing enamel surface

封闭的第一步必须清洁窝沟区，用装有小毛刷或橡皮杯的低速手机，并占有清洁剂，清洁剂可用乳石及不含氟的牙膏，不用含油质的清洁剂及过细磨料。清洁后，将窝沟处清洁剂冲洗干净。

（二）酸蚀 Acid etching

清洁后，酸蚀牙聆面隔湿，吹干牙面，用小棉球（或小海绵块）蘸酸蚀剂，置被酸蚀的牙面上，轻轻搅拌酸蚀面积为受封闭的范围，一般为牙尖斜面2/3。酸蚀剂用 30% ~ 40% 磷酸液或磷酸凝胶。酸蚀时间：恒牙 20 ~ 30 秒，乳牙 60 秒。要注意酸蚀剂不要溢到口腔黏膜处。

（三）冲洗及干燥 Wash and dry

酸蚀后用蒸馏水冲洗，常用水枪或注射器加压冲洗10～15秒，如果用磷酸凝胶酸蚀，则冲洗时间加倍。冲洗后用压缩空气吹干。也可用无水酒精辅助干燥，此时注意防湿。

酸蚀指证：酸蚀冲洗干燥后，呈白色雾状表现，如没有则重复酸蚀。

（四）涂布封闭剂 Painting sealant

自凝封闭剂　封闭前用等量的基质及单体（含有引发剂和促凝剂），混合调拌10～15秒，均匀混合后在45秒内涂布完毕，一般凝固时间为1～2分钟。

光固封闭剂　直涂布牙面上，涂布封闭剂时应尽量覆盖酸蚀面，使封闭剂向窝沟内伸入，并且有一定厚度。

（五）固化 Solidification

自凝封闭剂可自行在1～2分钟固化，光固化封闭剂涂后，立即照射可见光或紫外光，照射距离为1mm。时间根据产品要求而定，一般20～40秒，封闭剂凝固后，漱口或用棉签将表面氧化物清除。

（六）检查 Inspection

封闭固化后，用牙科探针检查固化情况，有无气泡，是否达到窝沟封闭，有无过多的封闭材料，有无咬𬌗过高，发现上述问题及时解决。

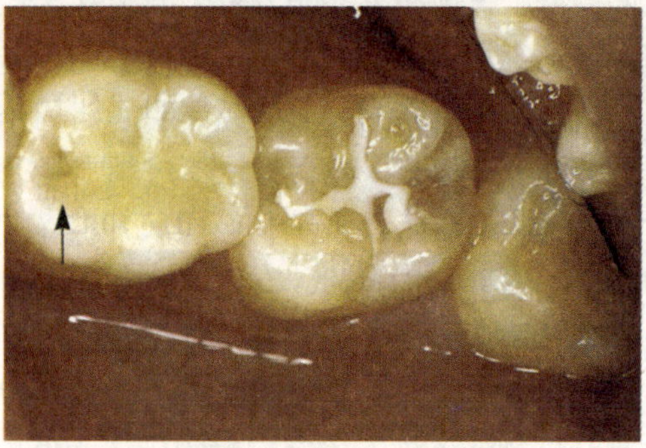

图 4-9　窝沟封闭定期复查

最后要求受封闭者定期（3个月、半年、一年）复查，脱落应及时重新封闭。

表 4-16　Six basic steps of performed sealant

Step	Method
1. Cleansing of the tooth	Teeth be cleaned by tooth brushing and pumicing then washing tooth surface
2. Acid etching	① The tooth should be isdated with coteon rolls or rubbes dam and etched
	② The ctching procedure is pertermed by dabbing the etching liquid lightly onto the occlusal surface by using cotton pledget for 60 second
	③ The etching liquied with 30% phosphoric acid
3. Wash and dry	The etching liquid should be remove from the tooth by flushing with water and drying
4. Painting sealant	① Light-cured sealant are painted onto the etched surface and cured by exposare to high-energy leght source
	② The chemically acitivated，sealants cure by mixing two or more component. The freshly mixed sealant is painted onto etched enamel
5. Solidification	① The chemically activated sealants solidified for 1 ～ 2minute
	② The light-cared sealants solidified for 20 ～ 40second
6. Inspection	① The examination should be done by using a sharp explorer
	② A properly applited sealant should be free of air bubbles，should fill the occlual pits and fissures

十、有关窝沟封闭效果的几个问题 Some problems on effectiveness of pit and fissure seanlant

1. 唾液污染酸蚀釉面　在进行封闭时，酸蚀后污染唾液是封闭剂脱落的主要原因之一。唾液污染酸蚀后的釉面，形成新的获得膜，阻止了封闭剂与釉质表面的化学及机械的结合。可溶性膜又形成了细菌及代谢产物渗入的间隙，造成了龋易感的条件及封闭剂脱落的原因。因此操作中出现唾液污染，应重新酸蚀，并加强防湿，再行封闭。

2. 酸蚀与龋病的易感　封闭剂脱落后，酸蚀面是否龋的使易感性增强，是防治人员是关注的问题。目前研究证明，封闭剂脱落后，局部釉质表面比未封闭处耐酸，患龋也较少。可能是釉质微孔中保留了树脂突的封闭作用。但不能就此不作处理，还应再次作封闭。

3. 早期龋的封闭　研究证明早期龋作封闭，可使龋停止发展。至于封闭剂是否可替代早期龋充填，还要进一步探讨。不过龋损是否长期停滞发展，还应看封闭后，龋损是否存留菌斑及酸性代谢产物不易清除，菌斑长期滞留仍有致龋危险。

4. 开展窝沟封闭，有效减少龋病发生　窝沟封闭是减少窝沟的有效措施。不需要特殊贵重设备，操作简便，对患者省时、省钱、无牙组织损伤。但这项工作还有待普级、加强。①提高口腔专业人员对窝沟封闭的认识；②大力培养初级技术专业人员；③健全社区防治，为窝沟封闭开展创造条件；④窝沟封闭应作为健康教育的内容。

十一、预防性树脂充填 Preventive resin restoration

预防性充填　是对窝沟早期及可疑龋，磨除少量龋损处组织，在酸蚀基础上，用树脂材料充填龋洞，并对 面涂封闭剂。充填材料一般用复合树脂材料或玻璃子水门汀作充填剂。两种材料与釉质的理化及机械性结合较好，辅以封闭剂，则可达到较好的防龋效果。

1. 适应证 Indication

①殆面窝沟粗糙（卡探针）；②窝沟较深；③变色（白垩色斑）。

2. 操作 Operation

（1）用圆钻除去窝沟龋坏组织，不作扩展磨除。

（2）冲洗干燥。

（3）酸蚀龋洞与殆面。

（4）龋洞内涂一层粘合剂后，再用树脂材料充填，材料凝固后，再涂一层封闭剂。

（5）检查充填是否完全及有咬殆高点。

十二、预防殆面龋的方法选择 Alternative method for occlusal caries prevention

1. 氟凝胶及氟泡沫方法，适用于无龋的乳牙及青年恒牙。

2. 窝沟封闭　适于：①萌出完全的乳牙及年青恒牙殆面沟。②窝沟较深，卡探针的窝沟及可疑龋。③充填过的窝沟龋，临近的无龋窝沟。

3. 预防性充填　适于：①殆面早期龋，可疑龋；②殆面限于釉质内小龋洞。

Option for protecting the occusal surfaces

Several options are now available to protect the occusal surfaces, with the selection depending on risk and professional's judgment. The first level of protection is simply to place a conventional sealant over the occlusal fissure system. This sealing preempts future pit-an fissure caries, as well as arrests incipient or reverses small overt lesions.

The second option reported by Simonsen in 1978, advocated the use of the smallest bur to remove the carious material from the bottom of a pit or fissure and then using an appropriate instrument to tease either sealant or composite into the cavity preparation. This he termed a preventive dentistry restoration.

The third option is use of glass-ionomers material for sealants, which is controversial. Due to their fluoride release and cariostatic effect, glass-ionomers have been used in place of traditional materials, as a pit-and-fissure sealant, however, resin sealants have shown much higher bond strength to enamel than glass-ionomers.

A fourth option reported by García-Godoy in 1986 involves the use of a glass-ionomers cement as the preventive glass-ionomers restoration (PGIR). The glass-ionomers cement (conventional or resin-modified) is placed only in the cavity preparation.

Each of these options requires a judgment decision by the clinician. That decision can well be based on the criterion that if an overt lesion cannot be visualized, it should be sealed;

The majority of all carious lesions that occur in the mouth occur on the occlusal surface. Which teeth will become carious cannot be predicted howerer; if the surface is sealed with a pit-and-fissure sealant, no caries will develop as long as the sealant remains in place.

第五节 非创伤性修复治疗
Section 5 Atraumatic Restorative Treatment, ART

Huge developments have occurred in oral health technology over the last few decades. However, the majority of the worlds population still suffers from untreated dental decay. The main reason for this is the continued dependency on traditional approaches to oral health care.

An innovative approach that brings safe and effective case for dental decay to communities without the need for expensive dental equipment is Atrumatic Restorative Treatment (ART). With this approach dental decay is removed solely with hand instrument and the cavity is filled with an adhesive, tooth coloured material which releaes fluoride. This material is also used to seal caries prone tooth surfaces. Thus ART is considered a combined preventive and restorative procedure to control dental decay This means that restorative case is no longer restricted to the dental clinic setting but can be delivered virtually anywhere. Even where traditional restorative care is available this approach brings care closer to all since injections are seldom required and dental drills are not used thereby making dental care more acceptable.

一、非创伤性修复治疗的建立基础 Established basis of ART

（一）龋的停止与发展 Stop and progress of dental caries

龋病的发生发展是致龋细菌的毒性产物与牙组织相互作用的过程。龋损的进展与停止，取决于致龋菌毒性物质量的持续。毒性物质不断增加，则破坏进展，减少或终止则组织自身出现再矿化或修复， 因此对龋洞进行充填或封闭处理，可使毒性物质减少，干预了龋的进展。多项研究证明：即使细菌毒性产物及腐质去除不完全，仍然可以使龋的破坏终止。

The development of dental caries

Caries begins on the enamel of the tooth. In the early stages there are no symptoms. The first sign that can be seen is a change in the colour of the enamel; it turm whitish.

If efforts to arrest the decay are not made, the dentine is then attacked. It becomes soft, spongy and yellow and the enamel becomes undermined.The decay then spreads through the dentine towards the pulp. At this stage the tooth may be painful when cold, hot or sweet food are eaten, or after biting on hard things. This is because the pulp is inflamed.

If a cavity is not treated with a restoration, the caries will continue to destroy the tooth; the hole will become bigger and the caries will rerach the pulp. The patient may then complain of toothache.

The destruction of the tooth crown can produce sharp enamel edges that hurt the tongue,cheeks or lips. The caries may destrory the tooth completely and it may have to be extracted.

However, not all decay. in dentine spreads further. There are ways to arrest decay. Arrested decay is dark in colour and is hard. However, the affected tooth may sill need to be restored to prevent the tongue or lips or cheeks from being cut on the sharp edges of the enamel.

Preventing and controlling dental caries

Caries can be prevented by the following 3 activities together:

by removing plaque completely, carefully and effectively at least once a day,

by restricting the frequency of eating and drinking sugary foods and drinks,

by increading the defense of the enamel, for example by using fluorides in toothpastes or mouthrinses.

Control of caries

A good way to do this is by placing an adhesive restorative material, such as glass-ionomer, into the cavity. This material will stick closely to the tooth and form a seal between the restoration and the tooth. It so prevents any more bacteria getting into the cavity. Glass-ionomeres also release fluoride into the surrounding tooth structures and make them stronger against further attack from bacterial acid.

（二）充填材料的发展 Development of filled materials

传统的龋洞修复方法是以合金材料的性能决定的，修复龋洞必须是固位型，因此要去除过多的牙组织，才能使汞合金与洞壁密合固位。充填后接触面是单纯机械性能接触，仍存在细菌及毒性物质渗入的间隙，因此充填不可能永久的。研究证明，汞合金充填寿命一般为6～10年。由于近代粘接材料的发展，龋洞修复使用了复合树脂和玻璃离子材料，使充填材料粘接密合加强。以 Black 原则，减少了充填牙体组织的损伤，并达到了修复治疗的效果。

20 世纪 80 年代，经过 Frencken 和 Phantumvanit 等人在不发达国家的连续临床观察，证实了 ART 技术可行，由此于 1994 年 WHO 正式提出在发展中国家推广 ART 技术。

The arrival of adhesive restorative materials has made it possible to develop tooth tissue-saving intervention techniques. These techniques, that include ART, have the potential to increase tooth life.

Buonocore introduced the first step towards a minimal intervention approach. He developed the acidetch technique in relation to composite resin. The historical development of adhesive restrative materials ispresennted in table 4-19.

表 4-17 Historical development of adhesive restorative materials

Resins	Macrofilled composites		Microfilled composites		Fine particle/hybrid composite
					Compomers
				Resin-modified Glass-ionomers	
Glass-ionomers		Conventional G.I`s		Metal containing GI`s	
	1955	1970	1980	1990	2000

Glass-ionomers

Dental glass-ionomers are supplied by the manufacturer as powder and liquid in separate bottles (hand-mix version) or in encapsulated form. The powder comprises a glass made up of a number of minerals, the most important being silicon oxide, aluminium oxide, and a fluorode glass. The liquid is usually a water-soluble organic aicd, commonly polyacrylic acid. Glass-ionomerrs bond to enamel and dentine without acid etching, leach fluoride into the tooth tissues and are pulp-friendly.

Resin- modified galss-ionomers

This type of adhesive restorative material was developed to improve the properties of conventional glss-ionomers. It is a combination of a glass-ionomers and a resin in the ratio of 80% to 20%. There materials have similar fluoride release patterns and antibacterial action to that of conventional glass-ionomers. Also the fluoride rechargeable effect is comprarable.

The differences between the two materials include the mechanism of adhesion that is both mechanism and chemical for resin-modified glass-ionomers. Resin-modified glass-ionomers have greater early physical strength that is attributed to the resin component. However, resin-modified glass-ionomers seem to wear more than conventional glass-ionomers.

Composite resins

This type of adhesive restorative material exists in many fomulation. Without an adhesive technique and chemicals, such as bonding and primer materials, a composite resin does not bond to tooth tissues.

Compomers

Compomers resemble composite resin in that they composed of filler particles and a resin. The filler particled are similar to those used in glass-ionomers.

Concluding comments

Table 4-18 presents strengths and weaknesses of the four adhesive dental restorative matrials according to requirements. It seems that conventional and resin-modifies glass-ionomers score high on the biological but low on most of the phydical requirements. The opposite is applicable for compomers and composite resin materials that score lowon the biological and high on most of the physical requirements. Conventional glass-ionomers and self-cured composite resins are available in hand-mix form and can therefore be used without light curing machines.

表 4-18 Strengths and weaknesses of four adesive dental restorative materials according to requirements

Strequirements	Glass-ionomers	Resin-modified Glass-ionomers	Compomers	Composite resins
Biological				
● biocompatible	+++	++	++	++
● encourages remineralization	+++	+++	+	−
● reduces demineralization	+++	+++	+	−
Physical				
● adhesion	++	++	+++	+++
● micro-leakage	++	++	++	++
● occlusal wear	+	−	++	+++
● fracture resistance	+	++	+++	+++
● thermal expansion	+++	++	+	+
● aesthetics	+	+	++	+++
● moisture tolerant	+++	++	−	−
General				
● hand-mix	+++	N/A	N/A	+
● self curing	+++	N/A	N/A	+
● ease of use	++	++	+	+
● cost	?	?	?	?
● shelf-life	++	++	++	++

+++ very good， ++ satisfactory， + could be better，−poor. N/A not available

二、适应证及禁忌证 Indication and Contraindication

（一）适应证 Indication

1. 乳牙及恒牙釉质及牙本质浅龋
2. 手动器械可进入的龋洞

（二）禁忌证 Contraindication

1. 龋患附近有肿胀（脓肿）或瘘管（脓肿开口于口内）。
2. 牙髓外露。

3. 牙髓有慢性炎症。
4. 龋洞明显，但手术器械不能进入。
5. 邻面洞不易操作。

In general, ART can be applied when:

there is a cavity involving the dentine and

that cavity is accessible to hand instruments.

ART should not be used when:

there is presence of swelling (abscess) or fistula (opening from abscess to the oral cavity) near the carious tooth,

the pulp of tooth is exposed,

teeth have been painful for a long time and there may be chronic inflammation of the pulp,

there is an obvious carious cavity, but the opening is inaccessible to hand instruments,

there are clear signs of a cavity, for esample in a proximal surface, but the cavity cannot be entered from the proximal nor the occlusal directions.

三、ART途径要求的器械及材料 Equipment and materials for the ART approach

1. 材料 Materials

玻璃离子修复材料（Adhesive restortive material glass-ionomers）

2. 器械 Instruments

（1）口镜（Mouth mirror） 暴露充填区视野。
（2）探针（Explorer） 探查龋洞范围及深度，除外髓腔暴露。
（3）牙科镊子（Pairv of tweezers） 用棉球清洁消毒龋洞，涂布封闭剂等。
（4）挖匙（Spoon excavator） 去除腐质，根据龋洞大小选择不同型号挖匙。
（5）牙用手斧（Dental hatchet）（或锄型器） 扩大洞口取出釉质悬突。
（6）玻璃盘（板）和调和刀（Mixing-pad and spatula） 用于混合充填材料。
（7）雕刻刀（Applier/carver） 扁平一端填洞，尖锐一端修正外形。
（8）树脂条和T形带（Petroleum jelly and plastic strip） 作邻面洞成形片。
（9）木楔（Wedges） 固定邻面树脂条。

Before applying the ART approach, it will be necessary to assemble all the equipment and materials required.This includes: appropriate supports for the patient and for the operator, dental instrument, restorative materials, relevant consumable materials and, a source of lighting.

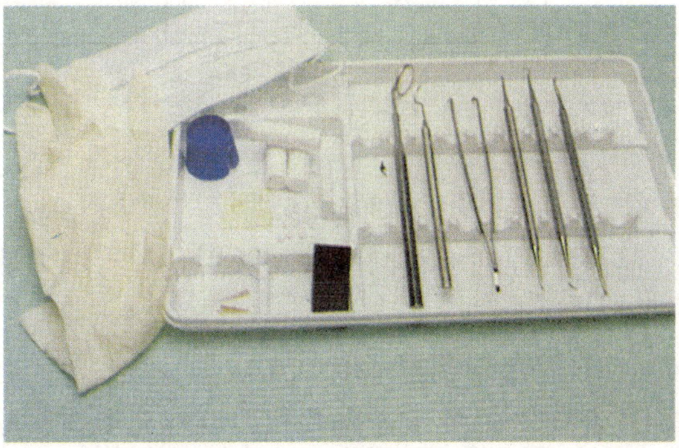

图4-10 ART的器械及材料

四、ART途径的操作步骤 The ART approach-step by step

1. 洞形准备 Preparation of cavity

（1）防湿、擦去菌斑、清洁牙表面、调整龋洞口大小，洞口小则用手斧扩大入口清理破碎釉片。

（2）用挖匙伸入龋洞，刮除腐质，接近髓腔腐质应保留，并保持龋洞干燥。

（3）令病人咬合，如对颌牙尖接触洞口，应作调𬌗。

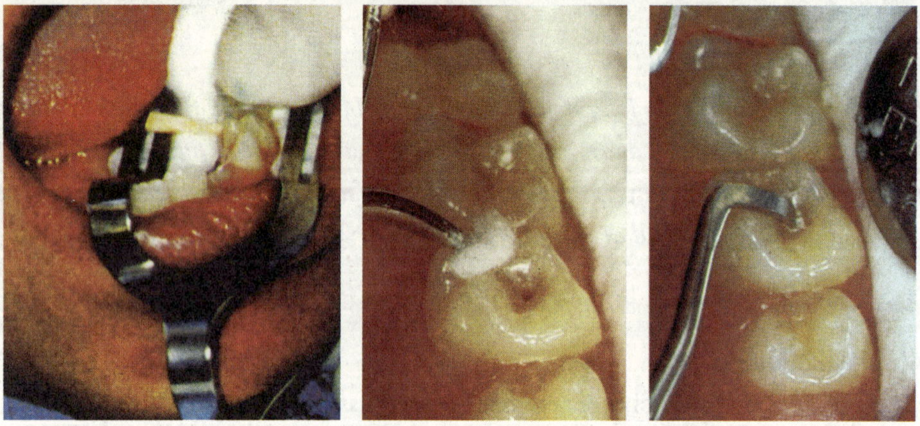

图 4-11 洞形准备

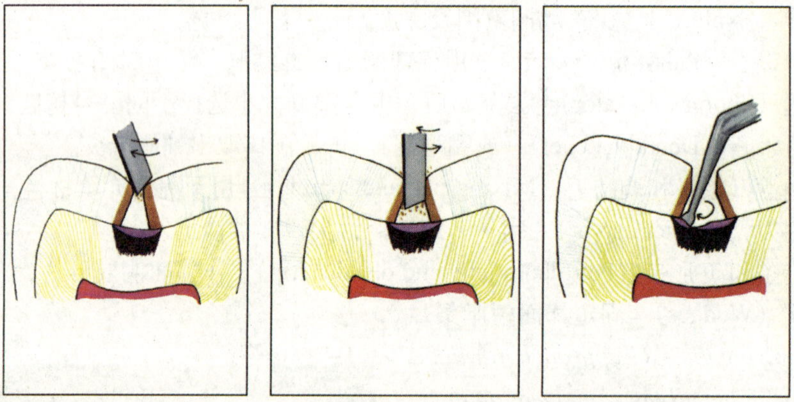

图 4-12 洞形准备

2. 清洁 Cleansing

用处理剂涂窝洞壁（一般用10%弱聚丙烯酸），用小棉球蘸处理剂涂布10秒后，立即冲洗两次，并干燥。

3. 混合与调拌 Mixture

根据产品要求，用调和刀调拌充填材料粉及液体，在20～30秒完成。

尽快将材料放入洞内。如果充填材料失去光泽变干，则重新调拌。

4. 充填 Filling

（1）单面洞　防湿、干燥龋洞，将调好的材料，用雕刻刀钝端将材料放入洞内，用挖匙凸面压紧玻璃离子，使材料稍高于牙面，充填材料应包括余下的点隙窝沟，注意避免气泡。然后带手套，手指涂少许凡士林放在充填物上压紧于洞内，使之充满，30秒后离开。用咬合纸检查有无过高点，用器械调整，然后再涂一层涂料。最后瞩病人漱口，一小时后进食。

（2）复面洞　充填方法与单面洞原则相同。不同之处是注意保持外形，特别是邻面。注意正确放置成形片。

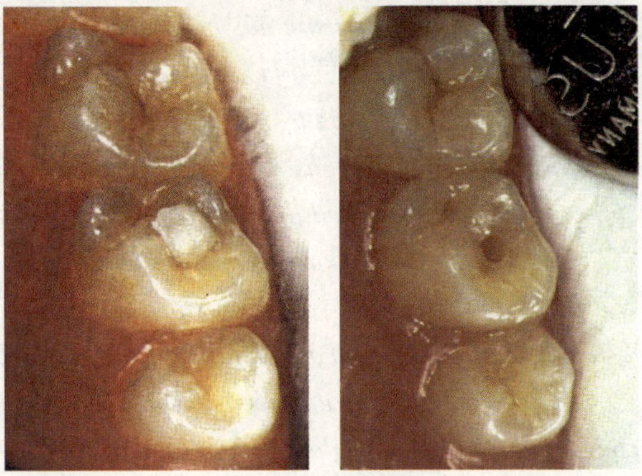

图 4-13　清洁

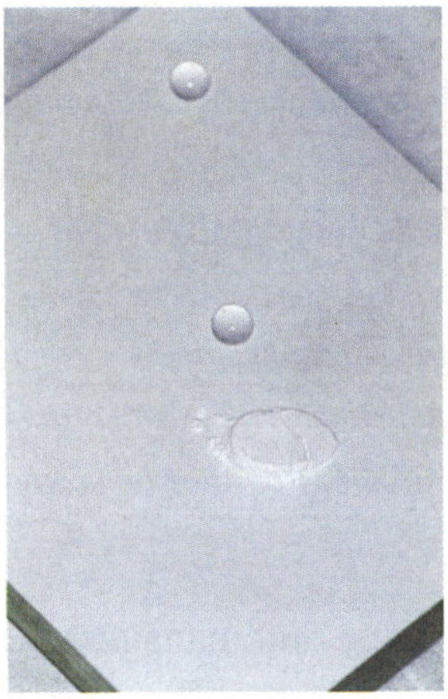

图 4-14　混合与调拌

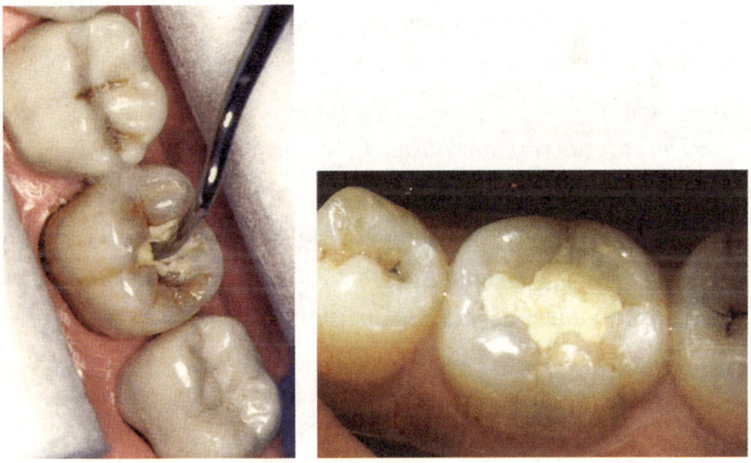

图 4-15　充填

A step-by-step guide to restoring single-surface cavities using ART

1. Preparation of the ART instruments and materials prior to cavity preparation

Before starting the cavity preparation ensure that all the instruments and materials that are likely to be required are laid out in a logical and ordered manner. The dental instruments should be arranged in the sequence that they are going to be used. A suggested layout is shown in 图 4-11

2. Isolation of the operating site

Isolation is an essential component in the placement of ART restorations as saliva must be controlled.

When placing ART restorations, isolation is usually achieved by means of cotton wool rolls.

For use in children, a cotton wool holder (图 4-11) can be used.

3. Examining the cavitated tooth

Once the operating site has been correctly isolated, the tooth and the extent of caries can be examined more easily. (图 4-11).

4. Gaining access to the carious lesion

In small carious lesions, where the opening to the cavity is small it is often necessary to widen the entrance for access. A dental hatchet can be used for this task.

5. Removal of soft, completely demineralized, dentine

Excavators are now used to remove soft dentine. (图 4-12).

6. Conditioning the cavity and adjacent pits and fissures

The use of hand instruments on the dentine surface results in a smear layer. In order to improve the chemical bonding of the glass-ionomer to the tooth tissues this smear layer must be removed by the use of a conditioner. (图 4-13).

7. Mixing the glass-ionomer

Mixing pad with one drop of liquid in the corner for conditioning and one drop in the centre for mixing with the powder. (图 4-14).

8. Restoring the cavity and filling the pits and fissures

The mixed glass-ionomer must be used promptly since any delay will compromise chemical bonding to the tooth surface.

The procedure si now finished. Ask the patient to avoid eating for at least an hour (图 4-15)

Restoring multiple-surface cavities using ART

As mentioned previously, the ART approach has only been validated for single-surface restorations using glass-ionomers. Since studies evaluating multiple-surface ART restorations with various adhesive materials are currently in progress, the clinical outcomes cannot be stated precisely.

五、ART修复失败的原因与处理 Failed ART restoratives: cause and management

1. 病例选择不当：①龋洞过大，洞壁薄、易断裂，而使充填物脱落；②露髓充填。
2. 洞内腐质去除不够。
3. 防湿不够，污染唾液，使充填材料与洞壁结合不好而脱落。
4. 充填前未涂处理剂，充填后结合不好，易脱落。
5. 材料调合时间过长，材料固化，则充填材料与洞结合不完全，而易脱落。

上述失败原因主要是违反操作原则，不恰当选择病例及操作不熟练。因此应严格操作，熟练充填技术，正确选择病例，提高充填效果。

what were the perceived reasons for failure of ART restorations?

A restoration may be considered to have failed for a number of reasons:

there has been marked wear of the resto-rative material

the restoration has fractured

the restoration is completely or partly missing

caries has developed at the restoration margin or in the adjacent fissure.

Material - related reasons included

the mechanical strength of the glass-ionomers that had fractured (most frequent use for failure)

excessive wear of the glass-ionomers, resulting in exposure of the enamel at the cavity margine of more than 0.5mm. This proved to be a rare cause for failure.

Operator - related reasons included

incomplete removal of dentine caries that inhibited proper bonding of the dental material, resulting in loss of the restoration

inadequate conditioning

inadequate isolation of the operating site

improper mixing of the glass-ionomer, resulting in the mixture being too dry or too wet

poor insertion of the glass-ionomer filling material into the cavity, particularly in small cavities, resulting in sub-surface voids which eventually became exposed.

How to manage a failed or defective ART restoration?

The options available to manage failed ART restorations are replacement or repair. If a replacement is indicated, the ART approach can be used again or another treatment modality could be used. If a repair is indicated for a glass-ionomer ART restoration using the same material, follow the description of the step-by-step approach. However, if a different material is required, follow the directions-for-use supplied by the manufacturer.

六、ART 的实际应用 ART as a practice builder

1. 优点及不足 Advantages

（1）ART 技术符合现代预防的基本观点。采用粘结材料充填，减少了牙体损伤。

（2）不用电源，不需昂贵口腔设备。充填器械便于携带，便于到条件差的社区及农村开展防治工作。

（3）操作简便，可推广使用。

（4）病人容易接受，并避免电机造成的恐惧心理。

（5）玻璃离子材料含氟离子，起到氟释放，促进再矿化作用。

2. 不足之处 Limitation

（1）材料在混合反应后出现体积收缩，则产生微漏。

（2）ART 的应用，长期效果还有待进一步观察、积累和改进。

从国内外实际临床证实，ART非常适合发展中国家及我国农村及边远小城镇条件简陋的地方开展防治工作，使更多人群得到初级口腔保健。

Advantages and limitations of ART

In summary, the advantages and limitations of the ART approach, are listed below:

Advantages

A biological friendly approach involving only the removal of soft, demineralized, tooth tissues. This results in minimal cavity preparations, which maximally conserves tooth tissue.

Not only is the cavity filled, but also the margin of the restoration and adjacent pits and fissures are filled with the same material. This results in a combined preventive and restorative procedure that is considered to prolong tooth life.

Little discomfort is experienced with this approach, thereby reducing the need for local anaesthesia to a minimum.

Anxiety, often found with traditional restorative procedures, is not induced.

Only easily available and inexpensive hand instruments are used, instead of expensive electrically driven dental equipment.

Infection control is straightforward and simple, since very few instruments are used, e.g. there is no need for sequentially autoclaved handpieces.

The cost is relatively low.

There is a high level of survival for single surface ART restorations after 3 years, placed using condensible glass-ionomer.

Limitations

Long-term results of ART restoration survival are not yet available.

Currently, it is recommended that the approach be restricted to single-surface restorations in permanent teeth, at least until studies in multiple-surface lesions and in primary teeth are completed.

七、ART 未来的发展方向 Future direction for ART

1. ART 技术的核心是材料，需改进材料体积收缩出现微漏的问题。另外，黏着性、压强及耐磨性还应不断增加，使 ART 充填技术，达到理想的远期效果。

2. 应广泛在边缘地区、广大农村及城镇开展，不断总结经验，完善 ART 技术，使之得到稳定及长期效果。

3. ART 技术适合我们的国情，应将它列为我们的口腔预防工作的范畴，列为防龋工作中重要措施。

The preceding context have described how the ART approach embodies the most current in scientific rationale relating to caries management. Thus, as has been shown, the ART approach to cavity cleaning and the choice of appropriate adhesive restorative materials is based on sound scientific research. The clinical outcomes resulting from applying this approach have shown extremely good results and point to a promising future. However, it must be remembered that the ART approach remains in its infancy. Despite this, the last five years have witnessed many new developments and an explosion of interest in the ART approach. As with any new approach, ART will be subject to further development and new directions for the approach will present themselves. These must, however, be subject to scientific evaluation and validation.

It is inevitable that the ART approach will be subject to further development and application. In spite of this, ART currently is an effective minimal intervention approach to the control of caries. It is anticipated that the principles adopted by ART, namely those of minimal intervention and maximal prevention will herald a new direction for the future of dentistry.

小结 Summary

1. Dental caries is a multifactorial, ubiquitous, plaque-related chronic infection of tooth. the main factors involved in the development of dental caries are the key oral bacteria, dietary carbohydrate, a susceptible tooth surface and saliva.

2. The earliest clinical evidence of dental caries is the "White spot" which is reversible; cavitation represents irreversible lesion.

3. The frequency of sucrose intake is more decisive than total consumption in the development of dental caries.

4. The major cariogenic bacteria are s.mutans, lactobacillus and a.naeslundii.

5. High salivary or plaque count of lactobacillus,or mutans streptococci are related in many cases to a high risk of disease.

6. The pit and fissure sealants are effective method on early caries lesions.

7. Prevental strategies of dental caries should be comprehenisne measure.

思考题 Review questions

1. Four factors of caries aetiology and the relations between them.
2. Main cariogenic bacteria and virulence factors of them.
3. Which risk factors of dental caries are in the mouth?
4. Idication of the pit and fissure sealants.
5. Indication of the ART.

参考文献 References

1. Phili Marsh and Michael V. Martin. Oral Microbiology. Fourth edition. MPG Book Ltd, 1999
2. Howard KK. et al. Oral Bacterial Eecology the molecular basis. Biddles Ltd, 2000
3. Bowden G.H.W. and I.R.Hamilton. Survial of oral bacteria. Grit Rev. oral Biol Med. 1998, 9:54～85
4. 杨圣辉. 龋活性试验 - 变形链球菌附着板方法的研究. 北京口腔医学, 1999, 7 (4): 163 ～ 166
5. 王伟健等. 北京儿童乳恒牙患龋状况八年纵向研究. 中华口腔医学杂志, 2003, 35 (4): 279 ～ 281
6. 郭继华等. 靶向融合防龋 DNA 疫苗的构件与体外细胞表达研究. 中华口腔医学杂志, 2003, 38 (4): 282 ～ 284
7. Fan M.W. et al. A DNA vaccine encoding a cellsurface protein antigen of streptococcus mutans protects gnotobiotic rats from caries. J Dent Res, 2002, 81: 784 ～ 787
8. Frencken JE, Holmgren CJ. Afraumatic Restorative Treatment for dental caries. Nijmegen STIbook, 1999
9. Massachusetts Department of Public Healtih. Prekenting pit and fissure caries: A guide to sealant use, 1986

（杨圣辉）

第五章　氟化物与人类健康

Chapter Ⅴ Fluoride and Human Health

概述 Overview

氟是人体所需的微量元素之一，应用氟化物预防龋病是 20 世纪预防口腔医学对人类的伟大贡献之一。半个世纪以来氟化物预防龋齿的历史表明，全球范围龋齿患病上升趋势受到遏制，发达国家龋齿患病水平显著下降，作为公共卫生措施的社区群体应用氟化物如饮水氟化和广泛使用含氟牙膏是主要因素。但是，摄入氟过量则会对人体健康产生危害，必须以科学的态度全面了解和认识氟化物对预防龋病的作用和对人体健康的影响，真正做到除氟害兴氟利。这是我们学习本章节的目的。

This part describes how the human physiology deals with fluoride when the material is ingested, fluoride's effect on our health, and how it works to prevent caries, and how it works to cause fluorosis. Achieving the best possible caries prevention usually requires the use of population-based programmes such as adding fluoride to drinking water and the widespread use of fluoride toothpastes.

要点 Key points

- 氟的防龋机制 The mechanism of fluoride for caries prevention
- 饮水氟化 Water fluoridation
- 含氟牙膏 Fluoridated toothpaste

第一节　氟化物与人体健康

Section 1 Fluorides and General Health

应用氟化物预防龋病是 20 世纪预防口腔医学对人类的伟大贡献之一。氟是人体所需的微量元素之一，人体摄入适量的氟可以预防和治疗龋病和骨质疏松症，特别是在儿童青少年时期牙发育生长和矿化阶段。人体摄入氟过少或过多则可能对健康产生影响或危害（主要是牙和骨骼等硬组织）。

一、氟的环境分布 Distribution of fluorides in the environment

氟是化学元素周期表中第 17 位卤族元素，由于化学性质活跃，自然界中常以化合物和络合物的形式存在。氟广泛分布在土壤和岩石中，约占地壳总量的0.06% ~ 0.09%（即地壳含氟量为600 ~ 900 mg/kg）。氟的成矿能力强，地壳中含氟的矿物近百种，主要有氟磷灰石、萤石、冰晶石、磷灰石、云母和电石等。各种岩石都含有一定量的氟，最高可达2500 mg/kg。生产磷肥的原料矿中含氟量可高达 42000 mg/kg。

虽然氟在自然界中丰富而广泛，但值得注意的是绝大多数都以矿物质和化合物形式存在，因此不具有生物活性作用。

Fluorine is seventeenth in the order of frequency of occurrence of the elements that it is the most electronegative of all chemical elements and combined chemically in the form of fluorides in nature. Fluorine represents about 0.06%~0.09% of the earth's crust. In rock and soil, fluoride may occur in a wide variety of minerals, including fluorspar, cryolite, apatite, mica, hornblende, and so on. Some kinds of rocks contain significant amounts of fluoride - up to 2500mg/kg. The rock phosphates used for the production of fertilizers, can have a fluoride content up to 42000 mg/kg.

There is an obvious abundance of fluoride in the world, but it should be remembered that most of it is firmly bound to minerals and other chemical compounds and is therefore not biologically available in its usual form.

表 5-1　含氟较多的矿物质

名 称	化学成分	氟 (%)
磷灰石	$Ca_5(PO_4)_3(OH, F, Cl)$	3.4
萤石	CaF_2	49
冰晶石	Na_3AlF_6	54

自然条件下大气中的氟主要来自土壤尘埃、工业废气、煤烟和火山灰等，含氟量约0.01mg/m^3，雨雪中的含氟量平均0.1mg/L，江河水中含氟量一般为0.01 ~ 0.3mg/L，有的要高些。地下水含氟量较地面水高，在大部分地区为0.2～4.7mg/L，各种植物普遍含有一定量的氟，以鲜重计平均为0.1mg/L。谷类一般在1mg/L以下（除氟污染外），蔬菜和水果很少超过0.3mg/L。海洋植物平均为4.5mg/L。茶叶以干重计含氟量范围可从10 ~ 1500mg/L，老叶比新叶高。陆地动物肉类含氟量以鲜重计约为0.3～3.6mg/L，海洋鱼类含氟量比陆地动物高。乳类含氟量很低，基本不受动物饮食含氟量的影响。

世界范围内，高山脚下和海洋地质沉积带水中的含氟量较高，如从叙利亚经约旦、埃及、利比业、阿尔及利亚、摩洛哥到非洲大裂谷。另一地质带由土耳其经伊拉克、伊朗、阿富汁到印度、泰国北部和中国。在美洲、中国和日本也有类似的地质带。

我国地下水含氟量超标地区主要分布在东北、华北和西北，此外在黄淮海平原的第四系沉积地质带水的含氟量也较高，南部各省多是零星分散的超标点。海水含氟量为0.8 ~ 1.4mg/L，温泉水含氟量常较高在3～6mg/L。个别冷泉水也较高。我国大城市自来水含氟量都较低，90%以上含氟量在0.5mg/L以下。

In natural situation, fluorides is widely distributed in the atmosphere (0.01mgF-/m^3), originating from the dusts of fluoride-containing soils, from gaseous industrial waste, from the domestic burning of coal fires, and from gases emitted in areas of volcanic activity.

In the world, waters with high fluoride content are usually found at the foot of high mountains and in areas with geological deposits of marine origin. Typical examples are the geographical belt from the Syrian Arab Republic through Jordan, Egypt, the Libyan Arab Jamahiriya, Algeria, Morocco, and the

Rift Valley. Another belt is the one stretching from Turkey through Iraq, the Islamic Republic of Iran, and Afghanistan to India, northern Thailand, and China. Similar areas can be found in the Americans and in China and Japan.

In China, the high fluoride content of underground water is mainly distributed in the north, northeast and northwest of China. The fluoride concentration in tap water is lower that 90% is less than 0.5mg/L in big cities.

二、人体氟代谢和排泄 Fluoride metabolism and excretion

（一）氟的吸收 Absorption of fluoride

每天随着饮水和食物经消化道进入人体的氟，主要在胃肠吸收，胃部吸收受胃液pH影响很大，小肠吸收比率高速率快，尤其是小肠上段以扩散作用的方式可很快吸收约75%～90%，液体吸收的比率要比固体的高而且吸收速率快。溶解度低的氟化物吸收率低，如骨粉中只有37%～50%的氟能被成人吸收。食品氟的吸收率取决于食品中的无机氟含量，食品中钙和铝含量高时，氟的吸收会降低。一般摄入氟后30分钟可达到吸收峰值，血浆峰值浓度可达30～60分钟。口腔黏膜吸收量很小，不足每日吸收量的1%。除了消化道外，呼吸道和皮肤也能有少量吸收。

Approximately 75% ～ 90% of fluoride ingested each day is absorbed from the alimentary tract, with higher proportions from liquids than from solids. The half-time for absorption is approximately 30 minutes, so peak plasma concentrations usually occur within 30-60minutes. Absorption across the oral mucosa is limited and probably accounts for less than 1% of the daily intake. Absorption from the stomach occurs readily and is inversely related to the pH of the gastric contents, and most of the remaining fluoride that enters the intestine will be absorbed rapidly. High concentrations of dietary calcium and other captions that from insoluble complexes with fluoride can reduce fluoride absorption from the gastrointestinal tract.

（二）氟的体内分布 The distribution of fluoride in the body

1. 在体液和软组织中 Fluoride in body fluid and soft tissues

氟在血液中以两种形式存在。一种是离子状态的氟，占血浆氟的15%～20%，它既不与蛋白质或其他血浆成分结合，也不与软组织结合。只有这种氟才参与生理反应，为医学、公卫和口腔专业所关注。另一种是与脂溶性有机质呈结合状态的氟，这种结合氟不像游离氟那样受摄入量的多少所影响。饮水中的氟是血液中氟的主要来源，在健康的青年和成年人中，饮水中氟含量（mg/L）与血浆中含氟量（μmol/L）的数值基本一致。血浆含氟量随年龄增长有增加的趋势。根据摄入氟对血浆氟浓度平衡的需要，婴儿出生后早期血氟可以是正平衡或负平衡。氟浓度在血浆和细胞外液及大多数软组织的细胞内液之间呈稳定分布状态，细胞内液较低，但可因血浆浓度的改变而同时发生相应的变化。随肾脏的排泄，肾小管内氟浓度在组织与血浆间的比值不到 1.0。氟浓度在几种特殊体液中如龈沟液、导管内唾液、胆汁和尿液，与血浆中也呈稳定分布状态。氟的转移是以氟化氢的形式通过膜渗透的扩散机制进行，因此任何改变膜的通透性和 pH 值的因素都可影响氟在组织间的分布。

There are two general forms of fluoride in human plasma. The ionic form, detectable by the ion-

specific electrode, is about 15% ~ 20% in the plasma that the one of interest in medicine, public health and dentistry. Ionic fluoride is not bound to proteins, to other components of plasma, or to soft tissues. The other form consists of several fat-soluble organic fluorocompounds, which can be contaminants derived from food processing and packaging. The concentration of ionic fluoride in soft and hard tissues is directly related to the amount of ionic fluoride intake, but that of the organic fluorocompounds is not.

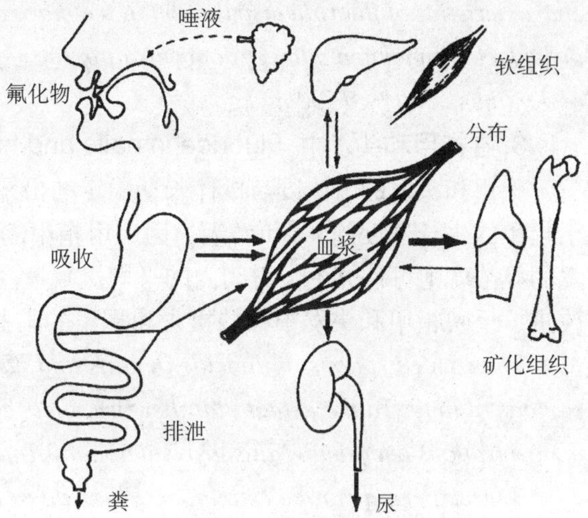

图 5-1　氟代谢示意图

Provided that water is the major source of fluoride intake, fasting plasma-fluoride concentration of healthy young or middle-aged adults, expressed as micromoles per liter (μmol/L) , are roughly equal numerically to the fluoride concentrations in drinking-water, expressed as milligrams per liter (mg/L) . Plasma-fluoride concentration tend to increase slowly over the years. Fluoride balance in infants can be positive or negative during the early months of life, depending on whether intake is sufficient to maintain the plasma concentration that existed at the time of birth.

2. 在骨和牙中 Fluoride in bone and teeth

骨骼和牙所积蓄的氟占全身氟的99%（主要在骨松质），正常人24小时摄入后吸收入血的氟约有50%沉积于钙化组织。儿童时期血氟主要向骨组织转移，骨氟随摄氟量和年龄而增加，老年时期则骨氟释放入血氟增加排泄。

牙中氟积蓄与骨骼基本相似，在牙形成和矿化时期以及矿化后进入牙组织，但主要在牙形成和矿化时期。萌出到口腔后可因环境氟的变化（唾液、菌斑、饮食等）牙氟也发生变化，主要在牙釉质表层（约50μm），牙本质髓腔面随着生理性继发牙本质的不断形成而有所增加。氟的分布在牙釉质表层最高（500 ~ 4000mg/kg），到牙釉质深层降低为50 ~ 100mg/kg。牙本质的氟浓度在 200 ~ 1500mg/kg。

Approximately 99% of the body burden of fluoride is in bone and teeth. Of the fluoride absorbed in blood each day, approximately 50% will be associated with calcified tissues within 24 hours and remainder will be excreted in urine. The distribution is shifted strongly in favor of greater retention in the very young and is probably shifted in favor of greater excretion in the later years of life.

The fluoride content of tooth tissues is same with bone that is reflects the biologically available fluoride at the time of tooth formation; in the bulk of the enamel, once formed, which continue to accumulate throughout lift. Post-eruptive change is reflected in the outer layer of enamel (about 50 μm) owing to diffusion of fluoride from the oral environment (saliva, dental plaque and ingested materials). The pulpal surface of dentine also shows post-eruptive change, with an increase in fluoride related to the final stages of dentine formation as well as to physiologically stimulated secondary dentine. The characteristics of fluoride distribution in teeth are a relatively high concentration of 500~4000 mg/kg in surface enamel and a lower concentration (50 ~ 100mg/kg) in deep enamel. Fluoride concentration of dentine is 200 ~ 1500mg/kg.

3. 在指甲和头发中 Fluoride in nails and hair

指甲和头发的氟浓度与机体长期稳定的摄氟量有关，可反映一定时期血氟的平均浓度。由于指甲的生长速度约 0.1mm/ 天，因此用指甲的氟浓度可以计算 1 ~ 3 周内的平均摄氟量。头发的氟浓度则可计算更长时间内的平均摄氟量。但指甲和头发的采样方法和检测技术尚需研究改进，反映指甲和头发中氟的摄入和积累的某些生理因素也需要进一步确定。

The concentrations of fluoride in nails and hair appear to be proportional to intake over longer periods of time. To the extent that they are, their concentrations reflect the average plasma fluoride concentrations over time. Nails grow at about 0.1mm/day so the average level of fluoride intake over a 1 ~ 3 week period can be estimated. Fluoride in hair could be used to estimate intake over longer periods. Refinements of the sampling methods for these human tissues and improved testing technology are needed. Additional research should clarify the physiological factors that can influence fluoride uptake and accumulation in these tissues.

4. 在唾液和菌斑中 Fluoride in saliva and plaque

（1）唾液中的氟　一般来说唾液中的氟浓度低于血浆氟浓度，约为血浆氟的 2/3，但在一定程度上可反映血浆氟浓度的水平，即血浆氟浓度升高，腺体分泌的氟浓度就增加。全唾液的氟含量不仅与腺体分泌有关，还与日常摄入的饮食以及氟制剂的使用有关。非刺激性唾液和全唾液的氟浓度高于刺激性唾液，分别为 0.018mg/L 与 0.013mg/L。尽管唾液氟浓度较低，但如果能保持人群有规律的暴露于低氟水平，对维持牙矿化物的稳定性，减少龋病发生，发挥防龋作用是十分有效的。

（2）菌斑中的氟　菌斑中氟含量为 5 ~ 10 mg/L（湿重），约是全唾液的 100 ~ 200 倍。其含量取决于外源性氟化物的使用频率和氟浓度的高低。在非氟化地区，菌斑中的氟主要来源于食物、唾液和龈沟液。在氟化地区，菌斑氟水平较高，部分原因可能由于血浆氟与唾液氟水平的轻度上升，也可能与直接接触氟化饮水有关。菌斑中的氟大部分以结合形式存在，少量的以离子氟形式存在。菌斑液中的氟与唾液的含氟量有关，菌斑液的氟含量较唾液高，这可能是与牙表面有较厚的唾液层，菌斑中氟离子排除较慢，或是菌斑中的氟化钙不易分解有关。唾液与菌斑和菌斑液直接接触，局部用氟后唾液中的氟很快会转移到菌斑或菌斑液中，使唾液和菌斑中的氟浓度适当升高。

The concentration of salivary fluoride is about two-thirds of the plasma fluoride concentration, and seems to be parallel to each other. The fluoride concentration in whole saliva is related not only to the fluoride excreted from the glands but also to dietary fluid intake and dental fluoride preparation.

Dental plaque (wet weight) contains a total of 5 ~ 10 mg/L fluoride that is about 100 ~ 200 times in saliva. Plaque fluid fluoride concentrations are much higher than salivary fluoride concentration. This may be due to slower elimination of the ion from the plaque, due to the thickness of the salivary film, or release of fluoride from sources of fluoride in the plaque such as calcium fluoride. Saliva is indirect contact with the plaque fluid and plaque. It appears that a transfer of fluoride from saliva to plaque or plaque fluid may occur during or immediately after topical fluoride procedures.

三、氟的排泄 Fluoride excretion

大约有10%～25%的摄入氟不被机体吸收经肠道排除体外。被机体吸收的氟几乎全部由肾脏排泄，最近的研究证明，汗液含氟量很低，与血浆氟相似约1～3μmol/L，因此，仅有微量氟经汗腺排泄。血浆氟的清除率与肾脏和钙化组织氟的清除率之和基本相同。正常人氯、碘、溴化物的肾脏清除率一般不超过1.0ml/min，而氟的清除率为35ml/min。在摄入氟3～4小时内可排出20%～30%，24小时可排出50%以上。在机体氟的摄入和排泄处于稳定的平衡状态时，日尿氟的排泄量基本可以反映氟的摄入量。肾功能不全的病人肾小球滤过率可降至正常人的30%，氟的排泄将受到影响以致软硬组织含氟量增加。氟可以自由滤过肾小球并经肾小管不同程度的再吸收，如胃的吸收和渗透膜转移一样，肾小管的再吸收是通过氟化氢扩散的机制。尿液pH值的变化（如食物、药物的影响或代谢紊乱等）可影响氟的肾脏清除率，某些情况下排尿量也会有影响，使氟在体内积蓄。

About 10%～25% of the daily intake of fluoride is not absorbed and is excreted in the faeces. The elimination of absorbed fluoride occurs almost exclusively via the kidneys. More recent data obtained with modern analytical indicated that sweat fluoride concentration are very low and similar to those of plasma (about 1 ～ 3μmol/l). Therefore, sweat is probably a minor route for fluoride excretion. The clearance rate of fluoride from plasma is essentially equal to the sum of the clearance by calcified tissues and kidneys. The renal clearance of chloride, iodide, and bromide in healthy adults are typically less than 1.0 ml but the renal clearance of fluoride is approximately 35 ml per minute. Fluoride excretion is expected to vary between 20%～30% after 3～4 hours of fluoride intake and more than 50% after 24 hours. At the stable balance situation between intake and excretion of fluoride, daily fluoride excretion is probably equal to fluoride intake. In patients with compromised renal function in which the glomerular filtration rate falls chronically to 30% of normal, fluoride excretion might decline sufficiently to result in increased soft- and hard-tissue fluoride concentration. Fluoride is freely filtered through the glomerular capillaries and undergoes tubular reabsorption in varying degrees. The renal clearance of fluoride is directly related to urinary pH and, under some conditions, to urinary flow rate. As in the cases of gastric absorption and transmembrane migration, the mechanism for the tubular reabsorption of fluoride appears to be the diffusion of hydrogen fluoride. Thus, factors that affect urinary pH, such as diet, drugs, metabolic or respiratory disorders, and altitude of residence, have been shown to affect, or can be expected to affect, the extent to which absorbed fluoride is retained in the body.

四、氟的毒性作用 Toxic effect of fluoride

氟化物的毒理作用 Fluoride toxicology

和其他人体必需微量元素一样，氟对人体的效应与剂量有关。低剂量无生理作用，适宜剂量有生理作用，大剂量有毒性作用。氟化钠的小鼠半致死量（LD50）是20～40 mg/Kg体重。

氟化钠的成人致死量为 5 ～ 10g，平均致死量为 4 ～ 5g，儿童服用 15 mg/kg 的氟可致死，而婴儿致死量仅为0.25g。由于平均致死量相差太大，whitford提出用很可能中毒剂量（PTD）作为确定需立即急诊住院治疗的指征。PTD很可能导致急性中毒，很可能引起中毒的氟摄入阈值为每公斤体重 5mg。超过 15 mg/Kg 体重则可能死亡。

过量氟可从四个方面对机体造成损害：①氟盐接触潮湿的皮肤或黏膜包括胃黏膜后形成氟氢酸，引起化学灼伤；②作为全身性原浆毒抑制酶的活性；③与神经活动所需的钙结合；④导致高血钾症引发心脏中毒。

Fluoride is also a toxic substance. Its acute ingestion in large quantities may be followed by rapidly developing signs and symptoms which may result in death. For example, the 24～hour LD50 value in the rat of administered NaF has been reported to be about 20～40 mg/kg. Because there are several variables that can affect the outcome of acute fluoride poisoning, it is concluded that 5～10 g of sodium fluoride would certainly be fatal for a person with a body weight of 70 kg. Based on the acute fluoride poisoning reports it may be concluded that if a child ingests a fluoride dose in excess of 15 mg F/kg, then death is likely to occur. A dose as low as 5 mg F/kg may be fatal for some children. Therefore, the probably toxic dose (PTD), defined as the threshold dose that could cause serious or life-threatening systemic signs and symptoms and that should trigger immediate emergency treatment and hospitalization, is 5 mg F/kg.

（一）急性氟中毒 Acute fluoride intoxication

人类发生急性氟中毒的情况比较少见，有时发生多为一次性大剂量误服造成的。急性氟中毒的症状是：流涎、恶心、呕吐、腹痛、肌无力，严重时肌痉挛、肌强直，血压下降，以致昏迷，或2～4小时内死亡。某些急性氟中毒的作用机制已经清楚，如：神经肌肉症状（痉挛），是由于氟与血浆中的钙结合，血钙下降造成的；胃肠道症状是由于氟与胃液中的盐酸（HCL）反应产生腐蚀性氟化氢（HF）和氟氢酸钠（$NaHF_2$）所致；还有一些是细胞毒性作用的结果。如果氟摄入量在 5mg/kg 以下，可服用一定量钙、铝、镁作为解毒剂；如果摄入氟量达到或超过 5mg/kg，应先迅速采用急救措施，然后住院观察；如果服用氟量接近或超过 15 mg/kg，应紧急将病人收入医院急诊室进行急救处理、心脏监护、抗休克疗法。急救处理的原则是：催吐、洗胃、口服或静脉注射钙制剂，补糖、补液及其他对症治疗。在社区预防工作中用氟防龋时，要严格掌握好剂量，并妥善保管氟化物，避免氟中毒。一旦接近或达到PTD要强制性采取急救措施，最简单易行的现场抢救措施之一是迅速让患者摄入适量牛奶，使牛奶中的钙与氟部分结合，从而减轻氟对机体的毒性作用，但仍需及时采取其他急救措施。

（二）慢性氟中毒 Chronic fluoride intoxication

慢性氟中毒主要表现为地方性氟中毒和职业性氟中毒。世界上许多国家的部分区域包括我国的一些地方都存在地方性氟中毒的危害，根据中国预防医学科学院近期的调查资料，我国有 29 个省（市、自治区）的 1054 个县有地方性氟中毒分布，病区人口 7226.32 万，现有氟牙症患者 2638.11 万人，氟骨症病人 128.7 万。地方性氟中毒以饮用水含氟量高为主，还有燃煤污染引起的地方性氟中毒在我国分布于云贵川鄂等省交界的边远山区。慢性氟中毒的临床表现为氟牙症和氟骨症，以及神经系统、骨骼肌和肾脏等非骨相慢性损害。职业性氟中毒可发生在工作与高氟物质材料长期接触的人员。

（三）氟牙症 Dental fluorosis

氟牙症又称氟斑牙或斑釉症，是牙形成和矿化过程中摄入过量氟所引起的一种牙釉质矿化不全。在地方性氟中毒的临床表现中，氟牙症是最敏感的流行病学监测指标，也是最容易发生的慢性氟中毒症状之一。

1. 临床表现 Clinical manifestation

氟牙症的临床表现，轻微程度仅有少量牙釉质白色斑纹或斑点，中等或重度则出现棕褐色染和坑凹状缺损，以致可能影响牙的整个外形。牙釉质和牙本质变脆，易磨耗。乳牙氟牙症比恒牙少见，程度也轻，原因是胎盘对氟有一定的屏障作用，母乳或牛乳含氟量很低。

Long-term intake of fluoride during enamel formation results in a continuum of clinical changes of the enamel varying from fine white lines in the enamel to severely chalky, opaque, enamel which breaks apart soon after tooth eruption. The severity of changes depends on the amount of fluoride ingested during the long period of tooth formation.

2. 病理表现 Pathological manifestation

氟牙症的病理改变主要在牙釉质，但牙本质也可出现矿化不全。正常成熟釉质是在釉质基质上形成釉质晶体，蛋白水解酶在过程中起重要作用（金属蛋白酶和丝氨酸蛋白酶降解釉质基质），氟的危害一是过量氟（具体剂量尚不清楚）可以作用于成釉细胞，在釉质分泌期抑制丝氨酸蛋白酶降解釉质基质；二是过量氟抑制溶酶体酶系统影响细胞吞噬作用，阻碍蛋白质和水分的消失，使晶体间隙不能完全关闭，成熟釉质出现微隙；过量氟也可影响釉质形成中的成核和晶体生长以及钙的体内平衡等。病变主要在釉质外层 1/3，呈现弥漫性矿化不全和多孔区。严重病例的微孔容积可达10%～25%。釉质矿化不全的程度（深度、面积）与病变程度有关。①轻度表现为白色条纹和斑点，条纹的分布与釉质生长线一致，条纹与正常釉质的界限不十分清楚。白斑多在牙尖部、切嵴和边缘嵴出现。②中度表现为釉质表面多孔，渗透性增加，由于口腔环境中的色素成分的沉着，可呈现黄、黄褐、褐、黑褐色的改变。③重度表现为多孔脆弱区域受损所形成的坑凹状缺损，部位主要在牙冠上 1/3，缺损的程度（深浅、大小）与氟牙症程度有关。

In principle, increased ingestion of fluoride during tooth formation leads to increase in enamel porosity that is along the striae of Retzius in the outer enamel surface. It is suggested that fluoride interferes with the complex process involved in protein removal and subsequent mineral acquisition during enamel maturation. Amelogenin (the major secreted enamel protein) is hydrolyzed and removed from matrix beginning in the secretory stage, and at a more rapid rate during the transition/early maturation-stage of enamel formation. A number of enamel matrix proteinases have been identified and include both metalloproteinases and serine proteinases. Beginning at the early-maturation stage of enamel development, a serine proteinases which is highly active against amelogenin is present in the enamel matrix. It has been suggested that fluoride may specifically alter the quantity and/or activity of the extracellular proteinases needed to degrade enamel proteins during the maturation stage of amelogenesis.

It appears that removal of protein during maturation is a critical step for final enamel mineralization. Therefore, a delayed withdrawal of amelogenin may be a critical mechanism in the formation of enamel fluorosis by delaying the growth of enamel crystals so that when the tooth erupts, the enamel remains incompletely mineralized.

五、氟的防龋机制 Mechanism of fluoride in caries prevention

氟的防龋机制

Laboratory research suggests that fluoride is most effective in caries prevention when a low level of fluoride is constantly maintained in the oral cavity. An important reservoir of this fluoride is in plaque, though some is also found in saliva, on the surfaces of the oral soft tissue, and in loosely bound form on the enamel surfaces. (WHO 1994)

氟的防龋效果是由以下几种作用机制所决定的：

（一）降低牙釉质溶解度和促进牙釉质再矿化 Reducing enamel solubility and promoting enamel remineralization

这是最早提出并可以简单地证明的作用机制，用浓度为1mg/L的氟溶液处理过的牙釉质，放入酸溶液，与未用氟溶液处理过的牙釉质相比较，可见到其溶解度降低。同样，牙釉质在含有0.1mg/L氟的酸溶液中其溶解度也降低。牙釉质溶解度降低是由于氟与釉质中磷灰石发生反应的结果。

全身用氟时，组织液中低浓度的游离氟进入正在形成和矿化的牙磷灰石晶体中，其反应方式有：①置换磷灰石晶体中羟磷灰石[$Ca_{10}(PO_4)_6(OH)_2$]晶胞的部分羟基(OH^-)、碳酸根(CO_3^-)和柠檬酸根($C_6H_5O_7^-$)等。其化学反应方程式是：

$$Ca_{10}(PO_4)_6(OH)_2+2F^- \rightarrow Ca_{10}(PO_4)_6F_2+2(OH^-)$$

由于F与OH的大小接近，F又有很强的结合力，所以置换是容易的。②F填补羟磷灰石晶胞中离子空缺位置。被置换和被填补的羟磷灰石晶胞变成氟磷灰石[$Ca_{10}(PO_4)_6F_2$]晶胞，使磷灰石晶体的结晶性、稳定性和硬度都得到增强。牙釉质的一个磷灰石晶体一般含有50万个以上的晶胞。

实验证明即使0.05mol/L的氟化物也可以使牙釉质的再矿化增加4.5倍。含有钙、磷、氟的矿化系统比单纯钙磷矿化液更迅速更有效地增加牙釉质的硬度。磷酸钙饱和溶液中加入低浓度的氟有利于沉淀和增加沉淀磷灰石的趋势。在氟的局部应用时，氟浓度相当高，除在釉质表层形成一定量的氟磷灰石外，主要形成氟化钙沉积层，其化学反应方程式是：

$$Ca_{10}(PO_4)_6(OH)_2+2F^- \rightarrow 10CaF_2+6(PO_4^-)+2(OH^-)$$

形成的CaF_2部分逐渐溶于唾液，部分进入菌斑。菌斑和多孔的脱矿牙釉质能富集氟，因此釉质表面和表层氟浓度很高。CaF_2释出的氟离子和菌斑释出的氟离子与磷灰石晶体反应，其反应方式有：①氟离子以弱静电结合方式吸附于磷灰石晶体表面。②通过与磷灰石晶体中羟磷灰石晶胞的OH^-置换。③与晶体表面溶解出来的Ca离子和PO_4^-结合为氟磷灰石再结晶到磷灰石晶体中。④与Ca离子和PO_4^-反应为氟磷灰石，结合在磷灰石晶体表面，使晶体长大。

用氟化物溶液浸泡方法观察对早期人工龋损的影响时，发现釉质表层的脱矿区变浅，趋向于完整和增厚，使龋损得到修复和重建。促进再矿化就是促进早期龋损愈合，达到防龋的目的。

（二）抑制细菌酶 Inhibitation of bacterial enzymes

研究证明0.2～190mg/L浓度的氟能抑制多种酶，如烯醇酶（enolase）、胆碱脂酶和某些转磷酸酶等。

1. 氟的抑酶作用

烯醇酶在细菌发酵的糖酵解和产酸中起重要作用。抑制烯醇酶从而抑制致龋菌的发酵产酸作用。抑制烯醇化酶 50% 活性的氟浓度为 0.5mg/L。抑制细菌产酸的最低氟浓度是 1 ~ 19mg/L。在糖酵解过程中烯醇酶需要二价金属镁离子激活。氟能够与 Mg^{2+} 形成 $Mg^{2+}-F-PO_4$ 复合物，竞争性地抑制烯醇酶的活性。烯醇酶是糖酵解过程中的一个重要酶，它可以使糖酵解过程中的中间产物 2 －磷酸甘油酸转化成磷酸烯醇式丙酮酸，进而生成丙酮酸，后者还原成乳酸。一旦烯醇酶受抑制，磷酸丙酮酸的转化就受到抑制，因此乳酸的形成也受阻。

2. 抑制细菌摄入葡萄糖

氟化物能抑制某些口腔致龋菌包括变链菌对葡萄糖的摄取、转化和利用，从而影响胞外多糖的合成、胞内多糖的储存，干扰细菌和菌斑在牙面上的堆积和粘附。

3. 抑制细菌产酸

氟可通过对胞内、外pH的影响抑制细菌的产酸能力。细菌糖代谢所产生的乳酸聚集在细菌胞浆内，胞浆内 H+ 浓度升高，细胞膜则将胞浆内的 H+ 主动向细胞外转运，从而使产酸过程得以继续进行。在低 pH 时，氟氢酸（HF）比氟离子更易扩散入细菌的细胞浆内，HF 则携带H+ 进入细胞浆，同时又抑制细胞膜向外转运H+，使胞浆内pH值降低，从而抑制了细菌的产酸。氟化物抑制细菌产酸的最低氟浓度为 1 ～ 2mg/L。

自然状态下口腔中的氟对龈上菌斑中的细菌不会产生明显的作用，但人为氟化后，体内氟化物可对细菌产生作用。当氟浓度增加时，所有细菌都会受到不同程度的影响，如抑制细菌的代谢（10mg/L），抑制细菌的生长（100 ~ 250mg/L），甚至杀死细菌（1000mg/L）。有文献报道，使用氟化凝胶治疗口干症病人时，菌斑中的氟浓度可达115mg/L，5年后1/3病人的口腔变链菌消失。

（三）影响牙体形态 Affection on the morphology of teeth

全身用氟除了使羟基磷灰石处于氟化状态、减少可溶解性并增加龋损的再矿化进程外，还可通过改变牙体形态增强牙的抗龋能力。大量的流行病学调查和动物实验的结果显示，生活在氟化地区儿童的牙有明显的形态学改变，即牙尖圆钝、沟裂变浅，而非氟化的低氟区儿童的牙则没有这种改变。氟化物影响牙形态学改变的可能机制是氟化物在牙发育期间产生的作用之一，这种形态的改变可以使牙易于自洁，抵抗力增强。目前普遍认为上述三个方面的联合作用是氟防龋的最重要机制。

近 30 年来，通过对氟防龋的作用机制的深入研究，目前普遍的观点是在牙发育形成时期氟对增加牙釉质硬度和降低其溶解度有一定作用。但是，氟防龋的主要作用是在牙萌出后的促进再矿化，即牙外环境（菌斑、唾液和口腔黏膜等）持续保持低浓度氟有利于牙釉质脱矿的再矿化从而起到预防龋齿的作用。

半个世纪以来氟化物预防龋齿的历史表明，全球范围龋齿患病上升趋势受到遏制，发达国家龋齿患病水平显著下降，作为公共卫生措施的社区群体应用氟化物如饮水氟化和广泛使用含氟牙膏是主要因素。

许多研究证明，采取社区群体用氟措施两年后即可取得良好防龋效果，时间越长效果越明显。青少年龋齿发病率减少，成年人患龋率下降。针对龋齿易感人群采取局部用氟措施也可收到理想效果。伴随氟防龋效果的唯一副作用是总摄氟量增加可能造成很轻或轻度的氟牙症，如美国饮水氟化取得了降低50%患龋率的效果同时伴随着10%的氟牙症患病率。WHO专家委员会认为，仅有专业人员才可检查到的在牙釉质表面有条状或斑状白色不透明区并不影响牙外观，不应影响氟防龋措施的应用，但应加强定期监测。

F works best to prevent caries when a constant, low ambient level of F is maintained in the oral cavity. Its most important caries-inhibitory action is post-eruptive, though a pre-eruptive role continues to be suggested. F's action in preventing caries is multifactorial; its effect comes from a combination of several mechanisms. Although some possible additional mechanisms have been hypothesized, three major mechanisms of action have been identified:

- *Promoting remineralization and inhibiting demineralization of early carious lesions.*
- *Inhibition of glycolysis, the process by which cariogenic bacteria metabolize fermentable carbohydrates.*
- *Some reduction in enamel solubility in acid by pre-eruptive incorporation of fluoride into the hydroxyapatite crystal.*

It has been held that pre-eruptive F exerts some degree of caries inhibition. In this model, F is thought to act by being incorporated into the developing enamel hydroxyapatite crystal and thus reducing enamel solubility. It has been argued that pre-eruptive benefits are especially important for reducing pit-and-fissure lesions. This is the "pre-eruptive" model of F's caries-preventive action assumed to be the primary effect for many years, but for which the actual supportive evidence is thin. If there is a pr-eruptive effect on caries inhibition, it is likely to be minor, the evidence for post-eruptive F action is much stronger. (Burt 1999)

Achieving the best possible caries prevention usually requires the use of population-based programmes such as adding fluoride to drinking water or salt or the widespread use of fluoride toothpastes. The question therefore arises whether the maximum caries preventive effect can be achieved without the appearance of some degree of very mild fluorosis in the target population. For example, in many parts of the United States of America much of the noticeable rise in the prevalence of very mild fluorosis can be accounted for children resident in fluoridated communities. In communities served with optimally fluoridated water supplies a small propotion of the population will continue to be affected by very mild fluorosis, evident as diffuse white lines and patches, which is not aesthetically damaging and which is usually cannot be seen by the untrained eye. (WHO 1994)

第二节 饮水氟化
Section 2 Water Fluoridation

一、饮水氟化的历史和现状 Development of water fluoridation

（一）饮水氟化的历史 A history of water fluoridation

早在1941年Dean通过对21个城镇的资料进行研究发现，当水氟浓度在1.0 mg/L这一最佳点时可获得最大防龋效果而氟牙症患病率处于很低的水平。于是在美国的小城 Grand

Rapids 从 1945 年 1 月 25 日开始了世界上第一个饮水氟化的防龋公共卫生措施，饮水氟浓度定为 1.0mg/L。在 50 多年来的发展历程中，适宜、安全摄氟剂量的研究表明，1.0 mg/L 水氟浓度并非适用于世界各地和不同季节。美国在 1962 年将饮水氟浓度的标准改为 0.7 mg/L ～ 1.2 mg/L，根据不同季节加以调整。但不同国家和地区实行此标准仍存在问题，尤其是亚洲和非洲。以香港为例，1961年香港开始实施饮水氟化，当时氟牙症流行状况为阴性，饮水氟浓度定为冬季 0.9 mg/L，夏季为 0.7 mg/L。1967 年将饮水氟浓度又调高至 1.0 mg/L。70 年代末出现了很轻度氟牙症流行，1978 年又将饮水氟浓度又下调至 0.7 mg/L。1988 年的口腔健康调查结果显示很轻度氟牙症仍有流行，便又将饮水氟浓度又下调至0.5 mg/L。尽管只下调了0.2 mg/L，氟牙症患病率有了明显下降而龋齿预防效果没有改变。近十年的情况表明香港地区饮水氟浓度为 0.5 mg/L 是适宜和安全的。1994 年世界卫生组织将饮水氟浓度的标准调整为 1.0mg/L 为绝对上限值，0.5 mg/L 为适宜下限值。

我国的广州市自 1965 年开始实施饮水氟化，氟化标准平均为 0.8mg/L，1975 年改为 0.7mg/L。因管理不善，广州曾一度出现氟牙症流行。11 年后 3 ～ 5 岁儿童乳牙患龋率降低 40%，7 ～ 12 岁儿童恒牙患龋率降低60%。广东省东莞市1974年开始实施饮水氟化，平均氟化浓度为0.6mg/L，没有出现氟牙症，10 年后 7 ～ 15 岁儿童恒牙患龋率降低 47%（两地于 1983 年和 1987 年相继停止饮水氟化）。

1.0mg/L was determined by epidemiological studies of Dean to the most appropriate fluoride concentration in drinking water because it was perceived that at this level the maximum caries reduction could be achieved with a minimal level of dental fluorosis. Subsequently, the formula was developed for the adjustment of the fluoride concentration in drinking water to vary according to the mean annual temperature of a community, and the 1.0mg/L F was modified into a range 0.7mg/L ～ 1.2mg/L presented later. This was adopted by the U.S. Public Health Service as its standards for fluoride concentration in drinking water, and these standards have been adopted world-wide.

However, by the 1990s, it has become clear that this formula may not be appropriate for all parts of the world. Even in the United States, the increased use of central air conditioning, consumption of processed soft drinks and foods, and inclusion of other dietary sources of fluoride, may have rendered obsolete the original assumptions of Dean. In tropical and sub-tropical areas in Africa and Asia, the variety of dietary practices of different races and cultures probably meant that the recommended range was completely inappropriate. It has been found, for example, in Hong Kong the prevalence and severity of fluorosis was extremely high since water fluoridation began in 1961. According to the formula, the most optimal concentration for Hong Kong should be 0.8 mg/L. This produced unacceptable high levels of enamel fluorosis. Consequently, the water concentration was reduced to 0.5mg/L in 1988. The current thinking for that the level of 1.0mg/L should be seen as an absolute upper limit, even in cold climate, and that 0.5mg/L may be appropriate as a lower limit for water fluoridation.

（二）饮水氟化的原则 Practical aspects of water fluoridation

在对氟牙症、饮水氟浓度及龋病三者之间的关系进行了大量研究后，Dean等学者认为：在预防龋病和预防氟牙症之间确实存在着一个可供选择的既安全又有效的饮水氟浓度范围。因人体氟的来源是多方面的，环境条件和生活方式不同，则人体氟的来源也不同，故在进行人工饮水氟化时，应综合考虑，不能单纯以饮水自然氟含量为依据，应参考当地龋病患病水平和氟牙症指数才能对饮水氟化的效果、安全性、可行性作出初步评价。

在Dean规定的三条原则基础上，刘大维等认为自来水氟化应遵循以下补充原则：①饮水的适宜氟浓度一般应保持在0.7～1mg/L之内。②低氟区饮水含量在0.5mg/L以下，在考虑氟化前，应首先调查该地区氟牙症的流行情况。如果氟牙症指数在0.6以上，则无氟化的必要。③饮水氟含量在0.5mg/L以下，氟牙症指数低于0.6时，可结合龋病的发病情况决定。应以15岁儿童的龋均为标准，如果超过1DMFT，可酌情适当增加饮水氟含量，如DMFT很低，则可考虑其他预防措施。④饮水氟含量超过1.5mg/L，则应采取措施消除过量的氟，但饮水氟含量在1.5mg/L以下，而氟牙症指数超过1时，应找出原因，采取措施，减少氟的摄入量。⑤饮水含氟量应按季节、气温的变化进行调整。⑥自来水氟化需要严格的管理和检测系统，保证安全有效。

二、饮水氟化的防龋功效 Efficacy of fluoridation for caries prevention

饮水氟化的防龋效果主要表现在龋齿数量减少和龋坏进程受到抑制。

1. 自出生时开始饮用氟化水的人防龋效果最佳。这种效果来自饮用氟化水的全身作用和口腔局部作用，牙萌出后的防龋效果主要来自局部作用，一生饮用可终生受益。从儿童到老年的不同年龄组都可见到防龋效果，预防根面龋的效果与冠部龋相似。40年来不同国家和地区的100多项科研报告表明，恒牙龋齿减少50%～59%，乳牙龋齿减少40%～49%。

More than 100 studies have been reported from many different countries over the past 40 years. These studies are remarkably consistent in demonstrating substantial reductions in caries prevalence as a result of water fluoridation. Where caries prevalence was high, the modal percentage reduction in caries over a period of years was 40%～49% in primary teeth and 50-59% in permanent teeth. (WHO 1994)

下表为澳大利亚Tansworth地区24年饮水氟化的防龋效果。

表5-2　饮水氟化的防龋效果（Tansworth，Australia）

年龄组	DMFT					
	1963	1967	1970	1973	1979	1988
6岁	1.3	0.9	0.5	0.4	0.1	0.1
9岁	4.0	3.2	2.9	2.0	1.1	0.3
12岁	8.4	7.0	5.6	4.3	2.4	0.9
15岁	12.5	11.2	10.2	7.7	4.6	1.5

（Sivaneswaran 1990）

2. 恒牙效果比乳牙好，可能与胎盘和乳腺的部分屏障作用和乳牙冠与组织液接触时间较短（牙冠矿化过程主要在出生前）有关。23个国家的152个饮水氟化研究报告的防龋效果见下图（图5-2）：

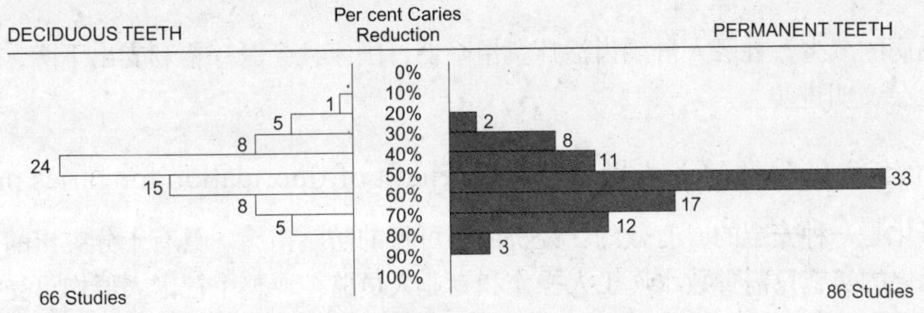

图 5-2 per cent caries reduction in 113 studies into the effectiveness of artificial water fluoridation in 23 countries. 66 studies gave results for the decidous dentition, and 86 studies gave results for the permancent.(from murray et al. 1991)

3. 儿童恒牙无龋率明显增加。美国 5 ~ 17 岁儿童无龋率 49.9%，饮水氟化社区无龋儿童是非饮水氟化社区的 6 倍（Brunelle 1990）。表 5-3 为美国两次全国性调查的儿童无龋率：

表 5-3 美国两次全国性调查的儿童无龋率

年龄组	1980 年	1987 年
5	95.4	97.3
6	89.7	94.4
7	96.5	84.2
8	58.6	75.0
9	50.6	65.5
10	37.9	55.7
11	33.7	45.0
12	26.9	41.7
13	21.1	34.0
14	19.6	27.7
15	14.9	21.8
16	11.8	20.0
17	10.7	15.6
平均	36.6	49.9

4. 龋均和患龋率明显降低，预防光滑面龋的效果要好于窝沟龋。以前的研究报告显示龋齿下降 50% ~ 60%，第一恒磨牙因龋丧失减少 75%，上前牙邻面龋减少 95%。20 世纪 90 年代以来有所变化，龋齿降低在20%～40%，这并不是饮水氟化防龋效果有所变化，而是现在多种氟暴露的因素在不断增加，非饮水氟化地区的某些氟暴露因素部分掩盖了饮水氟化的防龋效果。如在美国，70 年代以前市售含氟牙膏不多，现在已占牙膏市场的 98%。

5. 牙齿发育矿化好，氟的参与提高了牙齿矿化程度，釉质矿化不良和非氟斑减少，釉质表面更有光泽。由于第一恒磨牙丧失减少，乳磨牙早失和前磨牙早萌减少，错位牙和牙间接触不良减少。

6. 因龋病的减少，社区人群龋齿治疗费用降低，国家社会医疗福利支出下降，随之生活质量提高，社会文明进步。

三、饮水氟化防龋的成本效益 Cost-benefit of fluoridation for caries prevention

饮水氟化是一种安全的、有效的、经济的和可行的防龋措施。具有十分突出的公共卫生特征，饮水氟化的实施只需少数水厂工人操作和专业人员监控，整个社区人群均可受益，无论个人的经济状况、文化水平、健康程度以及口腔人力需求等。由于它的社会性较强，须由政府行为组织实施。它成本低效益高，在美国1万～20万人口的社区每年人均0.18～0.75美分，20万以上人口的城市每年人均0.12～0.21美分。在我国的广东省东莞市每年人均只需要4分钱。而通过饮水氟化产生的效益（如龋病减少，治疗费用降低，医疗福利支出下降等）所减少的医疗费用更可观。饮水氟化的不足和缺点是：没有集中供水系统的社区无法实施；饮用水在集中供水系统中只占2%，98%的水为工业和生活用水；只是龋齿预防的一项有效措施，但不能完全预防龋齿的发生。

Water fluoridation in the United States in 1989 was estimated to cost 51 cents per person per year on average, although in any one community the annual cost ranged from 12 cents to $ 5.41 per person per year. The health economists of U.S. in 1989 concluded that water fluoridation was one of the very few public health measures to demonstrate true cost savings, meaning that it actually saved more money than it cost to operate. Estimates from the workshop were that fluoridation cost $ 3.35 per carious surface saved, an estimate far less than the fee for any restoration. In 1992 the benefit-to-cost ratio was 80:1 that is, for every dollar spent on fluoridation, $ 80 in dental treatment costs was saved.

四、学校饮水氟化 School water fluoridation

学校饮水氟化适用于没有条件实施饮水氟化的低氟社区（如没有集中供水系统的村镇）。6岁以上的学龄儿童只有部分时间在学校，所以饮水氟浓度可以调节为水氟适宜浓度的4.5倍。学校饮水氟化的防龋效果与社区饮水氟化相似。学校饮水氟化也应专人负责，纳入学校卫生工作，要有相应的管理和监测制度。

到1983年，美国在13个洲的470所学校实施学校饮水氟化，共有17万学生受益。根据研究报告，6岁开始饮用学校氟化水12年后与基线相比DMFS减少40%，饮用学校氟化水时已经萌出的第一恒磨牙DMFS减少31%，接触氟化水后萌出的尖牙、前磨牙和第二恒磨牙DMFS减少57%，没有发现氟牙症问题（表5-4）。

在世界上，只有美国的部分学校在上世纪60年代起实行这一措施，虽然个别学校出现摄氟过量的问题并没有引发意外事故，但现在美国疾病控制中心（CDC）已经不再提倡学校饮水氟化。

In rural areas where community water fluoridation is not possible, the approach of fluoridating a school's drinking water was promoted for years. Relative to community water fluoridation, the disadvantages of school fluoridation were that children did not receive the benefits until they were old enough to begin school, and they drank the water only when school was in session. To compensate for this reduced exposure, the recommended concentration was 4.5 times the optimum for water fluoridation for the locality.

At its peak, school water fluoridation was introduced in 13 states in U.S.; data reported by CDC showed that in 1981, it was established in 470 schools, serving 170,000 children. The procedure was reported to reduce dental caries among school children by about 40%. There is no record of the procedure being used in countries outside US. Despite US CDC safety guidelines, a number of overspill mishaps have occurred, fortunately without lasting ill effects. CDC no longer promotes school water fluoridation.

表 5-4 学校饮水氟化 12 年后 DMFS 均数 **（Heifetz 等，1978）

研究地区	DMFS 均数 *	DMFS 均数 *	DMFS 均数差	与基线比较下降率 %
	1958	1970		
Elklake	13.12	7.94	5.18	39.5
	(*n*=1030)	(*n*=1149)		
	1968	1980		
Seagrove	12.39	6.49	5.90	47.6
	(*n*=766)	(*n*=758)		

*：两组学校基线年龄分布均经调查

**：儿童年龄 6 ~ 17 岁，Elk Lake，pa (5.0mgF)，Seagrove，NC (6.3mgF)

五、饮水氟化的安全性 Safety in water fluoridation

半个多世纪以来，对饮水氟hua1的安全性做了全面和系统的研究，包括天然适氟区和饮水氟化区的健康、疾病和死亡率统计，尸体解剖，以及氟的机体代谢和毒理学等方面。目前的结论是：饮水氟化达到适宜浓度对人类安全没有任何威胁，包括不会导致癌和肿瘤、畸形、心肝肾等脏器疾病和衰老的发生。最近的安全性研究报告是 20 世纪 90 年代初美国 CDC 关于饮水氟化作用利弊的研究报告。报告指出，氟的应用时间与肿瘤发病率之间没有明显的关系，包括骨、关节肿瘤及骨肉瘤。

In 1993, U.S. CDC concluded that the available laboratory data are insufficient to demonstrate a carcinogenic effect of fluoride in animals, and the weight of the evidence from more than 50 epidemiological studies dose not support the hypothesis of an association between fluoride exposure and increased cancer risk (the buccal cavity, kidney, and bones and joints) in humans.

第三节　其他系统用氟防龋措施

Section 3 Other Systemic Use of Fluorides for Caries Prevention

一、食盐氟化 Salt fluoridation

同饮水氟化一样食盐氟化一种可供选择的全身用氟防龋措施。由于人们每天摄入的食盐量比较恒定（5 ~ 10 克），摄氟量容易控制。氟化物用喷雾法加入食盐，可操作性强成本低，在瑞士等国家实行多年，防龋效果良好。我国湖北武汉曾进行过临床试验研究。

Salt fluoridation is the controlled addition of F to domestic salt for the purpose of preventing dental caries. Fluoridated salt uses the same public health principle as water fluoridation, namely that a small amount of fluoride in a dietary staple serves to inhibit dental caries with little conscious action by the individual.

（一）食盐氟化的历史 A history of salt fluoridation

世界上最早研究和应用食盐氟化的国家是瑞士。1946年正在研究食盐加碘的Wespi博士获悉 Dean 在美国饮水氟化的研究后，开始了食盐氟化的研究。1948 年 Rheinsalinen 盐业公司与之合作为规模生产氟化食盐进行了实验研究与探索。1955年Zurich洲首次在社区人群中应用含有5mg碘化钾和90mg氟化钠的食盐。1962年国家卫生专业委员会建议除实行饮水氟化的Basel市外普遍实施食盐氟化，使22个洲的氟化食盐市场占有率达到60% ~ 75%。1970年开始提高食盐含氟量到250mg/L浓度（按成年人每天摄入食盐 8 ~ 10 克计算）的防龋研究，随后哥伦比亚、匈牙利、芬兰和西班牙等国家也开展了食盐氟化的防龋研究。1981年瑞士医学会推荐袋状氟化食盐的氟浓度应统一为250mg/L。到 20 世纪 90 年代中期，法国和德国也开展了食盐氟化的防龋研究。泛美卫生组织采取了积极支持西半球发展中国家进行食盐氟化防龋项目的策略，哥斯达黎加、墨西哥和牙买加都进行了食盐氟化的防龋项目。

Fluoridated salt was first used in Switzerland in 1955. Fluoridated salt has been well accepted by the Swiss public, now holding 75% of the table salt market. The effects of fluoridated salt have also been studied in Colombia and Hungary, with generally favorable results, although neither country now markets fluoridated salt.

The material most commonly used to fluoridated salt is potassium fluoride (KF), although sodium fluoride (NaF) is also used. The early Swiss studies began with salt fluoridated to 90mg/L, but it became clear that this level was too low. In the early 1970s, the concentration was increased to 250mg KF/Kg salt (or 225mg NaF/Kg salt), which was based on adult salt consumption estimates of some 8 ~ 10g/day. 250mg KF/Kg salt now appears to be the standard in countries other than Switzerland as well.

By the mild-1990s salt fluoridation had become established in France and Germany as well as Switzerland. In the western hemisphere, it was established in Costa Rica, Mexico, and Jamaica. Further growth in Latin America is likely.

（二）食盐氟化的防龋效果 Effectiveness of salt fluoridation

食盐氟化的防龋效果与饮水氟化相似，瑞士 Vaud 洲 12 年食盐氟化的防龋效果见表 5-5：

表 5-5 瑞士 Vaud，2 年含盐氟化防龋效果

年龄组	DMFT 1970	1974	1978	1982	减少 %
8	2.2	1.9	1.6	1.8	17
10	5.4	3.7	3.6	4.3	19
12	10.4	7.3	6.6	5.0	52
14	16.2	12.6	10.5	8.2	49

Fluoridated salt raises ambient oral fluoride concentration throughout lift in a manner similar to water fluoridation. The first study in Swiss showed that those who had not benefited from fluoridated salt had 10.2 DMFT (n=153) while those from the canton of Vaud who had consumed fluoridated salt from the age of 5 years onwards showed only 7.1 DMFT (n=56).

匈牙利应用氟化食盐（250mgF/kg）8年后6岁儿童乳牙龋降低39%，对照组儿童乳牙龋上升了7%（Toth 1976）。在哥伦比亚的三个城镇，一项历时8年的食盐氟化（200mg/L）临床研究结果见表5-6：

表 5-6　哥伦比亚 8 年含盐氟化结果

	NaF 食盐	CaF_2 食盐	氟化水（1mg/L）	对照组
1964 年	3.7	3.8	3.8	4.3
1972 年	1.4	1.1	0.8	3.8
减少	2.3(61%)	2.7(72%)	3.0(78%)	0.5(13%)

我国武汉大学口腔医学院在进行了食盐氟化可行性实验研究以后，于1988年开始了在幼儿园实施200～250mg/kg食盐氟化的临床观察，并分别于1990、1994年报道了食盐氟化的防龋效果。结果表明，应用氟化食盐3年后，乳牙龋均和龋面均分别下降了49%和52%，第一恒磨牙龋均和龋面均分别下降了85%和86%。这提示200～250mg/kg氟化食盐在我国低氟区也有推广应用的前景。

（三）食盐氟化的优缺点 Advantages and disadvantages of salt fluoridation

实施食盐氟化除了具有饮水氟化类似的效果外，还有一些饮水氟化所没有的优点，主要包括：①覆盖人群广泛，不受地区条件限制可大规模的生产和供应；②不需要设备完好的供水系统；③与饮水氟化相比，减少了氟的浪费；④生产和控制方法简单，费用较低；⑤每个家庭可自由选择，无心理上的压力。

氟化食盐的不足之处在于：①防龋效果与大众接受程度和范围有关，因此，氟化食盐的推广需要加强对大众的宣传和教育；②难以精确控制每一个体的耗盐量，特别是对幼儿，存在着摄盐量过少而达不到良好的防龋效果。③食盐摄取量在不同地区与不同人群之间差异很大，WHO推荐每人每天6克摄入量，我国全国平均为13.2克，北方地区可高达20克以上，这对氟化食盐氟含量的确定带来一定困难；④氟化食盐的销售范围难以控制，如果进入高氟或适氟地区会造成危害。

The main advantages of salt as a vehicle for fluoride are that it does not require a community water supply and it permits individuals to accept or reject it; non-fluoridated salt, like non-iodized salt, can be made available to the population. Fluoridated salt is available at the same price as other kinds of salt, including iodized salt, so there is no extra cost to the consumer.

Difficulties arise with salt fluoridation when there are multiple drinking water sources which have a naturally optimal or excessive fluoride concentration. Also, salt fluoridation requires refined salt produced with modern technology and a level of technical expertise adapted from that used in adding iodine to salt.

The technical operations of salt fluoridation systems should be monitored and recorded regularly. In addition, the correct concentration and homogeneity should be periodically ascertained in the packages offered to the consumer.

二、牛奶氟化 Milk fluoridation

牛奶是天然营养食品，含有人体所需的多种营养素和微量元素。其中钙磷含量丰富，每100ml牛奶含钙125mg，磷96mg，对儿童骨和牙的生长发育有重要意义，对老年人预防骨质疏松症也非常重要。牛奶氟化是将适量的氟化物加入牛奶或奶粉中，氟化物不改变牛奶的味道、性质和消毒工艺，牛奶中氟的生物活性几乎不受影响，只是氟的生物利用率略低于饮水氟化(80%左右)。牛奶氟化经不同加工方法处理后氟离子浓度有所变化：5mg/L氟化牛奶经巴氏消毒（84℃ 4秒）后4℃保存3天，氟离子浓度仍为5mg/L（100%）；经超高温消毒（140℃ 4秒）后氟离子浓度为 4.40mg/L（88%），而且可以维持 3 个月之久；制成奶粉储存 2 个月后氟离子浓度为 4.65mg/L（93%）(Phillips 1991)。

牛奶氟化预防龋齿的临床研究也有35年的历史了。目前由英国Borrow基金会支持，世界卫生组织指导实施的国际氟奶项目正在十几个国家和地区进行。依据不同年龄儿童饮奶量的不同，牛奶氟化的剂量在 2 ～ 5mg/L，儿童摄氟量为 0.4 ～ 1.0mgF/ 日。文献中尚未见到引起氟牙症的报告。

牛奶氟化预防龋齿是WHO近年来推荐的一种可供选择的全身用氟措施，它与饮水氟化和食盐氟化一样，安全、有效和经济。牛奶氟化是1955年由Ziegler最早提出的，1960年Rusoff首次报告了美国牛奶氟化防龋研究的临床效果，1986年开始 WHO 和英国 Borrow 基金会指导和支持一些国家开展了国际牛奶氟化防龋的社区试点项目，临床防龋效果令人鼓舞。

Because milk is recommended as a good food for infants and children and is widely available both at home and in school in many countries it was considered, over many years ago, to be a suitable vehicle for supplementing children's fluoride intake. Strongly promoted by Ziegler, an influential pediatrician, the first project with fluoridated milk began in the Swiss city of Winterthur in 1955.

Milk was suggested as a vehicle for fluoride as a possible alternative to water fluoridation in the USA in the early 1960s, and in the UK from the late 1960s. Some clinical trials of fluoridated milk have been conducted, and caries levels were lower in groups consuming fluoridated milk. Children consume 200 ml of milk fluoridated at a level of 5 mg/L daily, have been introduced in Bulgaria, Chile, China and the Russian Federation; whilst in the UK an investigation into the epidemiological, organizational and legal feasibility of school milk as a vehicle for fluoride has been conducted.

氟化牛奶防龋效果的临床研究报告尚不多，不同年龄组儿童饮用氟奶不同年限后的防龋效果见表 5-7：

表 5-7 氟化牛奶的防龋研究效果

作者	报道时间	饮用年限	年龄（岁）	分组	DMFT	下降（%）
Russoff	1962	3.5	9 ~ 12	实验	0.34	80.0
(美国)				对照	1.70	
			12	实验	1.00	78.8
				对照	4.70	
Stephen	1981	4	8 ~ 10	实验	1.47	33.8
(英国)				对照	2.22	
	1984	5	9 ~ 11	实验	1.94	35.8
				对照	3.02	
Banoczy	1983	3	5 ~ 6	实验	0.29	74.0
(匈牙利)				对照	1.11	
	1985	5	7 ~ 10	实验	1.04	60.0
				对照	2.60	
Zahlaka	1987	3	7 ~ 10	实验	0.20	64.0
(以色列)				对照	0.55	

1988年在保加利亚开展的第一个社区范围的氟化牛奶防龋试点项目进行了5年，经WHO专家评估，6岁年龄组dmft实验组比对照组下降了53%；DMFT下降了89%。8岁年龄组dmft实验组比对照组下降了40%，DMFT下降了79%。目前大范围的氟奶防龋社区试点项目正在俄罗斯、英国、中国等十几个国家和地区进行。研究表明，每年饮氟奶200天以上防龋效果显著，低于150天则无明显效果。氟化牛奶防龋要成为一项公共卫生措施尚需进一步的研究和更大范围的社区试点。

北京氟化牛奶防龋社区试点项目（1994 ~ 1999）：

This was a community-based demonstration study carried out in 15 kindergartens (about 4000 children) in Haidian district of Beijing, China. On each weekday, each child in the participant kindergartens consumed 200ml of fluoridated milk at a concentration of 2.5mg F/L in kindergarten under a teacher's supervision. Every week, the children were given tow packs of fluoridated milk (250ml) for consumption at home in the weekend.

There was no statistically significant difference in the baseline mean dmft scores between the tow groups (表5-8). The difference between the mean number of new carious teeth in the test and control groups was found to be statistically significant (1.2vs. 1.8; P <0.001). There was also a statistically significant difference in the mean number of arrested carious teeth at the 21-month examination between the groups (0.3vs. 0.1; P <0.001). The mean numbers of examiner reversals were similar in the two groups (P =0.578) . The overall net caries increment over the 21-monthstudy period was 0.4 dmft in the test group and 1.3 dmft in the control group. This amounted to a 69% reduction, and was statistically significant (P <0.001).

表 5-8　The 21-month-results in milk fluoridation programme in Beijing

	试验组 (417 人)	对照组 (247 人)	*P* 值
基线龋均 dmft	3.2 (3.7)	3.5 (1.4)	0.312
基线患龋率	66	68	0.72
21 月后患龋率	72	82	0.003
新生龋均 dmft	1.2 (1.5)	1.8 (1.6)	< 0.001
新生龋率 (%)	51	73	< 0.001
误差龋均 dmft			
静止龋均	0.3 (0.9)	0.1 (0.5)	< 0.001
检查误差龋均	0.5 (0.9)	0.4 (0.9)	0.578
净增龋均 dmft	0.4 (1.9)	1.3 (1.2)	< 0.001

1996 年，世界卫生组织对开展氟化牛奶防龋措施进一步提出：

With experience gained on the development of milk fluoridation, WHO is now able to define three categories of projects which have already been introduced and which could be implemented in the near future. These are constituted by the WHO International Milk Fluoridation Programme as follows: (a) community level demonstration projects to evaluate the efficacy and organizational pattern of milk fluoridation for dental caries prevention as an alternative to other nonvoluntary means of fluoride delivery; (b) feasibility studies to explore whether milk could be used as a vehicle for fluoride intake at country or regional level; (c) clinical or laboratory studies relating to a specific research project whereby data obtained would facilitate the implementation of milk fluoridation for caries prevention.

三、氟片和氟滴剂 Fluoride tablets and fluoride drops

口服氟片适用于低氟区没有实施任何全身用氟防龋措施的儿童，特别是龋齿高危或易感儿童。氟片所用氟化物多为氟化钠，配以调味剂和赋形剂等制成含氟量为0.25mg、0.5mg和1mg的咀嚼片。由儿科或口腔科医师开处方后方可服用。处方前要了解当地饮水含氟量和多种氟暴露情况。每次处方总量不得超过120mgF，避免因一次性误吞引起急性氟中毒。医师要向儿童家长讲清每日剂量和用法，请家长监督儿童服用。由于多种氟暴露因素，氟片剂量和饮水氟浓度以及儿童年龄的关系应严格掌握（见安全控制一节）。家庭服用氟片不易长期坚持，托儿所和幼儿园有条件纳入工作计划，专人负责实施和监督，比较容易坚持。服用时应先将氟片咀嚼或含化后再吞咽，增加局部作用效果。氟片的防龋效果与饮水氟化相似，从婴儿到12岁坚持服用效果最好。Driscoll（1974）总结分析了欧美等国的21份研究资料，乳牙龋降低了 50% ~ 80%；34 份研究资料报告恒牙龋降低了 39% ~ 80%。它的成本低，目前主要用于龋齿高危或易感儿童。一般认为由于胎盘屏障作用，孕妇服用氟片对于预防胎儿出生后的龋齿意义不大。

类似氟片的有氟滴剂，用于无法应用氟片的婴儿每日滴入口腔。国外有将维生素A、D加入氟片或氟滴剂供儿童服用，同时补充维生素和氟素不影响氟防龋的效果。氟滴剂适用于2岁以下的幼儿。每日睡前将含氟溶液滴于颊黏膜或舌部，不漱口、不饮水，可获得全身和局部的双重作用。选择应用的原则和每天补充的氟化物量与氟片相同。使用氟滴剂可使龋病降低40%。

Fluoride dietary supplements were first introduced in the late 1940s, and were intended as a substitute for fluoridated water for children in non-fluoridated areas. Bacuase they are manufactured as (a) tablets or drops, intended to be swallowed (some drops are in fluoride-vitamin combinations for infants); (b) tablets for chewing; or (c) lozenges intended to be sucked slowly or permitted to dissolve slowly in the mouth, the term "supplements" is used to refer generically to all forms.

Supplements contain a measured amount of fluoride, typically 0.25 mg, 0.5 mg, or 1.0 mg, usually as sodium fluoride. They were, and still are, intended for use only in areas where there is little or no fluoride in drinking water, and where there is no other intentional use of ingested fluoride.

Obviously fluoride supplements have limited application as a public health measure. Fluorid3e tablets should be kept out of reach of young children, and should be packaged in child-proof containers. In some countries the number of tablets in a container is limited so that there can be no more than 120 mg of sodium fluoride in any one container; this seems a prudent safety precaution.

1994 年，针对容易摄入氟过量而引发氟牙症的危险，WHO 专家提出以下几点建议：

① 补充氟片（滴剂）作为预防保健措施应有限制的应用。

② 0.5 mg F/ 日的剂量只用于 3 岁以上龋病高危或易感儿童。

③ 氟片包装瓶上应注明 3 岁以下儿童须凭牙医处方服用。

The possibility of an increased risk of dental fluorosis has led WHO experts to conclude that:

① fluoride supplements have limited application as a public health measure.

② a dose of 0.5 mg F/day should be prescribed only for individuals at risk, and starting only at the a ge 3 years.

③ labeling should advise that fluoride supplements should not be used before 3 years of age unless prescribed by a dentist.

1991年在美国举行的有关氟摄入量问题的专家研讨会上又提出了新的补充氟素标准，除了年龄和水氟浓度因素外，还要考虑体重因素（表 5-9）。

表 5-9　儿童年龄、饮水氟浓度和体重关系

体重	年龄	饮水氟浓度 (mg/L)		
(kg)	(year)	<0.3	0.3 ~ 0.7	>0.7
3.14 ~ 12.4	出生至 2 周岁	0.25	0	0
12.14 ~ 16.4	2 ~ 4 周 岁	0.50	0.25	0
16.4 ~ 21.5	4 ~ 6 周岁	0.75	0.50	0
>21.5	>6 周岁	1.00	0.75	0

（Newbrun 1992）

1994 年 WHO 专家委员会推荐的氟片剂量标准见表 5-10。

表 5-10 儿童每日供氟剂量表（mg/ 天）

年龄	饮水氟浓度 mg/LF		
(岁)	<0.3	0.3 ~ 0.7	>0.7
0.5 ~ 2	0.25	0	0
2 ~ 4	0.50	0.25	0
4 ~ 16	1.00	0.50	0

出于对用药安全性的考虑，到目前为止，我国卫生医药主管部门尚未审核批准用于儿童龋病预防的氟片和氟滴剂。

第四节 含氟牙膏
Section 4 Fluoridated Toothpastes

含氟牙膏是世界上应用最广泛的局部用氟防龋方法，也是容易学习和掌握的自我口腔保健方法和公共卫生措施，适用于低氟和适氟地区的各年龄组人群。世界卫生组织认为，过去20年发达国家龋齿患病水平持续下降应主要归功于含氟牙膏的广泛应用。目前发达国家市场上的牙膏 90% 以上是含氟牙膏。

Toothbrushing with a fluoridated toothpaste is by far the most common form of caries control in use today. This method of using fluoride is the simplest and most rational way of combating caries in individuals of all ages. There is now increasing evidence that the decline in the prevalence of dental caries recorded in the most industrialized countries in the past 20 years can be attributed mainly to the widespread use of toothpaste that contain fluoride. In the most industrialized countries, 90% sold toothpaste is fluoridated.

一、含氟牙膏的发展历史 Development of fluoridated toothpastes

含氟牙膏的研究起始于 1942 年。最早被研究、试验和临床应用的是氟化钠牙膏，但不久便由氟化亚锡（SnF_2）牙膏取代，原因是摩擦剂为碳酸钙（$CaCO_3$）。牙膏中的氟离子与钙离子不断结合沉淀而使牙膏防龋作用很快丧失。氟化亚锡牙膏以焦磷酸钙（$Ca_2P_2O_7$）为摩擦剂取得了良好防龋效果，1955年成为第一种在美国批准上市的含氟牙膏，但长期应用氟化亚锡牙膏存在的产生牙齿着色问题而未能广泛应用。

20 世纪 60 年代初开始进行单氟磷酸钠牙膏的临床研究，以传统的磷酸二钙为摩擦剂，观察到其防龋效果与氟化亚锡牙膏相似。1963年开始研制的一种含氟牙膏使用的氟化物为单氟磷酸钠（Na_2PO_3F MFP），以难溶性焦磷酸盐为摩擦剂，由于MFP的氟离子存在于磷酸氟复合离子中，比较稳定，可以和多种摩擦剂配伍，使牙膏的游离氟含量长期保持稳定，1969年得到了美国牙医协会的认可，从此单氟磷酸钠牙膏开始广泛应用。随后在欧洲开发出氟化胺牙膏，把氟的防龋作用和胺类中阳离子表面活性剂的抗菌斑作用结合起来发挥作用。

早期临床试验认为氟化纳牙膏防龋效果差，其主要原因是由于碳酸钙摩擦剂与氟化纳相容性差。1967 年 Koch 等临床试验表明氟化钠与丙烯酸摩擦颗粒结合的牙膏有明显的防龋效果。

1981年Zacherl报告了氟化钠与二氧化硅（SiO_2）摩擦剂牙膏有显著的临床防龋效果。由于80年代研制出与氟化钠完全相容的摩擦剂，因而使含氟化钠的牙膏得以广泛应用。

近年来，牙膏中的氟离子还可以与菌斑抑制剂洗必泰和抗牙结石剂中的可溶性焦磷酸盐相容，又研究推出了复合型含氟牙膏以增强牙膏的防龋祛菌斑效果。目前常见的与氟化物配伍的牙膏摩擦剂见表5-11：

表5-11　可与各种氟化物配伍的摩擦剂

氟化物	NaF，SnF_2，Amine F	MFP
摩擦剂	Acylic	Aclic
	$(NaPO_3)_2$	$(NaPO_3)_2$
	$Ca_2P_2O_7$	$Ca_2P_2O_7$
	SiO_2	SiO_2
		$CaHPO_4$
		$CaCO_3$
		Al_2O_3

（Mellberg 1983）

目前，国外生产的牙膏基本都是含氟牙膏，占牙膏销售总量的80%～90%以上。我国含氟牙膏的生产和销售也逐年增加。许多专家的共识是含氟牙膏在世界范围的广泛应用是使龋病患病率出现大幅度下降的主要原因之一，特别是在发达的工业化国家。但由于含氟牙膏的价格较贵，影响在发展中国家的推广应用。因此，90年代以来，WHO的专家呼吁并推荐在发展中国家生产和应用大众能负担得起的含氟牙膏刷牙作为整个公共卫生措施的一个组成部分，以促进人类的口腔健康。

In 1942, the earliest attempts to add F to toothpaste were unsuccessful because of the incompatible abrasives used in the products that bound the F and thus made it biologically unavailable. The first successful clinical trials of an F additive used SnF_2 with a calcium pyrophosphate abrasive in 1955.

In all, more than 100 clinical trials have been conducted with various F compounds as the active ingredient: SnF_2, NaF, sodium monofluorophosphate (MFP), and amine fluoride have all been successfully tested. Even more abrasives have been developed and tried; insoluble metaphosphate, sodium trimetaphosphate, hydrated silica gel, calcium carbonate, dicalcium dehydrate, and calcium pyrophosphate are the main ones. New formulations are constantly under investigation and are soon marketed when found effective.

Serious marketing of F toothpastes was underway by the early 1970s, and public acceptance was immediate in virtually all of the economically developed nations. By the 1990s, F toothpastes accounted for well over 90% of the toothpaste market in developed countries. Their use in the developing world, where F toothpaste could potentially fill an important preventive role, is inhibited by their relatively high cost, poor distribution, and often by the relative absence of the oral hygiene culture taken for granted in the developed world. The development of the F toothpaste market in developing countries is a challenge to the manufacturers and to dental public health in general. WHO pointed out that every effort must be made to develop affordable fluoridated toothpastes for general use in developing countries.

二、含氟牙膏的防龋功效 Efficacy of fluoridated toothpastes in caries prevention

（一）防龋机制 Mechanisms of caries reduction

含氟牙膏刷牙时，大量的氟可在釉质表面形成氟化钙微粒并保持相当长的一段时间，这些氟化钙微粒构成了菌斑和牙釉质间的氟库，当菌斑 pH 值降低到 6 以下时便可释放出游离氟，这是由于氟化钙微粒上磷酸氢根（HPO_4^{2-}）的表面吸收作用形成的。这一化学反应过程可阻止氟化钙在中性pH值环境中的溶解，而pH值下降时，磷酸氢根就转变成磷酸二氢根（$H_2PO_4^-$），它不能阻止氟化钙微粒的溶解，游离氟便随之释放出来。由氟化钙微粒提供，为pH值变化所控制的游离氟在牙釉质表层脱矿 - 再矿化过程中起到促进再矿化作用。

When introduced into the oral cavity, F in toothpaste is taken up directly by demineralized enamel, although its retention on sound enamel is thought to be of relatively minor importance. It also increases the F concentration in dental plaque, thus leaving a store of F available for remineralization when pH drops. Salivary F levels, normally low in resting saliva, rise 100- or even 1000-fold after toothbrushing with an F toothpaste. This level drops over the next 1 to 2 hours, with some of the salivary F being taken up by plaque.

（二）氟浓度与防龋效果 Efficacy related to fluoride concentration

临床试验研究显示，牙膏氟浓度与其防龋效果呈正相关关系，由1000mg/L至2500mg/L之间每增加 500mg/L 可降低龋齿发病率约 6%，500mg/L 以下没有防龋效果。目前常用的牙膏含氟浓度一般以1000mg/L为标准，如0.22%NaF牙膏、0.76%MFP牙膏等，也有将两种氟化物联合配方制成双氟牙膏。WHO专家委员会认为长期应用含氟牙膏具有累加的防龋作用，其效果要远高于只有2、3年周期的临床实验结果。作为口腔预防策略，WHO推荐在发展中国家广泛应用含氟牙膏。

各种含氟牙膏防龋效果的临床实验结果相似，见表 5-12：

表 5-12 含氟牙膏的防龋效果

氟化物	研究报告数	平均龋齿减少率（%）
NaF	17	21.4
SnF_2	46	22.0
Na_2PO_3F	34	22.2
Amine F	4	22.5

（Mellberg 1983）

The possible benefit of using toothpastes containing more than 1000mg/L fluoride has been tested in clinical trials which have compared conventional 1000mg/L products with test pastes containing concentrations of 1500 ～ 2800mg/L. Use of toothpaste containing 1500mg/L resulted in statistically significantly lower caries increments. With 1500mg/L F against those with 2000mg/L F or more was a significant improvement with the highest fluoride concentration. Overall, the results of these studies show that there is a dose-response relationship in favor of using fluoride concentrations above 1000mg/L. As experience has accumulated, it has been shown that the cariostatic effect of fluoridated toothpastes in life-long use in entire populations is much greater than that reported from short-term clinical studies of 2 ～ 3years' duration.

三、儿童应用含氟牙膏的问题 The problem in use of fluoridated toothpastes in children

因含氟牙膏导致摄入氟安全性问题的文献报告主要集中在6岁以下学龄前儿童。文献报告普遍认为误吞含氟牙膏是发生氟牙症的危险因素之一，特别是 3 岁以下儿童误吞牙膏量可达70%以上。如果居住在适氟地区幼儿的吞咽反射机能完善，应用含氟牙膏每天刷牙两次，那么其来自含氟牙膏的氟摄入量与来自食物、饮水和饮料的氟摄入量基本相等。

但是6岁以下儿童的吞咽反射机能是不完善的。一项设计严谨的病例对照研究表明，不足2岁的幼儿应用含氟牙膏其发生氟牙症的几率是不用含氟牙膏幼儿的11倍（虽然以很轻度氟牙症为主）。Naccache 等1992年研究了学龄前儿童含氟牙膏用量与吞咽量的关系，结果表明年龄越小牙膏吞咽量越大（见下表）。

表 5-13　2-7 岁年龄组应用含氟牙膏的吞咽牙膏情况

年龄组	牙膏用量 / 每次刷牙 均值（克）	吞咽量 / 每次刷牙 均值（克）	吞咽率 / 每次刷牙 均值（%）
2	0.62	0.36	65
3	0.53	0.28	49
4	0.45	0.24	49
5	0.52	0.23	42
6	0.48	0.18	34
7	0.50	0.18	34

1997 年，英国 325 名 8 ～ 9 岁儿童参加的有关牙膏误吞与氟牙症关系的回顾性病例对照研究结论是：3 岁前用含氟牙膏刷牙与恒切牙氟牙症有高度的相关性；家长要监督幼儿刷牙方法和牙膏用量；儿童应使用 500 ～ 600mg/L 低浓度的含氟牙膏。1996 年英国儿童牙医协会提出 4 项建议：

（1）6 岁以下儿童使用的含氟牙膏浓度不超过 600mg/L。

（2）6 岁以下儿童每次刷牙使用的含氟牙膏用量为黄豆粒大小。

（3）家长监督 6 岁以下儿童使用的含氟牙膏用量。

（4）含氟牙膏包装上应表明含氟浓度和提示氟牙症的危险。

应用含氟牙膏导致氟牙症的文献报道很少，Holt 等报告 2 岁开始分别应用 550mg/L 和 1050mg/L 含氟牙膏的儿童，低氟浓度组恒切牙氟牙症明显低于高氟浓度组。Mascarenhas 也报告 2 岁就开始应用含氟牙膏的儿童氟牙症危险明显上升。

虽然现在尚无应用含氟牙膏导致氟牙症的报道，但对于学龄前儿童使用含氟牙膏应予注意。由于学龄前儿童吞咽功能发育尚不完善，使用含氟牙膏刷牙可误吞20%～50%的牙膏用量，这时期正是恒牙牙冠矿化阶段，易发生因吞咽过量氟致慢性氟中毒（氟牙症），因此，在低氟和适氟区或已全身用氟的学龄前儿童用含氟牙膏刷牙时应有家长或监护人的帮助和监督。含氟牙膏刷牙每天不超过3次，每次用量不超过0.5g或5mm（豌豆大小）。嘱刷牙时不要吞咽，刷牙后清水漱口要尽量吐干净。青少年和成人不存在误吞问题。

最近在北京完成的含氟牙膏防龋临床试验，1334名3～6岁儿童分为试验组和对照组，在24所幼儿园的老师监督下应用0.243%（1100mg/L）氟化钠牙膏和空白对照牙膏早晚刷牙两次，每次用黄豆大小膏体（用量约0.48克），2年后试验组与对照组相比dmfs减少20.7%。值得一提的是在试验的同时进行了尿氟安全监测，结果显示开始刷牙后尿氟排量试验组比对照组高出40%，一个月后至2年结束时两组儿童的刷牙后尿氟排量没有显著性差异，说明幼儿园老师监督学龄前儿童刷牙和控制牙膏用量的方法是可以解决学龄前儿童应用含氟牙膏刷牙预防龋齿可能引起摄入氟安全性问题。

Caries prevention in children with sodium fluoride dentifrice delivered through a kindergarten-based oral health program: It was a randomized, placebo-controlled, examiner-blind, two-year caries study. A population of 1,334 preschool children, three years of age, was recruited from 24kindergartens in Beijing. After the visual-tactile baseline examination, the children were randomly assigned to one of the two dentifrice groups: 0.243% sodium fluoride (1100mg/LF) or placebo (0mg/LF) that the children brushed twice a day at school under the supervision of the teacher. In the evaluable subset, the test group had a 20.7% reduction in dmft compared to the placebo group. The result demonstrate that fluoride in conjunction with increased dental awareness can deliver important reduction in caries in preschool children.

四、含氟牙膏的研究进展 Research progress of fluoridated toothpastes

20年来，为了保证儿童应用含氟牙膏的防龋功效同时降低发生氟牙症的危险，对低氟浓度的含氟牙膏进行了临床对比观察研究。Burt 回顾了20世纪80年代两个250mg/L与1000mg/L含氟牙膏的临床效果对比试验虽获得了相反的结果。但两个550mg/L与1000mg/L含氟牙膏的临床效果对比试验却取得了相似的防龋效果。Ammari 等最近总结了7个含氟牙膏的临床效果对比试验后认为250mg/L含氟牙膏对恒牙没有防龋作用，500mg/L含氟牙膏防龋效果仍需要更多的临床试验来验证。

牙膏是自我保健、维护口腔健康的必需用品，而含氟牙膏又是使用最广泛的个人防龋方法。因此含氟牙膏仍需要更多研究工作，例如婴儿的氟来源与其后恒牙可能出现氟牙症之间的联系；幼儿含氟牙膏用量的控制方法；儿童用低浓度含氟牙膏的防龋效果；含氟牙膏预防老年人根面龋的效果以及添加某些制剂增强含氟牙膏的防龋功效等。

A welcome development, alluded to already, would be the marketing of "children's toothpaste" of 500 to 550mg/L F separately from "adult strength" products, which might be 1500 to 2500mg/L F. Because the swallowing of toothpaste by children is a risk factor for fluorosis, if those children swallow high-F toothpaste, the prevalence and severity of fluorosis could get worse. On the other hand, high-F toothpastes are likely to be more beneficial for preventing coronal and root caries in adults than the first-generation products. Perhaps the market chould manage both forms of toothpaste with appropriate color-coding and warning labels on the high-F products.

第五节　其他局部用氟防龋措施

Section 5 Other Topical Use of Fluorides for Caries Prevention

用各种不同的方法使氟作用于牙齿表面，从而起到预防龋齿的作用称为氟化物防龋的局部应用。氟化物的局部应用适用于没有实施全身（系统）用氟措施的低氟和适氟地区，也可适当地与全身应用联合使用以增加防龋效果。现在普遍认为，口腔中长期持续保持低水平氟浓度可以不断促进釉质表面脱矿区域的再矿化，取得防龋的最佳效果。氟化物的局部应用依据制剂的氟浓度和使用方法可分为自我应用和专业人员应用两种方式，多用于学龄儿童及其以上各年龄组。氟化物局部应用的防龋效果略低于全身应用效果，对新萌出牙的效果明显好于萌出已久的牙（见表 5-14）：

表 5-14　局部用氟对已萌出恒牙和新萌出恒牙的效果比较

作者	氟化物	龋齿减少（%）	
		已萌出恒牙	新萌出恒牙
Averill（1967）	NaF	22.9	37.1
Horowitz (1969)	SnF_2	20.7	61.3
Muhler(1960)	SnF_2	44.2	84.0
Szwejda (1972)	SnF_2	20.4	44.4
Szwejda（1972）	APF	22.5	63.0

（Harris & Christen 1995）

氟化物的局部应用一般不存在产生氟牙症问题，因为恒前牙的矿化已经完成，但某些局部应用措施使用方法不当有可能产生儿童的急性氟中毒症状，应引起注意。

Topical fluorides for the prevention of dental caries are the most widely used dental products at home and in dental offices. Strong scientific evidence exists to support the efficacy of many topical fluorides in caries prevention. In general, high-fluoride concentration agents are applied professionally and low-fluoride concentration agents or products are applied by the individuals themselves. Topically applied fluorides do not increase the fluoride concentration of enamel greatly; rather, they intend to provide local protection at or near the tooth surface by incorporating and concentrating fluoride in plaque and the oral mucosa. This fluoride serves as a reservoir of available fluoride ions. During a cariogenic challenge, fluoride from these sources is mobilized to assist remineralization.

Individuals who are most likely to benefit from fluoride applications, both professionally or self-applied, are the following:

- *Caries-active individuals defined as those with past caries experience or those who develop new carious lesions on smooth tooth surfaces.*
- *Children shortly after periods of tooth eruption, especially those who are not caries-free.*

- *Individuals who are salivary flow-reducing medications, have diseases that decrease salivary flow or have received radiation to the head and neck.*
- *Patients after periodontal surgery, especially when the roots of teeth have exposed.*
- *Patients with fixed or removable prostheses and after placement or replacement of restorations.*
- *Individuals with an eating disorder or who are undergoing a change in lifestyle which may affect eating and oral hygiene habits conductive to good oral health.*
- *Mentally and physically challenged individuals.*

一、氟水漱口 Fluoride mouth-rinsing

氟水漱口是简便易行、经济有效的局部用氟措施，适用于低氟或适氟地区的学龄儿童和其他龋齿易感人群，特别适合纳入学校口腔保健和家庭口腔保健，在老师和家长的监督下进行。氟水漱口要防止误吞，学龄前儿童最好不用。

各种氟化物漱口液的剂量、用量和用法见表5-15：

表5-15 氟漱口液的剂量、用量和用法

氟化物	剂量浓度%	mg/L	用法	时间
NaF	0.20	900	10ml/1分钟	每周一次
NaF	0.02	100	10ml/1分钟	每日二次
NaF	0.05	225	10ml/1分钟	每日一次
APF	0.02	200	10ml/1分钟	每日一次
SnF_2	0.10	243	10ml/1分钟	每日一次

一般认为漱口液的氟浓度和漱口频率对防龋效果没有明显影响，氟水漱口可以减少龋齿发生20%～40%，如能配合口腔卫生指导，养成早晚刷牙，饭后漱口的保健习惯，效果更好。临床研究表明，中性氟化钠漱口液对口腔软组织无副作用，成本低，对光滑面的防龋效果最好，临床较为多用。APF漱口液体外实验可增进釉质表面脱矿区对氟离子的吸收，但临床效果与中性氟化钠漱口液无明显差异，而口味不佳不易被接受。氟化亚锡漱口液有减少牙面菌斑堆积的作用，不足的是对牙齿有轻度着色和对口腔黏膜有收敛作用，儿童也不易接受。NaF和APF漱口液的临床研究效果见表5-16：

表5-16 NaF和APF漱口液的临床研究效果

作者	氟浓度	开始年龄	人数	观察期	DMFS增加数			降低率
	(mg/L)	(岁)		(月)	对照	实验	△	(%)
Aasenden等	200NaF	8～11	114	36	12.3	9.0	3.3	27
	200APF	8～11	109	36	12.3	8.7	3.6	29
Heifetz等	3000NaF	10～12	126	24	7.5	4.7	2.8	38
	3000APF	10～12	133	24	7.5	5.5	2.0	27

对于某些特殊人群应用氟化物漱口液能收到良好的防龋效果，如经放射治疗或手术治疗等造成涎腺功能减退，唾液分泌减少的病人；配带正畸矫治器或可摘义齿造成菌斑堆积的患者；保持口腔卫生有障碍的残疾人；牙龈萎缩，根面龋易感的老年人；猛性龋病人等。各种氟化物漱口液要用塑料容器包装以保证有效氟浓度的稳定。

The idea of preventing caries by mouthrinsing with dilute F solutions has been around for decades, but it was some years before it became a standard procedure in preventive dentistry. A Swedish report in 1965 that found nearly 50% reduction in caries increment over 2 years naturally sparked interest in the procedure. Since then, NaF rinses have been extensively tested; others tested to a lesser extent include APF, SnF_2, ammonium fluoride, and amine fluoride. Its low cost. Convenience in handling, and pleasant taste have led to NaF becoming the most widely used of these products.

NaF has been tested as a weekly rinse at 0.2% F and for daily rinsing at 0.05%. Schoolbased public programs have been found the weekly regimen to be the most convenient; daily rinsing is most appropriate for individual use. F mouthrinsing is seen now as appropriate for high-risk groups as a "targeted" procedure rather than a population strategy.

The use of F mouthrinsing for caries prevention is essential in persons who have xerostomia or have received head and neck radiation that a dryness of the mouth from the lack of salivary secretions.

二、局部涂氟 Topical use of fluoride solution

涂氟是氟化物局部应用最早期的方法。所用氟化物有以下几种：

1. 2%NaF 溶液

常用的方法是先洁治而后用橡皮杯蘸摩擦糊剂抛光牙面，牙齿邻面可用无蜡牙线清洁，漱口、隔湿、吹干，用棉签涂布NaF溶液，湿润到全部牙面，保持3分钟待其干燥，也可用无蜡牙线将溶液带入邻面接触区，30分钟禁食水。每周涂布一次，连续4次为一个疗程。第二次涂布可省略清洁牙面的步骤，一次操作可进行 1 个象限或一侧半口牙。学龄儿童每两年一个疗程，直至恒牙全部萌出。研究报告可减少恒牙光滑面龋 30%。

2. 8% ~ 10%SnF_2 溶液

SnF_2 在水溶液中极不稳定，需要用时新鲜配制。8%SnF_2 溶液操作与 NaF 溶液基本相似，不同的是湿润牙面 4 分钟，每年涂布一次。10%SnF_2 溶液与 8%SnF_2 溶液的不同之处是湿润牙面时间 30 秒，每半年涂布一次。低氟区防龋效果可达 40% ~ 50%。值得注意的是在促进再矿化时可使脱矿区棕染（着色）。

3. 1.23%APF 溶液

操作方法与 NaF 溶液相似，防龋效果低氟区为 30% ~ 50%，适氟区为 20% ~ 30%。

涂氟方法繁复，学龄前儿童不易合作。操作应由专业人员在诊室中进行，不适宜作为公共卫生措施实施。

表5-17 三种氟化物溶液的特点和效果比较 Characteristics and effectiveness of NaF，SnF_2 and APF

Characteristics	NaF	SnF_2	APF
Percent %	2%	8%	1.23%
mg/L F	9200	19500	12300
Frequency of application	4 at weekly intervals at ages 3，7，10，13，	1 or 2/year	1 or 2/year
taste	Bland	Disagreeable	Acidic
stability	Stable	Unstable	Stable in plastic container
Tooth pigmentation	No	Yea	No
Gingival irritation	No	Occasional	No
Average effectiveness	29 %	32 %	28 %

三、含氟涂料 Fluoride varnishes

含氟涂料可以克服局部涂氟时氟化物在釉质表面停留时间短的不足，由50mg NaF加入1ml粘性涂料制成。用法较为简单，清洁牙齿、吹干，而后涂布含氟涂料。涂料很快凝固成为半透明薄膜，能保留数小时。氟离子逐渐释放到牙釉质表面，延长防龋作用。也有的窝沟封闭剂加入氟化物，在封闭窝沟的同时还有氟防龋的作用。

A theoretical advantage for varnishes over other methods of professional F application is that varnishes are adhesive, and hence should maximize F contact with the tooth surface. Varnishes are a way of using high F concentrations in small amounts of material.

四、含氟凝胶 Fluoride gels

含氟凝胶的优点是操作简便和氟与牙齿表面作用时间长，通过托盘可同时处理上下牙列，即可隔离唾液又可加压使氟凝胶布满牙面并挤入牙间隙，使氟较好地与牙齿邻面接触。氟化物常用APF，也有用氟化钠（2%）和氟化亚锡（8%）的。APF是由NaF（1.23%）加入0.1M的磷酸配制而成的，pH值为3.0。还有一种APF触变性凝胶，它实际上是一种粘性水溶液受力后可变为液体，使用时在托盘中不流淌，压入牙列后则成为液体容易进入牙间隙。上海研制的APF防龋凝胶含有NaF、KCL、KH_2PO_4和羟乙基纤维素等成分，pH值4.0。第一年每季度用一次，第二年起每半年用一次，幼儿乳牙龋齿发生率可减少57%。

使用含氟凝胶时先清洁牙面、隔湿、吹干，用大小适宜的泡沫塑料托盘装入适量含氟凝胶，压入上下牙列，轻轻咬动后固定4分钟，然后取出托盘，拭去粘附在牙面上和牙间隙里的凝胶，30 分钟内禁食水。含氟凝胶的缺点是成本较高，不宜大面积推广。

氟泡沫与氟凝胶相似，其优点一是用量少，每次只需0.9g（氟凝胶每次4g），相当于氟凝胶用量的22%（氟含量为 10.77mg）；二是用后口内氟化物滞留量比氟凝胶少 18% 左右；三是虽用量少但釉质氟沉积量相同。1994 年美国 ADA 批准临床使用作为氟凝胶的替代和选择用品。全国牙病防治指导组对国内氟泡沫的临床应用提出建议：鉴于氟泡沫的氟浓度高达12000mg/L（1.23%），pH 值又低（3.5），其口内滞留量每次仍达 1.26 ~ 1.27mg，目前适宜应用的范围与氟凝胶（1.23%）基本相同，即限于临床具有适应证的病人，并由口腔专业人员在临床必要的条件下严格操作使用。在尚未得到充分的科学证据证明其确实可以用于儿童群体预防龋齿之前，不宜作为儿童群体防龋的一项公共卫生措施。

氟凝胶（泡沫）在使用中要认真注意以下几点：

1. 严格限制用量，一次不超过 4 毫升。
2. 患者应保持垂直体位，头部略前倾。
3. 用托盘方法应使用排唾器。
4. 患者应用氟凝胶中和之后 30 秒钟不吞咽口水。
5. 应用氟凝胶过程中专业人员不得离开患者。

The proper use of topical fluoride should consider:

- *Use no more than 2 ml of gel per tray.*
- *Place patient in an upright position with the head inclined forward.*
- *Use suction device during and following treatment.*
- *Have patient expectorate repeatedly and thoroughly following treatment.*
- *Never leave the patient unattended.*

Fluoride gels were developed because it was apparent that their viscosity would make them easier to work with and would readily permit their application in trays, so that the entire dentition could be treated at one time. NaF and APF gels contain the same concentration of fluoride and pH as their respective aqueous solutions. In addition, the gels contain cellulose compounds for viscosity. Some gels are formulated to be thixotropic, that is, they tend to flow when under pressure but remain viscous when not. Theoretically, thixotropic gels may penetrate better interproximally and not drip from a tray as readily as non- thixotropic gels, but studies have not been done to confirm these attributes.

Fluoride gels may be considered to be as effective as their solution counterparts. Two studies have shown that caries-preventive effects have persisted for 2 years after discontinuation of applications of APF gels. Fluoride gel products have dominated the market for many years in the United States because of their desirable working characteristics compared with fluoride solutions.

A fluoride foam with a pH of 6 is marketed in some countries. Less fluoride retention may result following use of the foam than from a traditional gel, but efficacy of the foam has not been investigated.

五、其他 Others

1. 含氟充填材料 Fluoride containing filling materials

含氟充填材料是由玻璃离子粘固粉、聚羧酸盐粘固粉、银汞合金和洞衬剂等加入适量氟化物制成的。如非创伤性充填材料（ART材料）等。待充填凝固后，材料中的氟离子缓慢释放出来，起到促进再矿化和预防继发龋的作用。

2. 缓释氟材料 Fluoride releasing materials

缓释氟材料包括氟化物缓释片和氟化物控释药囊等，目前尚处于实验研究阶段。氟化物缓释片是由甲基纤维素形成氟化物的包衣制成，可嵌于修复体上使用，有报告氟化物缓释片可持续释放氟 24 小时。氟化物控释药囊是由药库内的氟化物和调节释放速率的多聚性膜构成，有效期可达数月之久。

A number of investigators have evaluated various ways to provide prolonged, sustained levels of fluoride in oral fluids in attempts to provide a ready source of fluoride for remineralization. These methods include devices applied to teeth, usually molars, that release low-levels of fluoride for prolonged periods, slow-release lozenges and bioadhesive tablets.

Fluoride has also been added to amalgam in an attempt to reduce the risk of recurrent caries at the margins of restoration. Glass-ionomer cements release fluoride and may also inhibit secondary caries. One difficulty with these materials is controlling the rate of fluoride release.

第六节 除氟害兴氟利
Section 6 Dialectical Conception for Fluoride

1994年，WHO氟化物与口腔健康专家委员会对世界各国应用氟化物预防龋齿提出了16点建议：

1. 绘制详细的有关氟化物的水文地质资料图；在氟牙症流行地区进行水质化学分析调查；制定开发水资源的明确规定，避免在高氟地带打饮水井。

2. 对于向大气层排放氟化物的工业企业和富含氟化物的矿业企业应建立和强化环境保护措施。

3. 明确哪些饮食习惯和方式可增加婴儿和幼儿过量摄氟危险，以适当方法加以避免。

4. 定期监测氟牙症以确定其患病状况是否增加或超过可接受水平，如果增加或超过应及时调节饮水、食盐或其他氟化措施的氟化物浓度。应用生化指标评价当前氟暴露状况以预测以后氟牙症的危害程度。

5. 分析某些地区中度以上氟牙症流行状况，研究开发适合的除氟技术在高氟区的社区和家庭推广应用。

6. 定期监测和评价各种氟防龋措施的效果。

7. 社区饮水氟化防龋是安全、经济和有效的，应在被接受和可行的社区推广应用。适宜的饮水氟浓度应在 0.5 ~ 1.0mg/L 范围以内。

8. 食盐氟化是可供选择的饮水氟化的替代措施，食盐氟化的最低氟浓度为 200mg/kg。

9. 牛奶氟化已取得令人鼓舞的防龋效果，但应进行更多的深入研究。

10. 氟片和氟滴剂作为公共卫生措施应限制使用。在中低患龋水平的地区应采取保守的策略，每天0.5mgF^-的剂量只给予3岁以上龋病高危或易感儿童。在高患龋水平的地区应使用推荐的剂量标准，给予 6 个月以上幼儿并应计算饮水摄氟量。

11. 在同一时期只实施一种系统（全身）用氟措施。

12. 含氟牙膏具有良好的防龋效果，在发展中国家应努力发展支付得起的含氟牙膏预防龋齿。含氟牙膏防龋作为一项公共卫生措施，国家应给予生产企业以税收等方面的优惠。

13. 含氟牙膏上应注明 6 岁以下儿童要在成年人监督下应用和每次只用很小量牙膏（少于 0.5mm）。用于儿童的具有防龋效果的低氟浓度含氟牙膏应研究生产。

14. 果味香型的含氟牙膏和氟浓度在 1500mg/L 以上的含氟牙膏不应用于 6 岁以下儿童。

15. 在低氟社区，在考虑儿童患龋状况和项目成本可行时，可采取学校集体氟化物刷牙和漱口的防龋项目。氟水漱口不易在 6 岁以下儿童中进行。

16. 应进一步研究氟化物预防根面龋的效果。

There is a need to carry out detailed fluoride mapping for existing water sources, as well as hydrological studies to show flow lines and hydrogeochemical surveys in areas where fluorosis is endemic. Governments in the affected areas should establish clear guidelines on exploitation of groundwater so that sinking boreholes in high fluoride zones can be avoided.

Countries that have industries that emit fluoride into the atmosphere or have mines of fluoride-rich minerals should introduce and enforce environmental protection measures.

Dietary practices that increase the risks of infants and young children being overexposed to fluoride from all sources should be identified and appropriate action taken.

Dental fluorosis should be monitored periodically to detect increasing or higher-than-acceptable lavels of fluorosis. Action should be taken when fluorosis is found to be excessive by adjusting fluoride intake from water, salt or other sources. Biomarkers should be used, where practical, to assess current fluoride exposure to predic further risk of fluorosis.

In view of the endemic nature of unsightly dental fluorosis in a number of regions, research on the development of affordable technology for partial defluoridation in households and communities is recommended.

The effectiveness of all caries-preventive programmes should be regularly monitored.

Community water fluoridation is safe and cost-effective and should be introduced and maintained wherever it is socially acceptable and feasible. The optimum water fluoride concentration will normally be within the range 0.5 ～ 1.0mg/l.

Salt fluoridation, at a minimum concentration of 200mg F-/kg, should be considered as a practical alternative to water fluoridation.

Encouraging results have been reported with milk fluoridation but more studies are recommended.

Fluoride tablets and drops have limited application as a public health measure. In areas with medium to low caries prevalence a conservative prescribing policy should be adopted: a dose of 0.5mg F-/day should be prescribed for individuals at risk from the age of 3years. In areas with high caries prevalence, a dosage regimen should be used, starting at 6months of age, that takes into account the fluoride content of the drinking-water.

Only one systemic fluoride measures should be used at any one time.

Because fluoridated toothpaste is a highly effective means of caries control, every effort must be made to develop affordable fluoridated toothpastes for use in developing countries. The use of fluoride toothpastes being a public health measure, it would be in the interest of countries to exempt them from the duties and taxation applied to cosmetics.

Fluoridated-toothpaste tubes should carry advice that, for children under 6years of age, brushing should be supervised and only a very small amount (less than 5mm) should be placed on the brush or chewing-stick. The caries-preventive effectiveness of toothpastes with lower levels of fluoride, manufactured especially for use by children, should be fully studied.

Fluoridated toothpastes with candy-like flavours and toothpastes containing fluoride at a concentration of 1500mg/L or more are not recommended for use by children under 6years of age.

In low-fluoride communities, school-based brushing and mouth-rinsing programmes are recommended, but their adoption should be based on the cost of implementation and caries status of the community. Fluoride mouth-rinsing is contraindicated in children under 6years of age.

Further research on the effectiveness of fluoride in preventing root-surface caries is recommended.

2002年8月15日，针对国内含氟牙膏有关争议，中华口腔医学会和全国牙病防治指导组发表了联合声明：应用含氟牙膏防龋安全有效。

最近有家报刊记者报道了某个国家买含氟牙膏也要凭医生的处方的消息，立即引起了一些传媒的关注，并询问有关专家，内容涉及的不只是含氟牙膏，还有其他一些含氟制品以及氟化物对人体健康的利弊问题。

为了使广大群众有一个正确的认识和判断，我们作为全国性专业机构，遵循循证医学的科学原则，有必要澄清以下事实：

氟是人体必需的一种微量元素，像任何一种微量元素一样，它有一个适宜而安全的应用范围。半个多世纪的科学研究和应用有充分的证据证明，适量应用氟化物能够有效地预防龋齿。

氟化物的应用分为两大类。一类是全身应用，包括饮水氟化、食盐氟化、牛奶氟化、氟片、氟滴剂等，目前国内还没有推荐这类应用。另一类是局部应用，包括含氟牙膏、含氟漱口水、氟保护漆等，目前国内含氟牙膏的应用比较广泛。

世界卫生组织及其他国际组织一直推荐使用含氟牙膏预防龋齿。应用合格的含氟牙膏是安全有效的，没有争议，不是“双刃剑”，不需要医生开处方，可以由消费者任意选购。但建议3岁以下的婴幼儿不能用，学龄前儿童使用含氟牙膏时控制用量，每次用“黄豆”大小的膏体即可。建议3岁以下的孩子不用含氟牙膏，以及学龄前儿童使用含氟牙膏时控制用量，就是因为年龄小的孩子自我控制力差，容易发生误吞。长期使用不安全。

根据中国预防医学科学院环境卫生研究所的研究，专家推荐我国成人每日最大安全氟摄入量是3.4mg，7～15岁儿童每日最大安全氟摄入量是1.9～2.1mg。我们用牙膏刷牙后都漱口，实际上通过含氟牙膏被吸收进入人体的氟非常少，即使长期使用也不会造成氟摄入量过多。

与国外相比，我国开展氟化物应用的时间短，范围小，除了含氟牙膏的应用较广泛外，其他用氟方法少，而且大多是在口腔专业人员操作和指导下应用的。造成慢性氟中毒（表现为氟牙症和氟骨症）的主要原因是人们生活在高氟区，高氟区主要是饮水中或燃煤中的氟含量很高，但是我国80%的地域是低氟区。

随着生活水平的提高，人们饮食中的甜食增加，患龋增加。第二次全国口腔健康调查结果显示5岁儿童的患龋率为77%，而发达国家特别是北欧70%的5岁儿童没有龋齿。为了增进我们的口腔健康和全身健康，我们应该遵循“兴氟利，除氟害”，“安全第一，效果第二”的原则，合理应用氟化物，特别是早晚两次使用含氟牙膏刷牙预防龋齿是安全有效的。

一、多氟源和总摄氟量 Multiple fluoride sources and total fluoride intake

1976年，魏赞道教授等贵州医学科研人员在地方性氟中毒的流行病学调查中发现，当地饮水氟含量不高，但食物、土壤等的氟含量较高，确定当地地方性氟中毒属于非水源性氟中毒(1979年，焦玉河等进一步证实这种非水源性氟中毒是燃煤污染所致)。在总结调查研究的基础上提出了“多氟源和总摄氟量”的概念。

总摄氟量是指氟的总摄入量为机体每日从空气、水、膳食等摄取氟量的总和（mg/d）。氟的总摄入量包括两个含义，一个是适宜总摄氟量，简称适宜摄氟量；另一个是安全总摄氟量，简称安全摄氟量。适宜摄氟量是指防龋和维护其他正常生理功能的生理需要量，是制定各种氟载体卫生标准的科学依据。因此在确定适宜摄氟量时，必须综合考虑机体摄氟的多种途径，才能使适宜摄氟量有比较准确的限定。安全摄氟量是指人体最大可能接受的量，长期超过此量将会导致慢性氟中毒的发生。

1994 年，WHO 氟化物与口腔健康专家委员会针对多氟源与氟防龋关系指出：

Most clinical trials involving the use of fluorides in caries prevention have tested a single product. In many parts of the world, however, exposure to fluoride from multiple sources is the rule rather than the exception: people in fluoridated areas brush their teeth with fluoridated toothpastes, and people anywhere can have a significant, but usually unknown, intake of fluoride from food and drinking in addition to their use of fluoridated toothpaste.

Exposure to multiple sources of fluoride can be beneficial or undesirable. It can be beneficial in the sense that fuller advantage is being taken of the several ways in which fluorides act to prevent caries, but it can also increase the potential for fluorosis. Some multiple exposure is controlled, as when a dentist applies fluoride gel to a caries-susceptible patient who is using a fluoridated toothpaste, but some exposure, for example to fluoride in food and drinks, is not. It is uncontrolled exposure to fluoride, sometimes from unsuspected sources, that is the principal public health concern. Periodic assessment of total fluoride intake in a population, as well as regular monitoring of fluorosis prevalence and severity in children, enables the public health administrator to determine whether further action is called for.

Use of more than one form of fluoride in a caries-prevention programme usually provides additive benefits, but sometimes the cost-effectiveness is low. For example, if fluoride mouth-rinsing is introduced to children with low to moderate caries activity who drink fluoridated water and brush regularly with fluoridated toothpaste, the minor additional benefit may be not worth the operational costs of the programme. By contrast, fluoride mouth-rinsing among children with high caries prevalence who have no other exposure to fluoride would clearly be cost-effective. Dental public health administrators should be aware of the total fluoride exposure in the population before introducing any fluoride programme for caries prevention. The likely cost-effectiveness of any such programme has to be judged in the light of existing exposure and caries prevalence in the target population.

对于氟防龋中的多氟源和总摄氟量问题的结论是：

1. Exposure to fluoride from multiple sources in young children, whether controlled or uncontrolled, can be both beneficial in terms of reduced caries and undesirable in terms of dental fluorosis.

2. Dental public health administrators should be aware of the total fluoride exposure in the population before introducing any additional fluoride programme for caries prevention, and the cost-

effectiveness of such programmes should be carefully considered.

二、高氟地区的除氟问题 Removal of excessive fluoride

高氟地区的除氟措施是预防地方性氟中毒危害的有效途径，可从以下三个方面着手：①寻找合适的水源和采取饮水除氟措施，选用适宜氟浓度的饮水来源；②改革炉灶和燃煤方式，消除因生活燃煤带来的氟污染；③合理处理工业“三废”，加强个体防护，改善工作环境，预防工业氟污染。

1. 高氟浓度饮水的除氟问题 Removal of Excessive Fluoride from drinking water

我国卫生防疫部门和地方病防治机构长期致力于地方性氟中毒的预防和控制工作，高氟浓度饮水的除氟措施主要是在地方性氟中毒危害地区寻找合适的水源，即打深井取适宜氟浓度的深层地下水取代高氟浓度的浅层地下水。

The first WHO publication dealing specifically with drinking-water quality was published in 1958 as International Standards for Drinking-Water. It was subsequently revised in 1963 and in 1971 under the same title. In 1884-1885, the first edition of the WHO Guidelines for Drinking-water Quality was published. In 2000, the first edition of Fluoride in Drinking water was published by WHO.

In cases where alternative sources are not available, defluoridation of water is the only measure remaining to prevent fluorosis. There are several different defluoridation methods recommended by WHO for both developed and developing countries to removal of Excessive Fluoride from drinking water.

表 5-18 Defluoridation methods recommended by WHO

Criteria	In developed countries	In developing countries
Set-up and water flow	Always continuous, often in columns	Often discontinuous in columns Fill and draw in batch
Scale and treatment site	Always at water works, often close to water source	At water works At village community level At household level
Treatment media/process	Contact precipitation Activated alumina Synthetic resins Nalgonda Reverse Osmosis Electrodialysis Bone charcoal	Bone charcoal Contact precipitation Nalgonda Activated alumina Clay Other naturally occurring media

2. 燃煤型氟污染的除氟问题 Removal of excessive fluoride from born coal

针对由燃烧高氟煤导致的燃煤型氟中毒，中科院地理科学与资源研究所和中国疾病控制中心（CDC）在国家‘十五’攻关计划支持下，开展了相关实验室模拟实验和现场中试试验。通过对高氟石煤和烟煤的氟释放规律研究，提出了不同温度下的燃煤氟释放率模拟公式，发现钙、镁、钾、钠等可不同程度地抑制煤氟的释放。在钙基物质固氟、固硫的技术原理基础上，研制出高效钙镁固氟、固硫剂。实验室研究结果显示其固氟率可达92.3%，现场中试效果中，蜂窝煤的固氟率达到86.6%，空气除氟率为73.6%，除硫率为86%，粉尘降低达47.3%。

三、氟防龋的安全与监测 Fluoride intake monitoring in caries prevention

氟化物防龋的效果与安全性监测与评价的目的是在应用氟化物防龋措施（全身或局部）时能取得最佳效果而避免因人体过量摄入氟所造成的任何不良反应（急慢性氟中毒）。氟化物防龋的效果与安全性是实施任何一项氟防龋措施所必须首先考虑的问题。也是氟防龋项目实施过程中必须定期监测与评价的主要方面。对此各国学者和研究机构进行了大量的试验研究工作。

1. 人体的适宜、安全摄氟剂量 Appropriate and safe dosage of human fluoride intake

1984年世界卫生组织根据大量科学研究资料提出了每日摄氟量的不同剂量范围：

表5-19 每日摄氟量的不同剂量范围

0.1 ~ 0.6mg	很低水平
0.7 ~ 1.4mg	低水平
1.5 ~ 4.0mg	适宜水平
5.0 ~ 12mg	高水平（可形成氟牙症和氟骨症）
20mg 以上	很高水平（如给予氟制剂治疗骨质疏松症）

同时指出成人每日适宜摄氟剂量在1.5 ~ 4.0 mg之间，最大剂量不超过6.0 mg/日。

1985年美国国家科学研究院（US NRC）推荐了不同年龄组每日摄氟剂量：

表5-20 不同年龄组每日摄氟剂量

年龄组（岁）	适宜摄氟剂量（mg/日）
0 ~ 0.5	0.1 ~ 0.5
0.5 ~ 1	0.2 ~ 1.0
1 ~ 3	0.5 ~ 1.5
4 ~ 6	1.0 ~ 2.5
7 ~ 10	1.5 ~ 2.5
11<	1.5 ~ 2.5
成人	1.5 ~ 4.0

1986年Anon分析了美国1942 ~ 1985年对食物氟含量方面的研究结果，提出了人体摄入

氟的适宜剂量：在牙矿化期为每日 0.05 ~ 0.07mg/kg 体重。此剂量既可以增强牙抗龋能力又不会导致氟牙症。而每日摄氟量超过 0.1mg/kg 体重将产生急、慢性氟中毒症状。

1995年刘原等调查了中国北方典型饮水型氟中毒流行区4个不同氟暴露水平地区的人群氟中毒和儿童龋齿患病率，并研究了它们与饮水氟浓度及总摄氟量的关系，提出了我国北方农村的适宜、安全饮水氟浓度分别为0.95 mg/L和1.21mg/L，7 ~ 15岁儿童适宜、安全摄氟量和总摄氟量为1.9mg和2.1mg/（人.日），成人最大安全总摄氟量为3.4mg/（人.日）。梁超轲等（1996）历时6年完成了我国人群总摄氟量卫生标准的研究，根据研究结果建议：①总摄氟量是指每人每天经饮水、食物和空气摄入氟离子（F^-）的总量。②总摄氟量标准值：8 ~ 15 岁为 2.0mg/（人.日）~ 2.4 mg/（人.日），15 岁以上为 3.0 mg/（人.日）~ 3.5 mg/（人.日）。

计算氟的总摄入量虽然理想，但较复杂。由于氟的适宜和安全总摄入量的标准难以统一，因此只提供一个范围，即每公斤体重的摄氟量在 0.05 ~ 0.07mg 之间为适宜的，一般不应超过上限。国外学者在广泛分析的基础上报告每日总摄氟量从婴儿的 0.2mg 到成人的 5.0mg，差别很大。每日从食物的摄氟量超过3.5mg，通常表明是特殊情况或者是不寻常的膳食习惯。中国营养学会常务理事会 1989 年通过推荐的每日膳食中营养素供给量的说明中，关于氟的摄入量见表 5-21。我国一些单位和组织建议氟的最大安全摄入量见表 5-22。

表 5-21　氟的适宜摄入量和安全摄入量

年龄	氟摄入量（mg/ 天 / 人）
初生 ~ 6 个月	0.1 ~ 0.5
6 ~ 12 个月	0.2 ~ 1.0
1 岁以上	0.5 ~ 1.5
4 岁以上	1.0 ~ 2.5
7 岁以上	1.5 ~ 2.5
11 岁以上	1.5 ~ 2.5
成人	1.5 ~ 4.0

表 5-22　我国部分单位和组织建议氟的最大安全摄入量

建议单位或组织	最大安全摄氟量（mg/ 天 / 人）
饮水氟卫生标准研制科研组	3.0
食品氟卫生标准研制科研组	3.5（未计入空气吸入氟量）
卫生部初级保健	4.0
中国预防医学科学院环卫所（1995 年）	3.4（成人） 1.9 ~ 2.1（7 ~ 15 岁）

国家氟化物卫生标准，见表 5-23

表 5-23 我国有关氟化物的卫生标准

项目	标 准	注
饮用水	不超过 1.0mg/L	见卫生部法监司 2001 年 6 月出版的《生活饮用水卫生规范》，2001 年 9 月 1 日起实施
环境空气	适用于城市地区： 日平均浓度：0.007mg/m^3（标准状态） 一小时平均浓度：0.02mg/m^3（标准状态） 适用于牧、农、林业区： 月平均浓度：1.8 ~ 3.0μg/（dm2.d） 植物生长季平均浓度：1.2 ~ 2.0μg/（dm2.d）	国家环境保护局 1996 年 1 月 18 日批准 GB3095-1996，1996 年 10 月 1 日实施
粮食		中华人民共和国卫生部 1984 年 12 月 22 日批准，GB4809-84； 国家标准局发布， 1985 年 9 月 1 日实施
大米、面粉	≤ 1.0mg/kg	
其他	≤ 1.5mg/kg	
豆类	≤ 1.0mg/kg	
蔬菜	≤ 1.0mg/kg	
水果	≤ 0.5mg/kg	
肉类	≤ 2.0mg/kg	
鱼类（淡水）	≤ 2.0mg/kg	
蛋类	≤ 1.0mg/kg	

2. 应用氟化物预防龋齿的适宜、安全剂量 Appropriate and safe dosage of use fluoride for caries prevention

作为公共卫生措施的全身用氟主要是饮水氟化，食盐氟化和牛奶氟化等。其安全问题主要是长期过量摄氟引起的氟牙症。

In 1984, WHO examined a large body of data and, among other points, concluded that there were no data adequate to concluded that fluoride produces cancer or birth defects. In addition, WHO noted that mottling of teeth (i.e., dental fluorosis) is sometimes associated with fluoride levels in drinking water above 1.5mg/L and crippling skeletal fluorosis can ensue when the fluoride level exceeds 10mg/L. WHO recommended a guideline value of 1.5mg/L, a level at which dental fluorosis should be minimal. In 1996, WHO re-evaluated the 1.5mg F/L guideline value that was set in 1984 and concluded that there was no evidence to suggest that it needed to be revised. It is to be emphasised that the WHO 1.5mg/L guideline is not a 'fixed' value but rather is intended to be implemented in the light of local conditions (e.g., diet, water consumption, ect.).

局部用氟预防龋齿的历史有 50 年了，局部用氟主要包括含氟的凝胶，泡沫，涂料和漱口水等。其安全问题主要是一次性摄入过量引起的急性氟中毒。

1987 年 Whitford 提出了儿童局部用氟的可能中毒量（PTD）问题（表 5-24）。可能中毒量为 5mg/kg 体重，是指儿童摄入氟的剂量达到或超过此剂量可能产生急性氟中毒的症状，需住院观察和准备急救措施。

表 5-24 应用氟凝胶与可能中毒量（PTD）的关系 *

氟凝胶	浓度		常用量		可能中毒量	
	化合物 / 氟素		毫升 / 毫克氟		体重 / 用量	
	%	%			10kg	20kg
2.72%NaF(APF)	2.72	1.23	5	61.6	4	8
0.40%SnF_2	0.40	0.097	1	0.97	50	100
8.0%SnF_2	8.0	1.94	1	19.4	2.5	5

* 表中 PTD 是以 1 岁儿童平均体重 10 公斤和 5 ～ 6 岁儿童平均体重 20 公斤计算的

由于幼儿的吞咽反射发育尚不完善，应用含氟牙膏和漱口水易发生氟中毒不良反应。因此，5 岁以下儿童最好不用氟水漱口。学龄前儿童刷牙最好用儿童含氟牙膏（氟浓度较低）。

根据上述人体适宜、安全摄氟剂量的研究，在我国，计划实施全身（或系统）用氟的社区应参考以下几点：①当地饮水氟含量应低于 0.5mg/L。如高于 0.5mg/L 而低于 1.0mg/L 则考虑局部用氟措施。②没有明显的氟污染（空气、食物等）或多种氟暴露（即在适合全身用氟的地区与人群中只能选用一种全身用氟的方法）。③ 5 ～ 6 岁儿童乳牙患龋率在 60% 以上，龋均在 3.0 以上。12 岁儿童恒牙患龋率在 40% 以上，龋均在 1.0 以上。④氟牙症指数（Dean）在 0.4 以下，其中很轻度氟牙症在 10% 以下。

在一个地区只推荐一种全身（或系统）用氟措施，用一种以上氟防龋措施有增加效益，但如果龋齿患病水平低，就可能出现成本高效果低而不合算。由于许多地方有多种氟来源，除牙膏外还有食物、饮料等，多种氟暴露可能有益但也增加了氟牙症的可能性。虽然只有专业人员才能辨认得出的很轻度氟牙症对健康无害和外观无碍，但必须进行定期的监测评估，保证人体摄氟量的适宜、安全。

3. 全身（系统）用氟防龋措施的安全监测 Monitoring the safety of systemic use of fluoride for caries prevention

开展氟化物防龋 50 多年来取得了令人瞩目的成就，目前氟防龋仍然是人类预防龋病的主要措施。在开展氟化物防龋项目的社区应同时进行氟化物防龋的效果与安全性的定期监测与评价。定期监测与评价的几个方面有：人体总摄氟量监测，环境氟监测，用氟剂量监测，氟牙症患病水平监测和尿氟监测等。

人体总摄氟量监测是最准确的监测方法，可以清楚的了解人体摄氟情况是否适宜安全。但具体操作困难较多，主要在科研课题而不是社区项目中应用。环境氟监测就是监控饮水、食物和空气等人体外环境氟的水平和污染状况，这是开展氟防龋措施的先决条件和基础资料。用氟剂量监测常参考环境氟监测资料用以不断调整用氟剂量以求适宜安全。氟牙症患病水平监测是与防龋效果的临床评价一起进行的，根据氟牙症患病水平监测结果调整用氟剂量的最大缺点是形成的氟牙症是不可逆的。尿氟监测是比较简便易行且行之有效的用氟监测方法。由于机体氟排泄的途径主要是由肾脏代谢随尿液排出，世界各国对于氟防龋的安全监测大多采用尿氟监测并且监测的技术方法也在不断完善。

综上所述，人体总摄氟量与安全性是开展氟防龋工作的重要前提。人体总摄氟量不应超过口腔健康与全身健康的适宜、安全剂量。通过定期检测尿氟排量监测总摄氟量，评估氟牙症流行状况及严重程度是口腔预防保健工作不容忽视的方面。

由于摄入氟素的量和时间的不同，一天中尿氟排泄率有很大变化，特别是以氟化牛奶和氟片形式全身一次性补充氟素或是用含氟牙膏刷牙时吞咽一定量的氟素等局部用氟措施均可加大尿氟排泄率的变化。因此，检测尿氟的留尿时间应尽可能达到24小时并最好连续48小时以监测尿氟排泄量及变化进而计算摄氟量是否安全适宜。

1. 氟牙症患病水平监测

氟牙症患病水平监测有几个问题应引起注意，以便保证氟防龋措施安全有效，也有助于公众正确认识氟防龋措施，克服疑虑和偏见。

（1）目前国内外文献报告的氟牙症患病水平监测中存在的主要问题是，所用数据是不同的调查者在不同的国家和地区使用不同的氟牙症指数（常用的就有3个）获得的，因此，文献中监测结果的可比性存在问题。就是同一地区同一项目因基线调查和后期评估的检查者没有使用同一指数的标准一致性检验，也影响数据的可靠性。

（2）氟防龋措施中因用氟过量或多种氟暴露所引起的氟牙症多为很轻度或轻度的。很轻度的氟牙症在诊断上比较困难，也是检查者自身和检查者之间最容易产生误差的。

（3）现在所使用的各种氟牙症指数并不是针对公众和专业人员所关心的因氟防龋措施或多种氟暴露造成的很轻度或轻度氟牙症引起的牙外观问题而设计的，使用上有一定的局限性。

考虑到上述情况，应重视氟牙症患病水平的监测，尽量避免调查偏性（误差）和干扰因素，客观准确的评价监测结果，应参考以下几点：

（1）比较分析的数据应是在同一地区，用同一指数和同一检查者（或检查者之间标准一致性检验是可靠的）所获得的。应有基线数据和定期（3 ~ 5 年）监测数据。

（2）与文献数据进行比较分析应使用与之相同的指数和监测条件。

（3）与文献数据进行比较分析应考虑氟防龋措施的可比性（氟浓度、特定人群、多种氟暴露因素等）。

2. 世界卫生组织推荐的尿氟安全监测方法

1996 年 WHO 推荐了国际牛奶氟化项目所采用的单位时间留尿法（time-controlled urine sample）的尿氟监测方法。通过成功的尿氟安全监测所获得的每日尿氟排量和每日摄氟量便可确定实施的氟防龋措施是否符合“兴氟利，除氟害”和“适当用氟预防龋齿”的原则。

表 5-25 为近年来文献报告的有关尿氟排量和尿氟浓度的数据，可作为参考。

表 5-25　尿氟排量（μg/L）和尿氟浓度（mg/L）数据表

尿氟排量 (μg/h)	高峰值 (昼)	低峰值 (夜)	24 小时均值	
3 ~ 5 岁	低氟区	8 ~ 13	6 ~ 11	7 ~ 12
食盐氟化		14 ~ 23	10 ~ 16	14 ~ 20
饮水氟化		16 ~ 20	14 ~ 18	16 ~ 20
6 ~ 7 岁	低氟区	10 ~ 14	8 ~ 12	8 ~ 13

续表

尿氟排量 (μg/h)	高峰值 (昼)	低峰值 (夜)	24 小时均值	
食盐氟化		25 ～ 40	18 ～ 26	20 ～ 30
饮水氟化		30 ～ 36	19 ～ 24	23 ～ 32
10 ～ 14 岁	低氟区	12 ～ 15	8 ～ 11	9 ～ 12
食盐氟化		31 ～ 48	18 ～ 26	24 ～ 34
饮水氟化		30 ～ 40	19 ～ 24	25 ～ 35
尿氟浓度 (mg/L)				
低氟区		0.3 ～ 0.5	0.2 ～ 0.4	0.2 ～ 0.5
食盐氟化		1.0 ～ 1.3	0.8 ～ 1.1	1.0 ～ 1.2
饮水氟化		0.8 ～ 1.2	0.7 ～ 0.9	0.9 ～ 1.2

(Marthaler 1992)

表 5-26 为适量、安全摄氟剂量表，可作为参考。

表 5-26　人体适量、安全摄氟剂量表

年龄 (周岁)	适宜摄氟量范围 (mg/ 天) 摄氟量 / 体重 最低	摄氟量 / 体重 最高	摄氟量 / 能量 最低	摄氟量 / 能量 最高
<1	0.16	0.33	0.39	0.78
1 ～ 3	0.30	0.60	0.66	1.31
4 ～ 6	0.45	0.90	0.87	1.75
7 ～ 9	0.63	1.25	1.06	2.12
10 ～ 12 (女)	0.85	1.70	1.13	2.26
10 ～ 12 (男)	0.82	1.65	1.25	2.51
13 ～ 15 (女)	1.11	2.23	1.20	2.39
16 ～ 19 (女)	1.21	2.43	1.12	2.23
成人 (女)	1.23	2.45	1.06	2.12
成人 (男)	1.45	2.90	1.45	2.90

(Marthaler 1992)

小结 Summary

通过本篇的学习，在全面了解和认识氟化物对预防龋病的作用和对人体健康影响的基础上，正确和灵活的运用氟防龋的原则和方法服务于临床和社区口腔预防保健工作。人体总摄氟量与安全性是开展氟防龋工作的重要前提。人体总摄氟量不应超过口腔健康与全身健康的适宜、安全剂量。无论开展任何一项全身或局部的氟防龋措施，都要符合“兴氟利，除氟害”和“适当用氟预防龋齿”的原则。

思考题 Review questions

1. 为什么说应用氟防龋是20世纪预防口腔医学对人类的伟大贡献之一?
2. 如何做到“兴氟利，除氟害”和“适当用氟预防龋齿”。

参考文献 References

1. 梁超轲等. 总摄氟量卫生标准的研究. 卫生研究, 1996, 25: 282
2. WHO. Fluorides and Oral Health. WHO Technical Report Series, 1994, 846
3. Murray JJ, Rugg-Gann AJ, Jenkins GN. Fluoride and Caries Prevention. Oxford, Wright, 1991
4. Murray JJ. Prevention of Oral Disease (Third edition). Oxford Univ. Express, 1996
5. Whitford GM. Acute and chronic toxicity. J Dent Res, 1992, 71: 1249-1254
6. Harris NO, Christen AG. Primary Preventive Dentistry 4th edition. Appleton & Lange, 1995
7. Burt BA, Eklund SA. Dentistry, Dental Practice, and the Community. 5th edition. W B. Saunders Company, 1999
8. 卞金有. 预防口腔医学 (第4版). 人民卫生出版社, 2003
9. Pine CM. Community oral health. Reed Educational & Professional Publishing Ltd, 1997
10. 全国牙防组. 第二次全国口腔健康流行病学抽样调查. 人民卫生出版社, 1998
11. Bian JY, Wang WJ, Rong WSH, et al. Caries prevention in Chinese children with sodium fluoride dentifrice delivered through a kindergarten-based oral health program in China. J Clin Dent, 2002, 13: 179-184
12. Ammari A B, Bloch-Zupan A, Ashley P F. Systematic review of studies comparing the anti-caries efficacy of children's toothpaste containing 600ppm of fluoride or less with high fluoride toothpaste of 1000ppm or above. Caries Res, 2003, 37: 85-92
13. Rolla G, Saxegaard D. Critical evaluation of the composition and use of topical fluorides, with emphasis on the role of calcium fluoride in caries inhibition. J Dent Res, 1990, 69: 780-5

（王伟健）

第六章　牙周病的公共卫生方面
Chapter Ⅵ Public Health Aspects of Periodontal Diseases

概述 Overview

本章从公共卫生的角度阐述了牙周病的病因、危险因素和流行特点。就社区群体的预防与控制，介绍了牙周病的三级预防、药物预防、专业保健和自我保健的各种方法等内容。强调了开展牙周病的社区公共卫生项目的特点和意义。

This chapter is deal with causes and risk factors of periodontal diseases and epidemic trends of periodontal diseases. It is introduced that three levels prevention; pharmacy prevention; methods of professional and self care for periodontal diseases. Community preventive program is emphasised.

要点 Key point

- 牙周病的危险因素和流行特点
- 牙周病的三级预防
- 牙周病的社区公共卫生项目

第一节　从公共卫生的角度认识牙周病
Section 1 Recognition of Periodontal Diseases From the Viewpoint of Public Health

牙周病是口腔常见病多发病之一，由于其在青少年、成年和老年人群中患病率高，又由于其病因复杂，与另一种口腔常见病多发病龋病相比，尚没有十分有效的治疗牙周病的方法，所以牙周病的防治成为口腔医学领域备受关注的研究课题。本章将从牙周病的公共卫生方面论述在人群中预防和控制牙周病的理论和方法。

一、牙周病的概念 Concept of periodontal diseases

牙周病是指发生在牙周组织（牙龈、牙周膜、牙槽骨）病变的总称。牙周病又分为牙龈病和牙周炎两大类。

Periodontal diseases is the expression for pathological changes of the periodontal tissues (the gingivae, periodontal membrane, alveolar bone and cementum). There are tow kinds of Periodontal diseases.

牙龈病（gingival diseases）是指发生在牙龈的疾病。从临床的角度可分为慢性缘龈炎（chronic marginal gingivitis），增生性龈炎（hyperplastic gingivitis），妊娠性龈炎（pregnancy gingivitis），青春期龈炎（puberty gingivitis），急性坏死性溃疡性龈炎（acute necrotizing ulcerative gingivitis），牙龈瘤（epulis）等。

牙周炎（periodontitis）是指发生在牙周组织以牙周附着丧失形成牙周袋为主要病理特点的疾病。从临床的角度分为成人慢性牙周炎（chronic adult periodontitis，CAP），青少年牙周炎（juvenile periodontitis，JP），快速进展型牙周炎（rapidly progressive periodontitis，RPP），青春前期牙周炎（prepubertal periodontitis，PPP），伴有全身疾病的牙周炎（periodontitis with Systemic diseases）等。

从公共卫生的角度看待牙周病的预防主要是针对慢性缘龈炎和成人慢性牙周炎。这是因为一方面这两种疾病都有明确的病因即慢性炎症，因此有比较有效的预防和控制的方法。另一方面这两种疾病患病率最高构成了牙周病各种类型的大部分。

Objects of periodontal diseases prevention from the viewpoint of public health are chronic marginal gingivitis and chronic adult periodontitis.

从公共卫生的角度看待牙周病的性质：牙周疾病是一种牙周组织缓慢进行的慢性炎症过程。

Characteristics of periodontal diseases from the viewpoint of public health are that periodontal diseases are slowly progressing inflammatory diseases.

二、牙周病的病因与危险因素 The etiology and risk factors of periodontal diseases

（一）牙周病的病因 The etiology of periodontal diseases

牙周病的病因是多因素的。包括局部因素和全身因素。在局部因素当中牙菌斑是始动因素，此外还有一些因素有利于牙菌斑的聚集而不利于牙菌斑的清除，称之为局部促进因素。全身因素则降低了机体的抵抗力或增加了机体对牙菌斑细菌的敏感性，从而促进牙周病的发生和发展。

The etiology of periodontal diseases are multi-factors which include local factors and systemic factors. Plaque act as the initiating factors in local factors, other local factors act as local promotive factors because these factors may improve plaque assembling or disturb plaque removal. Systemic factors may reduce the resistance of the body or promote the sensitivity to plaque so that promote periodontal diseases occurrence and progresst.

1. 始动因素 Initiating factors

牙菌斑（dental plaque）是黏附在牙齿表面的一层细菌性薄膜。根据黏附的部位分为龈上菌斑（supragingival plaque）和龈下菌斑（subgingival plaque）。龈上菌斑位于龈缘以上，主要分布在近牙龈1/3的牙冠处和其他不易清洁的部位，如窝沟、裂隙、邻接面等。龈下菌斑位于龈缘以下，分布在龈沟或牙周袋内。龈下菌斑又根据与牙面附着的关系分为附着性龈下菌斑（attached subgingival plaque）和非附着性龈下菌斑（unattached subgingival plaque）。附着性龈下菌斑是由龈上菌斑延伸到牙周袋内附着于牙根面。非附着性龈下菌斑位于附着性龈下菌斑的表面，不与牙根面接触而直接与龈沟上皮或袋内上皮接触。各种菌斑内的细菌成分不尽相同，其优势菌有G^+需氧菌和兼性菌，G^+兼性菌和厌氧菌，G^-厌氧菌和能动菌等。由于牙菌斑的致病性与菌斑中的优势菌成分有直接的关系，因此也有非特异性菌斑（non-specific plaque）和特异性菌斑（specific plaque）的说法。龈上菌斑与牙龈炎的发生发展关系密切，龈下菌斑特别是非附着性龈下菌斑与牙周炎的发生发展关系密切。

菌斑细菌的致病机制（etiologic mechanism of the bacteria in plaque）可通过细菌的抗原成分、酶、毒素、代谢产物（composition of its antigent，enzyme，toxin，metabolic products）进入或细菌本身侵入牙周组织，直接破坏牙周组织；或通过抑制宿主的防御功能而引发变态反应等，间接地损害牙周组织。

2. 局部促进因素 Local promotive factors

牙石（dental calculus），创伤𬌗（occlusal traumatism），食物嵌塞（food impaction），牙列不齐（dental crowding），不良修复体（unqualified dentures）等，有利于牙菌斑的黏附或不利于牙菌斑的清除，或造成对牙周组织的损伤，使牙周组织容易受到细菌的感染，因而对于牙周病的发生和发展起到促进作用。

3. 全身影响因素 Systemic factors

牙菌斑的致病性还与宿主对菌斑细菌的敏感性和宿主的防御功能有密切的关系。易感的宿主以及某些能增加宿主易感性降低宿主抵抗力的因素也是影响牙周病的发生发展的重要因素，例如某些内分泌异常（hormonal factors）、营养不良（malnutrition）、血液疾患（hematologic diseases）、药物（medicament）、放射线（X-rays）、精神紧张（mental stress）、增龄性变化（aging）、遗传因素（hereditary factors）、宿主的免疫炎症反应（immunity inflammatory reaction）等。在这方面比较熟知的像糖尿病患者往往伴有牙周炎，维生素C缺乏时牙龈出血，白血病或贫血病时伴有牙龈病，经常服用苯妥英钠会发生牙龈增生和牙龈瘤，放射性牙周炎，遗传性掌趾角化牙周综合征，艾滋病性牙周炎等都说明全身因素对牙周健康的影响。

值得指出的是，近十几年来，口腔医学研究进展还进一步揭示了牙周炎对全身健康的影响。牙周感染性菌血症可使机体产生相关抗体及凝集素，使血小板凝集形成血栓。此外，感染细菌的毒素激活单核细胞/成纤维细胞产生前列腺素E2、肿瘤坏死因子、白介素-1等，可以损伤血管内皮细胞，使血管内膜胆固醇沉积，从而诱发心肌梗死和冠心病发作。有报告称，有牙周感染者发生冠心病的几率为牙周健康者的1.4倍，发生脑卒中的几率为牙周健康者的2.1倍。患重症牙周炎的孕妇发生早产或娩出低出生体重儿的危险率为牙周健康的孕妇的7.5倍。

（二）牙周病的危险因素 The risk factors of periodontal diseases

这里牙周病的危险因素是指能影响牙周病发生和发展的，可以改变的一些因素。通过干预而改变这些因素，可以降低牙周病发生和发展的可能性。目前牙周病比较明确的危险因素有口腔卫生、吸烟和某些全身性疾病如糖尿病。

The means of the risk factors of periodontal diseases are that facts can affect occurrence and development of periodontal diseases. These facts can be changed so that can preventive and control periodontal diseases. It is clear that the risk factors of periodontal diseases are oral hygiene, smoking and some systemic disease such as diabetic.

1. 口腔卫生 Oral hygiene

口腔卫生的好坏实质上反映的是牙菌斑的多少，因此口腔卫生与牙周病有着密切的关系。一项研究显示，26～30岁的成年人，口腔卫生好的牙槽骨吸收14%，而口腔卫生不好的牙槽骨吸收25%。41～45岁的成年人，口腔卫生好的牙槽骨吸收22%，而口腔卫生不好的牙槽骨吸收40%。

Strong correlation between periodontal diseases and oral hygiene: A research results show that the rate of alveolar bone absorption among the adults of age 26～30 years with good oral hygiene are 14%, but the rate of alveolar bone absorption with bad oral hygiene are 25%. The rate of alveolar bone absorption among the adults of age 41～45 years with good or bad oral hygiene, the rate of alveolar bone absorption are 22% and 40% separately.

2. 吸烟 Smoking

许多研究都证明吸烟与牙周病的发生发展有密切的关系。

一项在泰国进行的关于吸烟与牙周健康状况的关系的研究。研究对象：泰国清迈124名，男（35～44岁）。根据牙周健康状况分为病例组：61人，CPITN = 3或4，对照组：63人，CPTIN＜3。根据问卷调查分为：吸烟组、不吸烟组和曾吸烟组。结果：病例组中90%为吸烟或曾吸烟者，对照组中61%为吸烟或曾吸烟者；吸烟组比不吸烟组有较高的牙周袋率和较高的CPITN为3或4的平均区段数（$P < 0.001$）；牙周疾病的严重程度直接与开始吸烟的年龄（$P < 0.05$）与吸烟的时间（$P < 0.001$）与吸烟的数量（$P < 0.05$）有关。结论：吸烟是牙周破坏的一项重要的高危因素。

The relationship between smoking exposure and periodontal status: Subjects: 124 male people aged 35～44 years in Thailand.Methods: Case group: 61, CPITN=3 or 4; Control group: 63, CPITN＜3. All subjects in case and control groups were interviewed about smoking habits and then reclassified into smoking, nonsmoking and exsmoking groups. Results: 90% of the case group and 61% of the control group were smokers or exsmokers; Compared to nonsmoker, smokers had significantly a higher prevalence of periodontal pockets and higher mean number of sextant with CPITN score 3 or 4 ($P<0.001$); The severity of periodontal disease was directly related to the age when starting to smoke ($P<0.05$), to the duration of smoking ($P<0.001$), and to the daily tobacco consumption ($P<0.05$). Conclusion: It is evident that tobacco smoking is an important risk factor for periodontal destruction.

吸烟导致和加重牙周病的机理尚不明了，一般认为是因为吸烟影响牙周组织血液循环、影响体液免疫、细胞免疫和炎症过程，尤其是削弱口腔中性粒细胞的趋化性和吞噬功能。吸烟者一般口腔卫生较差，容易使牙菌斑附着并形成牙石也是加重牙周病的一个因素。

3. 糖尿病 Diabetes

糖尿病与牙周病的密切关系已是口腔界的共识。目前公认糖尿病是牙周病的危险因素之一，而且牙周病和糖尿病之间具有双向影响的关系。

白求恩医科大学狄强等人进行了"四氧嘧啶致大白鼠糖尿病对牙周组织影响的实验研究"：分组：①正常大白鼠+粉末饲料；②咬殆创伤（银汞超填）+粉末饲料；③粪食；④咬殆创伤+粪食；⑤糖尿病+咬殆创伤+粪食；⑥糖尿病+粉末饲料。结果：①单纯糖尿病（6组）降低牙周组织抵抗力，但没见明显牙周病变；②咬殆创伤（2组与1组比较）牙周组织发生变化；③咬殆创伤+菌斑（4组）牙周组织有明显病理变化；④单一因素（创伤，2组）和双因素（创伤+菌斑，4组）第8天可见牙周膜破坏，牙槽骨和牙骨质吸收等变化，但第24天可见基本修复，而三因素（创伤+菌斑+糖尿病，5组）第24天时完全未见修复。结论：①菌斑和创伤是牙周疾病的致病因素；②糖尿病可大大促进牙周疾病的发生和发展。

Effects of experimental alloxan diabetic on the periodontal tissues of rats: Groups:Unoperated controls; Occlusal trauma alone; Coprophagy alone; Occlusal trauma plus coptophagy; Alloxan plus occlusal trauma plus coprophagy; Alloxan alone.Results: Alloxan diabetic reduced resistance of rat periodontal tissues,but no obvious diseases were causes in the periodontal tissues; Excessive amalgam filling groups compared with normal control groups, pathological changes of rat periodontal tissues were distinct; In the occlusal trauma plus coprophagy groups, distinct pathological changes of rats periodontal tissues were caured; In alloxan diabetic rats received excessive amalgam filling on the diet with feces, the disorganization of the periodontal ligament and the resorption of the alveolar bone and cementum were found at 8 days. These injures were not repaired at 24 days. However, in excessive amalgam filing rats and excessive amalgam filling rats on the diet with feces, the disorganization of the petiodontal ligament and the resorption of the alveolar bone and cementum were found at 8 days. These injuries were repaired at 24 days. Conclusions: This study shows that if the people who has traumatic occlusion and plaque suffer from physical diseases such as diabetic and etc. periodontal diseases may occur and become severe.

糖尿病促使牙周病发生和发展的机理可能是白细胞趋化和吞噬功能缺陷、组织内血管基膜的改变、胶原合成减少、骨基质形成减少以及免疫调解能力下降所致。而牙周感染会增加血清糖化（glycosylation）末端产物，使糖尿病的代谢控制复杂化。因此，控制糖尿病是保持牙周健康的有效措施，而有效的控制糖尿病患者的牙周感染又是控制糖尿病的重要手段。

（三）牙周病的预防策略

根据牙周病的病因与危险因素的理论，预防牙周病的策略应以保持口腔卫生为基础，彻底清除牙菌斑，采取戒烟和提高全身健康水平，积极治疗和控制糖尿病等全身性疾病的综合方法。

Strategy of periodontal diseases prevention: According to the theory of the etiology and risk factors of periodontal diseases, the strategy of periodontal diseases prevention should put in oral hygiene maintenance as its foundation thorough plaque removal and adoption of comprehensive measures including no-smoking, physical exercises actively and treatment or control diabetic.

三、牙周病的流行病学特点 Characteristics of epidemiologic studies of periodontal diseases

1. 牙周病的流行情况

有关牙周病流行情况的调查资料很多，有代表性的是我国分别于1983年和1995年完成的全国口腔健康流行病学调查。1983年的调查显示我国7、9、12、15、17五个年龄组的中小学生牙龈炎患病率城市为63.93%，农村69.68%；牙结石城市为41.87%，农村52.21%。1995年的调查显示，6个区段牙周健康的人数很少，12岁组占受检人数的24.96%，15岁为15.95%，18岁为22.75%，35～44岁为2.02%，65～74岁为0.33%。牙结石检出率较高，12岁为24.96%，15岁为67.91%，18岁为78.95%，35～44岁为94.15%，65～74岁为77.46%。

从牙周病的患病率可以看出，牙周病是影响口腔健康的最常见的口腔慢性疾病之一。

2. 牙周病是成年人丧失牙齿的主要原因

据北京医学院口腔医院的统计，门诊拔牙病例中有1/3是牙周病。

3. 早期没有明显感觉，容易被忽视

The prevalence of periodontal diseases indicate that periodontal diseases are one of the most common chronic oral diseases affecting oral health.

Periodontal diseases are the primary factor of missing teeth in adults: One cases evaluation for the extraction in the Dental Hospital Beijing Medical College show periodontal diseases cover 1/3 of extracted teeth.

No obvious sensation at the early stage, easily be ignored.

四、预防牙周病的意义－作为一项公共卫生措施 Significance in prevention of periodontal diseases-as a public health measure

由于牙周病患病的广泛性，对牙周健康已构成严重的危害，因此牙周病的预防已成为全球“2000 年人人享有口腔卫生保健”目标之一：

WHO 提出 18 岁前牙区段牙龈至少有 2 个不应在检查时出血，不应有 6mm 或更深的龈袋。

WHO 西太区提出 15 ~ 19 岁需洁治和口腔健康教育者不超过 25%。

我国提出 15 岁（农村和城市不同经济发展地区）至少 20% ~ 60% 有 3 个牙周健康区段（CPITN = 0）。

Prevention of periodontal diseases has become one of the objectives of “Oral Health for All by the year 2000” in the world :

WHO: (before 18 y) No bleeding of the gingivae at probing in at least 2 teeth of the front sextants, no periodontal pocket = or > 6 mm.

WHO (West Pacific Region) : (15~19 y) Need for scaling and oral health education should not exceed 25%.

China: (15 y) At least 20%~60% should have healthy periodontal tissues in 3 sextants (CPITN = 0).

第二节　牙周病的预防和控制

Section 2 The Prevention and Control of Periodontal Diseases

一、三期预防 Three stages of prevention

牙周病的预防和控制应遵循三期预防的原则。

一期预防是指牙周病损发生之前，应进行口腔卫生指导并采取有效刷牙自我清除牙菌斑。另外还要定期看牙科医生接受预防性清洁术，通过专业手段帮助彻底清除牙菌斑。

二期预防是指当发生牙龈炎或早期牙周病时，应在一期预防的基础上还应该进行洁治彻底清除牙结石。

三期预防是指当牙周病变发展到牙周病晚期时，应在二期预防的基础上还应进行刮治或其他牙周手术，通过牙周治疗手段控制牙周病的发展。

The Prevention and control of Periodontal Diseases should follow along the principle of three stages of prevention.

Primary prevention: Before occurrence of the lesion oral health instructions and plaque removal by the self-care of brushing teeth effectively should be carried out. And also it is necessary to check-up by dentist regularly to receive mechanical plaque removal by dental prophylaxis.

Secondary prevention: During gingivitis or early stage of periodontal diseases, apart from the primary prevention methods scaling or other periodontal treatment should be carried out so that to remove calculus thoroughly.

Tertiary prevention: During advanced stage of periodontal diseases, apart from the secondary prevention methods subgingival scaling or periodontal operation should be carried out so that to control the progress of periodontal diseases.

二、自我保健 Self care in oral health

预防牙周病的基本原则应该是一生中不断地彻底地清除牙菌斑，通过有效刷牙和应用牙线、牙签来清除牙菌斑是自我口腔保健预防和控制牙周病最主要的方法。

Constant and thorough plaque removal for a whole lifetime: It is the most important approach to prevent and control periodontal diseases by the way of removal plaque including brushing teeth effectively and using dental floss and toothpick.

1. 有效刷牙 Brushing teeth effectively

有效刷牙是指采用适当的方法最大限度地清除牙菌斑但又不损伤牙齿和牙龈。刷牙的目的是去除菌斑、牙面的食物残渣、软垢，按摩牙龈组织并作为牙膏的载体 。刷牙效果取决于三个因素：刷牙方式，刷牙频率和持续时间，以及牙刷的设计。其中，前两个因素最重要，因为采用好的刷牙方法并增加刷牙的时间可以更有效的去除菌斑。

The objectives of toothbrushing are to remove plaque, clean teeth of food debris and stain, stimulate the gingival tissues, and apply dentrifice.

Toothbrushing efficiency depends on three factors: brushing technique, brushing frequency and duration, and brush design. The first two factors are the most important since good technique combined with increased time spent brushing will improve plaque removal.

（1）刷牙方法 Toothbrushing techniques

学者们提出了许多的刷牙方法，这些方法每种都涉及水平法、垂直法、旋转法和颤动法的不同方式的组合（见表 6-1）。

A number of different toothbrushing techniques have been advocated, and each involves different combinations of horizontal, vertical, rotary, and vibratory motions (see Table click).

表 6-1 刷牙方法 Toothbrushing techniques

方法 Techniques	刷毛的位置 Bristle Position	动作 Motion	●效果 Effect
水平法 Horizontal Scrub	与牙面成 90° 角 90° to tooth	水平向的拉动 Horizontal Scrub	●龈上清洁 Supragingival cleaning ●牙龈按摩 Gingival stimulation
Fones 法	与牙面成 90° 角 90° to tooth	在牙面和牙龈上面划大圈 Large circles over teeth and gingiva	●龈上清洁 Supragingival cleaning
Leonard 法	与牙面成 90° 角 90° to tooth	垂直拉动 Vertical strokes	●龈上清洁 Supragingival cleaning ●牙龈按摩 Gingival stimulation
Smith-Bell	在殆平面 At occlusal surface	齿龈向横扫 Sweep gingivally	●龈上清洁 Supragingival cleaning
滚动刷法 Rolling Stroke	刷毛尖端接触牙龈 Apically at attached gingiva	殆面方向扫动 Sweep occlusally	●龈上清洁 Supragingival cleaning
Stillman 法	向根尖方向呈 45° 角；部分在龈缘，部分在牙间隙 45° to apex; pary on gingival margin and cervix of tooth	颤动 Vibratory pulsing	●牙龈按摩 Gingival stimulation
改良 Charters 法 Modified chartes	与根尖呈 90° 角 90° to apex	殆面方向扫动，环行颤动 Sweep occlusally Circular vibratory	●牙龈按摩 Gingival stimulation ●邻面清洁 Interproximal cleaning
改良 Bass 法 Modified bass	与根尖呈 45° 角，在龈沟中 45° to apex，in sulcus	殆面方向扫动 Sweep occlusallyVibratory horizontal jiggle	●龈上清洁 Supragingival cleaning

表中所描述的刷牙方法可以用来清除唇面、舌面和咬殆面的菌斑，但对于邻面效果较差。只有改良巴氏刷牙法可以有效的清洁龈沟，而改良charters刷牙法对于清洁固定矫治器很有用。

All the techniques described in the Table can be used to clean facial, lingual and occlusal surfaces, but are less effective for interproximal areas. Only the Modified Bass technique effectively cleans the sulcus, while the Modified Charters technique is useful for cleaning fixed orthodontic appliances.

刷牙可以导致牙龈组织的创伤，这取决于不同的刷牙方法。采用水平刷牙的患者，过度的压力和牙膏中的摩擦剂会导致牙龈退缩和牙体组织的损伤。使用fones和leonard刷牙法，压力过大也可以引起牙龈的创伤，而且，牙刷的滚动可以损伤膜龈联合部和牙槽黏膜。如果已经出现了损伤，医生应该帮助患者调整其刷牙方法避免进一步的损伤。

Depending on the technique used, toothbrushing can cause trauma to gingival tissues. For patients who use a horizontal scrubbing technique, excessive pressure and abrasive toothpaste will lead to gingival recession and tooth damage. The Fones and Leonard techniques, with vigorous pressure, can also cause gingival trauma, and the rolling stroke can traumatize the mucogingival junction and alveolar mucosa. If trauma is present, practitioners should help patients adapt their existing technique to avoid further injury.

如果有规律的使用，所有的刷牙方法都是有效的。如果患者可以有效的清除菌斑而不导致创伤，那么应该继续使用原来的刷牙方法。

If used regularly, all of the toothbrushing techniques are effective. Patients who successfully remove plaque without causing trauma should continue using the same technique.

（2）牙刷的设计 Toothbrush design

不同设计的手动牙刷因为刷牙时间、刷牙方式和压力以及存留牙齿的数目和形状的不同，其临床优点缺点很难评价。然而，软刷毛和较小的刷头可以更好的清洁邻面，长的牙刷柄可以更舒适并改善依从性。最近出现的新型的带角度或复合平面（取代了水平）的刷毛牙刷可以更有效地到达邻面区域，并更有效地去除菌斑。

The clinical advantages of different manual toothbrush designs are difficult to substantiate due to large variations in toothbrushing times, styles and pressures, and in the shape and number of teeth. However, softer bristle texture and a smaller brush head have been related to interproximal efficacy, and longer handles are more comfortable and may improve compliance. Recently, a novel head design with angled or multilevel (instead of horizontal) bristles has shown increased penetration of interproximal areas and increased potential for plaque removal.

电动牙刷在去除菌斑，减轻牙龈炎症，减轻对牙龈的损伤，减少细菌的黏附和生存，减少着色方面优于手动牙刷。另外，电动刷牙可以有效的去除邻面牙菌斑，这种牙菌斑积聚迅速，并且难于用人工刷牙方法去除。最近，许多低成本的使用电池的电动牙刷已问世。

Powered toothbrushes are consistently superior to manual toothbrushes for removing plaque, and reducing gingivitis, gingival abrasions, bacterial adherence and viability, and staining. In addition, powered toothbrushes are particularly useful for removing interproximal plaque, which accumulates quickly and is difficult to remove with a manual brush. Recently, a number of low cost battery-powered toothbrushes have become available.

（3）刷牙步骤 Toothbrushing procedure

常规的刷牙模式应该是避免漏掉任何一个区域，理想刷牙时间是3分钟。尽管刷牙可能导致牙龈创伤，不刷牙所带来的问题要比不适宜的刷牙技术造成的创伤严重。最后，彻底刷牙和合适的刷牙的频率较刷牙方法更加重要。

A routine brushing pattern should be established to avoid exclusion of any areas, and a three minutes brushing time is ideal. Although toothbrushing may cause gingival trauma, the problems produced by failure to brush are more serious than the damage caused by improper brushing techniques. Ultimately, throughness and brusheng frequency are more important than a specific toothbrushing technique.

2. 应用菌斑显示剂评价菌斑控制的效果 Assessment of plaque control by using plaque disclosing

由于牙菌斑是薄而无色的，紧密地附着在牙齿表面，正常情况下肉眼不易看清，只有通过特殊的染色才能显示出来而被肉眼所辨认。常用的菌斑显示剂用中性品红和四碘荧光素钠制成溶液或片剂。使用时将菌斑显示液滴布在，或用棉球轻轻涂布在牙的颊舌面，如果是菌斑显示片，则将其嚼碎，然后用舌尖舔牙的各个面，让菌斑显示剂均匀地涂布在牙表面。通常染色后的菌斑呈现红色。

用菌斑显示剂显示菌斑可以用来评价菌斑控制的效果，可用以下公式计算菌斑百分率。

$$\text{菌斑百分率}=\frac{\text{有菌斑牙面总数}}{\text{受检牙面总数}}\times 100\%$$

受检牙面数＝受检牙总数× 4

评价：10% 或少于 10% 可认为菌斑控制良好，20% 以下认为菌斑基本被控制。

$$\text{plaque}(\%)=\frac{\text{tooth surface with plaque}}{\text{tooth surface examined}}\times 100\%$$

tooth surface examined = tooth × 4

assessment: 10% or <10% show good result, <20% show plaque control basically.

3. 掌握判断牙龈是否健康的标准

牙龈出血是牙龈炎早期表现，也是自我判断牙龈炎的标准。如果发生牙龈出血，应使用软毛保健牙刷进行有效刷牙。一般来说，经过一周认真的刷牙，一旦牙菌斑得到有效的清除，牙龈出血就会得到控制。

Criteria for healthy gingivae: Gum bleeding is the early symptom of gingivitis and the criteria for self-diagnosis of gingivitis. When gum bleeding occurrence brushing teeth effectively using qualified toothbrush with soft bristle should carry out. As soon as dental plaque be removed effectively in one week brushing gum bleeding will be controlled.

北京大学口腔医学院的孟焕新等曾做过“牙周探诊出血的组织学和细菌学背景”的研究：研究对象为牙周健康者8例，边缘性龈炎12例，青少年牙周炎5例，成人牙周炎15例共40例。采用探诊出血指数（BI），改良Mazza法分6级：0＝牙龈健康，外观正常；1＝龈炎有颜色改变无探诊出血；2＝探诊点状出血；3＝出血流满龈沟但不溢出龈沟；4＝出血溢出龈沟；5＝牙龈自发出血。结果：① BI 与牙龈结缔组织的炎症程度密切相关，BI 值高说明炎症程度重。②探诊出血是龈炎早期指征。③出血病损的龈下螺旋体和能动菌比例显著高于不出血病损，BI 值与此菌呈正相关。

Professor Meng huanxin, School of Stomatology Beijing Medical University did the research “Histologic and microbiologic background of gingival bleeding on probling”. Subjects: Gingival tissue specimens and bacterial plaque samples were obtained from 40 subjects with clinically healthy gingival (8), marginal gingivitis (12), juvenile periodontitis (5) and adult periodontitis (15). Bleeding Index, modified Mazza:0. clinically healthy gingival 1. gingival with color change and no bleeding 2. spot bleeding 3. bleeding within gingival groove 4. bleeding out of gingival groove 5. bleeding automatically. The results showed that 1. significant positive correlation between BI scores and the percentage of infiltrated connective tissue. It means the BI scores increased in parallel with the increase of infiltrated connective tissue; 2. Bleeding is the indication of gingivitis in the early stage; 3.The proportion of subgingival spirochetes and motile bacteria in bleeding lesions was greater then in nonbleeding lesions. There was posiive correlation between BI and subgingival spirochetes, motile bacteria.

4. 定期检查，接受教育，发现疾病，及时治疗

要养成每半年或一年到医院作一次口腔检查的习惯，做到无病早防有病早治。

Regular check-ups, oral health instructions, finding diseases early, in time treatment.

5. 增加营养，增强体质，积极治疗和控制全身疾病

牙菌斑无时无刻不附着在牙面，清洁过的牙齿1～2个小时后就会有新的菌斑形成。虽然菌斑是牙周病的始动因素，但并不是只要有菌斑存在就会发生牙周病。现代研究认为，易感的宿主以及某些能增加宿主易感性的因素对于牙周病的发生和发展也是十分重要的。一方面是菌斑中细菌的致病作用和某些增加这种致病性的全身疾病，另一方面宿主自身的免疫功能始终都在对抗着这种致病作用，这两方面的作用处于平衡状态或增强宿主的健康状态牙龈健康就能得以维护。

Nutrient supplementation, health build up, positive medication and control of systemic diseases

6. 认识吸烟对牙周健康的影响远离烟草 Recognition of the smoking effect on periodontal health and no-smoking

三、专业性保健 Professional oral health care

预防牙周病的发生和发展，维护牙周健康还必须寻求口腔专业人员的帮助，做到自我保健与专业保健相结合。发达国家取得的牙周病防治的成绩就是建立在群众自我口腔保健的基础上，国家为老百姓提供了许多专业保健措施。防治牙周病的专业保健措施包括：

1. 通过预防性清洁术（Dental prophylaxis）机械性清除牙菌斑

个人清除牙菌斑的能力和效果是有限的，牙齿的有些部位如邻面、最后一颗磨牙的远端等是很难清洁干净的。预防性清洁术就是口腔专业人员用专业的口腔器械帮助受捡者彻底地清除牙菌斑。通常是用特制的牙齿邻面清洁器或牙线先清除牙齿邻面菌斑，然后用橡皮杯蘸上打磨膏清洁牙齿的光滑面。经过这样的专业处理就能做到彻底的清除牙菌斑。

2. 通过洁治清除牙石（Calculus removal by scaling）

牙石是一种沉积于牙面或修复体表面的钙化或正在钙化的菌斑及软垢，由唾液或龈沟液中的钙盐逐渐沉积而成，形成后不易去除。去除龈上牙石的方法叫洁治（scaling），去除龈下牙石的方法叫刮治（subgingival scaling）。洁治属于牙周病群体防治的公共卫生措施范畴，而刮治则属于临床牙周病治疗的一种方法。洁治有手用器械洁治和超声波洁治两种方法。近年来又有喷沙洁牙的方法问世。洁治应该定期进行，泰国在全国范围内推行农村卫生员经过培训后定期为农民进行手用器械洁治取得了很好的效果。还有一点需要强调的是，洁治或刮治后一定要用有效刷牙进行维护，有效刷牙结合定期洁治才能维护牙龈健康。

3. 去除促进牙周疾病发生的局部因素如食物嵌塞、创伤𬌗、不良修复体、错𬌗畸形等

Removal of local promotive factors: i.e. food impaction, traumatic occlusion, unqualified dentures, malocclusion etc.

四、药物方法 Medicine approach

应用0.1%或0.2%葡萄糖酸洗必太含漱，每天2次，每次10毫升，每次一分钟。亦可应用甲硝唑（灭滴灵）含漱。此外也可局部或全身应用抗生素如四环素、红霉素、螺旋霉素等。

Medicated mouthwash with 0.1% or 0.2% chlorhexidine gluconate 10 ml for 1 minute twice per day or with metronidozole. Antibiotics 1.e. tetracycline, erythromycin, spiramycin can also be used locally or systematically.

五、应用自我保健和专业保健相结合的方法，在人群中开展口腔卫生项目

Implementation of oral health programs among the population using the approach of integration of personal and professional oral health care. Here are some examples:

根据牙周病的病因和预防的理论，要在社区中开展群体预防项目，以下是几个实例。

北京大学口腔医学院杨是教授开展的“学校初级口腔保健措施对提高学生口腔健康的研究”：该研究在北京3所小学4年级学生（9～10岁）中进行。分为3组：第1组接受口腔卫生和刷牙教育，每天在校监督刷牙1次并使用含氟牙膏，每学期洁治1次；第2组不进行洁治，其余与第1组相同；第3组为对照组只接受口腔卫生和刷牙教育。1年后结果显示：①提高了学生的口腔卫生知识：懂得每天应刷2次牙的人数：试验组增加39.9%，对照组增加32.0%。懂得应该使用含氟牙膏：试验组增加92.2%，对照组增加12.9%。②改进了牙周健康状况：龈沟出血指数下降：1组0.49/0.37，2组0.58/0.45；菌斑指数下降：1组0.92/0.87，2组1.12/1.06。

Effects in improving oral health status by developing school-based primary oral health programs: Subjects: 4th grade (9～10 years old) students from 3 primary schools in Beijing. Methods: Group 1: received oral health and toothbrushing instruction, supervised daily toothbrushing with fluoridated toothpaste, and prophylaxis once a semester. Group 2: same with group 1 without prophylaxis.Group 3 (control group): only received oral health and toothbrushing instruction.Results (one year later): 1. A rise in oral health knowledge. The increase that both in test and control groups understand that one should brush their teeth twice a day are 39.9% and 32.0% respectively. But understanding to use fluoridated toothpaste are significantly different (test group 92.2%, control group 12.9%, $P<0.01$). 2. Improvement of periodontal health. Girls and boys in test 1 and 2 groups showed a significant reduction in BI (0.49, 0.58 and 0.37, 0.45) and PI (0.92, 1.06 and 0.87, 1.12).

日本E. Kishimoto等开展的“牙科卫生教育项目对社区居民牙周健康的作用”的研究：选择112名成人（平均46岁），分别在0、1、2、12月时检查CPITN，牙龈红肿，牙齿松动度、软垢指数；进行口腔卫生教育，方法是1小时口腔卫生幻灯宣教，教刷牙和牙签的使用法，牙间隙清洁法；结果显示：1. 第2个月检查时，牙龈红肿，探诊出血，软垢指数明显下降（$P<0.01$）。2. 一年以后，90%以上的人仍按宣教的方法刷牙。说明定期口腔检查和宣教相结合对公众保持牙周健康是有效的。

The effect of dental health education programon the periodontal health of residents in community: Subjects: 112 adults with average 46 years old in 2 communities. Methods: 1. CPITN, redness and swelling of gingival, tooth mobility, debris Index and bleeding Index. 2. Examination at 0, 1, 2, 12 month.

3. Oral health instruction: one hour slides; toothbrushing, tooth pick and cleaning interdental area method. Results: 1. The redness and swilling of gingival, bleeding Index, debris Index decreased significantly (P<0.01) at the 2 month examination. 2. One year later, more than 90% of subjects brushed their teeth based on our instruction. Conclusion: The program combined the examination with the instruction is useful in public.

瑞典Per-Osten Soder等开展的“在儿童和青少年时期的预防项目对成人的牙周健康状况的影响”的研究：方法：同一组牙医，1970年随机选择247名成人（31～40岁），都没有参加过任何预防项目。1985年随机选择1681名成人，在儿童和青少年时期都参加了预防项目。结果：1970年有47.9%需要牙周治疗，而1985年只有13.9%需要牙周治疗。说明在儿童和青少年时期的预防项目改善了成年人的牙周健康状况。

The influence of the preventive program at youngsteron the periodontal health condition at adult: Method: 247 randomly selected persons with age 31 ~ 40 years old, were examined for periodontitis in 1970. The person had not participated in any prevention program. 1681 young adults who had participated in prevention programs during their childhood and adolescence. randomly selected in 1985. Results: 47.9% of young adults need periodontal treatment in 1970. But in 1985 the periodontal treatment need of young adults was 13.9% only. Conclusion: preventive programs in childhood and adolescence improve periodontal health of adults.

小结 Summary

1. 牙周病的预防主要是针对缘龈炎和成人慢性牙周炎这两种慢性炎症疾病，以彻底清除牙菌斑为基础，通过自我保健和专业保健相结合的综合措施，来控制疾病的发生和发展。

2. 探诊出血是早期牙龈炎的指征。

3. 有效刷牙是保持牙周健康的最主要方法。

4. 洁治是专业性牙周保健的主要内容。

5. 教育群众知道良好的口腔卫生及定期的专业保健对于预防和控制牙周病的重要性。

1. Prevention of periodontal diseases is mainly focused on 2 chronic inflammatory diseases i.e.: marginal gingivitis and chronic adult periodontitis. Its foundation is thorough plaque removal through comprehensive measures of integrating personal and professional care to control the occurrence and development of the diseases.

2. Gingival bleeding on probing is the criterion of the early stage of gingivitis.

3. Brushing teeth effectively is the most principle measure for maintaining periodontal health.

4. Scaling is the main substance of professional periodontal health care.

5. Tell the people the importance of good oral hygiene and regular professional health care to the prevention and control of periodontal diseases.

思考题 Review questions

1. 牙周病三级预防的内容。
2. 如何开展牙周病的社区公共卫生项目。

参考文献 References

1. 郑麟蕃, 张震康主编. 实用口腔科学. 北京: 人民卫生出版社, 1993
2. 曹采方主编. 牙周病学. 北京: 人民卫生出版社, 2000
3. 张震康, 樊明文, 傅民魁主编. 现代口腔医学. 北京: 人民卫生出版社, 2003
4. 张震康. 口腔医学科学研究的重要进展和方向. 北京大学学报 (医学版), 2002, 34 (2): 97-98
5. loe H. E. Theilade, Jensen S B. Experimental gengivetis in man. J Periodontol, 1975, 46: 10-26
6. Arnim S S. The use of disclosing agents for measuring tooth cleanliness. J Periodontol, 1963, 34: 227-245
7. American Dental Association, Council on Scientific Affairs. Acceptance program guidelines for toothbrushes, 1996
8. Cynthia M Pine. Community Oral Health. Butterworth-Heinemann, 1997
9. Axelssoner P. Diagnosis and Risk Prediction of Periodongtal Diseases. Quintessence Books, 2002
10. Axelssoner P. Preventive Materials, Methods, and Programs. Quintessence Books, 2004
11. Axelssoner P, Nystrom B, Lindhe J. The long-term effect of a plaque control program on tooth mortality, caries and periodontal disease in adults. Results after 30 years of maintenance. J Clin Periodontol, 2004, 31: 749-757

（张博学）

第七章　自我口腔保健技术和方法

Chapter Ⅶ Techniques and Methods for Oral Self-Care

概述 Overview

本章主要叙述牙刷、刷牙与洁牙剂，包括手动与电动牙刷，洁牙剂的组成成分和各种牙膏。此外，还介绍了其他洁牙用品及其使用方法，如牙线、牙间刷与口腔含漱剂等。

This chapter briefly describes toothbrushes, toothbrushing and dentifrices, including manual and electric toothbrushes, various methods of toothbrushing and assessment of their efficiencies, the ingredients and composition of dentifrices, other cleansing aids and techniques are also introduced, beside them, such as dental flosses, and flossing techniques, interdental brushes and mouth rinses, etc.

要点 Key points

- *manual toothbrushes and toothbrushing methods and their effectiveness*
- *electric toothbrushes and its role, advantages and limitation*
- *dentifrices and its functions*
- *dental floss and flossing techniques*
- *mouth rinses and its functions*

第一节　牙刷与刷牙

Section 1 Toothbrushes and Toothbrushing

成功地去除牙菌斑和控制疾病的最关键的方面之一是人们对菌斑作用的理解，同样重要的是对其表现的认识。对个人进行菌斑的临床表现与部位的教育与个人用机械或化学清除牙菌斑的方法和作为预防和治疗牙周病的基础。同样重要的还有个人了解牙龈出血与牙周病之间的关系－能够观察到应该仔细去除菌斑的部位将会帮助人们有效地清除。

One of the most critical aspects of successful plaque removal and disease control is comprehension by the patient of the role of plaque and, equally important, its appearance. Educating the patient on the clinical appearance and location of plaque is as essential to preventing and treating periodontal diseases as the mechanical or chemical debridement techniques the patient uses. It is also important for the patient to understand the relationship of bleeding gums and periodontal diseases-being able to visualize the target of plaque control efforts will give direction to those efforts.

对于没有经过教育或指导的人来说，要了解菌斑沉积的概念是难以理解的。这些人可以刷牙但并不理解需要清除的菌斑部位，甚至他们不知道健康的牙周组织是怎么样或者一个清洁的口腔感觉如何。与受过教育的人比较，他们就有口腔组织结构的知识，能够确定龈上菌斑沉积的困难部位可能是一个问题。

To the uneducated or uninspired patient, the concept of plaque accumulation is difficult to comprehend. These patients may brush their teeth without comprehending the goal of their plaque control efforts. They may not even know how healthy tissue or a clean mouth feels. This is in contrast to the motivated patient, who has knowledge of the structures of the mouth and can identify difficult areas where supragingival plaque accumulation may be a problem.

一、牙刷 Toothbrushes

刷牙是最普遍应用的去除殆面与光滑牙面龈上菌斑的机械方法，然而，刷牙只能去除平均每个人约50%的牙菌斑。为了提高效率，已经对牙刷的构成，大小与形状还有其刷毛进行了各种评价。已经发现符合一定的标准的牙刷是一种有效的牙刷或称之为保健牙刷，这些牙刷是软毛，多束刷毛的刷头与末端磨圆的刷毛。研究已经发现，软毛，尼龙丝，多束刷毛，比硬毛更能有效地去除牙菌斑，即使当用力较轻时。还指出磨圆的刷毛比直接横切的刷毛对牙龈的损伤较少。

Toothbrushing is the most commonly used mechanical method to remove supragingival plaque from the occlusal surfaces and broad, flat tooth contours. However, the average person removes only about 50% of the plaque present when brushing their teeth. In efforts to improve this, various evaluations of the composition, size, and shape of toothbrushes and their filaments have been conducted. It has been found that certain standard criteria are present in an effective toothbrush. These are soft bristles, a multitufted head, and end-rounded filaments. Research has found that soft, nylon, multitufted bristles removed more plaque than hard bristles, even when applying less pressure. It has also been noted that brushes that have end-rounded filaments produce less gingival abrasion than filaments cut straight across.

直到近来，最普遍的牙刷设计是平面刷毛，与此相反，一种波浪型刷毛的选择性设计近年来已出现，它可以增加去除牙邻间部位菌斑的效果。牙刷的其他部位可以有各种各样的设计，包括刷头、刷柄与把柄的形状，角度，长度与直径。虽然这些变化对去除牙菌斑和组织健康的直接影响较小，但它们可以影响一个人控制牙刷的能力，并使其适合于在口腔内。人们的需要与优先选择决定了哪种牙刷最适合于某个人。这可能有必要应用一种以上的牙刷，主要取决于难以达到的部位或者具体的牙周状况。

Until recently, the most common brush design has been flat plane bristles (2-1). In contrast, an alternative design with a rippled bristle pattern has been recently introduced that may increase the efficiency of plaque removal in interproximal areas (2-2).

Other parts of a toothbrush may display various designs. These include the shape, angulation, length, and dimeter of the head, shank, and handle. Although these variations may have less of a direct impact on plaque removal and tissue health, they may influence a patient's ability to control the brush and adapt it within their mouth. Patient needs and preferences determine which brush is best for an individual. This may necessitate the need for more than one type of brush, depending on difficult-t-reach areas or specific periodontal conditions.

牙刷的更换时间一般取决于牙刷的使用情况。刷毛倒斜表明需要更换，刷牙习惯与存放方式影响牙刷使用的时间长短。为了提供指导，推荐每3个月更换一把牙刷以便保持最佳的洁牙效果。

Timing of toothbrush replacement generally depends on the condition of the brush. Splaying and matting of bristles indicate the need for replacement. Brushing habits and storage influence toothbrush longevity. In an effort to establish a guideline, it is recommended that toothbrushes be replaced every 3 months to maintain optimal cleaning ability.

（一）牙刷的发展 Development of toothbrushes

用天然材料制作的牙签，大概是用来剔除嵌塞的食物，相信是最早发明的洁牙工具。在美索巴达米亚的出土文物发现精心制作的金制牙签是大约公元前 3000 年苏美尔人所用的。最早记载的“牙刷”（口香藤）（chew-stick）认为是原始的牙刷，其年代追溯到约公元前1600年的中国文献。口腔保健与宗教仪式有关。如佛教有牙签，伊斯兰教用“miswak”或“siwak”。原始牙刷是用各种适口的木材，一端轧成像牙刷样的松散的纤维，现在许多亚非人中还在应用。Ebers papyrus 在公元前约 1500 年编著的，很可能追溯到大约公元前 4000 年包含的参考文献情况与牙周病相似，用的制剂为漱口液与牙膏。Hippocrates的著作（公元前300年）包括描述与牙石有关的牙龈病以及治疗不健康口腔的复杂制剂。认为第一把牙刷在早期的中国文献中提到是用猪鬃制作的。Pierre Fauchard 于 1728 年在“牙外科学”（Le chirurgien Dentiste）一书中描述了口腔健康的许多方面。他反对用马尾制作牙刷，因为粗糙对牙有损伤建议用海绵状物或草根。Fauchard推荐洁牙并制作器械与夹板固定松动牙，还有牙膏与漱口剂。大约在1780年英国的 William addis 制作了一把较早期的牙刷。到 19 世纪早期，各国欧洲国家的工匠们用金、象牙或乌木制作刷柄为放置牙刷刷头。19 世纪中叶在美国 H.N. Wadsworth 获得了第一把牙刷的专利。

到了 1900 年左右，当赛璐珞（假象牙）可以用来制作牙刷柄时产生了各种新的牙刷，在 1919 年，美国牙周病学会规定了牙刷设计与刷牙方法的规范试图作出标准化的专业推荐。到 1938年，尼龙开始用于牙刷的构造。由于二次世界大战开始阻碍了中国的猪鬃出口，改用合成材料取代天然鬃毛。自那以后，改进了合成材料，生产厂家的规格标准化，现代的许多牙刷都应用合成材料。动力牙刷，虽然产生较早，但是直到 1960 年并没有得到积极的推动。关于牙刷的关键词见 Table7-1。

Development of toothbrushes

Crudely contrived toothpicks, presumably used for relief from food impaction, are believed to be the earliest implements devised for the care of the teeth. Excavations in Mesopotamia uncovered elaborate gold toothpicks used by the Sumerians about 3000B.C.

The earliest record of the “chewstick”, which has been considered the primitive toothbrush, dates back in the Chinese literature to about 1600B.C. the care of the mouth was associated with religious training and ritual: the Buddhists had a “toothstick”, and the Mohammedans used the “miswak” or “siwak”. Chewsticks made from various types of tasty woods by crushing an end and spreading the fibers in a brush-like manner are still used by many Asiatic and African people.

The Ebers Papyrus, compiled about 1500 B.C. and dating probably at about 4000 B.C., contained reference to conditions similar to periodontal diseases and to preparations used as mouthwashes and dentifrices. The writings of Hippocrates (about 300 B.C.) include descriptions of diseased gums related to calculus and of complex preparations for the treatment of unhealthy mouths.

Early toothbrushes

It is believed that the first brush made of hog's bristles was mentioned in the early Chinese literature. Pierre Fauchard in 1728 in Le Chirurgien dentiste described many aspects of oral health. He condemned the toothbrush made of horse's hair because it was rough and destructive to the teeth and advised the use of sponges or herb roots. Fauchard recommended scaling of teeth and developed instruments and splints for loose teeth, as well as dentifrices and mouth washes.

One of the earlier toothbrushes made in England was produced by William Addis about 1780. By the early nineteenth century, craftsmen in various European countries constructed handles of gold, ivory, or ebony in which replaceable brush heads could be fitted. The first patent for a toothbrush in the United States was issued to H.N. Wadsworth in the middle of the nineteenth century.

Many new varieties of toothbrushes were developed around 1900, when celluloid was available for the manufacture of toothbrush handles. In 1919, the American Academy of Periodontology defined specifications for toothbrush design and brushing methods in an attempt to standardize professional recommendations.

Nylon came into use in toothbrush construction in 1938. World War II complications prevented Chinese.

表 7-1　Key words: toothbrushes

Abrasion (gingival)	lesion of the gingival that results from the mechanical removal of the surface epithelium.
Abrasion (tooth)	loss of tooth structure produced by a mechanical cause (such as a hard-bristled toothbrush used with excessive pressure and an abrasive dentifrice) abrasion contrasts with erosion, which involves a chemical process
Bristle (bris'l)	individual short stiff natural hair of an animal; historically, toothbrush bristles were taken from a hog or wild boar, but current toothbrush bristles are made of nylon and are called filaments
End-rounded	characteristic shape of each toothbrush filament; a special manufacturing process removes all sharp edges and provides smooth, rounded ends to prevent injury to gingival or tooth structure during use
Filament (fil'ah-ment)	individual synthetic fiber; a single element of a tuft fixed into a toothbrush head
Mechanical plaque control	oral hygiene methods for removal of bacterial plaque from tooth surfaces using a toothbrush and selected devices for interdental cleaning; contrasts with chemotherapeutic plaque control in which an antimicrobial agent is used
Power-assisted toothbrush	a brush driven by electricity or battery; also called automatic, electric, or mechanical (in contrast with manual)

续表

Abrasion (gingival)	lesion of the gingival that results from the mechanical removal of the surface epithelium.
Stiffness	the reaction force exerted per unit area of the brush during deflection; the term stiffness is used interchangeably with firmness of toothbrush bristles or filaments; the stiffness depends primarily on the length and diameter of the filaments
Sulcular brushing	a method in which the end-rounded filament tips are activated at and just below the gingival margin for the purpose of loosening and removing bacterial plaque from the gingival sulcus
Toothbrush head	the part of the toothbrush composed of the tufts and the stock (extension of the handle where the tufts are attached)
Tuft	a cluster of bristles or filaments secured together in one hole in the head of a tooth-brush

（二）手动牙刷的设计研究 Design of studies on manual toothbrushes

为了研究手动刷牙对菌斑控制的作用已经对牙刷进行了各种设计研究。受试者可以是牙科学生或者各种不同程度牙龈健康与疾病状况的病人，有些菌斑研究允许牙面菌斑沉积在24至72小时然后用各种方法来评价菌斑沉积的量与局部记载分布。随后，要求参与者在监督之下用牙刷或刷牙方法按一定的时间刷牙（属于单一的刷牙研究），紧接着作菌斑评估。取代由病人进行的有监督或无监督刷牙，还有专业人员（牙科助理员或卫生士）完成的单一用牙刷洁牙的研究，试图使刷牙步骤标准化。研究的结果使我们认识到用一种单一的刷牙方式进行的筛选实验并不能提供对牙龈作用的可靠信息。

通常用单盲（检查者）交叉试验设计，在两个研究周期之间有一个静止期比较不同的牙刷/刷牙方法。其他研究方案提供参与者开始前的洁牙与指导，然后让他们按研究的要求用一种牙刷/刷牙方法，应用较长的时间（短期1～4周，长期2～6个月）为家庭护理的一部分。这种长期研究有减少任何一种新用品（新奇的作用）对结果可能产生的任何影响的优点，在每天的环境中测试手动牙刷。然而同时控制混杂因素的影响如依从性，得以减少。

1986年美国牙医学会（ADA）制订了与控制菌斑和减少牙龈炎效果有关的化学治疗产品的临床研究指南。与化学治疗药品比较，牙刷是减少牙菌斑与牙龈炎的更普遍应用的手段。然而，在科学文献中，关于长期检测牙刷对减少牙菌斑与牙龈炎效果的资料很少。鉴于在指南中检测6个月的化学治疗制剂，ADA接受标准牙刷的新内容只要求提供牙刷构成的信息和实验室毛束一般不尖锐或锯齿状的终端，即使没有标准结构的手动（与电动）牙刷，要求有一个30天的临床研究，证实临床安全性，以及与基线数据比较，菌斑与牙龈炎的评价有15%统计学显著的减少（council on scientific affairs 1996）。当进行文献检索时，只发现有5项研究比传统的30天的评估要长的。

Design of studies on manual toothbrushes

A variety of research designs have been employed in order to study the effects of manual toothbrushing on plaque control. Subjects were either dental (hygiene) students or patients with various stages of gingival health or disease. For some studies plaque was allowed to accumulate on the teeth for a period of between 24 and 72 hours before its amount and topographical distribution were evaluated using a variety of methods. Subsequently, the participants were asked to brush their teeth under supervision for a certain time with the toothbrush/toothbrushing method under study (single-use brushing study). This was followed by another assessment of plaque. Instead of supervised or unsupervised toothbrushing by the patient, cleanings in single-use studies have also been performed by professionals (dental assistants or dental hygienists) in an attempt to standardize the brushing procedure. Studies employing a single brushing have to be considered screening experiments and cannot provide definite proof of superiority of a certain type of toothbrush or toothbrushing technique. In addition, it is obvious that such studies cannot provide data on the effect on gingival parameters.

When different brushes/methods were compared, usually a single (examiner) blind crossover study design was employed, with a washout period interposed between the study periods. Other study protocols provided participants with baseline prophylaxis and instructions and had them use the toothbrush/toothbrushing method under study for a longer period of time (short-term: 1～4 weeks; long-term: 2～6 months) as part of their home care. Such longer-term studies have the advantage of reducing any possible influence of new devices (novelty effect) on the outcome, and of testing manual toothbrushes in the everyday environment. At the same time, however, the control of confounding variables such as compliance is reduced.

Clinical study guidelines were defined by the American Dental Association (ADA) in 1986 for chemotherapeutic products relative to efficacy in plaque and gingivitis reduction (Council on Dental Therapeutics 1986). Compared to chemotherapeutic products, the toothbrush is a much more common means for reducing plaque and gingivitis. However, in the scientific literature there is a paucity of data on long-term clinical testing of toothbrushes for plaque and gingivitis reduction effectiveness. Whereas chemotherapeutic agents are tested for 6 months under the guidelines, the newly issued ADA Seal of Acceptance for standard toothbrushes requires only composition information and laboratory studies documenting that bristles are "generally free of sharp or jagged edges and endpoints". Even for nonstandard configuration manual (and electric) toothbrushes, one 30-day clinical study, demonstrating clinical safety and a 15% statistically significant reduction in plaque and gingivitis assessment compared to baseline, is all that is required (Council on Scientific Affairs 1996). When a literature search was conducted in the preparation of this paper, only five studies could be identified that were longer than the traditional 30-day assessments. All of these studies will be reviewed below.

（三）牙刷的设计 Toothbrush design

在过去有多种手动牙刷的设计声称各个品牌清除牙菌斑的优越性，然而关于菌斑控制与口腔卫生实践的世界专题学术讨论会作出一致的结论没有充分的证据证明任何一种牙刷设计优于另一种（Frandsen，1986）。

还有近年来，研究继续介绍新型牙刷设计以便证实其优越性，然而，这些新产品的研究只发表了一篇报告（Soparkar et al. 1991，Benson et al. 1993，Yankell et al. 1993，Hanioka et al. 1995. Table 1，2）。同时，最近的其他研究评价新的牙刷设计与传统的设计进行比较并没有显示出去除牙菌斑的优越性（Stabble et al. 1988，Emling & Yankell 1994，Claydan & Addy 1995，Yankill & Emling 1995 Table 2）。

1. 手动牙刷 Manual toothbrushes

（1）一把有效牙刷的特点 Characteristics of an effective toothbrush

1）在大小，形状与质地上符合个人需要；

2）易于有效进行灵活操作；

3）易于清洁，通气；不受潮湿影响；

4）耐久与便宜；

5）具备有弹性，柔软，刷毛直径，强度，硬度以及刷柄的轻度的主要功能特点；

6）毛端磨圆；

7）设计实用，有功效与整洁。

Conforms to individual patient requirements in size, shape, and texture

Is easily and efficiently manipulated

Is readily cleaned and aerated; impervious in moisture

Is durable and inexpensive

Has prime functional properties of flexibly softness, and diameter of the bristles or filaments, and of strength, rigidity, and lightness of the handle

Has end-rounded filaments or bristles

Is designed for utility, efficiency, and cleanness

Toothbrush design

There are numerous manual toothbrush designs, and claims of superiority for plaque removal by individual brands have been made in the past. However, world workshops on plaque control and oral hygiene practices have consistently concluded that there is insufficient evidence to prove that any one toothbrush design is superior to another (for review see Frandsen 1986).

（2）牙刷规格的全面描述 General description

1）各部分 parts (figure 1)

①刷柄 handle　刷牙时手握住的部位。

②刷头 head　工作端，由刷毛束（簇）与固定毛束的孔组成。

③刷颈 shank　连接刷头与刷柄的部分。

2）长度 dimensions

①总刷长度，15 ~ 19cm，幼儿与儿童的尺寸可以较短。

②刷头，只应长至适合于毛束排列。

③刷面长度 25.4 ~ 31.8mm，宽度 7.9 ~ 9.5mm，刷毛高度 11mm。

3）刷柄 handle

几乎所有现代的牙刷刷柄均为塑料，结合耐久，不受潮湿影响，外形合意，价格低，充分的硬度，与质地光滑。

4）形状 shape

①选择的特点　易于把握住；用时不滑动或转动；无锐角或突起，重量轻，与强度一致。

②变异　刷颈部弯曲，呈凹线或成角形，有或者没有放拇指的部位可以帮助调节牙刷到难以达到的部位，轻度的改变不会增加操作的复杂性或者影响到控制牙刷的位置与压力，弯曲或厚的刷柄对某些手不灵巧的人有帮助。

5）刷头 head

①设计 design

毛束排列：长为5～11束刷毛，宽为2～4排，留有空隙使牙刷易于清洁。

多束毛排列：长为10～12束刷毛，宽为3～4排，空隙紧密提供光滑刷面，允许毛束彼此支撑。

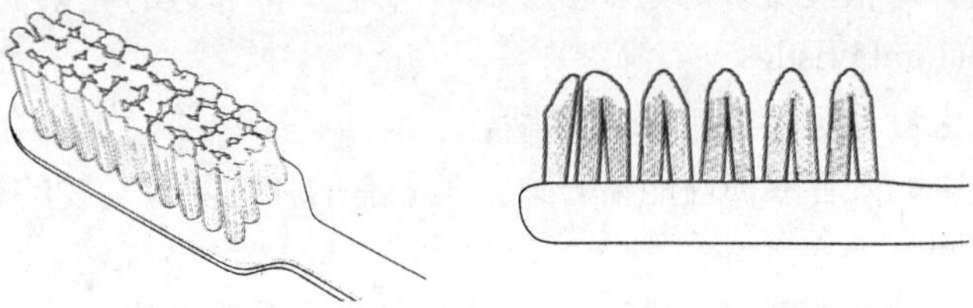

图 7-1

②刷面 brushing plane (profile)

牙刷有各式各样形状的毛束外形，刷面整洁，在刷面顶部刷毛的安排有特点，刷面整洁可以是同等的长度，长度也可有变化，如拱形波形或U/V形。所有毛束应软，毛端磨圆，对口腔软组织与牙结构无伤害，应用适当时都能减少菌斑与牙龈炎，有效地清洁难以达到的部位如向邻面扩展，错位牙，或暴露的根面，取决于个人的技能与理解程度。

Brushes are available with variously shaped filament profiles. The brushing plane is also referred to as the trim, which is the characteristic arrangement of the tips of the filaments at the brushing surface.

The trim may range from filaments of equal lengths (flat planes, figure) to those with variable lengths, such as dome-shaped, rippled, or bi level. All filaments should be soft and end-rounded for safety to oral soft tissues and tooth structure. When used properly, all can reduce plaque and gingivitis. Efficiency for cleaning the hard-to-reach areas, such as extension onto proximal surfaces, malpositioned teeth, or exposed root surfaces, depends on individual patient abilities and understanding.

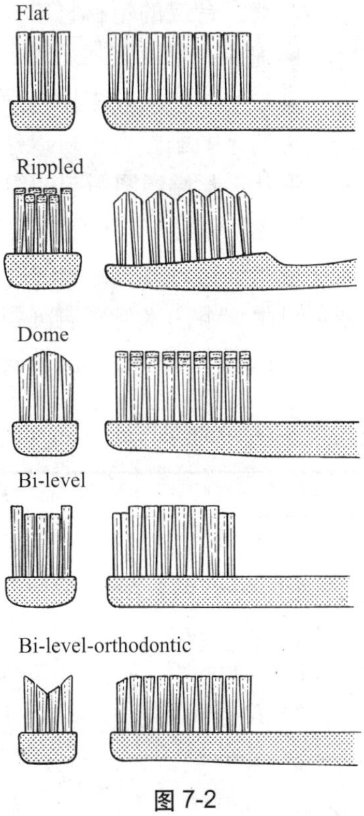

图 7-2

A variety of filament profiles are available. In addition to the classic flat planed brush, other trims include the rippled, dome, and bi-level. Brushes for use over orthodontic appliances are made with various bi-level shapes.

6）刷毛与细丝 bristles and filaments

现在大多数牙刷为尼龙丝。天然刷毛相对不卫生，其物理条件不能标准化，硬度取决于丝的直径与长度，牙刷分为软、中、硬三种，厂家之间的一致性是不可比较的。

①影响硬度的因素 factors influencing stiffness

直径：较细的丝较软，有较大的回弹力。

长度：丝较短则较硬，弹性较小。

一束毛的丝数：每根丝支撑邻近的丝。每一束毛支持邻近的毛束。

②天然刷毛 natural bristles

来源：从历史上看，天然刷毛来自猪鬃

均匀性：刷毛质地或者磨损性能不一致，其固有的弹性随着动物的种类，还有地理部位以及产毛的季节而不同。

直径：直径大小从 0.087 ~ 0.475mm 不等，取决于毛的部位、动物的年龄与寿命。

形状：毛有缺陷，不规则，毛端常有开口。

缺点：不推荐用天然毛制作的牙刷是因为：不能标准化；更易损坏更不规则；有孔，有微生物与碎屑沉积；吸收水分（水使毛变软）。

③细丝 filaments

构造：合成的塑料材料，主要是尼龙。

均匀性：可以控制。

直径：丝的直径可以从超软到硬。直径从 0.15 ~ 0.3mm。

小的牙间刷丝直径可以达到 0.075mm。

形状：丝端磨圆引起的组织损伤最小，研究显示，牙龈损伤与丝端没有磨圆直接有关。图 3 显示丝端磨圆与未磨圆的实例。

尼龙丝与天然毛比较的优点：不用时洗刷清洁，快速干燥；更耐用，保持形态更多；丝端磨圆封闭，不沾水与碎屑沉积；更能抵抗细菌与真菌的沉积。

根据国人的口腔情况，我国保健牙刷的设计标准于 1978 年由卫生部等制订。

表 7-2 我国各型保健牙刷的设计标准

	幼儿	7-12 岁	13 ~ 18 岁	成人
牙刷全长 (mm)	120 ~ 130	140 ~ 150	155 ~ 160	160 ~ 180
刷头长度 (mm)	16 ~ 18	20 ~ 24	25 ~ 30	30 ~ 35
刷头宽度 (mm)	7 ~ 8	9 ~ 10	10 ~ 11	11 ~ 12
毛束高度 (mm)	8.5 ~ 9	9.5 ~ 10	10.5 ~ 11	11 ~ 12
毛束排数 (mm)	2 ~ 3	3	3	3 ~ 4
刷毛直径 (mm)	不超过 0.18	不超过 0.18	不超过 0.2	不超过 0.2
刷毛尖端 (mm)	圆纯形	圆钝形	圆钝形	圆钝形

(3) 新型牙刷的设计 Novel toothbrush designs

近年来，有一种新型牙刷，刷毛呈扇形向刷头外展已经在一些国家上市，有几项单纯用这种牙刷刷牙的研究显示比另外二种牙刷效果更好，这些研究设计集中于用 Rustogi 等（1992）改进的修正navy指数（Elliot等1972）强调龈缘与邻面部位的牙菌斑。在后来的二项单纯用牙刷刷牙的研究singh等（1993）与Balanyk等（1993）证实这种牙刷比另一欠毛牙刷效果更好。但是其他人的研究（Reardon等1993，claydon等1996）。未发现新型牙刷有显著性差异。而Keiser等（1997），sharma 等（1994）的 30 天与 3 个月的研究发现新型牙刷有显著性差异。相反，Grossman 等（1994）的研究发现新型牙刷的效果还不如其他牙刷。

因此，新型牙刷在减少牙菌斑与牙龈炎方面的效果其说不一。

(4) 双头与三头牙刷 Double-and triple-headed toothbrushes

有几项研究已表明双头（三头）牙刷可能改善菌斑控制，尤其在舌侧。Bastiaan（1984）用双头牙刷与单头平面牙刷比较。结果表明双头牙刷舌侧清除菌斑的效果优于单头牙刷，但颊侧发现无差异。Gibson等（1988），Agerholm（1991）的研究与传统牙刷比较，双头牙刷清除舌侧菌斑的效果明显地好。Yankell 等（1996）测试一种新的三头牙刷与传统的标准平面牙刷比较，实验室检测在邻面进入优于二种手动牙刷，Yankell等（1994，1995）二项单纯用牙刷的6个月研究在减少舌面龈炎方面其效果明显地比平面刷头的牙刷好。

(5) 牙刷柄 Toothbrush handle

有几项研究在于探讨不同的牙刷柄的设计对去除牙菌斑的差异。Davies 等（1988）发现，在监督刷牙的情况下，长波浪形刷柄的牙刷比短柄、无波浪形的设计去除菌斑的效果明显地好。Kanchanakamd 等（1992）评价新设计的“45 度概念”的牙刷去除儿童的牙菌斑，后来在成人进行的研究（1993），刷柄的设计有利于巴斯法，结果显示这种牙刷比传统牙刷的标准刷柄能够去除更多的牙菌斑。Kieser等（1997）评价了另一种新型设计的刷柄与刷颈成双角形的牙刷，在一项 30 天的平行设计研究中，这种牙刷显示比二种对照的牙刷去除牙菌斑的水平更高，舌侧部位减少最多。

(6) 牙刷头 Toothbrush head

对非传统的平头牙刷头作了评价。Scopp等（1976）研究过一种凹面牙刷，报告菌斑的水平比传统的牙刷低（$P<0.10$）。Wasserman（1985）用一种深槽形设计的牙刷看到菌斑沉积在统计学上显著减少。相比之下，Thevissen等（1987）发现传统的平面多束毛的牙刷比凸型牙刷更有明显效果。

(7) 牙刷毛 Toothbrush bristles

Bergenholtz等（1969）比较了四种标准牙刷，其刷毛的硬度与密度不同（硬与软，多束毛与空束毛）。在牙科学生中进行的一项单纯刷牙应用研究发现无明显差异。Finkelstein等（1984）在比较了七种设计不同的牙刷之后得出结论：设计的特色而不是毛的质地说明了机械性清除牙菌斑的效率。相比之下，pretara-spanedda等（1989）证实了刷毛的密度较大在单纯刷牙之后去除牙菌斑的效果更明显。

Vowles等（1977）观察过细毛牙刷，虽然含有3倍以上的刷毛与粗毛牙刷比较，其洁牙能力较差。相比之下。

Beatty等（1990）证实在学校儿童中较细的刷毛效果较好，然而在护士与牙科卫生学生组中二种牙刷效果相当。

Bergenholtz等（1984）在平直多束毛与V形牙刷之间当在无监督下应用时去除牙菌斑的能力并未发现有差异，而在专业人员使用时，V形牙刷去除邻面菌斑的效果比平直形牙刷好。V形牙刷趋于有较好的去除菌斑的效果，但没有统计学的显著性，Chong等（1983）也报告了这一结果。当用一种新的交叉毛束设计的概念牙刷与标准的垂直毛束牙刷作比较时没有发现差异。

（8）光能转化型与离子型手动牙刷 Light energy concersion and ionic manual toothbrushes

两项最近的研究介绍了另外的手动刷牙的新途径。Hoover等（1992）调查了一种新的光能转化型牙刷带有一种平导体（Tio2）具有对牙菌斑光电化学作用的特点。另一种不带半导体的类似牙刷作对照，3 周之后在一组 73 名学校儿童的研究中显示颊面牙菌斑显著减少。作者推测，平面面与舌面比较，更可能允许光到达半导体。报告的半导体光反应的特性可能与看到的菌斑减少有关系。然而，如果真是这样，这种设计同时也限制了它的用处。

Van Swol 等（1996）评价了一种小的极细微的电流在手动刷牙期间对确立的牙菌斑与牙龈炎的作用，在 64 名成人中进行了 6 个月的研究，Quigley & Hein 菌斑指数记分显示从基线调查到 6 个月，实验组与不带电的对照牙刷比较有更为显著的改善。

Two recent studies intrpdced another novel approach to manual toothbrushing. Hoover et al (1992) investigated the plaque-removing potential of a new light energy conversion toothbrush incorporated with a semiconductor (Tio2) to take advantage of the suggested photo-electro-chemical effect on dental plaque. A similar toothbrush without the semiconductor served as control. After a period of three weeks the new toothbrush showed significantly more reduction of plaque on the buccal surfaces in a group of 73 school-children. The authors speculated that "as the buccal surfaces are more likely to allow light to reach the semiconductor during brushing than the lingual areas, it was possible that the reported photocatalytic property of the semiconductor may be involved in the observed reduction of plaque. However, if this was indeed the case, it would at the same time limit the usefulness of this design.

Van Swol et al. (1996) evaluated the effect of a small, imperceptible electric current on established dental plaque and gingivitis during manual toothbrushing in 64 adults over a period of 6 months. The Quigley & Hein Plaque Index scores showed significantly more improvement from baseline to 6 months for the test over the uncharged control brush.

2. 电动牙刷 Electric toothbrushes

电动牙刷的作用：优点与限制 The role of Electric toothbrushes: Advantages and limitations

用手动牙刷清除牙菌斑对大多数人来说仍然是保持良好口腔卫生的主要方法。然而，对大多数病人来说，不是这些标准所能完成的。与手动牙刷有关克服这一限度的一种可能方法是发展一种机械性刷牙工具，正如早在 1855 年瑞典钟表匠 Frederick Wilhelm Tornberg 取得一把机械性牙刷的专利（Scutt & Swann 1975）。第一把电动牙刷闻世较晚，首次在 20 世纪 60 年代介绍过提供的刷头通过一种能源能完成多种动作。随着时间的推移，这一用品作为一种有价值的选择已得到确认。

第一把电动牙刷模仿手工牙刷普遍用的前后动作。当首次介绍时，有许多这种用品的效果报告，然而，早期的权威性报告评价了这方面的研究，认为手动牙刷与电动牙刷在去除菌斑方面同样有效（Ash 1963）。由于缺少明显的优点和存在许多机械性故障，对动力牙刷没有好感。20世纪60年代后期逐渐从市场消失，然而，动力牙刷继续推荐给残疾人以及手的灵巧性差的人。

1966年在世界牙周病学专题研讨会一致认为没有口腔知识的人，对口腔卫生保健没有经过高度激励的人，还有那些掌握适当的用手刷牙方面有困难的人，“用带有标准动作的电动牙刷刷牙可以使牙齿更经常地保持清洁”（Greene 1966）。自那以后研究与开发继续开始进行电动牙刷的设计已经作了许多改进。这些改进包括振动或转动牙刷以及高频率动作牙刷（Fishman 1997）。认为这种取代手动牙刷的直线性与颤动样的动作可以在较短的刷牙时间内更有效地去除牙菌斑与色斑。这种新一代产品的牙刷显示出比传统的手动牙刷能更好地去除牙邻面部位的牙菌斑，这样在1996年的世界牙周病学大会上谨慎地作出结论，有限的证据提出电动牙刷比手动牙刷提供额外的效益（Hancock 1996）。关于现代电动牙刷的知识集中在6个方面：研究方法，效果、磨损、刷牙力量、要求（顺从性）、特殊病人群。

The role of electric toothbrushes: advantages and limitations

Mechanical plaque removal with a manual toothbrush remains the primary method of maintaining good oral hygiene for the majority of the population. When performed well for an adequate duration of time, manual brushing is highly effective. However, for most patients, neither of these criteria is fulfilled. One possible way to overcome the limitations associated with manual brushing was to develop a mechanical brushing device, and as early as 1855 the Swedish clockmaker Frederick Wilhelm Tornberg patented a mechanical toothbrush (Scutt & Swann 1975). The first electric toothbrushes came much later, and were first introduced in the 1960's. They provided a brush head capable of a variety of motions driven by a power source. Over time such devices have become established as a valuable alternative to manual methods of toothbrushing.

The first electric brushes mimicked the back-and-forth motion commonly used with a manual toothbrush. When first introduced there were many reports of the effectiveness of such devices. However, an early authoritative report reviewed such research and stated that both manual and electric toothbrushes were equally effective in removing plaque (Ash 1963). Because of the lack of clear superiority and many problems of mechanical breakdown, powered toothbrushes fell out of favor, and during the 1960's they gradually disappeared from the market. However, powered brushes continued to be recommended for the handicapped and for persons with reduced manual dexterity.

At the World Workshop in Periodontics in 1966, the consensus was that in non-dentally oriented persons and persons not highly motivated to oral health care, as well a those who have difficulty in mastering a suitable handbrushing technique, "the use of an electric brush with its standard movements may result in more frequent and better cleansing of the teeth"(Greene 1966). Since then, research and development have continued, and many modifications to electric toothbrush design have been made. These include oscillating or rotating brushes and brushes which move at a high frequency (Fishman 1997). It was believed that this substitute for the linear, vibratory hand motion applied to manual toothbrushes would lead to more effective plaque and stain removal over shorter brushing times. It has been shown that this new generation of brushes remove plaque significantly better in the approximal area than do conventional manual toothbrushes. This led, in 1996 World workshop in Periodontics, to the careful conclusion that limited evidence suggested that electric brushes provide an additional benefit compared to manual brushes (Hancock 1996).

This position paper will discuss the current knowledge with respect to modern electric toothbrushes, and will focus on six aspects: Research methodology; Effectiveness; Abrasion; Toothbrushing force; Compliance; Special patient groups.

（1）研究方法的影响 Impact of research methodology

在电动牙刷的试验中，所有的受试者都是人。这种明显的事实引出的许多实际考虑到的问题之一是可能影响到一个临床试验的过程与结果。纯粹的事实是仔细评价人们存在着牙菌斑与牙龈炎能够影响其口腔卫生的水平（overholser，1988）任何一个受试人群暴露于临床试验步骤有时会引起改善，那是由于心理作用而不是检测的物质或器具的物体作用。这种作用称之为“霍桑效应”（即受人关注带来的进步）。如果有对照的临床试验是正确平衡的，那么，这种作用不应该引起实验组与对照组有任何差别的改变（Cowell 等 1975）。

在检测牙刷的效果中，双盲研究实际上不可能，因此在一项研究电动牙刷的作用设计中必须考虑电动牙刷的新奇效应（Owen，1972），可能是一种好奇心的简单表示但是一般病人对电动牙刷表示较大的兴趣而渴望用它（Muhler，1969），减少这种新奇效应的一种方法是通过相当长的周期来检测牙刷为了使这种效应减弱或消失。由于新奇效应，因而短期的研究特别容易有错误的倾向（Ash，1963）。一项涉及Sonex牙刷的研究说明了这个问题的存在。刷牙6周之后出血指数与龈炎指数显著减少有利于超声牙刷（Terezhalmy等，1995a）。然而，6个月的研究，并没有显示出手动牙刷有任何差异（Terezhalmy等，1995b）。所以，开始时的阳性作用可能是参与者意识到新牙刷，因而热心应用，这一反应随着时间而谈化，这可能很好地解释为什么6个月以上的试验周期，sonex 牙刷明显地超过手动牙刷的优势消失了。

在荷兰阿姆斯特丹的ACTA试图解决与牙刷去除牙菌斑与改善牙龈健康能力有关这些问题的比较研究，设计了一项短期菌斑模式，试图尽可能地控制多种变量，包括刷牙周期，手的灵巧性，动员程度，刷牙次数以及“新奇效应”（Van der weijden，1993a）。简而言之，要求受试者 24 ～ 48 小时不刷牙，评价刷牙前后的菌斑水平。在一项分别在口腔进行试验的设计中，刷牙可以由专业人员或者受试者本人进行。其他研究组已经成功地应用了这一相同的模式用于检测不同的牙刷（Rapley 等，1994，Dejager 等 1998）。

由于短期牙龈炎研究面临的问题，为了从刷牙获得最大的效益，需要由专业人员来指导和培训如何使用牙刷（例如，Van der Weijden 等，1994）。这种指导也对参与研究的受试者牙龈炎水平会有影响，大多数可能变得比较健康。因此，最近提出了一个模型，在短期研究中包括有一个实验性牙龈炎期，即在培训之后，重新造成牙龈炎（Van der weijden等，1998）这一模型允许经过适当培训的受试者有充分水平的牙龈炎，研究结果显示重新开始刷牙4周内牙龈炎消退，因此，在检测与牙龈健康有关的牙刷方面，这一模式看来是一项有价值的研究设计。

（2）效果 Effectiveness

①动作方式 mode of action

1986年国际口腔卫生专题研讨会作出结论直到那个时期为止，不论哪种刷牙方法，电动的或者是手动的牙刷都不会清除更多的牙菌斑（Löe 等 1986）。那时，只有我们所称呼的传统的电动牙刷。第一代电动牙刷的刷头设计像手动牙刷那样的横竖动作两个方向（水平与垂直方向）。

在过去的10年中，新一代电动牙刷已经出现它们分别可以分成两种不同的类型。第一种牙刷有更多的（振动）旋转动作取代了传统的往返动作（Walmsley 1997）。旋转动作可以是单个牙刷的动作或者是单个毛束反时针方向的动作。第二种牙刷刷头动作频率较高的各种牙刷（Johnson 等 1994）。

In 1986, an international workshop on oral hygiene concluded that up to that time neither powered nor manual toothbrushes removed more plaque, regardless of the brushing method (Löe & Kleinmann 1986). At that time, only what we now call conventional electric toothbrushes were available. This first generation of electric toothbrushes had a brushhead designed as a manual toothbrush which made a (combined) horizontal and vertical motion.

Over the last decade a new generation of electric toothbrushes has become available, and they can be conveniently categorized into two distinct types. First, there has been a move towards more (ocillating) rotary action brushes instead of the traditional side-to-side motion (Walmsley 1997). The rotary motion can be either the motion of a single brush or of the individual tufts moving in a counter-clockwise direction. Second, there are brushes which operate with a brush head motion at a higher frequency (Johnson & Mclnnes 1994).

②刷牙时间 toothbrushing duration

一般来说，病人不愿意花费口腔专业人员所推荐的刷牙与用牙线洁牙的时间，大多数病人刷牙的时间少于1分钟（Hawkins等，1986）。在清洁牙面时，电动牙刷可能比手动牙刷要快，在大多数成人的菌斑控制项目中，效果可能有提高。例如，临床上已经证明，Rotadent电动牙刷去除同等量的牙菌斑所花费的时间为手动牙刷的一半（Preber等，1991）。有两项研究专门集中在刷牙时间与去除菌斑的效果之间的关系（Van der Weijden等1993b，1996a）。这些研究显示在相同的刷牙时间内手动牙刷去除的牙菌斑比电动牙刷少。即使在6分钟之后由专业人员用手动牙刷只能去除用电动牙刷1分钟之后牙菌斑的75%。随着时间的增加达到6分钟，手动牙刷的效果随之增加，但看来是要达到最佳的作用效果，至少用电动牙刷要2分钟之后。用电动牙刷2分钟之后大约可去除85%的牙菌斑，而6分钟之后能去除93%。

In general, patients are not willing to spend the time dental professionals recommend to brush and floss, and most patients brush their teeth for less than 1 minute (Hawkins et al. 1986). Electric toothbrushes are potentially faster than manual brushes at cleaning tooth surfaces, and the efficiency could potentially improve the plaque control regimen for most adults (Boyd et al. 1997b). The Rotadent, for example, has been clinically demonstrated to need only one half as much time as a manual brush to remove an equal amount of plaque (Preber et al. 1991) two studies have focused specifically on the relationship between toothbrushing duration and plaque-removing efficacy (Van der Weijden et al. 1993b, 1996a). These have shown that a manual toothbrush removes less plaque than an electric toothbrush given the same brushing time. Even after 6 minutes, the manual toothbrush in the hands of a professional removes only 75% of the plaque which is removed after 1 minute with the electric toothbrush.

With increase in time up to six minutes, the efficacy of a manual toothbrush increases, but there appears to be an optimum effect after at least 2 minutes with the electric toothbrushes. After 2 minutes with an electric toothbrush approximately 84% of the plaque has been removed, whereas after 6 minutes 93% has been removed.

③去除色斑与控制牙石 removal of stain and control calculus

除了去除牙菌斑的效果外，少数研究者调查了去除牙色斑的效果。Grossman等（1996）采用一种实验模型引起色斑，通过4天用一种浓洗必太茶方法含漱（不允许用其他形式的口腔卫生方法）。结果显示用电动牙刷刷牙比手动牙刷更有效地去除外源性牙色斑，这个实验证实了Schemehorn等（1996）的体外实验发现。他们也采用洗必太引发色斑模型处长至4周。两种电动牙刷（Braun Oral-B Plaque Remover 与 Somicare）在去除色斑的效果方面都优于手工牙刷(Mclnness 等 1994，Moran 等 1995)。

也用二项研究对电动牙刷控制牙石的效果进行了调查，Moran等（1995）评价了21天内产生的牙石。没有看到电动牙刷与手动牙刷有差异，van der Weijden等（1994）评价了一项8个月产生的牙石研究也没有看到两种牙刷之间的显著差异。

Besides plaque-removal efficacy, a few researchers have investigated stain removal. Using an experimental model to induce stain by rinsing for 4 days with an intense chlorhexidine tea regimen (no other form of oral hygiene was allowed), Grossman et al. (1996) showed that electric toothbrushes were more effective in removing extrinsic dental stain than manual brushes. This confirmed the "in vitro" findings of Schemehorn & Henry (1996). Also, using the chlorhexidine-induced stain model for an extended period up to 4 weeks, both the Braun Oral-B Plaque Remover and Sonicare have been shown to be superior to a manual toothbrush with respect to stain removal (Mclnnes et al. 1994, Moran & Addy 1995).

The effectiveness of the electric toothbrush incontrolling calculus has been investigated in two studies. Moran & Addy (1995) evaluated the development of calculus over a 21-day period. No differences between the electric toothbrushes and the manual brush were observed. Van der Weijden et al. (1994) assessed calculus development in an eight-month study and also did not observe a significant difference between the manual and electric toothbrush.

④电子牙刷 electronic (ionic) toothbrushes

一种电子牙刷输送 0.15mA 电流通过刷头作 5 个月的评价试验（Van der Weijden 1995a）对菌斑分值或探针检查出血指数均未发现明显的作用。而另有一项6个月的双盲试验看到“离子”手动牙刷比常规手动牙刷导致菌斑与牙龈炎的显著下降（Van Swol等1996)。这些矛盾的结果需要进一步评价。

对电动牙刷已经进行了多次评价，看到电动牙刷有较好的效果，主要是改善了邻间部位的清洁状况。一种情况可能有争议受试者用手动牙刷，再加用一些邻间清洁用具，电动牙刷就会没有优越性。然而，Axelsson（1993）就此问题作过讨论，认为邻间清洁在欧洲并不普遍。在今天的工业化国家约 15% ~ 20% 的人在定期刷牙的基础上最好的完成邻间口腔卫生。因此，通过改善邻间部位的清洁状况，电动牙刷在预防牙周病方面能起到重要作用。

为从电动牙刷得到最大效益，专业人员的口腔卫生指导是重要的。许多研究已看到这一点。调查预先没有专业人员的指导或者录音指导，发现没有或有很少的差异（Barmes等1993，Stoltze等1994），而当研究包括用电动牙刷和专业人员指导时，发现有明显好的结果（Vander Weijden等1993a，1994，Grossman等1995）。Ainame等（1997）进行的一项12个月的研究仅在开始时给予指导，并且不再重复，发现电动牙刷优于手动牙刷。

An "electronic"(ionic) brush which sends a 0.15 mA current through the brushhead was subjected to a 5-month evaluation (Van der Weijden 1995a). no effect on either plaque scores or bleeding upon probing was evident. In another double-blind 6-month study, a significant reduction in plaque and gingivitis was observed for the "ionic" manual toothbrush s compared to a regular manual toothbrush (Van Swol et al. 1996). These conflicting results need further evaluation.

With the above review of electric toothbrushes it has been mentioned a number of times that the better efficacy observed with the electric toothbrushes is mainly the result of improved approximal cleaning. One could argue that subjects who use a manual toothbrush and in addition some interproximal cleaning device will not benefit from an electric toothbrush. However, as has been discussed by Axelsson (1993), interproximal cleaning is not a comoon practice in Europe. In industrialized countries today 15%~20% of the population at most perform interdental oral hygiene on a regular basis. Therefore, the electric toothbrush cn play an important role in the prevention of periodontal diseases through improved approximal cleaning.

In order to get the maximum benefit from the electric toothbrush, professional oral hygiene instruction appears to be important. This has been observed in a number of studies. Investigations of toothbrushing with no prior professional instruction, or taped instruction, have found no or only minimal differences (Barnes et al. 1993, Stoltze & Bay 1994). However, when studies included professional instruction in the use of the electric toothbrush, significantly better results were found (Van der Weijden et al. 1993a, 1994, Grossman et al. 1995). Although in a twelve-month study by Ainamo et al. (1997) instructions were given only at the outset and were not repeated, the electric toothbrush was found to be superior to the manual.

3. 刷牙方法不当致不良反应 Detrimental effects of improper toothbrushing

（1）磨损 Abrasion

在口腔疾病的预防中，适当的口腔卫生有着最重要的价值，然而，当进行彻底的口腔卫生时遇到几个问题，由于刷牙方法不当，牙膏有摩擦剂，刷毛硬，以及有定期刷牙习惯的人有时牙龈，牙本质或釉质受到损害。可以发展成牙龈缘溃疡，牙龈萎缩，根面外露以及美观问题（Sandholm 等 1982，Vehkalahti 等 1989），这些发现中最为普遍的是龈缘局部萎缩（Sandholm 等 1982，Khocht 等 1993）。

In the prevention of oral diseases, proper oral hygiene is of foremost value. Unfortunately, several problems are encountered when thorough oral hygiene is performed. Due to improper brushing techniques, abrasive toothpaste and hard bristle filaments, people with regular toothbrushing habits sometimes damage the gingival, the dentin or enamel. They may develop marginal ulceration of the gingival, gingival recession, exposure of root surfaces and esthetic problems (Sandholm et al. 1982, Vehkalahti et al. 1989. the most ecommon of these findings is the local recession of the gingival margin

(Sandholm et al. 1982, Khocht et al. 1993).

（2）硬组织的磨损 Abrasion of hard tissues

硬毛牙刷与软毛牙刷的争论是口腔医生的一个老问题。Hirshfield在他的著作《牙刷－它的应用与滥用》提出两种情况。在 20 世纪开始时，许多文章集中于牙刷的副作用，甚至对定期应用的安全性以及普遍接受性提出疑问，相比之下，也有许多报告支持口腔卫生需要用牙刷。在20世纪开始时，刷牙并不普遍，因为新奇，与担心有关系。硬度的变化，天然刷毛的存在，直到 30 年代后期，当塑料（作刷柄）与尼龙（作刷毛）变成为广泛应用时，到 60 年代后期，逐渐认识到釉质磨损与牙龈萎缩的危险，软毛尼龙牙刷变成为推荐选用（Fishman1997）。

单纯从牙上清除沉积物需要用牙膏具有一定的磨损。在口腔内有四种组织受到刷牙磨损作用的影响，它们是釉质、牙本质、牙龈组织与牙槽黏膜。直至今天，有少量的科学资料帮助我们了解与牙刷磨损有关的风险，特别是研究硬组织的磨损是困难的，因为这种影响通常要经过多年才能看得到；各种因素，在磨损过程中起到作用，包括刷牙所用的力量，刷毛的硬度，刷牙次数，牙膏的磨损性，以及所消耗的食物的侵蚀（Davis等1980），一把特殊的牙刷所用的牙膏的量也可能对牙体组织的磨损有影响，这些因素难以对牙刷的作用进行临床研究。Slop（1986）用一种体外模型研究刷牙的结果对釉质磨耗的程度。虽然看到一定程度的磨耗，但对组织广泛的磨损可能没有危险。对牙本质的磨损也知道的很少。这对手动牙刷与电动牙刷都一样。有一种途径体外评估相对的牙本质磨损。在美国印第安纳进行的几面研究的结果表明振动／旋转的电动牙刷对牙本质的磨损是安全的。然而，最近在苏黎世进行的研究（Imfeldt 等，1998），显然用同样的模型，出现相互矛盾的发现。这些差异的来源可能是原来的模型的微小差异的结果是进一步研究的课题。

The hard versus soft bristle brush controversy is an old one among dentists, and Hirshfield, in his book the Toothbrush-Its Use and Abuse, quotes advocates for both positions (Walmsley 1997). At the beginning of the 20th century, many published papers focused on the side effects of toothbrushes and even questioned the safety of regular use and general acceptance. In contrast, there were also many reports in support of the need for oral hygiene. At the start of this century, toothbrushing was not common and was correlated with fear because of its newness (Saxer & Yankell 1997). Variations on hard, natural bristles existed until the late 1930's, when plastic (for handles) and nylon (for bristles) became widely available. By the late 1960's, with the growing awareness of the dangers of enamel abrasion and gingival recession, toothbrushes with soft nylon bristles became the recommendation of choice (Fishman 1997).

The simple act of cleaning away dental deposits from teeth requires that the toothbrush-dentifrice combination possess some level of abrasivity. In the oral cavity four tissues are at risk from the abrasive effect of toothbrushing. These are the enamel, dentine, the gingival tissues and alveolar mucosa. Up till now, few scientific data have been available to help us understand the risks associated with toothbrush abrasion, and in particular, research into the abrasion of hard tissues is difficult. First of all the effect usually takes years to become visible. Second, various factors play a role in the process of abrasion, including the force with which the brush is used, the stiffness of the bristles, the frequency of toothbrushing, the abrasiveness of the toothpaste, and the erosiveness of the food which is consumed

(Davis & Winter 1980). The amount of dentifrice applied to a particular brush may also contribute to the potential abrasion of dental tissues (Harte & Manly 1976). These factors make it difficult to perform clinical research into the effect of the toothbrush itself.

(3) 牙龈损伤 Gingival abrasion

Epstein等（1943）描述了几种影响牙刷磨损的变量，刷牙用力与刷毛种类直接与刷牙本身有关。牙刷毛的硬度与不利的形态认为是牙龈受损伤来源的一种病因因素（Hirshfeld 1931，Lange 1977）。

经常刷牙的颊侧牙龈与龈缘线角部位有更明显的创伤性牙龈操作的表征。这些损伤可以产生牙龈萎缩（Serino等1994，Joshipura等1994）。首次报告电动牙刷的安全性集中在那些往返动作的牙刷。研究观察应用传统电动牙刷产生的牙龈损伤的数量，并与手动牙刷可能产生的损伤进行比较（Niemi 等 1986），肉眼观察受损伤侧的数量，检查者首先对损伤的解释预先进行培训。Walsh（1989）发现在牙龈软组织损伤方面电动牙刷与手动牙刷之间无差异。

Sonicare 电动牙刷用狗进行安全性检测（Engel 等 1993）。2 个月内每天刷牙 7.5 分钟，在临床上与组织学上没有明显损伤。最近Danser等（1998）进行一项研究以刷牙的结果，确定牙龈损伤的发病率采用手动牙刷与 Braun Oral-B D9 电动牙刷，这项调查显示作为刷牙的结果电动牙刷与手动牙刷都引起少量的牙龈损伤。

有 2 项纵向调查用一种电动牙刷引起的牙龈损伤，研究对牙龈组织的间接影响（Van der Weijden 等 1994，Wilson 等 1993），没有看到一种电动牙刷比手动牙刷引起更多的牙龈损伤。Wilson等（1993）还测量了牙龈的萎缩，在一年的研究期间，他们并没有看到手动牙刷或电动牙刷对牙龈萎缩的水平产生明显的改变。用Rotadent电动牙刷进行的一年研究，用电动牙刷的人颊侧牙龈附着水平丧失0.12mm，而用手动牙刷的人仅丧失约0.05mm（Boyd等，1989a）。这些差异并没有统计学意义，虽然一年内附着丧失0.1mm比一项洁治项目中病人的流行病学平均值要高（saxer 等 1997）。

Epstein & Tainter (1943) described several variables that affect toothbrush abrasion, of which brushing pressure and bristle type were directly related to the brushing itself. The stiffness and unfavorable shape of toothbrush bristles have been claimed to be an etiologic factor in the origin of gingival injury (Hirshfeld 1931, Lange 1977).

Frequent brushers tend to show more signs of traumatic gingival lesions buccally and on the line angle of the marginal gingival. These injuries may produce recession of the gingival (Serino et al. 1994).

First reports on safety with electric toothbrushes have focused on those brushes with a side-to-side motion. Studies have looked at the number of gingival abrasions that have occurred with the use of the Braun Oral-B D3 (conventional electric toothbrush) and compared their occurrence to the potential damage caused by manual toothbrushing (Niemi et al. 1986). Visual scoring of the number of abrasion sites was made, the examiner being pre-trained in the interpretation of abrasions. Results demonstrated a greater amount of abrasions following use of the manual brush. Walsh (1989) found no differences between electric and manual toothbrushes with respect to gingival abrasion of the soft tissues.

The Sonicare brush has been subjected to safety testing in dogs (Engel et al. 1993).

Following brushing for 7.5 minutes daily for 2 months, no damage was evident on clinical or histological examination.

(4) 刷牙用力 Toothbrushing force

几项实验与临床研究支持这样的假设，刷牙时用力过度，对牙刷引起的创伤有部分作用（Arnim 等 1961，Alexander 等 1977，Niemi 等 1986）。Mierau 等（1984）观察到一组没有牙龈萎缩的受试者平均刷牙用力为 2.12N（± 0.31），而有多种龈萎缩的一组平均用力为 3.75N（±0.47）。Abbas等（1990）研究显示机械性口腔卫生基本上是一个创伤性程序。他们观察到在口腔卫生结束之后很快用探针检查出血指数分值增加了。

有些电动牙刷通过达到一定压力程度之后给予刷牙者反馈信息，试图限制或减少刷牙用力，其中研究之一是 Van der Weijden 等（1995）进行的与没有反馈系统的牙刷作比较显示压力控制在 350 克不能减少所用的力。

一项最近的研究评价习惯性刷牙用力的人应用各种牙刷（Van der Weijden 等 1996c）。除了一种手动牙刷之外，检查了三种电动牙刷，结果显示用手动牙刷比电动牙刷所用的力量更大，差异在100克以上。Danser等（1998）研究刷牙用力与牙龈损伤之间的关系，没有看到两者之间的相关性，表明其他因素（就是刷牙本身，牙体解剖，刷毛形态）看来比电动牙刷所用之力更加重要。

Several experimental and clinical studies support the assumption that excessive force in brushing is partly responsible for the origin of toothbrush trauma (Arnim & Blackburn 1961, Alexander et al. 1977, Niemi et al. 1986). Mierau & Spindler (19840 observed that in a group of subjects without recession the mean brushing force with a manual toothbrush was 2.12N (±0.31), whereas a group with multiple recession had a mean force of 3.75 N (±0.47). Abbas et al. (1990) showed that mechanical oral hygiene basically is a traumatic procedure. They observed increased bleeding upon probing scores shortly after oral hygiene procedures.

With some electric brushes it has been attempted to limit or reduce the brushing force by giving feedback to the brusher that a certain threshold has been reached. One of these systems was investigated in a study by Van der Weijden et al. (1995b), in which it was shown that a pressure control at 350 grams was not able to reduce the force used, compared to a brush without this feedback system.

A recent study evaluated the habitual brushing force individuals use with various toothbrushes (Van der Weijden et al. 1996c). In addition to manual toothbrush, three electric toothbrushes were examined; The Rotadent, the Interplak and the Braun D7. the results showed that with a manual brush considerably more force was used than with the electric brushes, the difference being more than 100 grams. Danser et al. (1998) studied the relation between force and gingival abrasion. No correlation was observed, which indicates that other factors (e.g., brushing it self, tooth anatomy, bristle form) appear to be more important than the force used with an electric brush.

(5) 依从性 Compliance

多项研究比较了电动牙刷（Van der Weijden 等 1993 ~ 1997）但这些研究资料都不是结论性的，资料表明，按照现时的标准，4种电动牙刷都是很有效的牙刷。因此，选择不应该依据去除牙菌斑的效果。

选用电动牙刷应考虑到使用舒适。最好的牙刷是适合病人使用的牙刷。关于电动牙刷的选用情况，有一项2个月使用的调查，结果表明25%的人不喜欢而停止使用。另有一项6个月的调查，发现大多数人不能做到一天2次使用。最近一项研究评价牙周病人使用电动牙刷的次数，62%每天使用刷牙。

文献表明刷牙时间越长，去除牙菌斑效果越好。大多数人刷牙只用60秒钟（Van der Weijden 1993b，1996b）理想的刷牙时间至少2分钟。因此应强调增加定期刷牙的时间。在同样的时间内，电动牙刷去除牙菌斑的效果比手动牙刷好，而且应用舒适。

但是选择电动牙刷，有几个影响因素，不只是科学数据而是实际起作用的方面，如刷头大小，刷柄大小与重量以及电池功率。

（6）特殊病人的选择

维持牙周健康的病人，用电动牙刷对口腔卫生依从性差的人控制牙菌斑的沉积特别有好处。Hellstadius等（1993）报告一组依从性差的牙周治疗病人，治疗前接受过广泛的口腔卫生指导，经过40个月，仍保持较少的菌斑控制48%，而用手动牙刷菌斑减少仅12%，这项研究观察了3年。

儿童使用电动牙刷，早期的一项研究显示电动牙刷比手动牙刷去除牙菌斑较多，另一项交叉设计研究发现二组之间无统计学显著性差异，最近的一项研究比较一种新的电动牙刷与手动牙刷（Grossman等，1995）结果显示电动牙刷组去除菌斑效果显著。电动牙刷特别有助于家长帮助儿童刷牙或专业人员帮助儿童刷牙效果很好（Van der Weijden 等 1993 ~ 1996）。

电动牙刷对残疾病人特别有用。然而有对照的临床试验研究很少。有两项研究表明对精神失常与手灵巧性差的儿童电动牙刷有价值（Kelner，1963，Bratel等1964）。近来的少数研究显示电动牙刷对残疾成人有价值（Bratel 等 1991，1998，Blahut 等 1991），Martin 等（1987）报告对手活动受限制的众议院老年病人的研究，病人没有给予任何口腔卫生指导，评估用电动牙刷前后的口腔清洁与牙龈健康结果提出效果增加，用电动牙刷保持对住院老年人的口腔健康有价值。

另外，还显示专业人员用电动牙刷刷牙高度有效（Van der Weijden等，1993a，b，1996b）护理儿童的口腔卫生，电动牙刷是有用的工具。

青少年正畸病人经常显示控制菌斑无效，因为固定矫正器难以去除菌斑（Boyd 1997），Yankell 等（1985）与 Wilcoxon 等（1991）调查正畸病人应用电动牙刷的效果。2个月交叉研究20个正畸病人显示其效果超过手动牙刷，另一项一个月周期的研究有牙龈炎的正畸病人经过口腔卫生指导之后用电动牙刷显示菌斑与出血状况均比手动牙刷好。（Ha1997）。一项3个月的研究（white 1996）也得出结论，电动牙刷可以帮助正畸病人增进口腔健康。不过，这项研究没采用盲法。唯一的一项长期临床试验评价电动牙刷对正畸病人牙周健康的效果，18个月的结果显示电动牙刷比手动牙刷更有效果。

在评阅了过去20年发表的之后，得出的结论是电动牙刷与老的设计比较，去除龈上牙菌斑与控制牙龈炎的效果更好。

- 手动牙刷与电动牙刷之间的差异主要是电动牙刷去除邻面牙菌斑的能力增加
- 专业人员指导与强化应用动力牙刷对达到理想的结果，看来是重要的
- 虽然硬软组织损伤的原因不完全了解，刷牙是其影响因素之一。长期应用（8 ~ 12个月）电动牙刷与手动牙刷进行比较，没有发现电动牙刷对软硬组织有反应或者创伤

◆ 在过去10年的临床试验显示有对照的电动牙刷临床试验看来比手动牙刷有优势，现代设计的特点起到这方面的作用

In reviewing many of the published reports over the past two decades, one comes to the conclusion that the electric toothbrush has become, compared to the old design, more effective in the removal of supra-gingival plaque and controlling gingivitis.

◆ *the difference between manual toothbrushes and electric toothbrushes is primarily in the increased ability of the electric brushes to remove plaque from the approximal area.*

◆ *professional instruction and reinforcement in the use of powered toothbrushes seems important to achieve optimal results.*

◆ *although the etiology of hard and soft tissue abrasion is not fully understood, toothbrushing is one of the factors involved. No adverse reactions or trauma involving either oral soft or hard tissues have been attributed to the long-term (8-12 month) use of electric brushes when compared to manual toothbrushes.*

◆ *clinical trials over the past 10 years show that in controlled trials electric toothbrushes appear to be superior to manual brushing. Modern design features are responsible for this.*

二、刷牙方法 Brushing techniques

向病人全面进行刷牙指导包括讲授what，when，where and how四个方面。除了描述具体的刷牙方法之外，其次考虑牙刷的掌握，刷牙的顺序与次数，受限的部位等。

Complete toothbrushing instruction for a patient includes teaching what, when, where, and how. In addition to descriptions of specific toothbrushing methods, the succeeding sections consider the grasp of the brush, the sequence and amount of brushing, the areas of limited access, and supplementary brushing for the occlusal surfaces and the tongue. The possible detrimental affects from improper toothbrushing and variations for special conditions are described. The care of toothbrushes is outlined.

（一）刷牙要领 Key points for toothbrushing

1. 掌握牙刷 Grasp of brush

（1）目标 objective

为了成功地去除牙菌斑，牙刷的操作与手的把握方式有关。如何把握和放置牙刷病人需要具体指导，当开始刷牙时去除的牙菌斑是用染色剂浸染的，菌斑的粘性、压力的控制是能够领悟的。牢固而舒适的掌握有几点：在整个刷牙期间要控制好牙刷；在每次刷牙动作开始时，放置于有效的部位，整个刷牙动作坚持到底，再放置下一个刷牙部位；对用力的大小要敏感。

A. Objectives

Manipulation of the brush for successful removal of bacterial plaque can be related to the manner in which the brush is held. Patients may need specific instruction in how to hold and place the rush. When they start to brush to remove the bacterial plaque that has been colored with a disclosing agent, the tenaciousness of the plaque and the need for controlled pressure can be realized. With a firm, comfortable grasp, the following can be expected:

a. control of the brush during all movements; b. effective positioning at the beginning of each brushing stroke, follow-through during the complete stroke, and repositioning for the next stroke; c. sensitivity to the amount of pressure applied.

（2）步骤 procedure

把牙刷柄握在掌中，拇指对准刷颈，紧靠刷头，这样能有效地控制；当牙刷损伤有妨碍或手指能触及前牙当刷头达到后牙区时，不要太靠近刷头；

直毛放置在牙上所需的方向，取决于刷牙所用的方法；

整个操作过程中，适应于掌握刷头在牙面的各个部位，允许调整腕臂自由移动；

去除菌斑用力适当，用力太大，刷毛弯曲成曲面离开所需刷牙的部位。

B. procedure

Grasp toothbrush handle in the palm of the hand with thumb against the shank.

a. near enough to the head of the brush so that it can be controlled effectively; b. not so close to the head the brush that manipulation of the brush is hindered or that fingers can touch the anterior teeth when reaching the brush head to molar regions.

Direct filaments in the direction needed for placement on the teeth; direction depends on the brushing method to be used.

Adapt grasp for the various positions of the brush head on the teeth throughout he procedure; adjust to permit unrestricted movement of the wrist and arm.

Apply appropriate pressure for removal of the bacterial plaque. Too much pressure, however, bends the filaments and curves them away from the area where brushing is needed.

2. 顺序 sequence

（1）用任何方法，刷牙的步骤应确保完全覆盖每个牙面。

（2）从与对侧相对的一个牙弓的一个磨牙区，随后回到舌侧或唇侧，重复对侧牙弓。

（3）每次牙刷放置的部位必须与前一次完全覆盖有重叠（见图 7-3）。

（4）鼓励病人从最需要刷的部位开始。

最经常遗忘的部位

最难刷或最难损伤的部位，如用右手刷牙的右侧或者用左手刷牙的左侧。

（5）建议改变顺序至少一天一次，当时间有限，菌斑去除不完全时不会使同一个部位总是轮到最后刷。

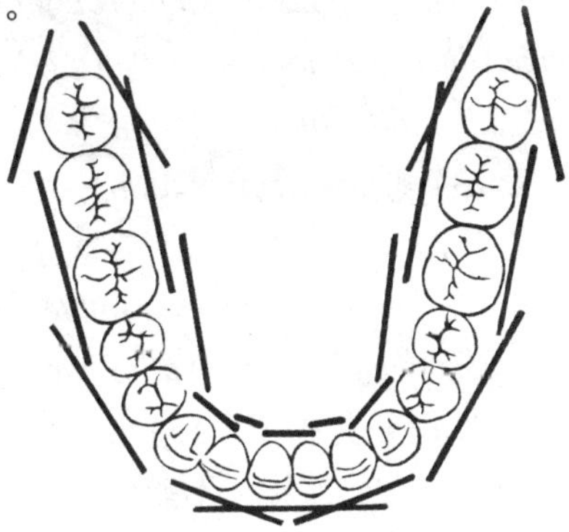

图 7-3

A. the procedure in brushing, for any method used, should assure complete coverage for each tooth surface.

B. start brushing from a molar region of one arch around to the opposite side, then back around the lingual or facial. Repeat in the opposing arch.

C. each brush placement must overlap the previous one for thorough coverage (figure).

D. encourage the patient to begin by brushing one of the areas of greatest individual need.

Areas that are most frequently missed;

Areas that are most difficult for brush placement and/or manipulation, such as the right side for the right-handed brusher or the left side for the left-handed brusher

E. suggest that the sequence be varied at least once each day so that the same areas are not always brushed last when time may be limited and plaque removal may be less complete.

3. 刷牙数量 Amount of brushing

（1）计数系统 The count system

为了一致地分配刷牙的次数，确保完全覆盖，帮助病人专心于完成刷牙过程一种计数系统是有用的。

每个部位计数 6 次颤动（或 5 或 10 次，最适合于特殊病人)，改良 stillman 法或其他方法用一种颤动动作。

巴斯，Charters 或其他振动法，在每个牙刷部位，牙刷刷毛端缓慢振动 10 次计数。

To ensure thorough coverage with an even distribution of amount of brushing and to help the patient concentrate on the performance, system of counting is useful.

Count 6 strokes in each area (or 5 or 10, whichever is most appropriate for the particular patient) for modified Stillman or other method in which a stroke is used.

Count slowly to 10 for each brush position while brush is vibrated and filament ends are held in position for the Bass, Charters, or other vibratory method.

（2）钟表系统 The clock system

有些病人刷牙完全靠看中一个鸡蛋计时器3或4分钟，定时步骤不能保证完全覆盖，因为最适合于进入的单个部位可能花费更多的刷牙时间

Some patients brush thoroughly while watching a clock or an egg timer for 3 or 4 minutes. Timed procedures cannot assure thorough coverage, because single areas that are most accessible may get more brushing time.

（3）联合 Combination

许多人用计数系统与钟表系统相结合产生最彻底的去除牙菌斑的效果

For many patients, use of the "count" system in combination with the "clock" system produces the most complete removal of bacterial plaque.

4. 刷牙次数 Frequency of brushing

由于个体差异，不能用一套次数规定。对病人进行教育时，强调每天彻底清除牙菌斑，而不是刷牙次数。

为了控制菌斑与口腔卫生，预防口臭，至少每天刷牙2次，伴随着适当的牙间保健。细菌保持不受干扰的时间越久，菌斑致病的可能性就越大。鼓励睡前有一个清洁的口腔。细菌在黑暗，温暖与潮湿的口腔环境中生长旺盛，病人用漱口液等应在清除牙菌斑之后用。

Because of individual variations, one set rule for requency cannot be applied. The emphasis in patient education should be placed on complete plaque removal daily rather than on number of brushings.

For the control of bacterial plaque, and for oral sanitation and halitosis prevention, at least two brushings accompanied by appropriate interdental care, are recommended for each day. The longer the

bacteria remain undisturbed, the greater the pathogenic potential of the plaque.

A clean mouth before going to sleep should be encouraged. Bacteria thrive in the dark, warm, moist climate of the oral environment. Patients who use a chewable fluoride tablet, mouthrinse, or gel application before going to bed should complete their plaque removal before fluoride application.

（二）刷牙方法 Toothbrushing methods

根据牙刷的动作与部位可以把大多数刷牙方法分为8组，除了有些方法用人名之外，其他方法部分或全部的步骤用指定的动作，有些方法只是为了描述性、比较性和历史性的目的而记载的，并不是现在推荐的。少数方法甚至显示是有伤害的。

Most toothbrushing methods can be classified into one of eight groups based on the motion and position of the brush. Noted beside certain categories that follow are names of methods that utilize the designated motion as part or all or their particular procedure. Some of these methods are recorded for descriptive, comparative, or historic purposes only, and are not currently recommended. A few even have been shown to be detrimental.

（1）龈沟动作：Bass 法

（2）转动：旋转颤动，改良 Stillman 法

（3）振动：Stillman，Charters，Bass 法

（4）环状动作：Fones 法

（5）垂直动作：Leonard 法

（6）水平动作法 Horizontol

（7）生理动作：Smith 法

（8）牙刷擦洗法 Scrub-brush

1. 巴斯刷牙法 The Bass methods

巴斯刷牙法（the Bass method）又称水平颤动法或龈沟法。作为一种有效的清除龈缘附近以及龈沟内菌斑的方法，Bass 法最为广泛接受，因为这个部位对控制牙龈牙牙周感染最为重要。能去除龈缘附近与龈沟内的牙菌斑，特别是邻间区，牙颈部与暴露的根面区，适用于所有人群以及实施过牙周手术的病人。

（1）刷牙要领：手持刷柄，刷毛指向根尖方向（上颌牙向上，下颌牙向下），虽然刷毛呈45度角，但通常对病人较容易和较安全的是先与牙长轴平等，然后稍作旋转，与龈缘呈45度角（图7-4A）。刷毛角度：把牙刷刷毛端放在直指龈沟的位置，刷毛约与牙长轴呈45度角（图

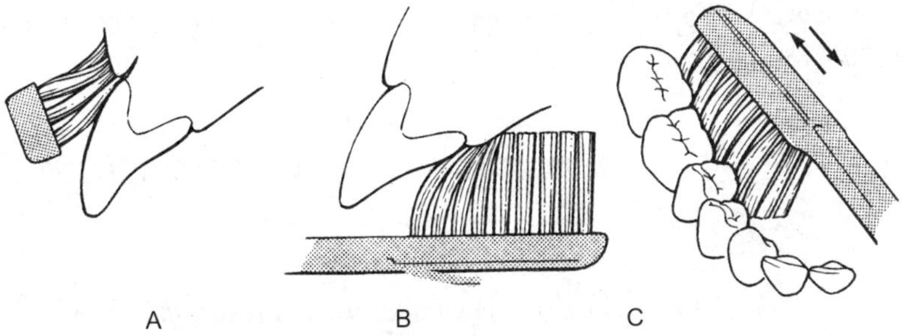

图 7-4

7-4B)。勿使刷毛屈曲：轻度加压使刷毛端进入龈沟。以短距离（2 ~ 3mm）水平拂刷颤动牙刷，勿使毛端离开龈沟，至少颤动 10 次。重新放置牙刷：将牙刷移至下一组 2 ~ 3 颗牙，注意重叠放置（图7-4C）在上颌下颌牙弓唇舌面的每个部位重复全面拂刷。牙刷舌腭侧前牙面位置将牙刷竖放在前牙，使刷毛垂直并指向和进入龈沟。

（2）缺点：刷牙用力过猛可使短距拂刷变成为强力摩擦而损伤龈缘。敏捷的要求对某些人可能太高，45度角难以看到。当病人相信旋转刷牙法可以帮助洁牙时，可以先刷龈沟，但两种方法应分开，而不是像改良 Bass 法那样合在一起。

The Bass method: sulcular brushing

The Bass method is widely accepted as an effective method for bacterial plaque removal adjacent to and directly beneath the gingival margin. This area around the tooth is the most significant in the control of gingival and periodontal infections.

1) Purposes and indications

a. For all patients for bacterial plaque removal adjacent to and directly beneath the gingival margin.

b. Particularly for open interproximal areas, cervical areas beneath the height of contour of the enamel, and exposed root surfaces.

c. For the patient who has had periodontal surgery.

2) Procedure

a. Grasp brush handle

Direct the filaments apically (up for maxillary down for mandibular teeth). Even though the brush placement calls for directing the filaments at a 45° angle, it is usually easier and safer for the patient to first place the sides of the filaments parallel with the long axis of the tooth. From that position the brush can be turned slightly and brought to the gingival margin to the 45° angle.

b. Angle the filaments

Place the brush with the filament tips directed straight into the gingival sulcus. The filaments straight into the gingival sulcus. The filaments will be directed at approximately 45° to the long axis of the tooth, as shown in figure.

c. Press lightly without flexing

Press lightly so the filament tips enter the gingival sulci and embrasures and cover the gingival margin. Do not bend the filaments with excess pressure.

d. Vibrate the brush

Vibrate the brush back and forth with very short strokes without disengaging the tips of the filaments from the sulci. Count at least 10 vibrations.

e. Reposition the brush

Apply the brush to the next group of two or three teeth. Take care to overlap pplacement, as shown in figure.

f. Repeat stroke

The entire stroke (parts A through D) is repeated at each position around the maxillary and mandibular arches, both facially and lingually.

g. Position brush for lingual and palatal anterior surfaces

Hold the brush the long narrow way for the anterior components as described for the rolling stroke method. The filaments are kept straight and directed into the sulci.

3) Problems

a. An overeager brusher may convert the previously mentioned "very short strokes" into a vigorous scrub that causes injury to the gingival margin.

b. Dexterity requirement may be too high for certain patients. A 45° angle can be difficult to visualize.

c. Rolling stroke procedure may precede the sulcular brushing when a patient believes it helps to clean the teeth. The two methods should be performed separately rather than trying to combine them in what has been referred to as a "modified bass."

The procedure of rolling the brush down over the crown after the vibratory part of the sulcular brush stroke has several disadvantages: (1) too often the brush is hastily and carelessly replaced into the sulcus position, or the opposite is true, and considerable time is consumed in the attempt to replace the brush carefully; (2) gingival margin injury by the constant replacement of the brush can result; and (3) patient may tend to roll the brush down over the crown prematurely, thereby accomplishing very little sulcular brushing.

2. 旋转法或旋转颤动法 The roll or rolling stroke method

清洁牙龈从牙上去除牙菌斑、牙垢，与食物残渣不强调龈沟。用于牙龈相对健康，组织外形正常，掌握龈沟方法有困难的儿童，同时用振动方法作一般性清洁（charters，stillman）。第一次开始指导刷牙时用改良stillman法，因为开始的牙刷放置相同。这种方法对难以掌握复杂刷牙方法的人特别有帮助。

刷牙操作步骤：①手握刷柄，刷毛指向牙尖方向，上颌牙向上下颌牙向下；②刷毛一侧放在附着龈上。刷毛指向牙尖方向，当刷头的塑料部分与𬌗平面或切牙平面平行时，一般为牙刷的高度适当；③轻压使刷毛屈曲，刷毛一侧放置在牙龈上，牙龈会发白；④牙刷缓慢在牙上旋转，因为牙刷转动，手腕稍作转动，刷毛保持屈曲，随着牙外形，而可以清洁牙颈部，部分刷毛可以到达牙间隙部位；⑤重复与反复转动5次或5次以上。重复全部动作（以A到D），每个牙或每组牙至少5次。当牙刷移动与换位时，转动手腕，牙刷离开牙面，用刷头北部把颊部向面侧拉长。当牙刷转动到起始部位时，注意刷毛尖端一定不要拖拉超过龈缘（图7-5）；⑥重叠动作，当牙刷移动至邻近部位时，牙刷放置重叠；⑦舌侧或腭侧面的牙刷放置，用牙刷长窄的方向，在切端托住牙刷的跟部，轻压（上颌牙向下，下颌牙向上）直至刷毛与牙及牙龈平行，轻压与拉动（下颌牙曲面向上，上颌牙曲面向下），以刷毛宽度重复与反复5次。

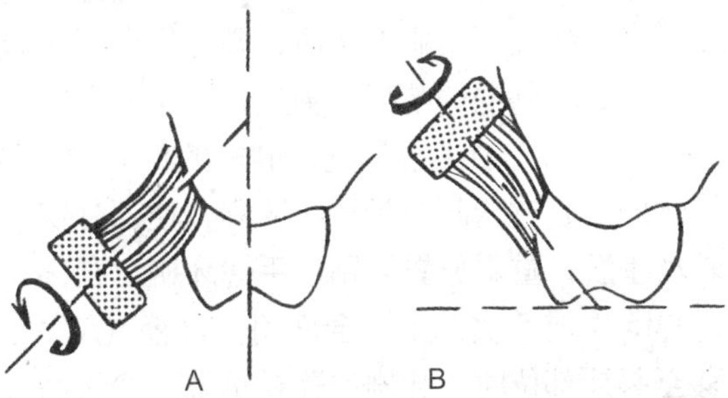

图 7-5

缺点：开始放置的部位太高，刷牙时能够损伤牙槽黏膜，如果倾向于快速大弧度动作刷不到牙颈部1/3，因为刷毛端掠过这一部位而没有进入这一部位，同样地还有牙间隙部位也有这种可能。把牙刷毛端对准牙龈进入能产生点状损伤。

Purposes and indications

a. Cleaning gingiva and removing plaque, material alba, and food debris from the teeth without emphasis on gingival sulcus.

- *For children with relatively healthy gingiva and normal tissue contour when a sulcular technique may seem difficult for the patient to master.*
- *For general cleaning in conjunction with the use of a vibratory technique (charters, stillman).*

b. Useful for preparatory instruction (first lesson) for modified stillman method because the initial brush placement is the same. This can be particularly helpful when there is a question as to how complicated a technique the patient can master and practice.

3. 改良 Stillman 法 The modified Stillman method

这一方法最早由stillman记述，为按摩与刺激而设计的，还有清洁牙颈部，刷毛端部分放在牙龈上，部分放在牙颈部，稍指向根尖方向，加压使牙龈发白，刷柄稍作转动动作刷端保持在牙面位置上，刷动数次后，移至邻牙。改良stillman法常在振动之后再结合转动。改良法减少了牙龈创伤的可能，增加祛除菌斑的效果。

This method, as originally described by stillman, was designed for massage and stimulation, as well as for cleaning the cervical areas. The brush ends were placed partly on the gingival and partly on the cervical areas of the tooth and were directed slightly apically. Pressure was applied to effect a blanching. The handle was given a slight rotary motion, and the brush ends were maintained in position on the tooth surface. After several applications, the brush was moved to the adjacent teeth.

A modified stillman, which incorporates a rolling stroke after the vibratory (rotary) phase, frequently is used. The modifications minimize the possibility of gingival trauma and increase the plaque removal effects.

目的与指征：清除牙冠外形高点以下颈部及暴露的邻面部位的牙菌斑，一般用来清洁牙面并按摩牙龈。

Bacterial plaque removal from cervical areas below the height of contour of the crown and from exposed proximal surfaces.

General application for cleaning tooth surfaces and massage of the gingival.

操作步骤：①手握刷柄，刷毛指向根尖（上颌牙向上，下颌牙向下）；②牙刷一侧放置于附着龈上，刷毛对准根尖方向，当刷头的塑料部分与颌平面或切端平面平行时，一般牙刷的高度适当；③轻压使刷毛屈曲，刷毛侧向牙龈施以轻压，使牙龈发白；④刷毛角度：转动手腕使刷柄旋转，刷毛约与牙长轴呈45°角方向；⑤振动牙刷，轻而稳地振动，保持刷毛受压，保持毛端处于不变的接触位置，刷柄的振动动作缓慢计数 10 次；⑥旋转并振动牙刷，转动手腕，缓慢向下越过牙龈与牙振动牙刷，使部分刷毛到达牙间隙部位；⑦使牙刷重复反复动作，通过转动手腕，重新放置牙刷。手握牙刷，稍离开牙面，避免拖动刷毛回到越过游离龈缘；⑧重复动作 5 次或 5 次以上。全部动作过程（从 A 到 F）。在每个牙或每组牙至少反复 5 次。当牙刷移至邻牙部位时，牙刷位置要重叠；⑨舌面与腭面牙刷放置：牙刷放置与前牙呈垂直方向，如旋转动作法所描述。加压与振动，旋转与重复（图 7-6）。

缺点：用磨毛牙刷不小心放置，可以引起组织损伤，施压要轻。如果转动刷牙动作太快，振动对祛除龈缘菌斑可能无效。

4. Charters 法

在他长期的职业生涯中，Dr. W.J. Charters强调预防的重要性。他以传授邻间刷牙法为目标，通过祛除邻面“粘蛋白膜”来清洁，以及通过机械性刺激按摩牙龈。在他发表的许多文章中，Charters 记述两种牙刷放置，一种是与牙长轴呈直角，另一种是与向㐬平面毛端呈45°角。直角放置主要有意用于邻间牙周组织丧失的病人，允许刷毛进行楔状间隙部位。

每一种牙刷放置指导施力于毛端使其进入邻间区。在两牙之间的刷毛，尽可能施加压力，给牙刷几次轻度转动或振动动作。这样可使刷毛侧与龈缘接触，产生一种理想的按摩作用。

经典的牙周病学教科书Charters法为刷毛指向㐬平面与牙长轴呈 45° 角。

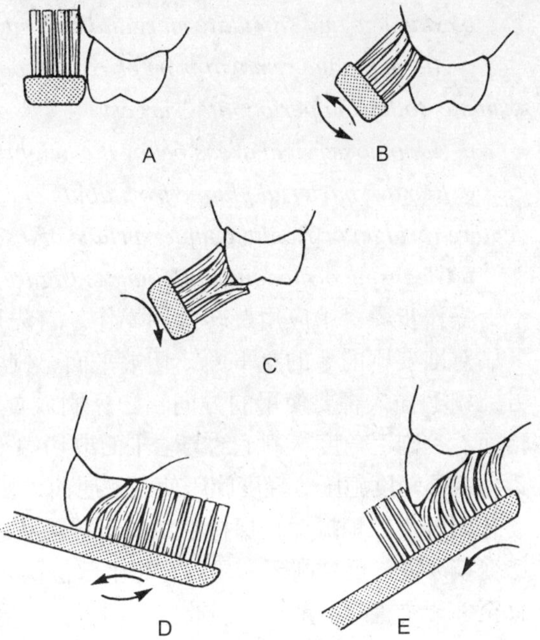

图 7-6

The charters method

During his long productive dental career, Dr. W. J. Charters emphasized the importance of prevention. The interproximal toothbrushing method that he taught had as its objectives cleanliness through removal of the “film and mucin” from the proximal surfaces and gingival massage through mechanical stimulation.

Among his many published papers, Charters described two brush positions, one at a right angle to the long axis of the tooth and another at a 45° angle with the tips of the bristles toward the occlusal plane. The right-angle position might have been intended primarily for patients with interdentl periodontal tissue loss, where access permitted the bristles to enter the embrasure.

For either brush position, the instructions were to force the tips into the interproximal area. “With the bristles between the teeth, as much pressure as possible is exerted, giving the brush several slight rotary or vibratory movements. This causes the sides of the bristles to come in contact with the gum margin, producing an ideal massage.

The classic periodontal textbooks have described the Charters method with the bristles directed toward the occlusal plane at a 45° angle with the long axis. This method is described as follows.

目的与指征：松散食物残渣与菌斑，按摩与刺激龈缘与邻间牙龈，当邻间组织丧失时，帮助去除邻面牙菌斑。例如，在牙周手术之后。适合于牙冠外形高点以下的颈部与暴露无遗的根面部位。去除基牙，固定桥龈缘以下或者卫生桥的下面的牙菌斑，清洁矫正器。

Purposes and indications

a. Loosen debris and bacterial plaque

b. Massage and stimulate marginal and interdental gingiva

c. Aid in plaque removal from proximal tooth surfaces when interproximal tissue is missing, for example, following periodontal surgery

d. Adapt to cervical areas below the height of contour of the crown and to exposed root surfaces

e. Remove bacterial plaque from abutment teeth and under the gingival border of a fixed partial denture (bridge) or from the undersurface of a sanitary bridge

f. Cleansing orthodontic appliances (figure)

操作步骤：①应用旋转擦刷操作。首先用基本旋转擦刷法作一般性清洁。②手握刷柄把牙刷对准要刷的牙的殆平面或切端平面，刷上颌牙时毛端指向正文，刷下颌牙时毛端指向上方。刷毛插入将要使用的方向；③牙刷放置　刷毛一侧对准釉质，刷端朝向殆平面或切端平殆面；④刷毛角度　刷毛约与殆平面或切端平面呈45°角，牙刷滑动至靠近游离龈缘与牙面的集团；⑤轻度施压，轻度施压使刷毛屈曲，使毛端力量在两牙之间，毛端一侧压迫龈缘；⑥振动牙刷轻而稳地振动，保持毛端处于接触状态。通过刷柄的旋转动作，牙刷缓慢振动 10 次；⑦变换牙位，反复刷牙，牙刷在每个部位刷牙数次，直到完成所有的牙；⑧重叠擦刷　当牙刷移至邻牙位置时，重叠牙刷放置；⑨舌侧与腭侧牙刷放置因为 Charters 法难以在舌侧面完成，因此经常建议采用改良 Stillman 法。如果偏爱 Charters 法，牙刷放置设定如下：后牙　刷毛端对准殆面，延伸刷柄，通过所刷牙对侧的尖牙切端。将刷头前部刷毛端对最后的后牙远中面，然后是每个牙间的楔状区，施压与振动刷牙。前牙　刷柄与牙长轴平行，将刷毛前部刷毛端放置于牙邻间楔状区，施压并振动刷牙；⑩固定修复体的牙刷使用　放置牙刷时，使毛端指向修复体龈缘下方。（图 7-7、图 7-8）缺点：牙刷刷毛不能进行龈沟，去除龈下菌斑沉积。某些部位，正确的牙刷放置受到限制或不能放置因此，必须调整，结果增加了刷牙操作的复杂性，需要手指灵巧度高。

5. Fones 法，又称圆弧法

许多病人，特别是学校儿童很可能以这种方法为指导。因为Fones发现这一方法首先在口腔卫生教科书内作了叙述，在美国口腔卫生师中应用了多年，这种方法可能是年幼儿童首先容易学习的。选择刷毛直径为 0.006 ~ 0.008 英吋的细丝软毛牙刷。操作如下：在牙闭合的情况下，牙刷进入口腔放置在颊部内侧轻轻接触牙龈超过最后上颌磨牙，用一种快而宽的圆弧动

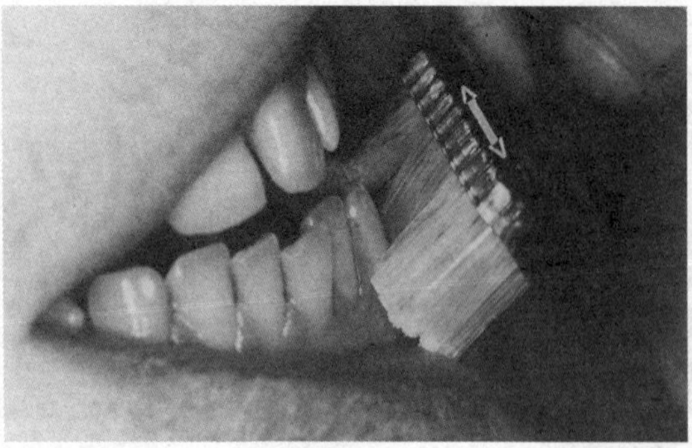

图 7-7

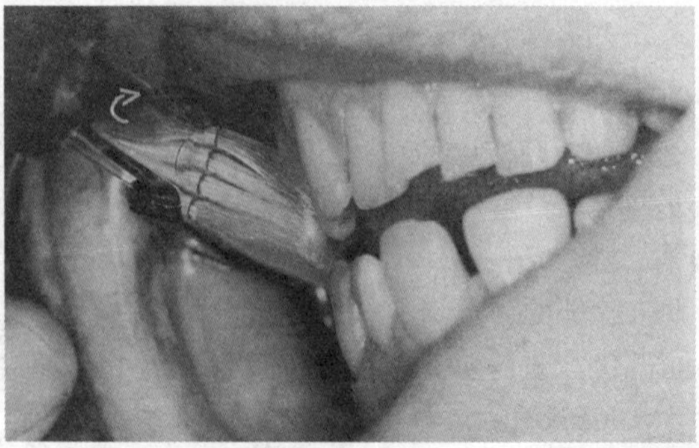

图 7-8

作，很轻的压力从上颌牙龈刷到下颌牙龈，使前牙切端对切端接触，让开唇部，作连续的圆弧动作，舌侧与腭侧牙面需要往返动作，牙刷通过上颌牙弓腭侧刷到下颌牙弓的磨牙，前后往返动作。(图 7-9)

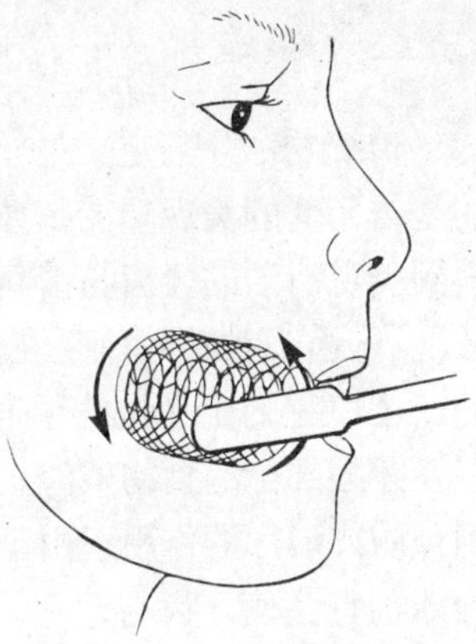

图 7-9

Circular: the fones method

Many patients, especially schoolchildren, probably received instruction in this method because it was advocated by fones, who founded the first course for dental hygienists. He described the technique in the first dental hygiene text, which was used for many years by dental hygiene students throughout the United States. Although now considered possibly detrimental for adults, particularly when used by a vigorous brusher, this method may be recommended as an easy-to-learn first technique for young children. A soft brush with 0.006 to 0.008 inch filament diameter is selected. In abbreviated form, the technique described by Dr. Fones includes the following:

a. With the teeth closed, place the brush inside the cheek with the brush tips lightly contacting the gingival over the last maxillary molar.

b. Use a fast, wide, circular motion that sweeps from the maxillary gingival to the mandibular gingival with very little pressure (figure).

c. Bring anterior teeth in end-to-end contact, and hold lip out when necessary to make the continuous circular strokes.

d. Lingual and palatal tooth surfaces require an in-and-out stroke. Brush sweeps across palate on the maxillary arch and back and forth to the molars on the mandibular arch.

6. 其他刷牙方法 Other toothbrushing methods

旋转振动法，改良Stillman法与Bass法很可能是病人最常用的方法，其他几种方法垂直法(Leonard 法)，水平法，生理法（Smiths 法）还有牙刷擦洗法。

Ⅰ垂直法，又称竖刷法。当用一种原始的天然树枝制作的牙刷刷牙时，采用上下动作，真正的垂直动作以一种有力的擦刷动作从上颌牙龈到下颌牙龈。Leonard 叙述和提倡的垂直动作是上下牙分开刷，其方法如下：使牙尖对尖或端对端，牙刷的刷毛放置与牙长轴成直角；用力刷，但不用太大的压力，大多为上下牙面上的动作，在刷牙力量到达龈缘之后稍作转动或圆弧动作；用足够的压力使刷毛进入楔状区，但不足以损伤牙刷；用同一套动作不刷上下牙，而保持牙的尖对尖，保持牙刷从𬌗面或切面滑动。

Ⅱ水平法。水平或交叉刷牙法一般认为是有伤害的，一种没有限制的水平擦刷动作使牙承受压力，大多倾向于唇面，加之用一种有摩擦剂的牙膏，这种方法可以产生牙损伤，因为邻间区不接触这种方法，邻面菌斑得不到清除。

Ⅲ生理法，又称Smiths法。其原则是牙刷顺着食物自然咀嚼时流过的组织通道。用一种有 4 排刷毛，长度一样的软毛牙刷从下牙的牙龈到上牙，在龈沟部位增加少许水平动作。

Ⅳ牙刷擦洗法是以有力的水平、垂直与圆弧动作相结合，有些部位有旋转动作，不注意用力擦刷能引起牙龈萎缩，用有摩擦剂的牙膏，能引起牙损伤。

三、洁牙剂及其作用 Dentifrices and the functions

传统的洁牙剂定义是一种与牙刷同时用于清洁可以达到的牙面的物质。这个定义主要考虑的是洁牙剂的美观功能，涉及去除牙面的牙垢、“膜”、食物残渣以及着色。这样一个人就可以得到美观清洁的牙齿与清新的口气。进而表明应用洁牙剂还对龋病与牙龈疾患提供“第二种功效”。这第二种功效就是在洁牙剂中加入一种药物，可以得到实际的治疗作用。现在对洁牙剂的一个广泛的定义是洁牙剂是一种与牙刷或其他用具一起使用的物质以便去除牙菌斑、牙垢，以及牙龈部位的食物残渣，以及为了牙齿美观与卫生的目的，并且应用特殊的制剂到达牙面起到预防或治疗的作用。由于研究取得的结果，能够应用现代的知识，帮助病人选择一种合适的洁牙剂将会使牙齿与牙龈获益，帮助其保持在一种健康状态。

这样，洁牙剂的功效可分成为三种（美观，美观－治疗，治疗）。分述如下：

（1）美观 cosmetic这一功效涉及用一种美观的洁牙剂（不含药物）以一种常规的非特殊的方式试图从牙面去除像牙垢，膜（唾液、薄膜、菌斑）与色素这些物质，这种洁牙剂的纯功效是提供一副美观清洁又健康的牙列以及清新的口气。

（2）美观－治疗 cosmetic-therapeutic这一功效涉及用一种美观的洁牙剂（不含药物）以这样一种方式提供有效而彻底的物理-机械的方法去除牙菌斑，这种洁牙剂的纯功效，除了与用美观的洁牙剂有关的那些功效之外，对龋齿牙石与牙龈疾患有“治疗”作用。

（3）治疗 therapeutic这一功效涉及应用一种治疗性洁牙剂（含一种药物）能把药物传递到牙面或牙周围环境中（菌斑、唾液、牙龈组织等），这种洁牙剂的纯功效是提供药物的化学或药理学的作用，如临床表现为菌斑，牙石，龋或牙龈疾患减少。

这样，洁牙剂的一个扩展的定义修正如下：洁牙剂是一种物质与牙刷一起用于清洁可以达到的牙面。还可以提供以下一种或多种作用：①主要的美观作用包括：清洁，抛光与口气清新；②美观－治疗作用，通过有效而彻底的物理－机械方法去除牙菌斑；③治疗或药理学作用，通过把药物传递到牙面或者牙周围环境之中。

Traditionally, a dentifrice has been defined as a substance used with a toothbrush for the purpose of cleaning the accessible surfaces of the teeth. This definition primarily concerned the cosmetic functionality of a dentifrice and involved the removal of material alba, "film", food debris, and stain from the tooth surfaces. Thus, one obtained a cosmetically clean dentition and a fresher breath.

It was further indicated that the use of a dentifrice also provided "secondary beneficial effects" upon the incidence of dental caries and gingival disease. These secondary beneficial effects, in contradistinction to an actual therapeutic effect obtainable by the incorporation of a drug substance into a dentifrice.

A dentifrice is a substance used with a toothbrush or other applicator to remove bacteria plaque, material alba, and debris from the gingival and teeth for cosmetic and sanitary purposes, and for applying specific agents to the tooth surfaces for preventive and/or therapeutic purposes. As a result of research, current knowledge can be applied to aid the patient in the selection of an appropriate dentifrice that will benefit the teeth and gingival and help to maintain them in a healthy state.

Thus, the functions of a dentifrice can be threefold (cosmetic, cosmetic-therapeutic and therapeutic) and described as follows:

1. Cosmetic. this function involves the use of a cosmetic dentifrice (not containing a drug substance) in a routine, nonspecific manner in an attempt to remove materials such as material alba, film (pellicle and plaque), food debris, and stain from the tooth surfaces. The net effect of this dentifrice function would be to provide a "cosmetically clean and healthy dentition" and a fresher breath.

2. Cosmetic-therapeutic. This function involves the use of a cosmetic dentifrice (not containing a drug substance) in such a manner as to provide for the efficient and thorough physical-mechanical removal of dental plaque. The net effect of this dentifrice function would include, in addition to those already associated with the use of a cosmetic dentifrice, a "therapeutic" effect upon the incidence of caries, calculus, and gingival disease.

3. Therapeutic. This function involves the use of a therapeutic dentifrice (containing a drug substance) so as to transport the drug substance to the tooth surface or the tooth environment (plaque, saliva, gingival tissues, and so on). Thus, the net effect of this dentifrice function would be the providing of the specific chemical or pharmacologic action of the drug substance, as manifested clinically by a reduction in the incidence of plaque, calculus, caries, or gingival disease. Additionally, depending upon the efficiency of the toothbrushing procedure, secondary cosmetic or cosmetic-therapeutic effects could be provided.

The previous discussion has been utilized as a basis for an expanded definition of a dentifrice. The revised definition is as follows:

A dentifrice is a substance used with a toothbrush to clean the accessible surfaces of the teeth so as to provide one or more of the following effects: (1) primarily cosmetic, including cleaning, polishing, and breath freshening; (2) cosmetic-therapeutic, through the efficient and thorough physical-mechanical removal of dental plaque; and (3) therapeutic or pharmacologic, by means of conveying a drug substance to the tooth surfaces or the tooth environment.

（一）洁牙剂（牙膏）的组成成分 Ingredients and composition of dentifrices

虽然世界上洁牙剂有多种物理形式（膏剂、粉剂与液剂），但主要的物理形式还是膏剂。这样，洁牙剂的组成成分基本上是一种膏剂的形式（普遍称之为牙膏）。洁牙剂的基本成分：①粉状洁牙剂含有摩擦剂、洗涤剂、芳香剂与甜味剂；②膏状或凝胶状洁牙剂含有上述相同的成分，再增加胶粘剂，润湿剂，防腐剂与水，或者可能有着色剂。在商业上现有的洁牙剂各种成分的含量范围如下：

洗涤剂	1% ~ 2%
清洁与磨光剂	20% ~ 40%
胶粘剂	1% ~ 2%
润湿剂	20% ~ 40%
芳香剂	1% ~ 1.5%
水	20% ~ 40%
治疗剂	1% ~ 2%
防腐剂，甜味剂，着色剂	2% ~ 3%

一种治疗性洁牙剂有一种药物或者化学制剂，增加了一种特殊的预防或治疗作用。在厂家生产产品的过程中，一个主要问题是结合的制剂彼此之间的相容性。

Although dentifrices are available in various physical forms (paste, powder, and liquid) throughout the world, the predominant physical form is the paste. Thus this discussion of the ingredients and composition of dentifrices basically concerns dentifrices that are in a paste form (commonly referred to as toothpaste).

Dentifrices are composed of a variety of materials, each of which has a specific function. These materials include cleaning and polishing agents, detergents (or surface-active agents,) binding agents, flavoring agents, sweetening agents, preservatives, water, and in the case of therapeutic dentifrices, a drug substance. Additionally, miscellaneous ingredients such as coloring materials, corrosion inhibitors, and whitening agents are often utilized in the dentifrice formulation. The approximate amounts of these ingredients that are present in typical dentifrice formulations are shown in table 7-3.

表 7-3　Approximate ranges of basic ingredients in dentifrice formulations

Ingredient	Approximate per cent of formulation
Cleaning and polishing agents	20 to 60
Detergents (surface-active agents)	1 to 2
Humectants	20 to 40
Binding agents	1 to 2
Flavoring agents	1 to 1.5
Water	20 to 40
Colors, preservatives, sweeteners, stabilizers, etc.	1 to 3
Therapeutic (or drug) substance	1 to 2

A therapeutic dentifrice has a drug or chemical agent added for a specific preventive or treatment action. In manufacturing products, a major problem is to combine agents that are compatible with each other.

（二）牙膏的基本化学成分 The essential chemical composition of dentifrice

1. 洗涤剂（发泡剂或表面活性剂）Detergents (foaming agents or surfactants)

（1）用途：降低表面张力，浸松牙面沉积物与色素，乳化残渣，用牙刷易于清除，有助于许多人喜欢的发泡形成。

（2）使用标准：无毒性，中性反应，在酸或碱的媒介中有活性，稳定与其他洁牙剂成分相容，无明显的芳香剂，以及形成泡的特点。

（3）所用物质　合成洗涤剂：月桂醇硫酸钠usp，月桂酰肌氨酸钠，椰子单酸甘油酯磺酸钠。

2. 清洁剂与磨光剂 Cleaning and polishing agents

在一个摩擦剂系统中牙膏可以有联合制剂以便起到清洁与磨光的作用。

（1）用途：一种摩擦剂为了清洁，磨光剂产生光滑，磨光牙面保持无着色，无细菌沉积与滞留。

(2) 使用标准：理想的摩擦剂有很好的清洁作用又不损伤牙面，提供一种高度光亮能够防止或延缓色素与沉积物的沉积。

(3) 所用摩擦剂：碳酸钙，正磷酸钙，双氢磷酸二钙，无水磷酸二钙，不溶性偏磷酸钠(IMP)，水合氧化铝。

二氧化硅，硅酸盐，脱水硅凝胶，凝胶牙膏，合成非晶形零点凝胶，合成非晶形复合硅铝酸盐。

3. 胶粘剂（增稠剂）Binders (thickeners)

(1) 用途：在储存期间防止固体与液体分离。

(2) 标准：稳定，无毒与其他成分相容。

(3) 所用种类：有机亲水胶体：藻酸盐，合成纤维素衍生物。

有机胶体需要一种防腐剂防止微生物生长。

4. 润湿剂 Humectants

(1) 用途：保持水分，防止暴露于空气而硬化，稳定制剂。

(2) 标准：稳定、无毒。

(3) 所用物质：甘油，山梨醇，丙二醇。

这些制剂需要防腐剂，防止微生物生长。

5. 防腐剂 Preservatives

(1) 用途：防止细菌生长，延长储存期限。

(2) 标准：与其他成分相容。

(3) 所用物质：酒精，苯甲酸盐，甲醛，二氯化酚。

6. 甜味剂 Sweetening agents

(1) 用途：给予病人能够接受的愉快芳香。

(2) 标准：与其他成分相容。

(3) 所用物质：人工非致龋性甜味剂。

山梨醇与甘油，用作润湿剂，有助于甜味感觉。

7. 芳香剂 Flavoring agents

(1) 用途：使洁牙剂成为所希望的、调节其他可能味觉不太好的成分。

(2) 标准：在生产与储存期间保持不变与其他成分相容。

(3) 所用物质：基本油类（薄荷油，肉桂油，冬青油，丁子香）薄荷醇，人工非致龋性甜剂。

8. 着色剂 Coloring agents

(1) 用途：引人注目。

(2) 标准：不使牙及其他口腔组织着色。

(3) 种类：植物性染料。

（三）牙膏的基本作用 The basic function of dentifrice

牙膏配方的基本成分及其相互之间的相容性和稳定性决定了牙膏的基本作用在于口腔保健，即在刷牙时作为刷牙的辅助剂，其作用如下：

(1) 有助于通过刷牙的机械方法，增强牙刷去除食物残渣、软垢和牙菌斑的效果，保持清洁、美观、健康。

（2）有助于消除或减轻口腔异味，使口气清新，有爽口作用。

（3）如果在牙膏膏体中加入其他有效成分，如氟化物、抗菌药物，或控制牙石与脱敏的化学制剂，则具有某种特殊功效，如防龋，减少菌斑与牙石形成以及脱敏作用等。

（四）药物牙膏 Drug containing dentifrice

通过机械性方法，彻底去除牙菌斑对大多数人来说实际上都很难做到。因此，20 世纪 70 年代以来提出了在牙膏中加入一定的抗菌剂。虽然有大量的抗菌斑存在，但只有很少数与牙膏配方相容，并在口腔内表面停留较久。药物牙膏是这一类牙膏的统称。在国外，一般称为预防性或治疗性牙膏（prophylactic or therapeutic dentifrices），即具有预防或者辅助性治疗功效的牙膏，还有处方与非处方药物牙膏之分。另外，也并非所有有功效成分的制剂都归属于药物（例如氟化物），在国外已正式进入药典作为药物，但在我国至今尚未被纳入。但是这些有特殊功效成分的药物或化学制剂都应该是安全和无明显副作用的。

1. 定义与含义 Definition and implications

一种治疗性牙膏可以叙述为含有一种药物结合到配方中，对口腔组织会产生一种功效。这种功效可以是对硬组织（牙表面），也可以是对软组织（牙龈），通过化学的、生理学的或者是药理学的手段来达到。两种最重要的口腔健康功效可以归咎于一种治疗性牙膏或药物牙膏：a.预防或减少龋齿形成的发病率；b. 预防或转化牙龈疾患。当一个厂家在考虑在牙膏配方中放入一种药物，目的是为了得到一种治疗作用时，那么所用的这种药物的性质很重要。如果专家认为这种药物一般来讲是安全有效的，那么这种牙膏就可以在一定的合理期间内，以合理的经费花费而上市。然而，对感兴趣的药物，如果专家认为一般不安全和有效的话，厂家就需要努力确定这种含有新药的牙膏的安全性与有效性，并且要提供证据文本。在美国必须通过FDA审批。就要花费很长的时间，很多的经费。

A therapeutic dentifrice may be described as one that contains a drub substance that has been incorporated into the formulation in an effort to produce a beneficial effect upon the oral tissues. This beneficial effect can be produced upon either the hard tissues (tooth surfaces) or the soft tissues (gingival) and can be achieved by chemical, physiologic, or pharmacologic means. The two most important and beneficial oral health effects that can be attributed to a therapeutic dentifrice are (1) the prevention or reduction of the incidence of dental caries formation and (2) the prevention or reversal of gingival disease.

When a manufacturer is considering the incorporation of a drug substance into a dentifrice formulation for the purpose of obtaining a therapeutic claim, the nature of the particular drug substance to be utilized is very important. If the drug substance is one that would be generally regarded as safe and efficacious by experts (in respect to a particular formulation and a particular therapeutic claim), then the marketing of this dentifrice probably can be accomplished within a reasonable period of time and with a reasonable financial expenditure.

However, if the drug substance of interest is one that would not be generally regarded as safe and efficacious by experts, then the material is classified as a "new drug substance." As such, the manufacturer is required to comply with stringent Food and Drug Administration (FDA) regulations in an effort to establish and document the safety and efficacy of the dentifrice containing the new drug substance.

The FDA regulations require that extensive laboratory and clinical evaluations be conducted and the results submitted as part of a New Drug Application. This New Drug Application must be approved by the Food and Drug Administration prior to the marketing of the dentifrice.

2. 药物牙膏的开发 Development of a therapeutic dentifrice

一种药物牙膏（新药）的开发一般要经过以下的评价程序：a. 体外实验室筛选步骤，确定物质的特殊活性（例如：抗微生物，酶，釉质溶解减少）；b. 动物实验在一个实验动物模型系统内，确定物质减少或预防口腔疾病的能力（如龋病，牙龈炎）；c. 动物实验研究，确定物质的相对毒性，这样可以确定是否在短期内存在任何严重的问题，或者是可以预料得到的问题；d. 短期人体研究（仔细监测）确定物质的药理学与代谢方式；e. 实验室实验产生一种可以接受的，稳定的配方（例如，牙膏，漱口液）；f. 短期人体临床研究评价特殊的活性，例如，配方减少菌斑形成的能力，减少釉质溶解度，防止菌斑 pH 值下降以及抑制特殊微生物的能力等；g. 短期人体临床研究评价配方对于一种特殊疾病参数的作用如牙龈炎；h. 附加的（与长期）的动物毒理学评价以便确定是否可以在人体安全地进行更广泛的临床研究；i. 长期的人体临床试验，以便确定和以文件证明配方的安全性与有效性。

The development of a therapeutic (containing a new drug) dentifrice, in general, is a very expensive and lengthy endeavor. When a material is either obtained from a natural source or synthesized and is suspected to be of oral disease preventive value, it is generally subjected to the following evaluation sequence:

a. Laboratory in vitro screening procedures to determine the specific activity of the material (for example, antimicrobial, enzymatic, enamel solubility reducer).

b. Animal in vivo experiments to determine the ability of the material to reduce or prevent oral disease (such as caries or gingivitis) in an experimental animal model system.

c. Animal in vivo investigations to ascertain the relative toxicity of the material so as to determine at an early stage whether any serious problems exist or can be anticipated.

d. Short-term (carefully monitored and supervised) in vivo human studies to determine the pharmacologic and metabolic pattern of the material.

e. Laboratory experiments to produce an acceptable and stable formulation (for example, dentifrice, mouth rinse).

f. Short-term in vivo human clinical studies to evaluate a specific activity, such as the ability of the formulation to reduce dental plaque formation, to reduce the solubility of enamel, to prevent plaque pH decreases, to inhibit specific microorganisms, and so on.

g. Short-term in vivo human clinical studies to evaluate the effect of the formulation on a specific oral disease parameter such as gingivitis.

h. Additional (and long-term) animal in vivo toxicologic evaluations so as to determine whether more extensive clinical investigations can be safely conducted in humans.

i. Long-term in vivo human clinical studies to establish and document the safety and efficacy of the formulation.

美国ADA对药物牙膏的分类 American dental association classification

美国ADA牙科治疗委员会（CDT）对用于口腔疾病的诊断，治疗与预防的所有药物与化学品，包括牙膏与漱口液。采用接受（accepted），临时接受（provisionally accepted）和不接受（unaccepted）三种分类。如果在用途、成分、广告宣传与标识方面符合接受标准，接受期限为3年，接受可以更新延续，以及任何时候可以重新考虑。

接受的产品包括适当的安全性与效果的证据，接受的产品将会列在表内，可以用接受印章。

临床接受的产品包括有合理的用途与安全性的证据，但是在口腔方面的用途缺乏充分的证据来作出接受的判断。

不接受的产品没有可靠的用途证据存在以及安全性存有问题的产品。

The council on dental therapeutics of the American dental association will consider for evaluation dentifrices and mouth rinses that make a therapeutic claim. Commercial products are examined either upon the request of the manufacturer or distributor or upon the initiative of the council. Any firm may submit its appropriate products to the council for consideration for acceptance. Products will be listed in accepted dental therapeutics and described in suitable reports in the Journal of the American Dental Association if they meet standards of acceptance with respect to usefulness, composition, advertising, and labeling. Products are usually accepted for three years. Acceptance is renewable and may be reconsidered at any time. After consideration of a new product has been completed, the Council will classify the product as accepted, provisionally accepted, or unaccepted.

Accepted products include those for which there is adequate evidence of safety and effectiveness. They will be listed in accepted dental therapeutics and may use the seal of acceptance.

Provisionally accepted includes those products for which there is reasonable evidence of usefulness and safety but which lack sufficient evidence of dental usefulness to justify being accepted.

Unaccepted products include those for which the council has determined that no substantial evidence of usefulness exists and those for which a question of safety exists.

牙膏中药物制剂的作用（action of therapeutic agents）：

氟化物沉积 fluoride deposition；菌斑抑制 bacterial plaque inhibition；控制牙石沉积 calculus deposition control；脱敏 desensitization。

美国ADA于1988年接受含氟牙膏准则和1986年制订并与1994年修正的接受控制菌斑与龈炎的化学治疗产品准则都规定了临床试验的设计标准和效果评价标准。

这两个条文明确规定被接受的产品必须符合规定的最低标准要求。厂家对产品的所有陈述词必须有科学证据，广告宣传材料必须得到同意方可传播，并规定产品的评价周期为4个半至6个月，每3年重复一次。对药物性牙膏等产品的规定是必须证实其防治效果，包括氟防龋，所用化学治疗制剂必须能证明其活性成分对作用部位在生物学上可以利用，与配方中的其他成分没有相互作用或者干扰作用。1985年前只要求提供临床研究报告。现在经过修订的新准则要求同时提供实验研究报告，包括产品研究、效果与安全性研究。

当前，牙膏中除加入有明显防龋效果的氟化物外，其他加入的药物或化学制剂有洗必太、三氯羟苯醚（triclosan，又称玉洁纯），可溶性焦磷酸盐、柠檬酸钠、氯化锶、硝酸钾、氟化亚锡等，研究证明都具有各自的辅助治疗价值。国内的牙膏中则有的加入某种单味中草药，如两面针、黄芩、厚朴等，也有一定的临床效果。

（1）氟化牙膏 Fluoridated toothpastes

在氟化物牙膏出现以前的年代里，曾经研究过多种防龋牙膏，例如，叶绿素牙膏，含氨牙膏，含酶抑制剂牙膏，如n-月桂酰肌氨酸钠，脱氢乙酸钠，以及抗菌素，如青霉素，混合短杆菌肽。现在的研究表明氟化物牙膏的防龋效果最好。

应用含氟牙膏一般推荐所有年龄组的人，指令性的是儿童和有龋倾向的成人，在牙龈萎缩之后，以及牙周手术之后根面暴露，为预防根面龋有必要用含氟牙膏。

Over the years, research on chlorophyll dentifrices, ammoniated dentifrices, dentifrices containing such enzyme inhibitors as sodium n-lauryl sarcosinate and sodium dehydroacetate, and antibiotics, such as penicillin and tyrothricin contributed to the search for a major break into dental caries prevention. Research has shown that fluoride dentifrices contribute the greatest benefits at present.

Problems with dentifrice formulation have been related to finding compatible constituents to combine with the active ingredient in the dentifrice formula.

The use of a fluoride-containing dentifrice is generally recommended for all age groups and is mandatory for children and caries-prone adults. Fluoride for prevention of root caries is necessary after gingival recession and root exposure after periodontal therapy.

虽然20世纪50年代最早出现的氟化亚锡（SnF_2）牙膏的主要作用是降低釉质在酸中的溶解度和增强釉质再矿化，预防龋发生。但是原来的SnF_2牙膏不理想，稳定性差，配方灵活性不佳（调味系统、摩擦剂等）。因此到80年代开始选择其他氟化物，如单氟磷酸钠（SMFP）、氟化钠（NaF）取代SnF_2。

最近5～10年中，由于龈炎患病率高，重点转向既能防龋又能控制龈炎的口腔局部使用制剂，又重新开始评估SnF_2的可能作用。因为它有内在抗微生物作用，比香精油（essential oils）与三氯羟苯醚的作用强，含有效防龋成分，无需加稳定剂，有控制龈炎作用，对根面反应明显，可减少牙本质过敏，现在经过改进的SnF_2配方牙膏性质稳定，是因为在配方中提供自身腐蚀的锡盐作为“抗氧化剂”，与氟反应以保护氟化亚锡，加入的锡盐如焦磷酸锡，作为储存源，全和提供，并加入螯合剂，结合金属，保护SnF_2以免水解和氧化。新配方可使SnF_2水平在理论上达到100%，并达到防龋和控制龈炎所需要的水平。

据Beiswanger等报告，SnF_2牙膏的临床效果为减少龈炎14.6%～18.8%，龈出血为20.3%～30.5%，其作用机制主要是抗微生物作用，特别是改变与菌斑毒力有关的细菌代谢。微生物学研究证实SnF_2不产生机遇性病原的过度生长，也不使口腔微生物在整个抗微生物作用过程中产生抗性。

（2）抗菌剂牙膏 Dentifrices containing antimicrobial agents

一种与牙膏相容的制剂是三氯羟苯醚，基于它是一种广谱抗菌剂，最近已有几种产品上市。临床研究显示，它只有中等抗菌斑活性，有三种方法可以提高它的临床效果：一种是与共聚物（Gantrez）联合，增加其口腔保留时间，一种是与抗牙石制剂（焦磷酸钠）联合，或者与第二种补充性抗菌剂（枸橼酸锌）联合。把这些制剂用于牙膏配方中进行的第一次人类志愿者研究显示枸橼酸锌－三氯羟苯醚牙膏比共聚物或焦磷酸盐－三氯羟苯醚牙膏有更多的三氯羟苯醚牙膏保持在口腔表面。同时它在菌斑的水平也比三氯羟苯醚／共聚物产品要高。锌在口腔内保留的时间比三氯羟苯醚要长。而焦磷酸盐似乎缺乏直接针对性，因而可能降低了这种制剂抗菌斑的意义。

含有抗菌斑制剂的牙膏不应干扰氟化物的抗龋功效。实验表明枸橼酸锌／三氯羟苯醚并不降低氟化物的生物利用率。

长期应用含抗菌剂的牙膏也不破坏口腔自然的微生物生态环境。临床研究显示在没有监督的情况下用含三氯羟苯醚／枸橼酸锌或共聚物牙膏6个月没有导酸产生微生物的抗药性，也没有使口腔的真菌过度生长，也没有外源性微生物在口腔内定殖。

因此，就总体而言，微生物学、化学与药物动力学以及临床的资料显示：定期，无监督使用含0.30%三氯羟苯醚，0.75%枸橼酸锌牙膏刷牙将会减少牙菌斑，牙石，以及增进牙龈健康，同时不干扰牙菌斑的自然生态环境，同时，保持氟化物的抗菌特性。

One dentifrice-compatible agent is Triclosan, and several products have been marketed recently, based on this broad spectrum antimicrobial agent. Clinical studies have shown Triclosan by itself to possess only moderate antiplaque activity. Three strategies have been adopted in attempts to increase its clinical effectiveness, these involve combining Triclosan with: a copolymer (Gantrez(r)) to increase its oral retention; an antitartar agent (sodium pyrophosphate); or a second complimentary antimicrobial (zinc citrate).

The first comparative studies of human volunteers using these agents formulated in toothpastes showed that significantly more Triclosan was retained on oral surfaces from the zinccitrate Triclosan dentifrice, compared to the copolymer or pyrophosphate-Triclosan toothpastes. The Triclosan/zinc citrate dentifrice also gave significantly higher Triclosan levels in dental plaque than the Triclosan/copolymer product. Zinc was retained in the mouth for even longer periods than Triclosan, whereas pyrophosphate appeared to lack substantivity, and this may reduce the potential antimicrobial significance of this agent in vivo.

Dentifrices contining antimicrobial agents should not interfere with the beneficial anticaries properties of fluoride. Laboratory and in situ caries studies have been carried out to compare a non-fluoride (negative) control paste with a conventional (positive) control dentifrice, and a test toothpaste containing 0.30 per cent Triclosan + 0.75 per cent zine citrate. The zinc citrate/Triclosan toothpaste did not reduce the bioavailability of fluoride.

The long-term use of a dentifrice containing antimicrobial agents shouldalso not disrupt the natural microbial ecology of the mouth. Clinical studies showed that the unsupervised use of dentifrices containing Triclosan with either zinc citrate or copolymer for six months did not lead to the development of microbial resistance, nor to overgrowth of the oral flor by yeasts, nor to colonization of the mouth by exogenous microorganisms.

Collectively, therefore, the microbiological, chemical, pharmacokinetic and clinical data presented at this symposium show that regular, unsupervised use of a dentifrice containing 0.30 per cent Triclosn and 0.75 per cent zinc citrate will reduce dental plaque and calculus, and improve gingival health without disrupting the natural ecology of dental plaque while, at the same time, maintaining the anticaries properties of fluoride.

（3）脱敏牙膏 Dentifrice for desensitization

有几种制剂对降低牙本质过敏有作用。市场上广泛使用的两种脱敏牙膏含氯化锶和硝酸钾。硝酸钾（potassium nitrate）直接作用于感觉神经细胞疼痛，当疼痛加重加，神经细胞释放钾作为对大脑的一种信号。因为用硝酸钾牙膏刷牙时，加入的钾作用于神经细胞外部，抑制神经传送疼痛信号。氯化锶（strontium chloride）通过阻塞牙本质小管缓解疼痛。

Thomas Schiff等（1998）进行了一项双盲有对照的临床试验证实了每天2次用含5%的硝酸钾和1500ppm的单氟磷酸钠在一种沉淀碳酸钙基的牙膏有明显的降低牙本质过敏的作用。

Desensitization

Fluorides, potassium nitrate, strontium chloride, and sodium citrate are among the agents shown to be effective. Because most tooth sensitivity is related to areas of exposed dentin and cementum, attention must be paid to the abrasiveness of a dentifrice to avoid products that may uncover the dentinal tubules and cause additional sensitivity.

This eight-week clinical study was conducted to assess the effect of a dentifrice containing 5% potassium nitrate and 1500 ppm sodium monofluorophosphate in a precipitated calcium carbonate (PPC) base on dentinal hypersensitivity, as compared to a placebo dentifrice without the potassium nitrate.

The dentifrice formulation in this clinical study contains an agent to reduce dentinal hypersensitivity (potassium nitrate). This dentifrice also provides protection against dental caries since it contains sodium monofluorophosphate, a clinically proven anticaries agent. It has also been demonstrated in previous clinical studies that sodium monofluorophosphate may contribute to a reduction in dentinal hypersensitivity, thereby possibly contributing to the results obtained in this study.

The results of this independent, double-blind and controlled clinical study demonstrate that the twice daily use of a dentifrice containing potassium nitrate and 1500 ppm sodium monofluororophosphate in a precipitated calcium carbonate (PCC) base over an eight-week period provides a statistically significant and clinically beneficial reduction in dentinal hypersensitivity, measured as tactile and thermal, as compared to a placebo dentifrice without potassium nitrate.

（4）增白牙膏 Whitening dentifrice

从美观的角度考虑，大多数人把牙齿洁白作为清洁、年轻、美丽的社会指标来考虑。因为随着年龄增长，人牙倾向于变成更黄一些以及着色增加，现在越来越多的人对口腔保健品增白牙齿感兴趣。

现在市场上出现的非处方牙膏加入1% ~ 3%浓度的过氧化物可能对牙龈有益。这些含过氧化物的口腔保健品经常使用也提供牙齿的增白作用。例如，Sharma等（1997）用一种碳酸氢钠／过氧化钙牙膏每天刷牙2次与没有含过氧化物的碳酸氢钠组比较，共用1个月在临床上观察到明显的增白作用。1998年，C. J. Kleber等的一项实验室研究用一种含碳酸氢钠与1%稳定的过氧化氢的牙膏经过8小时或8小时以上的局部处理之后，明显地减少了人牙的内源性黄色。提出定期使用这样产品，经过较长一段时间，在临床上有牙齿的增白作用。

From a cosmetic standpoint, most people regard white teeth as a social indication of cleanliness, youth, and beauty. Since human teeth have a natural tendency to become more yellow and discolored with age, perhaps the increasing interest by the population in dental products that help whiten the teeth is in step with the advancing average age of that population. When the concept of tooth whitening came into common use, it was limited to severely discolored teeth and achieved by an in-office procedure using 30% ~ 35%.

Today, there are over-the-counter (OTC) dentifrices and mouthwashes currently marketed with 1% to 3% concentrations of peroxide added, presumably for gingival benefits. These peroxide-containing dental products may also provide a tooth whitening effect following regular usage. For example, Sharma et al. observed a clinically significant tooth whitening effect for subjects using a baking soda/calcium peroxide dentifrice twice daily for 1 month compared to a baking soda dentifrice without peroxide.

After a total of eight or more hours of topical treatment, a dentifrice containing baking soda and stabilized 1.0% hydrogen peroxide significantly decreased the intrinsic yellow color of human teeth compared to a control dentifrice containing baking soda or a conventional silica dentifrice in this laboratory study. These data suggest that perhaps regular use of such a product, over an extended period of time, may contribute to a clinical improvement in tooth whiteness and this certainly warrants further in vivo research efforts.

（5）中草药牙膏 Dentifrice containing herbs

在国内市场上中草药牙膏品种逐渐增多，是一个值得关注和研究的重要领域，有些中草药牙膏经抑菌试验证实有一定的抑制牙周致病菌的作用，但尚缺乏作用机制的研究，以及符合RCT 标准的临床试验研究，中草药牙膏的研究与开发应该是很有前途的。

过去用牙膏刷牙只是为了美观与社会的原因，然而，在最近的几十年中，氟化物、抗生素、氨化合物，霉抑制剂以及碳酸氢盐加进牙膏之中试图抑制龋齿，在这些制剂中，只有氟化物，其防龋的安全性与效果通过临床试验得到确认。现在许多厂家把其他治疗性或预防性制剂加至牙膏之中以减少牙菌斑、牙龈炎与牙石的形成，也已逐渐变得很普遍。少数牙膏还含有脱敏制剂。虽然，美观与治疗作用之间的分界线并不容易划清，大多数市场销售的牙膏有类似的目标。清洁与磨光可进入的牙面给口腔提供舒适的感觉与气味。还起到一种载体的作用，为牙齿提供氟化物。

In the past dentifrices were used in conjunction with a toothbrush solely for cosmetic and social reasons. However, in the last decades fluorides, antibiotics, ammonium compounds, enzyme inhibitors, and bicarbonate have been added in attempts to inhibit dental caries. Of all these agents only fluoride has stood up to clinical testing for safety and efficacy in caries prevention. It is also becoming increasingly common for manufacturers to add other therapeutic or preventive agents to reduce plaque, gingivitis and calculus formation. A few toothpastes also contain desensitizing agents. Although the line between the cosmetic and therapeutic actions is not drawn easily most dentifrices currently on sale have similar objectives. They clean and polish the accessible surfaces of the teeth and provide a pleasant sensation and odour to the oral cavity. They also act as a vehicle for applying fluoride to tooth structure.

第二节 其他洁牙用品与方法

Section 2 Other Cleansing Aids and Techniques

虽然用牙刷有可能清洁某些牙邻间区，但是有效地去除牙菌斑仅用牙刷是达不到的。因为牙刷的刷毛不可能完全进入牙邻间区这样的看法是普遍都能接受的。已经有几种不同的用品帮助清除牙邻间菌斑，但是在推荐一种用品之前，必须先对牙邻间区作出评价。这种评价必须考虑这些因素：①病人用牙刷去除牙邻间菌斑做得怎么样？②病人手的灵巧程度是否能操作牙间清洁用品？③有什么样的不利因素，例如，解剖学的变异，桥体、种植体、矫正器、活动矫正器或者其他修复体存在，可能使清洁牙邻间区比较困难；④牙齿拥挤程度如何，有无脱矿化或邻面龋的证据？⑤牙间隙的大小与形态怎么样－牙间乳牙是否有炎症、肿胀，或者变钝成坑状，或者高度降低？

在评价了这些因素之后，可以个别地针对病人的特点作出推荐，帮助病人有效地去除菌斑，在提出的调整计划中改变或者重新评价这些因素。

在牙周病的起始与控制过程中，牙邻间区的解剖学，还有对牙间清洁用品的选择是一个主要因素。因此，牙邻间区的适当清洁是关键。因为这个部位对牙周病的发生非常容易受到影响。

Although some cleaning of interdental areas is possible with a toothbrush, it is generally accepted that effective plaque removal is not accomplished with a toothbrush alone, since it is impossible to get the toothbrush bristles completely into the interdental region. Several different types of devices have been developed to assist interdental plaque removal. Before recommending one of these devices, the clinician must evaluate the interdental region. This evaluation must consider such factors as: 1) how well does the patient's toothbrushing method remove plaque from the interdental area? 2) how much manual dexterity does the patient have for manipulating interdental cleansing aids? 3) what contributing factors, such as anatomic variations, bridges, implants, orthodontics appliances, removable appliances or other restorations, are present that may make interdental cleansing more difficult? 4) how crowded are the teeth, and is there evidence of demineralization or interproximal decay? And 5) what is the size and shape of the interdental space-is the interdental papillae inflamed and bulbous, or is it blunted, cratered, or reduced in height?

After evaluating these factors, the clinician can individualie the recommendations made to the patient to aid in effective plaque removal. Adjustments in the suggested regimen are made as these factors change or are re-evaluated.

Anatomy of the interdental area is a major factor in the initiation and control of periodontal disease, as well as in the selection of an interdental cleaning device. Proper cleaning of the interdental area is therefore critical, since this area is most susceptible to the initiation of periodontal disease.

一、牙线及其用法 Dental floss and flossing techniques

牙线是最一致广泛推荐的牙间清洁用品。牙线有各种类型，从有蜡到无蜡，从圆到扁平到海绵样，有不同的大小，芳香剂与颜色。不论其种类，广泛的推荐的力度如何，研究显示只有约18%的成人定期用牙线。虽然许多口腔医生可能偏爱某一种牙线，但有几项研究显示不同种类的牙线可能的清洁作用并没有差异。Smith 及其同事进行的一项研究评价 4 种不同的牙线对不同牙面的清洁效率，虽然发现有蜡牙线对粗糙的牙面更有效，但是不同的牙线之间对光滑牙面与根面并没有明显差异。病人的偏爱是最终决定选用哪种牙线。

牙线是现有的几种能够进入牙龈沟并完成龈下菌斑去除的用品之一。在健康的有适当外形的邻间龈组织中，牙线能正确地深入到龈乳牙顶部以下2到3.5mm而不引起牙周韧带或牙龈的损伤。然而，重要的是仔细监督病人的龈下操作方法，因为龈沟上皮的分离有可能发生。还可能有与牙线使用不当的其他创伤。牙线的放置以及用牙线动作的启动是重要的，因为猛烈的或者没有控制的移动或者用力太大能够引起组织的撕裂。牙线通过接触区时不应突然折断。反复的创伤能够引起软组织裂口。有控制的移动对保持牙龈健康是基本的（图 7-10）。

有牙周炎病史与软组织萎缩而引起牙间区开放的病人，使用牙线洁牙的效果降低。这是由于在牙根解剖学中存在着凹面、凹槽、窝与其他变异，特别是磨牙与前磨牙的近中面，使牙线无法进入这些牙面区。优质牙线（super floss）遗留49.9%的菌斑，有蜡牙线留下54.7%的菌斑。

即使牙线有能力去除牙间区的菌斑，公众常规使用牙线仍然有限，这种有限的使用是由于：①难以掌握这种方法；②操作花费时间；③损伤牙间龈组织，引起不舒适。

特殊病人与特殊的解剖学考虑有必要采用不同的方法或用品作邻间清洁。手灵巧性差的病人或者不能有效地掌握用牙线洁牙方法的病人可以选用一种牙线支架，一种弹弓样的工具在两个分叉的指间伸展牙线能够用来把牙线插入牙接触区之间进行洁牙，在牙的邻面刮擦。必须指导病人小心使用牙线支架，避免牙线用力过度可能引起组织裂口或牙龈损伤。使用这种用具很可能发生，因为牙线围绕着弯曲的牙外形包裹比较困难。

可以用其他适合的用品来提高牙间清洁的效果，包括用纱布带来清洁更开放的，暴露的牙

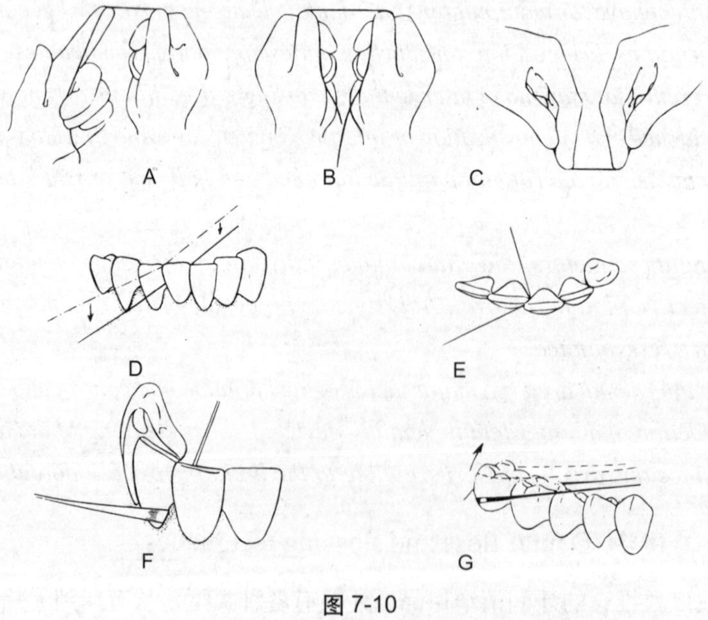

图 7-10

面。牙线也能够有效地用来清洁冠桥的楔状隙，已经联合的或固定的和围绕固定矫正器的两牙之间的部位。

Dental floss is the most consistently and widely recommended interdental cleaning aid. Various types of floss are available, ranging from waxed to unwaxed, round to flat to spongy, and in different sizes, flavors, and colors. Despite the assortment available and its wide recommendation, studies show that only about 18% of adults use floss regularly.

Although many clinicians may develop a preference for one type of floss, several studies have shown that there are no differences in the cleaning potential of different types of floss. A study by Smith and associates evaluated the cleaning efficiency of four different types of floss on different tooth surfaces. No significant difference was found between the different types of floss on smooth tooth and root surfaces, although waxed floss was found to be more effective on rough surfaces. Patient preference should ultimately determine the choice of which type of floss to use.

用牙线洁牙的方法 Flossing technique

用牙线洁牙可以在刷牙前，或者在刷牙之后，取决于病人的偏好。正确地用牙线洁牙确实有一定的难度，病人试图掌握这一方法常常会有失败的教训。通过指导病人截取一段 12 ~ 15 英吋长的牙线缠绕在每只手的一个或两个手指上（通常用中指），用拇指与食指抓住牙线，两手之间的距离（仅 1 英吋），正好允许在两牙之间进行牙线操作（图 ABC）牙线也可以打结形成圈形使用比较方便。

使牙线进入接触区以轻柔往返拉锯式动作移动直到通过接触区。然后针对一个牙的邻面，轻压牙线，使牙线接触牙面的颊侧线角至舌侧线角。由于牙线连续地用于牙邻面上下移动刮除菌斑。牙线上下移动的程度决定于牙龈组织的阻抗力。一旦感觉到有阻抗力，就不应再用力使牙线进入龈沟，然后使牙线移动过龈乳头到邻近牙面，重复刮除动作。完成两牙之间两个牙面的清洁之后，牙线通过接触区退回（图DEFG）上颌牙线的进入方式是把牙线放在一只手的拇指与另一只手的食指之间，把一个手指放在上颌牙弓对侧的牙上以提供平衡与支点。下颌牙线的进入方式是把牙线放在两只手的两个食指之间，一个食指在舌侧面，另一个食指在颊侧面，把舌侧的食指一侧放在口腔对侧的牙上起到支点或支持的作用（图 7-11）。

虽然已经显示用牙线清除牙间菌斑相当有效，然而这一操作方法是能引起刺激反应的。仔细监测与调整这种方法对长期有效的使用牙线是基本的。

Flossing can be done before or after brushing, depending on patient preference. Flossing correctly is a definite challenge and often a frustrating experience for patients attempting to master the technique. Patients are usually instructed to wind the floss 12-15 inch around one or two

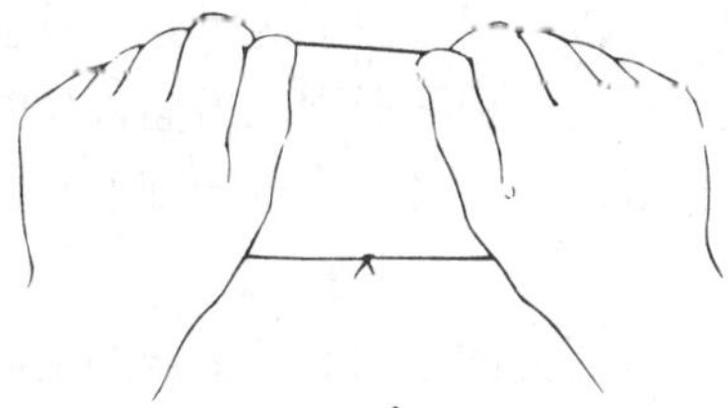

A

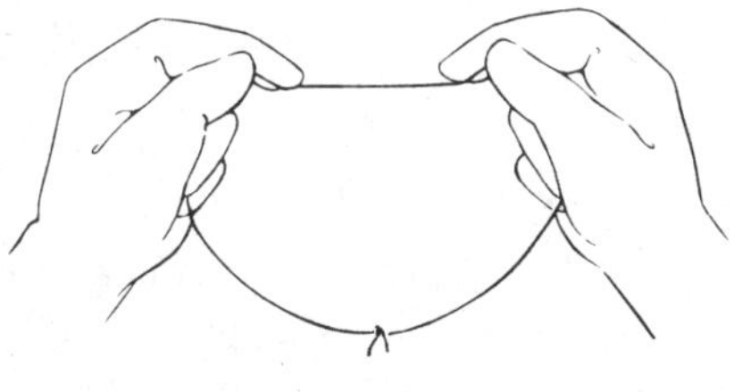

B

图 7-11

fingers on each hand (usually the middle fingers), grasping the floss between thumbs and index fingers, with the distance between hands just enough 1/2 inch to allow for manipulation of the floss between the teeth.

The floss is introduced into the contact area, and moved back and forth in a gentle sawing motion until it is through the contact. The floss is then pressed against the interproximal surface of one tooth so that it contacts that surface from buccal line angle to lingual line angle (fig). As the floss is continually applied to the interproximal surface it is moved up and down, scraping off the plaque. The extent of the downward motion of the floss is determined by resistance of the gingival tissue. Once resistance is felt, the floss should not be forced further into the crevice. The floss is then moved over the papillae to the adjacent tooth surface, and the scraping motion repeated (fig). The floss is removed by drawing it back through the contact.

Maxillary teeth. Direct the floss up by holding the floss over two thumbs or a thumb and an index finger as shown in figure 23-1A and B. rest a side of a finger on teeth of opposite side of the maxillary arch to provide balance and a fulcrum.

Mandibular teeth. Direct the floss down by holding the two index fingers on top of the strand. One index finger holds the floss on the lingual aspect and the other on the facial aspect (figure 23-1c). The side of the finger on the lingual side is held on the teeth of the opposite side of the mouth to serve as a fulcrum or rest.

Although dental flossing has been shown to be relatively effective in removing interdental plaque, it is a procedure that is technique sensitive. Careful monitoring and adjustment of this technique is essential for effective long-term use of dental floss.

二、牙间刷及其应用 Interdental brushes and techniques

牙间根面暴露的病人，用牙线去除菌斑可能比较困难或者效果不好。设计的牙间刷就是为了在这些情况下克服去除邻面牙菌斑的困难，这些牙刷由尼龙刷毛组成，双股拧绞在一根金属丝上形成一把锥形刷（像圣诞树样）或者不形成锥形刷（瓶口刷）(P29) 刷毛呈直角套在金属丝上伸展，形成一种圆形刷，当插入牙间隙时，刷毛弯曲更完全地与根面接触，达到牙线不能进入的部位 (P29)，现在有各种刷形与刷柄的设计并且可以制作成适合病人的需要的形状（图 7-12）。

除了那些暴露的根面有解剖学的变异之外，还有开放的牙间隙，牙间刷能够用来清洁暴露的分叉部位，这是其他用品难以达到的。其他可以用牙间刷清洁而得益的部位是义齿，桥体楔状区，以及固定矫正器。这种牙刷结构最近的改变把尼龙套在金属轴上使这种用品用于种植体保持清洁。

Interdental brushes and techniques

In patients with exposed interdental root surfaces, plaque removal with dental floss may be more difficult or less effective. Interdental brushes have been designed to alleviate the difficulties of interproximal plaque removal in these situations. These brushes consist of nylon filaments, twisted onto a wire to form a tapered (Christmas tree) or nontapered (bottle-neck) shape (fig). Filaments extend from

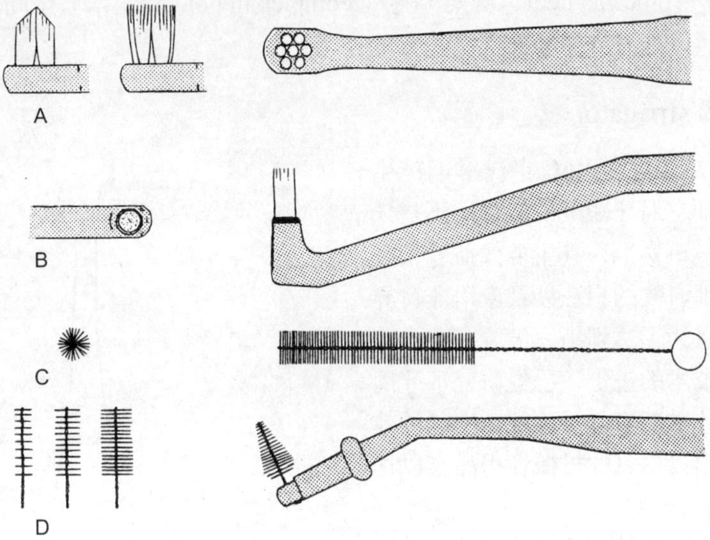

图 7-12

this coated wire at right angles, forming a circular shape that, when pushed into the interdental space, distort to more fully contact the root surface and reach regions inaccessible to floss (fig). Various brush sizes and handle designs are available and may be tailored to meet the patient's needs.

In addition to these exposed root surfaces with anatomic variations and open interdental spaces, interdental brushes can be used to clean exposed furcation areas that are difficult to reach with other devices. Other regions that may benefit from cleaning with an interdental brush are under pontics, bridge embrasures, and fixed orthodontic appliances (fig). Recent changes in the construction of the brush and the coating of the metal core with nylon make this device useful in implant maintenance.

单束毛牙刷 single-tufted brushes

一种单束毛牙刷已经证明对其他用品不易达到的部位是有用的。这些部位的案例包括围绕在移植牙或错位牙周围的不规则龈缘，一把正常大小的牙刷引发恶心反射的舌侧与腭侧组织，最后磨牙的远中区，矫正器，义齿，以及与冠桥或种植体基牙有关的精密附着体。这些特殊情况常常只能在对病人进行仔细的评价之后才能确定。这些努力再次强调在对病人进行教育与指导中需要一种长期的策略，非常灵活地适合于病人的变化需要。

A single-tufted brush has proved to be useful in those regions not easily reached with other devices. Examples of such regions include irregular gingival margins around migrated or malposed teeth, lingual and palatal tissues that elicit a gag reflex with a full-size toothbrush, distal areas of the most posterior molars, orthodontic appliances, pontics, and precision attachments associated with crown and bridge or implant abutments (fig). These special circumstances are often only identified after careful patient evaluation. These efforts again underscore the need for a long-term strategy in patient education that is flexible enough to meet the patient's changing needs.

其他牙间清洁用品还有纱布条（knitting yarn），纱布带（gauze strip），牙间头（interdental tip)，管状清洁器（pipe cleaner)，支架牙签（toothpick in holder)，木质牙间清洁器（wood interdental cleaner）等对清洁牙邻面都有一定的作用。

三、冲洗器 Irrigator

口腔冲洗器是20世纪60年代早期产生的，原来由于验证它对牙龈炎的效果而不是牙菌斑而受到质疑，事实上，其主要效益看来是去除食物残渣，那时候的想法涉及应用非特异性菌斑的假设并且为了达到组织健康应减少菌斑量，由于科学技术的进步，已经研究了牙周病的多方面特点，重新考虑了口腔冲洗器的效益。特别是在以前讨论过的机械性用品难以达到的龈下间隙有菌斑存在。

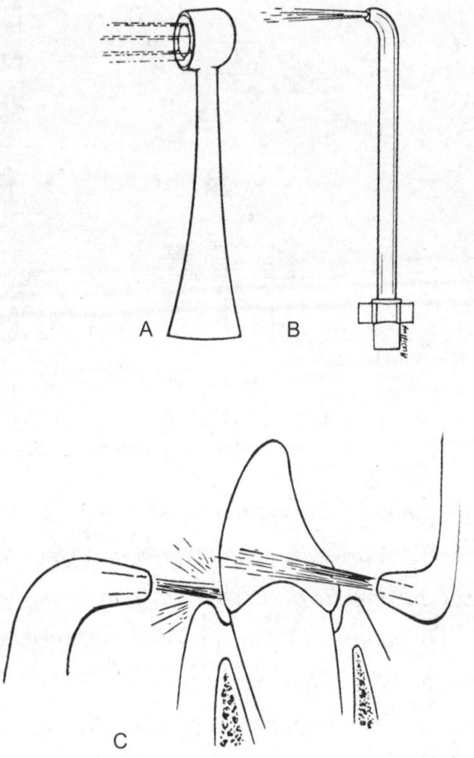

图 7-13

口腔冲洗是停止与控制牙龈感染的一种辅助方法，控制牙龈与牙周感染需要阻断微生物的繁殖与定殖，冲洗可以阻止微生物的定殖，机械性用品包括牙刷与牙间用品能够达到祛除龈上菌斑并且可以稍许进入龈缘以下，有的病人需要较好的进入龈下，冲洗能够补充其他方面的努力，需要有口腔专业人员提供指导与监督。

冲洗龈上牙龈，用一个标准喷射头，可以提供一种冲洗液约达到浅牙周袋一半的深度，可以影响病人的龈下环境。应该指导病人把喷射头放置在与牙长轴呈90°角的位置（不直接针对龈沟)，以低压开始充洗。喷射头应缓慢沿着龈缘移动，每个邻面区停留5～8秒钟。已经生产出了专门为龈下冲洗设计的喷射头，增加了冲洗液在龈沟内的渗透作用，加入了抗微生物或抗菌斑制剂，现在的冲洗器可以能够减少或抑制菌斑还有牙龈炎。然而，由于制剂的渗透有限，看来冲洗并不能去除或者解除所有的龈下菌斑。需要专业洁治和根面平整来达到和去除中度至深度牙周袋内的龈下菌斑。

当把一种口腔冲洗器或者任何附加的用品给有亚急性细菌性心内膜炎危险的病人，或者有急性情况，像急性坏死性溃疡性牙龈炎或者牙周脓肿的病人时一定要小心谨慎。

Oral irrigator, developed early in the 1960s, originally received questionable reviews due to their demonstrated effectiveness against gingivitis but not plaque, and the fact that their primary benefit was seen as removal of food debris. Thinking at that time involved the application of the nonspecific plaque hypothesis and the need to reduce plaque quantity to achieve tissue health. As scientific technology has advanced and the multifaceted character of periodontal diseases has been investigated, the benefits of oral irrigation have been reconsidered. This is particularly the case when one considers that the previously discussed mechanical devices have limited access to the subgingival space and the plaque that is present there.

Supragingival irrigation, using a standard jet tip, may deliver an irrigant approximately one-half the depth of a shallow pocket, allowing the patient to influence the subgingival environment (fig). Patients should be instructed to place the tip at a 90-degree angle to the long axis of the tooth (not aimed directly into the crevice) and start at low pressure. The tip should be slowly moved along the gingival margin, pausing 5 to 8 seconds at each interproximal region. Tips designed specifically for subgingival irrigation have been developed that increase the penetration of the irrigant into the crevice. With the addition of antimicrobial or antiplaque agents, irrigators may now be able to reduce or inhibit plaque as well as gingivitis. However, due to the limited penetration of agents, it does not appear that irrigation is able to remove or detoxify all subgingival plaque. Professional scaling and root planning is required to reach and remove subgingival plaque in moderate-to-deep periodontal pockets.

Care must be taken when recommending an oral irrigator or any adjunctive aid for patients at risk for subacute bacterial endocarditis or those with acute conditions such as acute necrotizing ulcerative gingivitis or a periodontal abscess.

四、口腔含漱剂及其作用 Mouth rinses and functions

1. 口腔含漱剂的定义 Definition of a mouth rinse

口腔含漱剂可以简单规定为一种物质在口腔内含漱，然后吐出为了使口腔与口气清新。这样，它的目的主要是美观。最流行的形式是一种液体，此外，还有片剂、糖块，浓缩剂以及喷雾剂。口腔含漱液体，进入口腔的材料或者是一种全浓度的或者是一种稀释的形式。

按照这个标准，水和生理盐水可以认为是最简单的口腔含漱剂。然而最广泛采用的口腔含漱剂是加香料的配方，含有多种特殊的成分与特点的香料，像肉桂，丁香，薄荷油与冬青。口腔含漱剂还常有其他名称，漱口剂，口腔杀菌剂以及含漱剂。

A mouth rinse may be defined simply as a substance that is swished around the oral cavity and then expectorated in order to freshen the mouth and breath. Thus, its purpose is primarily cosmetic. The most popular form is a liquid, although mouth rinse troches, lozenges, concentrates, and sprays are also available. In the case of the liquid mouth rinses, the material may be introduced into the oral cavity in either a fullstrength or a diluted form.

By these criteria, water and saline solution could be considered to be the simplest mouth rinses. However, the most widely purchased and utilized mouth rinses in the United States are flavored formulations that contain a variety of specialized ingredients and characteristic flavors, such as cinnamon, clove, peppermint, and wintergreen. Mouth rinses are also often referred to by other names, such as mouthwashes, oral antiseptics, and gargles.

2. 口腔含漱剂的成分 Composition of mouth rinses

一种液体口腔含漱剂配方的基本成分是水、酒精、芳香油与染色材料。其他成分可能包括润湿剂、收敛剂、乳化剂、抗菌剂，甜味剂以及治疗性物质。

虽然水是任何口腔含漱剂配方的最大部分，乙醇也有相当高的浓度（约15%～30%），酒精的存在主要是增加芳香油以及其他难溶于水的化合物的可溶性。

润湿剂的利用包括甘油与山梨醇以及收敛剂，通常以锌盐或铝盐的形式存在。乳化剂像聚氧乙烯山梨糖醇脂肪酯与由聚氧乙烯与聚氧丙烯组成的阻断共聚物用于减少表面张力以及有助于稳定其他成分。普通磨碎剂（主要用于片剂或糖块中）是苯佐卡因与苯甲醇。

口腔含漱剂配方的一种重要成分是抗菌剂。这是因为口腔含漱剂的作用之一是通过抑制口腔细菌的活性起到除臭的作用，虽然像芳香油，酒精这些材料能起到某些抗菌作用。但与特殊的抗菌成分相比其作用是小的。最普遍应用的抗菌剂是季铵类化合物，酚类化合物。现在常用于口腔含漱剂的抗菌剂有洗必泰，香精油，氟化亚锡，血根碱与氧化剂。

The basic ingredients in a liquid mouth rinse formulation are water, alcohol, flavoring oils, and coloring materials. Other components may include humectants, astringents, emulsifiers, antimicrobial agents, sweeteners, and therapeutic substances. These ingredients are described in detail in three excellent publications.

Although water makes up the greatest part of any mouth rinse formulation, ethyl alcohol is also present in fairly high concentrations (approximately 15 to 30 per cent). Alcohol is primarily present to enhance the solubility of flavoring oils and other compounds of low solubility in water.

The humectants utilized include glycerin and sorbitol, and the astringents, when present, are usually either zinc or aluminum salts. Emulsifiers, such as polyoxyethylene sorbitan fatty acid esters and block copolymers consisting of olyoxyethylene and polyoxypropylene, are used to reduce surface tension and assist in the stabilization of other ingredients. Saccharin is a widely used sweetening agent. Common anesthetics (used mainly in the troches or lozenges) are benzocaine and benzyl alcohol.

An important ingredient in the mouth rinse formulation is the antimicrobial agent. This is due to the fact that one of the means by which mouth rinses can exert their "deodorizing" effect is by inhibiting bacterial activity in the oral cavity. Although such materials as certain flavoring oils and alcohol can exert some antimicrobial effect, their action is minor compared to that of the specific antimicrobial ingredients.

The most commonly used antimicrobial agents are the quaternary ammonium compounds and the phenolic compounds, chlorhexidine, essential oils, stannous fluoride, sanguinarine and oxygenating agents.

3. 口腔含漱剂的功能 Functions of a mouth rinse

(1) 美观功能 cosmetic function

最初，应用口腔含漱剂的主要目的是美观，由此使口腔与口气清新，在这方面，可以认为口腔含漱剂具有一种社会功能，通过体外微生物评价，人体微生物取样，以及临床观察与临床试验研究已经证实了口腔含漱剂对口气的作用。

As previously mentioned, the primary objective in suing a mouth rinse is a cosmetic one whereby the mouth and breath are freshened. In this respect, mouth rinses could be considered to serve a social function.

Substantiation of the effect of mouth rinses on the incidence of objectionable breath odor (and other oral parameters) has generally been obtained through the use of four types of investigations. (in vitro, in vivo)

（2）治疗功能 Therapeutic function

像洁牙剂一样，一种治疗性口腔含漱剂是规定为一种含有药物的配方，用作为一种载体把药物传递到口腔的软硬组织，这种药物赋予一种化学的、生理学的与药物学的作用，在临床上表现为减少牙菌斑、牙石与牙龈疾患的发生率。

许多（含药物）治疗性口腔含漱剂的配方，有关它们对菌斑、牙石、龋或牙龈疾患已经作出了评价。

As was the case with dentifrices, a therapeutic mouth rinse can be defined as a formulation containing a drug substance and used to transfer this drug substance to the hard and soft tissues of the oral cavity. This drug substance then imparts a chemical, physiologic, or pharmacologic action that is manifested clinically as a reduction in the incidence of plaque, cries, calculus, and gingival disease.

As previously mentioned, claims in reference to the relief of sore throats and the prevention of the common cold would also be considered therapeutic, but primarily from a medical aspect, rather than a dental aspect.

Many therapeutic mouth rinse formulations (containing drug substances) have been evaluated with regard to their effect on plaque, calculus, caries, or gingival disease.

（3）含氟口腔含漱液 Fluoride-containing mouth rinses

自20世纪60年代以来，已有大量的临床试验，使用了多种配方，证实了含氟口腔含漱液的防龋效果（其范围从27%～60%）。有三种氟化钠含漱液是安全有效的：

a. 0.2% 氟化钠水溶液（900 ppm F−）pH 值为 7.0，每周或每两周一次含漱在降低龋齿发生率方面是安全有效的。

b. 0.05% 氟化钠水溶液（230 ppm F−）pH 值为 7.0。每天一次含漱，降低龋齿发生率也是安全有效的。

c. 酸性磷酸氟化钠水溶液，pH 值约 4.0 产生约 0.02% 氟离子的浓度，每天一次含漱，降低龋齿发生率也是安全有效的。

在过去几十年中，氟化物口腔含漱液已经广泛用作防龋的公共卫生措施之一，a.b两种配方已被采纳作为病人保健项目或学校保健项目的标准。除了6岁以下儿童禁忌使用外，其他各个年龄组的人都可以推荐使用，但是以酒精为基础的氟含漱液，由于每天使用，有意或无意的摄入因而强烈劝阻使用。

Since 1960's, many clinical studies have been conducted with fluoride mouth rinses. For the most part, sodium fluoride has been the most widely utilized and investigated substance. The data indicate that mouth rinses containing sodium fluoride (at various concentrations and frequencies of use) are safe and effective with regard to reducing the incidence of caries.

There were three formulations:

a. Aqueous solutions of 0.2 per cent sodium fluoride with a pH of approximately 7.0 are safe and effective in reducing the incidence of dental caries when applied to the teeth as a rinse once a week or once every two weeks.

b. Aqueous solutions of 0.05 per cent sodium fluoride with a pH of approximately 7.0 are safe and effective in reducing the incidence of dental caries when applied to the teeth once daily as a rinse.

c. Aqueous solutions of acidulated phosphate sodium fluoride with a pH of approximately 4.0 that yield a fluoride ion concentration of approximately 0.02 per cent are safe and effective in reducing the incidence of dental caries when applied to the teeth once daily as a rinse.

Over the past several decades, fluoride mouthrinsing has become one of the most widely used caries-preventive public health methods. Two regimens (a, b) have been adopted as standard for individual programmes of patient care or for school-based programmes.

Except for children under 6 years of age, it is contraindicated and the fluoride containing mouth rinses could be recommended to others age groups to use. However, the daily use and the inadvertent or intentional ingestion of an alcohol-based fluoride rinse are to be strongly discouraged

（4）洗必太口腔含漱剂 Chlorhexidine containing mouth rinses

洗必太，一种双胍，浓度为0.2%的局部凝胶与含漱液。在欧洲已经研究和应用了几十年。1986年作为一种处方制剂0.12%浓度的含漱液在美国出现。在口腔医学中仅次于氟化物，这种抗菌斑、抗牙龈炎已经经历了广泛的研究。对减少菌斑与牙龈炎是最有效的可以利用的制剂。它有广谱活性，而且表明不产生抗药性，短期研究已经证实平均减少菌斑与牙龈炎为60%，而三项长期的研究，检查了 700 以上的受试者，报告菌斑减少平均为 55%，牙龈炎为 45%。

洗必太的作用机制是针对牙与细菌的。在与牙的关系中，洗必太使牙面的表膜形成减少，改变细菌的滞留与生长机制，导致牙面细菌定殖减少。细菌细胞壁的改变是由于吸收洗必太的结果，引起细胞内成分的渗漏与溶解，洗必太效果的关键特征是它的直接性，直接性是一种制剂在较长的一段时间内保持在口腔内，并且缓慢释放其活性形式。在口腔内的保持是与一种带正电的制剂对带负电的细菌细胞或牙面的亲和力有关。洗必太是带正电的，有高度的直接性。

洗必太的副作用包括牙与复合染色的严重程度与病人消耗咖啡，茶与红葡萄酒还有吸烟有相互关系。在应用洗必泰之后有味觉改变也已引起关注。在美国市场上有一种peridex（浓度为0.12%，酒精11.6%，pH值5.5的含漱液）。推荐每天用2次。已经显示洗必太作为一种辅助性应用不仅对控制牙菌斑与牙龈炎有效，而且在口腔内外科术后使用，预防根面龋，而且作为一种龈下充洗剂都能显示出明显的积极作用。当与氟化亚锡一起用于预防项目时，应该指导病人在用洗必太含漱之后半小时到 1 小时再用氟化物产品，可以减少可能导致两种制剂同时使用，效果降低的一种竞争性的相互作用。

Chlorhexidine

Chlorhexidine, a bis-guanide in a 0.2% concentration topical gel and rinse, has been used and studied extensively in Europe for decades. In 1986, a 0.12% concentration rinse was made available as a prescription agent in the United States. This antiplaque, antigingivitis agent has undergone extensive research, second in dentistry only to fluoride. Chlorhexidine appears to be the most effective agent available for the reduction of plaque and gingivitis. It has a broad spectrum of activity, yet development of resistance has not been shown. Short-term studies have demonstrated plaque and gingivitis reductions averaging 60%, while three long-term studies, examining over 700 subjects, reported plaque reductions averaging 55% and reductions in gingivitis of 45%.

The mechanism of action of chlorhexidine is tooth-directed and bacteria-directed. In relation to the tooth, chlorhexidine produces a reduction in pellicle formation and an alteration in bacterial retention and growth mechanisms, resulting in reduction of bacterial colonization on the tooth. An alteration in the bacterial cell wall, resulting from absorption of chlorhexidine, results in leakage of intracellular components and lysis. The key feature of chlorhexidine's effectiveness is its substantivity. Substantivity is the ability of an agent to be retained in the oral cavity and slowly released in its active form over an extended period of time. Retention in the oral cavity is related to the affinity of a positively charged agent to the negatively charged bacterial cell or tooth surface. Chlorhexidine is positively charged and has high substantivity.

Adverse effects of chlorhexidine include tooth and composite staining the severity of which has been correlated to the patient's consumption of coffee, tea, and red wine as well as tobacco smoking. Alteration of taste following chlorhexidine use has also been noted. Chlorhexidine is marketed in the United States as peridex (0.12% concentration mouth-rinse, 11.6% alcohol, pH 5.5), with a recommended usage of twice daily. Adjunctive use of chlorhexidine has been shown to be effective not only in the management of plaque and gingivitis, but has also shown significant positive effects when used following intraoral surgical procedures, in a root caries prevention regimen, and as a subgingival irrigant. When used in a preventive programme in conjunction with stannous fluoride, patients should be advised to use the fluoride product 30 minutes to 1 hour after rinsing with chlorhexidine to reduce a competivitive interaction that could reduce the effectiveness of both agents.

（5）香精油 Essential oils

是一种非处方性酚类化合物，商品名称为施德林（Listerine）（21.6%与26.9%酒精，pH值为5.6），含有香精油：麝香草酚0.064%，薄荷醇0.042%，桉油精0.092%以及甲基水杨酸盐0.060%。短期研究报告菌斑，牙龈炎平均减少35%，长期研究显示平均菌斑减少25%，牙龈炎减少29%，牙菌斑减少范围为22%～36%，牙龈炎为23%～36%，最长为9个月周期，Charles等（2001）的一项6个月的研究报告，菌斑减少56.1%，牙龈炎减少22.9%。N. Sharma等（2004）最新的一项6个月的研究报告菌斑减少51.9%和56.3%，牙龈炎减少15.8%和22.3%。香精油是一种不带电的化合物，它的直接性低。这种制剂的作用机制表现为破坏细胞壁和抑制其酶的活性而杀死微生物（Fine，1988，Kubert等1993）。阻止革兰阳性先驱菌种的聚合，减慢细菌的繁殖从革兰阴性病原体浸出内毒素，预期能够减少细菌数量，减慢菌斑成熟，减少菌斑量与致病性（Fine 1988）。

最近的研究工作提出当微生物从浮游（或流动）状态到固着状态（即作为生物膜的一部分）时，细菌的表现型可以改变，这种改变可能与生物膜基质的分离作用有联系，对抗微生物制剂能引起易感性改变（Pan等，2000）。因此，任何杀菌含漱液不只是取决于常常在体外证实的对微生物的特性，而且还要看它在人体内对菌斑生物膜渗透的能力。

为了检测香精油含漱液对生物膜中细菌的作用，最近进行了两项研究：一项是由Pan等进行的随机单盲交叉试验研究，这项研究的发现证实，香精油含漱液的抗菌斑作用，部分地归咎于它的快速杀灭细菌与菌斑的渗透能力。另一项研究（Fine等，2001）采用一种模型，测试二种临床分离的两种放线共生放线杆菌同基因株的每一种。两种临床"生物膜一型"菌株能在体外形成坚韧的生物膜，鉴于它们自然产生的变化，总是浮游地生长。针对这四种菌株评价几种口腔含漱液的抗微生物活性。

研究支持这种的观察结果，生物膜的形成赋予对抗微生物制剂的抗药性。它证实，三种抗微生物口腔含漱液都能杀灭几乎所有的浮游型微生物，而对生物膜内的微生物证实是可以变化的，这一与杀菌口腔含漱液的效果有关的信息非常有价值。

综合上述研究，支持这样的概念，香精油口腔含漱液能够穿透菌斑生物膜。这一作用表明，这种含漱液减少菌斑与牙龈炎能力的部分意义。

但是口腔含漱液只能少量地穿透龈下区，龈沟液的外流（每小时40次更换整个袋液）将会在几分钟内稀释龈下所用的杀菌剂（Binder等，1987）。因此，不能期望现时的口腔含漱液对牙周炎的治疗提供治疗效益，即使在用于龈下之后，也没有证实对牙周炎的杀菌作用（quirynen et al. 2002）。

关于使用香精油口腔含漱液的安全方面的问题，许多流行病学研究调查了用含酒精的漱口液与口腔癌之间的可能联系缺乏证据支持。pH值低于5.5是否可以引起牙侵蚀症，研究结果显示，用香精油含漱液漱口之后，唾液pH值很快上升，也没有发现菌斑的Ca_2+与磷酸含量有任何明显影响，只是这种制剂的副作用对舌与口腔黏膜有烧灼感，有点苦味。酚类产品的着色状况比洗必太少。不推荐在醒酒过程中应用，也不推荐用甲硝哒唑或戒酒硫的病人应用，可能引起胃肠功能紊乱。

Listerine (21.6% and 26.9% alcohol, pH< 5.5) is a nonprescription phenolic compound containing the essential oils: thymol 0.064% menthol 0.043%, eucalyptol 0.092%, and methylsalicylate 0.060%. short-term studies have reported plaque and gingivitis reductions averaging 35% and long-term studies have shown an average plaque reduction of 25% and an average gingivitis reduction of 29%.

Similarly designed studies for essential oils mouthwash showed plaque reductions ranging from 22%~36% and gingivitis reductions ranging from 23% to 36%, with the longest study being 9 months. A 6 months study (charles et al. 2001) showed 56.1% plaque reduction and 22.9% gingivitis reduction. Another new study (N. Sharma et al.) reported 51.9% and 56.3% plaque reduction, and 21% and 29.9% gingivitis reduction.

Listerine is an uncharged compound and has low substantivity. The mechanism of action for this agent appears to kill micro-organisms by disrupting their cell walls and by inhibiting their enzyme activity (Fine 1988, Kubert et al. 1993). They prevent bacteria from aggregating with Gram-positive pioneer species, slow bacterial multiplication, and extract endotoxins from Gram-negative pathogens. This can be expected to reduce bacterial load, slow plaque maturation, and decrease plaque mass and pathogenicity (Fine 1988).

About the safety in application of Eos mouthwash, a number of epidemiological studies have sought to investigate a possible association of the use of alcohol-containing mouthwashes and oral cancer, there is lack of evidence to support. Whether a pH below 5.5 may cause tooth erosion or not, the results showed that rinsing with this EO mouthwash actually significantly raised salivary and plaque pH levels at the measured time of 2 and 5 min postrinsing, and salivary pH remained above baseline values through 15 min of postrinsing (Steinberg et al. 1996). Listerine also does not appear to exert any significant influence on plaque Ca_2+ and phosphate contents, thereby suggesting that no enamel demineralization occurs (Nazari & Lynch 1997). Adverse effects of this agent are a burning sensation on the tongue and *oral mucosa, and a bitter taste. Phenolic products are available over the counter and produce less stain than chlorhexidine. However, alcohol-containing mouthrinses are not recommended in recovering alcoholics because its presence may create the desire for alcohol. Nor are they recommended in patients taking metronidazole or disulfiram, as inadvertent sallowing can cause gastrointestinal upset.*

(6) 氟化亚锡 Stannous fluoride

虽然氟化物对口腔医学的主要功效是减少釉质在细菌酸中的溶解度，增强釉质的再矿化，氟化亚锡已经显示出抑制微生物菌斑沉积的第二种功效。短期研究已经证实菌斑减少，但在长期研究中还缺乏统计学上的显著减少以及一致的结果。锡离子本身可以有助于氟化亚锡的作用机制，它被认为是干扰细菌的生物化学合成，代谢与聚合。表现为氟化亚锡有中等程度的直接性，0.4%浓度最为有效。副作用与味觉有关，保存期短，以及牙上有黑线样着色形成。氟化亚锡最常用作为一种水凝胶，建议每天用 1 ~ 2 次，氟化亚锡有美国 ADA 接受的抗龋能力，但这种认可并没有扩大到包括牙菌斑与牙龈炎减少方面。

Stannous fluoride

Although fluoride's major benefits to dentistry have been to decrease the solubility of enamel to bacterial acids and enhance enamel remineralizaiton, stannous fluoride has shown a secondary benefit of inhibiting microbial plaque accumulation. While short-term studies have demonstrated plaque reduction, statistically significant reductions and consistent results are lacking in long-term studies. The stannous ion itself may contribute to the mechanism of action of stannous fluoride, which is attributed to interference with bacterial biochemical synthesis, metabolism, and aggregation. It appears that stannous fluoride has moderate substantivity, with the 0.4% concentration being the most effective. Adverse effects are related to taste, a short shelf life, and the formation of black line stains on teeth. Stannous fluoride is most often available as an aqueous gel and suggested usage is one to two times daily. Stannous fluoride products have ADA acceptance for their anticaries ability, but this approval does not extend to or include their plaque or gingivitis reduction properties.

(7) 血根碱 Sanguinarine

一种自血根植物的生物碱提取物，血根碱（benzophenathradine）在短期研究中，证实有某种程度的菌斑与牙龈炎减少。有 viadent 牙膏（pH5.2）与口腔含漱液（11.5% 酒精，pH4.5）。这个配方含 0.01% 氯化血根碱。长期研究证实其效果为当受试者用含漱液与牙膏时菌斑减少 17% ~ 42%，牙龈炎减少 18% ~ 54%。提出的作用机制是改变菌胞的附着机制，其直接性程度不清楚。副作用包括口腔组织的烧灼感。美国 ADA 并未认可。

An alkaloid extract from the bloodroot plant, sanguinarine (benzophenathradine) has, in short term studies, demonstrated some plaque and gingivitis reduction. It is available as Viadent dentifrice (pH 5.2) and mouthrinse (11.5% alcohol, pH 5.4). This formula contains 0.01% sanguinarine chloride. Long-term studies demonstrate effectiveness when subjects used both the mouthrinse and the dentifrice with plaque reductions of 17% to 42% and gingivitis reductions of 18% to 54%. The mechanism of action is proposed to be an alteration of bacterial cell attachment mechanisms and the degree of substantivity is unclear. Adverse effects include a burning sensation of the oral tissues. It is has not been approved by the ADA.

（8）氧化剂 Oxygenating agents

病人用氧化剂漱口的短期研究产生的结果不一致，长期研究与对照组比较显示对菌斑或牙龈炎的减少无作用。1989年美国牙周病学会的一份意见书引证了许多与应用过氧化氢，还有与食盐和碳酸氢钠一起应用的副作用。这些副作用包括组织损伤，延迟伤口愈合，可能的致癌或协同致癌作用，还有白色念珠菌过度生长。虽然看到的大多数副作用与高浓度和长期应用有关，临床医生需要考虑与这些产品有关的可能的安全问题。现在 ADA 没有认可这些产品。

Short-term studies of patients using oxygenating rinses yield inconsistent results and long-term studies show no benefits when compared with control subjects, for plaque or gingivitis reduction. A 1989 American Academy of Periodontology position paper cited numerous adverse effects relating to the use of hydrogen peroxide alone as well as a combination with salt and baking soda. These effects include tissue injury, delayed wound healing, potential carcinogenic or cocarcinogenic effects as well as Candida albicans overgrowth. Although most adverse effects are seen with respect to high concentrations and chronic use, clinicians need to consider the potential safety questions related to these products. There are currently no ADA-approved products.

（9）季铵化合物 Quaternary ammonium compounds

短期研究已经显示用季铵化合物之后平均菌斑减少35%，混合有牙龈炎减少的结果，氯化十六烷比啶（CPC）是这个组的活性成分，一般浓度为0.05%（Cepacol）或0.045%（Scope）。Scope还含有0.005%的度米芬。CPC的作用机制与增加菌胞壁的渗透性，降低细胞代谢，改变细菌对牙面的附着，直接性低，副作用包括牙着色，口腔组织烧灼感。这些产品的酒精含量为14%～18%，pH 范围 5.5～6.5。推荐使用每天 2 次，减少菌斑与牙龈炎，ADA 没有认可。

Short-term studies have shown an average plaque reduction of 35% following use of a quaternary ammonium compound with mixed gingivitis reduction results. Cetylpyridinium chloride (CPC) is the active ingredient in this group, known to consumers as Cepacol (0.05%) or Scope (0.045%). Scope also contains 0.005% domiphen bromide. The mechanism of CPC's action is related to increased permeability of the bacterial cell wall, decreased cell metabolism, and alteration in attachment of the bacteria to the tooth surface. Substantivity is low and adverse effects include tooth staining and a burning sensation of the oral tissues. The alcohol content of these products ranges from 14% to 18% and pH ranges from 5.5 to 6.5. recommended usage is twice daily. They are not ADA approved for reduction of plaque or gingivitis.

（10）金属盐类 Metal salts

金属盐类能够杀灭口腔细菌，还具有抗菌斑活性并且能够抑制细菌酶。已经显示金属离子有抗微生物效果，其减少的程度按下列顺序：Ag+ ＞ Cu_2+ ＞ Sn_2+ ＞ Zn_2+ ＞ AL^{3+}[ref38]锡离子是应用最为普遍的金属离子，已经有多种机会评价了锡。虽然有感觉方面的问题，还有与外源性牙着色有关系。但是已经表明稳定的氟化亚锡含漱液，凝胶与牙膏在短期与长期临床试验中，在减少菌斑与牙龈炎方面是有效的。

锌盐也广泛用于牙膏与口腔含漱液，锌的优点超过其他金属离子主要因为它不着色，也没有像其他金属盐有损伤软组织或全身性作用。多年来已经证实了锌作为菌斑抑制剂的可能性，锌离子在口腔的作用是直接的，Afseth等显示，在5次用水溶液漱口之后锌滞留的增加在10倍以上，重复应用在菌斑内的浓度增加。在口腔内的活性，滞留是一个很重要的因素，锌是一种有效的抗微生物制剂，有多种抑制作用。然而，它也是一种有效的菌斑抑制剂，在不全致死水平上，目标针对细菌的代谢，锌活性的一个主要方面是：抑制微生物如同胰蛋白酶那样的蛋白酶活动，例如porphyromonas gingivalis还有是一种有效的由变形链球菌产酸的抑制剂从一个好的含锌牙膏配方中能提高相当高水平的锌，例如锌/三氯羟苯醚系统，人体试验显示其抑制糖酵解以及其后酸的产生的结果。

Metal salts can be bacteriocidal against oral bacteria and also possess anti-plaque activity and can inhibit bacterial enzymes. Metal ions have been shown to be antimicrobially effective to a decreasing extent in the following order: Ag+ > Cu^{2+} > Sn^{2+} > Zn^{2+} > Al3+ref38. Stannous (Sn^{2+}) is one of the most common metal ions used, usually as stannous fluoride. Stannous has been reviewed on a number of occasions and although there are sensory issues, s well as association with extrinsic tooth staining, it has been shown that stable stannous fluoride rinses, gels and pastes are effective in reducing plaque and gingivitis both in short-term and long-term clinical trials.

Zinc salts are also widely used in toothpastes and mouth rinses. Zinc has advantages over other metal ions, mainly because it does not stain or have detrimental soft tissue or systemic effects as other metal salts can. The potential of zinc as a plaque inhibitor has been demonstrated for many years. Zinc ions are substantive in the mouth. Afseth et al. showed that the retention of zinc increased more than 10-fold after five rinses with aqueous solutions, concluding that the concentration increases in plaque with repeated application. As has been discussed, retention is a very important factor for activity in the oral cavity. Zinc is an effective antimicrobial agent, having multiple inhibitory actions. However, it is also an effective plaque inhibitory agent, targeting bacterial metabolism at sub-lethal levels. Two of the main areas of zinc activity are in inhibiting the trypsinlike protease activity of organisms such as Porphyromonas gingivalis, as well as being an effective inhibitor of acid production by mutans streptococci. Relatively high levels of zinc can be delivered to plaque from well-formulated zinc containing toothpastes, such as the zinc/Triclosan system described below and the consequence of this on inhibition of glycolysis and subsequent acid production has been shown in vivo.

（11）三氯羟苯醚 Triclosan

a. 三氯羟苯醚是一种广谱抗菌剂

它是非专利标准附属物2，4，4′-3氯-2羟基-2苯醚。其抗菌作用的主要部位是细菌的胞浆膜。在抑菌浓度（0.1 ~ 10 mg/ml）上，阻止基本氨基酸的摄取，在杀菌浓度上，引起细菌胞浆膜的解体，使细胞内容物外漏。它是有效的针对各种革兰阳性与革兰阴性细菌，作为一种抗菌剂以非处方的消费者产品，如除臭肥皂棒，液体肥皂，以及腋下除臭广泛用于世界各国。含有三氯羟苯醚的皮肤擦洗消毒剂用于医院环境。

正如Linche指出的，还发现三氯羟苯醚作为一种有用的抗菌剂结合到口腔保健品中，因为它的广谱活性，发现对口腔内细菌的作用，与口腔产品成分的相容性以及长期用于消费者产品的历史。

1989年Desalva等回顾了所有有关三氯羟苯醚的药理学与毒理学的信息并得出结论：认为“它用于牙膏及口腔含漱液产品是安全的”。1990年Gaffar等报告它对发现的各种口腔细菌体外的抗菌活性，对各种口腔细菌的最低抑制浓度（MIC）为< 0.29 ~ 6.25的范围。

现在，三氯羟苯醚是最广泛地用于抗微生物的口腔保健品之中，已与枸橼酸锌和一种共聚体一起加入到口腔含漱液与牙膏之中。它有对真菌、革兰阳性与革兰阴性细菌的广谱抗菌活性，已显示其作用方式有多种功能。不仅如此，它还显示无着色能抑制几种重要的牙龈炎症的介体。因此有双重作用，抗菌和抗炎症性质。然而它本身只具备中度的抗微生物／抗菌斑性质。所以，通过试图增加它在口腔的保留时间，或者用共聚物或者通过联合其他补充性抗微生物／抗菌斑制剂如枸橼酸锌来增强其抗微生物与抗菌斑活性。

Triclosan is a broad-spectrum antibacterial agent manufactured by the Ciba-Geigy Corporation and marketed for use in oral products under the tradename Irgacare MP. It is the nonproprietary designation pertaining to 2,4,4′-trichloro-2′-hydroxydiphenyl ether. The primary site of antimicrobial action of triclosan is the cytoplasmic membrane of bacteria. At bacteriostatic concentrations, triclosan prevents the uptake of essential amino acids. At bacteriocidal concentrations, triclosan causes disorganization of the cytoplasmic membrane of bacteria and leakage of cellular contents.

Triclosan is effective against a variety of both Gram-positive and Gram-negative bacteria, and is widely used in most countries of the world as an antibacterial agent in such over-the-counter consumer products as deodorant soap bars, liquid soaps and underarm deodorants. Antibacterial skin scrubs containing triclosan are used in hospital environments.

As indicated by Lindhe, triclosan has also been found to be a useful antibacterial agent for incorporation into oral products because of its broad spectrum of activity, effect on bacteria found in the oral cavity, compatibility with oral product ingredients and a long history of use in consumer products.

DeSalva, Kong and Lin in 1989 reviewed all the available pharmacological and toxicological information concerning triclosan and concluded that "Triclosan can be considered safe for use in dentifrice and mouthrinse products."

In 1990 gaffar, Nabi and co-workers reported on the in vitro antibacterial activity of triclosan on various bacteria found in the oral cavity. The minimum inhibitory concentrations (MIC) for triclosan with regard to various oral bacteria are presented.

Triclosan is the most widely used antimicrobial in oral care products. It has a broad spectrum of antimicrobial activity against yeasts, Gram posivive and Gram negative bacteria and has been shown to be multi-functional in its mode of action. Not only this, it has also been shown to cause no staining and can inhibit several important mediators of gingival inflammation, thereby having a dual effect, both as an antibacterial but also having anti-inflammatory properties. However, Triclosan has only moderate antimicrobial/anti-plaque properties by itself. Accordingly, attempts to boost the antimicrobial/anti-plaque activity of Triclosan have been made by attempting to enhance either its oral retention either using copolymers or by combination with other complementary antimicrobial/anti-plaque agents such as zinc citrate.

b. 三氯羟苯醚／共聚物 triclosan/copolymer

一种含有三氯羟苯醚与一种聚乙烯甲基醚（PVM）与顺丁烯二酸（马来酸）(MA）的共聚物的系统（商品名Gantrez）已上市多年。虽然在这一系统中，三氯羟苯醚是仅有的活性剂，但是它在口腔内存留的时间改进了，由于共聚物的存在，虽然这一概念的许多方面已在体外得到证实，但是人体试验的结果也表明了共聚物提供系统的效果，增强了三氯羟苯醚抗菌斑，牙龈炎以及与菌斑有关的疾病的效果。Volpe 等总结了许多短期的还有 6 个月的临床试验。检测产品的临床功效与安慰剂对照组比较，明显地减少了龈上菌斑与牙龈炎。

A system containing triclosan with a co-polymer of polyvinyl methyl ether (PVM) and maleic acid (MA) (trade name Gantrez (r) *has been marketed for a number of years as Colgate Total (Colgate-Palmolive) and has been reviewed extensively.*

In this system, although Triclosan is the only active agent present, it is claimed that retention is improved within the oral cavity due to the presence of the co-polymer, although much of this concept has been demonstrated in vitro. However, results of in vivo studies have also indicated the efficacy of the copolymer delivery system, enhancing the efficacy of Triclosan against plaque, gingivitis and plaque related diseases. A number of short term as well as six month clinical studies have been completed and these have been summarized by Volpe et al. the clinical benefit of the test product was significant for reducing supragingival plaque and gingivitis compared with a placebo paste.

c. 三氯羟苯醚 / 枸橼酸锌 Triclosan/zinc citrate

枸橼酸锌与三氯羟苯醚联合，已经多次作了评价，其增进口腔健康的效果已在许多研究中显示出来。1980年代后期的两项1年的研究以及随后的许多6个月的研究表明这个系统减少菌斑沉积与保持牙龈健康的可能性，事实上，在一项 7 个月的比较研究中，发现 0.3% 三氯羟苯醚 / 0.75%的枸橼酸锌系统在减少牙龈出血，牙石形成还有减少龈上菌斑方面，其作用明显地超过三氯羟苯醚 Gantrez 系统以及三氯羟苯醚焦磷酸产品。已经在短期的人体试验中证实了它具有减少菌斑沉积以及延缓牙龈炎发展的作用。这一系统保持牙龈健康的效果也在一种口腔含漱液系统中显示出来。

实验室研究已经显示锌与三氯羟苯醚一起有补充和添加抗菌与抗菌斑的性质，导致减少细菌生长，抑制葡萄糖摄取，以及抑制龋菌种的代谢，降低毒力因素，如牙周病菌蛋白酶的表达。

药物动力学研究已经证实，同等水平约有 25% ~ 30% 的锌与三氯羟苯醚的剂量，在用枸橼酸锌 / 三氯羟苯醚牙膏刷牙之后即刻保持在口腔内，大部分与口腔软组织有关联。事实上，体外实验已经证实牙龈组织与覆盖于牙面的表膜可能起到储存抗微生物制剂的作用。许多临床研究已显示出锌与三氯羟苯醚在口腔内是真实存在的。

虽然体外研究已经显示由于一种共聚物的存在，三氯羟苯醚的吸收激剧增加，同时人体试验提供的资料显示三氯羟苯醚 / 枸橼酸锌牙膏比三氯羟苯醚与共聚物或焦磷酸牙膏提供明显多的三氯羟苯醚并保持在口腔表面。牙菌斑中的水平也比其他配方高。这一信息与其他研究的结果一致提出单纯增加三氯羟苯醚浓度的效果，不如与其他补充性抗微生物 / 抗菌斑制剂联合应用的效果好。

The combination of zinc citrate and Triclosan, marketed under the Mendadent, Aim, Signal and Pepsodent brands (Unilever Oral Care) has been reviewed on a number of occasions and the effectiveness of the combination to improve oral health has been shown in numerous studies. Two one-year studies were completed in the late 1980s, and these, together with a number of subsequent six-month studies, showed the potential of the system to reduce plaque accumulation and maintain gingival health.

in fact, in a direct seven-month comparison study, a 0.3 per cent Triclosan/0.75 per cent zinc citrate system was found to have a significantly superior effect at reducing gingival bleeding and calculus formation as well as being directionally better at reducing supragingival plaque compared with a triclosan, Gantrez system and a Triclosan, pyrophosphate product. Reduced plaque accumulation and delayed development of gingivitis has also been demonstrated in shorter in vivo studies. The effectiveness of the system for maintaining gingival health has also been shown as a mouthrinse system.

Laboratory studies have shown that zinc and Triclosan together have complementary and additive antibacterial and anti-plaque properties, resulting in reduced bacterial growth, inhibition of glucose uptake and metabolism by cariogenic species and reduced expression of virulence factors such as proteases by periodontal pathogens.

Pharmacokinetic studies have demonstrated that equivalent levels, approximately 25 ~ 30 per cent of the zinc and Triclosan doses, were retained in the mouth immediately after tooth brushing with the zinc citrate/Triclosan dentifrice, the bulk being associated with the oral soft tissues. In fact, in vitro studies have demonstrated the potential of gingival tissues and pellicle-coated teeth to act as reservoirs for these antimicrobials any many clinical studies have shown that both zinc and Triclosan are substantive in the mouth.

第三节　口臭的预防与治疗
Section 3 Prevention and Treatment of Bad Breath

口臭或称口腔异味（oral malodour，或 halitosis）是由人的口腔呼出的污秽难闻而令人讨厌的气味。是个古老而又现代的口腔公共卫生问题。之所以古老，是因为口臭是一个历史久远的老问题；之所以现代，它又是影响现代人际交往，只是在最近十几年来才引起人们关注的口腔公共卫生问题。因为口臭在人群中很常见。据估计在美国有 2500 万人因口臭而去口腔保健机构寻求诊断和治疗。据 Miyazaki 等调查报告，在日本有 25% 的人有口臭。在我国口臭也十分常见而又普遍，并且很少引起人们的关注。

一、口臭形成的原因 The causes of bad breath

口臭形成的原因是复杂的，由多种因素引起。但在大多数情况下，口臭源于口腔。其他来源包括鼻道，上颌窦，饮酒，吸烟，以及肾功能不全引起的尿毒症和代谢紊乱等，还有来自一些食物，如葱、蒜等原因引起的短暂性口臭。

Bad breath is of major importance socially and economically. It may be caused by a number of factors and can occasionally be linked to more serious underlying medical etiologies. In most cases, bad breath originates within the oral cavity. Examples of other sources include: the nasal passages, alcohol ingestion, uremia associated with kidney dysfunction and metabolic disorders. Although these may be potentially important signs, they will not be discussed here.

Oral malodour caused by smoking and food intake, such as garlic, onions, and other foods is a distinctly different problem and is not the subject of this section.

（一）口臭与牙周病的关系 The relationship between oral malodour and periodontal diseases

大多数寻求治疗的病人多有口腔内的原因。然而，正如 Rosenberg 指出的，口臭与牙周病的关系是一种复杂的关系。许多病人主诉口臭都有某种程度的牙龈或牙周的病理状况。因此，病因是充分的。但是，明确的牙周病理状况并不是先决条件或者是产生口臭所必需的。不过，这种牙周炎的范例是认识逻辑的扩展。由于口腔内微生物的作用，特别是与牙周炎有关的微生物，引起牙周袋内食物残渣的腐败与蛋白质降解而产生挥发性硫化物。口臭与口腔卫生很差以及坏死性口腔病损有关联。如患有急性坏死性溃疡性龈炎的人有口臭。因此，很久以来，就有一种看法，口臭总是有一种牙周病方面的原因。检查病人的口腔状况，总会发现一种或多种可疑因素，如龋齿破坏大，坏死牙髓组织为外露，食物嵌塞，不良修复体等均可使细菌与食物残杂存留，以至于口臭的产生。

The vast majority of patients who seek treatment for oral malodour in the dentist or periodontologist`office have an intraoral `etiology. However, as Rosenberg point out, "the relationship between oral malodour and periodontal diseases is a perplexing one". Many patients with a chief complaint of oral malodour have some level of gingival and or periodontal pathology sufficient to be the etiology, but clearly periodontal pathology is not a prerequisite or is it necessary for the production of oral malodour. This periodontitis paradigm is a logical extension of the recognition that putrefaction of food debris and degradation of proteins in the periodontal pocket occurs from the action of the oral microbiota and in particular the microorganisms associated with periodontitis. Associations of very poor oral hygiene and necrotizing oral lesions such as acute necrotizing ulcerative gingivitis inpeople with oral malodour, have perpetuated the idea that there is always a periodontal etiology.

Examination of the status of the patient's restorative dentistry in a individual who complains of oral malodour may reveal one or a number of the following factors which can be prime "suspects": large carious lesions, exposed necrotic pulp tissue, open margins, sites of food impaction, tight embrasures, washed out cement, abraded or eroded restorations, and retentive clasps, bars and attachments. All of these findings can contribute to the production of malodour because they can retain bacteria and debris. Systematic repair and/or replacement often improves the chances of success when the etiology is a dental problem. From a practical view, it is often necessary to prioritize and sequence the treatment since time and expense do not permit patients to get all their work done at once.

1. 牙周炎有助于产生口臭 Priodontal associations

（1）牙周炎是由厌氧条件与特定蛋白质利用细菌所引起；

（2）这些细菌存在于牙周袋及陈旧菌斑内，其机质含有硫化物；

（3）龈下厌氧菌，如龈卟啉菌，普氏菌及其他许多微生物产生挥发性硫化物（VSC），它来自硫化氢（H_2S），甲硫醇（CH_3SH）和二甲基硫化物（CH_3SCH_3）。这种硫化物是某些特异细菌代谢的副产品。许多不同宿主的机质含有：龈沟液组成成分，白细胞，牙龈出血，上皮细胞，其他细菌及其组成成分；

（4）当与呼气混合时，VSC 在口内释放，成为臭气；

（5）硫化物可能有助于牙周炎的病理形成。因为它对多种宿主细胞与过程有致病的可能；

（6）菌斑与牙周炎病损有关，导致细菌在其他口腔部位，如舌背定植，形成完全的口臭状态。

Periodontal associations

Commonly held clinical opinion suggests the following (greatly simplified) ntenets about how periodontitis might contribute to the development and production of oral malodour:

- *periodontitis is caused by anaerobic and facultative protein utilizing bacteria.*
- *These bacteria are located in periodontal pockets and older established plaquenwhere sulphur containing substrates are available.*
- *Subgingival anaerobes, such as Porphyromonas gingivitis, Prevotalla spp., and many others, reduce sulphur containing amino acids to hydrogen sulphide H_2S, methyl mercaptan, CH_3SH and dimethyl sulphide CH_3SCH_3 referred to as VSC (volatile sulphur compounds). Volatile sulphur compounds are some of the specific by-products of bacterial metabolism of many different host substrates including but not limited to: crevicular fluid constitutents, leucocytes gingival bleeding, epithelial cells, other bacteria and their constituents (table7-4).*
- *These VSC are released into the oral environment where they mix with expired air and contribute to malodour.*
- *VSC might contribute to the pathogenesis of periodontitis because they have pathogenic potential on a variety of host cells and processes.*
- *The plaque associated with periodontitis lesions lead bacterioa to other oral sites such as the tongue dorsum where they colonize and contribute to the total oral malodour status.*

Table7-4 Microbiologic targets for anti-malodour treatment

Target →	reduction or elimination of specific bacteria capable of Producing VSC's
Chronic Adult Periodontitis (CAP)	
	Porphyromonas gingivitis
	Prevotella intermedia/nigrescens
	Actinobacillus actinomycetemcomitans (Aa)
	Campylobacter rectus
	Fusobacterium species
	Peptostreptococcus micros
	Bacteroides forsythus
	Eubacterium species
	Treponema species
Refractory Adult Periodontitis	
	CAP + Various exogenous species
	Pseudomonas species
	Enteric rods
	Candida species
	Miscellaneous other microorganisms frequently encountered

续表

Target ->	reduction or elimination of specific bacteria capable of Producing VSC's
Acute Necrotizing Periodontitis	Same as Refractory Adult Periodontitis + Spirochetes
Acute Necrotizing Ulcerative Gingivitis	Same as Acute Necroyizing Periodontitis
Tongue and Tonsil Flora	Same as CAP + Capnocytophaga sp. And Rothia sp

许多牙周病人并不诉说口臭，即使这些人常常口臭较严重。还发现有牙周病的人有其他口臭的致病因素，例如，唾液流速低，舌苔厚。但并没有确定是否有较多引起口臭的细菌。Bosy等认为，仅有牙周炎可能与口臭没有关联。在牙周情况稳定时，没有查出无牙颌或健康人有牙的原因。口臭的产生可能与蛋白质降解有关。舌面上、扁桃体，以及唾液中的细菌和宿主酶的有机物含硫。许多口腔状况健康的人有口臭，是因为呼气带有硫与鼻后分泌物含有丰富的蛋白质所引起。

Many patients who have periodontitis do not complain about oral malodour even though these individuals often have higher levels of VSC. Many other oral malodour etiologic factors can be found in patients with periodontitis, for exsample a low saliva flow rate and the quantity of tongue coating they have. Yaegaki and Sanada found more wet weight of tongue coating in patients with periodontitis but they did not determine whether the coating contained higher numbers of odour causing bacteria. Indeed, Bosy et al suggests that periodontitis alone may not be associated with oral malodour.

In periodontally stable, edentulous or healthy individuals with no detectable dental cause, oral malodour production may be associated with degradation of proteins, sulphur containing compounds on the surface of the tongue, tonsils and in saliva by bacteria and host enzymes. Many patients with a healthy oral status have oral malodour caused by expired air passing over sulphur and protein rich mucous secretions associated with post-nasal drip

（二）口臭与牙龈炎的关系 Gingivitis associations

口臭与牙龈问题有关系，是由于细菌降解基质引起臭气。由于口腔卫生差，菌斑的细菌成分含有大量革兰阴性细菌，利用多种来源的蛋白质作为营养素，由于代谢的结果，产生硫化物，在正常呼吸与谈话的环境中释放出来。当菌斑长期滞留时，发生龈炎，进而形成口臭循环。炎症与肿胀通过提供宿主蛋白质与氨基酸，产生龈沟液以及牙龈肿胀增加牙周袋深度，转而增加滞留细菌引起的臭气，促进口臭的循环过程。在少数情况下，牙龈病理改变与坏死，肉芽肿增生，或溃疡形成，可以引起臭气。急性牙龈问题，如急性疱疹性龈炎，持续的牙龈出血与血质不调，牙龈纤维瘤及其他情况，可以形成整个臭气状态。所有这一切状况都需要明确诊断与适当治疗。

环境因素，如吸烟加剧菌斑滞留，减少牙龈代谢，这些因素降低局部环境的氧张力，有助于利用蛋白的厌氧菌生长。

Gingival associations

Oral malodour associated with gingival problems appears to be due to the bacteria degradation of odour causing substrates. The bacteria composition of plaque which is allowed to build up due to inadequate oral hygiene contains larger number of Gram-negative bacteria which utilize proteins from a variety of sources as nutrients. As a consequence of metabolism, volatile compounds are produced and released into the environment during normal respiration and talking. When plaque is retained for a period of time, gingivitis develops and further contributes to the oral malodour cycle. Inflammation and swelling contribute to the process by furnishing host protein and amino acids through the production of crevicular fluid and the swelling of gingival increases the volume of the pocket which in turn increases the amount of odour causing bacteria which are retained.

Environmental factors such as smoking exacerbate plaque retention and decrease gingival metabolism. Both factors reduce the oxygen tension in the local environment which favours growth of anaerobic protein-utilizing bacteria.

二、诊断与治疗 Diagnosis and Treatment

诊断病人口臭有几种方法：①直接找口腔医师或牙周专家；②由其他医务人员转来。在口腔诊所作出诊断。实际诊断有一系列主观与客观的步骤。出发点必须是综合和全面的诊断。

（一）诊断工作步骤 Diagnostic procedure

1. 一旦病人要求诊断，首先必须采集一份完整的医疗与口腔科病例并作出评价。如发现病人有医学方面的原因，必须转诊找内科医生。治疗这些病人多采用多学科途径，提供医学咨询，包括耳鼻喉科专家。

2. 未发现全身问题，则找口腔医生或牙周病专家检查，寻找口臭发病的原因，以避免不完全的治疗。

3. 检测 VSC 是诊断治疗的一部分，以客观手段确定臭气水平。

（1）气相色谱技术（Gas chromatography technique）已正式采纳作为臭气研究。但不便于在临床应用。

（2）口气检测仪（BB checker）（Tokuyama corp. Tokyo，Japan）是一种二氧化锡半导体气体探测仪，它对还原气体敏感，目的是用于估计还原气体的检测阈。它体积小（1.7kg inweight and 22 × 16.6cm width and 8.6cm height），气体通过一次性小管自动吸入探针部位。气体水平以ppm 值表示。菌斑指数较高，则口气浓度倾向于较高。Sulser指出，47%主诉有口臭的病人与他们的口腔情况有关。据 Tonzetich 报告，通过清洁改善口腔状况能够消除口臭。这个仪器还可以用于辨别心理性口臭的病人。

The gas chromatography technique has been normally adopted for the experimental studies on malodour. Since it is unconvenient to use at chairside, some simpler device is desirable. A tin dioxide semiconductor gas sensor which is sensitive to reductive gases, has been developed by Tokuyala Corp., Tokyo, Japan (the BB checker). The aim is to estimate the detection threshold for the reductive gases with this device.

BB checker has a compact feature. Since the gas is automatically via a disposable tube into the sensor probe portion. The gas level is displayed on the monitor as ppm value.

Although, the data did not reach significance levels, the oral gas concentration tended to become higher with higher plaque scores. As pointed out by Sulser, 47% of patients complaining about halitosis can be related to their oral condition. Thus, the improvement of the oral condition by cleansing procedures as reported by Tonzetich can eliminate the malodour.

Patients with psychogenic halitosis also often visit the dental clinics. Therefore, this device could be useful to discriminate the psychogenic patients by demonstrating them the objective levels at the chairside.

（二）口臭的治疗和预防 Prevention and treatment

1. 治疗牙龈与牙周有关疾病。
2. 用锌与玉洁纯（triclosan）系统联合治疗口臭证明可以有效减少口臭。
3. 常规应用牙膏与漱口液两种产品，效果增加，特别是用牙膏刷牙。
4. 刷牙和刷舌是减少口臭的有效方法。玉洁纯是一种广谱抗菌剂，它能阻止基本氨基酸的摄取，对多种革兰阳性、阴性细菌有作用。在牙膏中含有锌与玉洁纯可以减少菌斑和龈炎。
5. 漱口液含锌盐（枸橼酸锌）或洗必太（0.2%）可以有效地减少口臭。

The incidence of oral malodour in the general population is high, with many people experiencing problems such as "morning mouth". Mass marketed dentifrice and mouthwash can play an important role in helping to reduce both the incidence and the extent of oral malodour.

- *The combination of zinc and triclosan has been demonstrated to be effective in the reduction of oral malodour. The efficacy was measured using studies involving assessment of the reductions in volitile sulphur compounds in mouth air, thiol levels in saliva and mouth odour levels.*
- *Regular use of products containing the dual active system increased the efficacy of both the dentifrice and mouthwash. The increase in efficacy is especially noticeable for the dentifrice.*
- *Although after a single use mouthwash has higher efficacy than a dentifrice, the benefit of the dentifrice could potentially be increased by stopping post brushing rinsing, swilling the toothpaste around the oral cavity and regular use of the product. The last point is important because mouthwash is often used on an irregular base whereas dentifrice is commonly used on a daily basis.*

小结 Summary

From evidence-based point of view, there are two approaches recommended for personal oral hygiene practices. The first approach is mechanical removal of plaque by the individual, the old rule of brushing twice a day still has merit, together with the recommendation to use additional cleaning aids once a day. Such as flossing, interdental brushing, other mechanical aids, and irrigation. The second approach is chemotherapeutic removal of plaque and calculus.

Mechanical plaque control procedures are the established mainstay for controlling dental disease. However, these efforts vary individually and depend on a number of influences that after result in the outcome being less than completely successful. In light of this, more recent research efforts have been directed at developing methods of enhancing plaque removal efforts.

As scientific advancements have confirmed the bacterial nature of plaque, antimicrobial agents have been developed and incorportated into therapeutic approaches.

There are presently numerous antibacterial/anti-plaque systems are available commercially. Chlorhexidine, Triclosan and metal ions are among the most common agents in commercial products and it is generally believed that these actives, together with combinations of essential oils, have shown the greatest clinically efficacy in the majority of non-prescription oral care products.

The most successful approach to date appears to be using broad spectrum antimicrobial/anti-plaque agents to reduce plaque growth and in consequence, plaque metabolism. The degree of success is dependent on the agent concerned.

思考题 Review questions

1. how man-y factors must be considered before recommending one of dental cleansing devices?
2. which means of interdental cleaning have been proven effective?
3. what are the main functions of a mouth rinse?
4. desrible the main functions and its adverse effects of chlorhexidine?
5. why is Triclosan the most widely used as an antimicrobial agent in oral care products?
6. which metal salts are also widely used in toothpastes and mouth rinses and why these are?

参考文献 References

1. David L. Cochran, et al. Plaque & Calculus removal. Quintessence publishing Co, Inc, 1994
2. Edwina A. M. Kidd, et al. Essentials of dental caries. Oxford University Press, 2002
3. B M G. rading, et al. The Oral environment: the challenge for antimicrobials in oral care products. International Dental Journal, 2003, 53: 353-362
4. J O P. uhayoun. Penetrating the plaque biofilm: impact of essential oil mouth wash. J clin Periodont, 2003: 30 (suppl. 5) 10-12
5. S A.antus. Evidence-based control of plaque and gingivitis. J Clin Periodont, 2003: 30 (suppl. 5) 13-16
6. Esther M. Wilkins Clinical practice of the dental hygienist 7th edition. Williams & Wilkins, 1994
7. Richard E. Stallard. A textbook of preventive dentistry, 2nd edition. W. B. Saunders company, 1982
8. Niklaus P. Lang, et al. Proceedings of the European workshop an mechanical plaque control. Quintessence publishing Co, Inc, 1998
9. 卞金有等. 预防口腔医学. 第 4 版. 人民卫生出版社, 2003

（卞金有）

第八章 营养、膳食与口腔健康

Chapter Ⅷ Nutrition, Diet and Oral Health

概述 Overview

本篇主要分为三个部分：第一部分叙述营养与口腔健康，包括营养与口腔组织的生长发育，营养与钙化过程，牙齿发育的阶段（关键期的概念），营养与牙周组织，牙齿在营养中的价值，以及营养、膳食与儿童和成人的口腔健康。第二部分叙述营养与口腔疾病主要涉及龋病，牙周病，口腔癌，感染，牙侵蚀症，创伤以及与营养不良有关的口腔表征，第三部分，介绍口腔疾病防治中的营养指导方针，包括糖的消耗，健康促进，膳食指导的一般原则。

This chapter is to be basically divided into three parts: The first part describes nutrition and oral health, including nutrition and the growth and development of oral tissues, nutrition and calcification process, diet and oral health of children and adults; The second part describes nutrition and oral diseases, such as dental caries, periodontal diseases, oral cancer, oral infection, trauma , dental erosionand some oral manifestations related to malnutrition. The last part introduces the nutritional guidelines in the prevention and management of oral diseases, including sugars consumption, health promotion, general principles of dietary counseling.

要点 Key points

- *Calcification process and nutrition*
- *Stages in tooth development: concept of critical periods*
- *Enamel hypoplasia (ehp) and development defects of enamel (dde)*
- *Sugar and dental caries*
- *Dental erosion*
- *Dose-response relationship*
- *Adequate nutrition and diet counseling*

口腔与人体其他器官一样，其生长发育和健康维持都受着遗传、行为和环境因素、包括营养还有感染的影响。人类从环境中摄取的营养素大约有 50 种，膳食是主要营养来源。食物的主要作用是：(1) 提供成为人体物质基础的结构成分；(2) 维持机体内部环境恒定；(3) 调节机体的各种过程；(4) 提供机体生存与活动能量。然而，没有一种食物能够提供人体功能所需要的所有营养素，因此，理想膳食只有通过动植物食品的适量混合与搭配，才能达到适当平衡。不仅营养缺乏能影响人体的正常生长发育，造成某些细胞的活性障碍，而且过量和不平衡也会对生长发育产生不利影响，损害人体健康，为疾病提供契机。

许多流行病学与动物实验研究已经提出了膳食中的营养素能够以下列方式影响口腔疾病：(1) 通过改变负责组织形成的细胞的系列化环境，如釉质，这样在牙萌出前改变牙结构及其成分以及物理化学特性；（2）通过改变生物合成反应（蛋白质、蛋白多糖与脂肪）以及由此改变矿化组织机质钙化的性质；（3）通过直接或间接影响钙激素，涉及矿化过程的细胞活性；（4）通过改变唾液的流量及其物理，化学或免疫特性；（5）通过增强或抑制正常发生于萌出的牙釉质表面的矿化过程；（6）通过影响牙面或龈沟内菌斑菌落的植入、定殖与代谢活性。

不认识营养素的不同的系统影响的重要性就不明白膳食对口腔疾病病因学与发展的总体影响。像依赖于菌斑的龋病与牙周病，其结果通常取决于宿主，微生物与营养因素之间的相互作用。在膳食营养成分及其他因素的影响下，例如，以蔗糖为代表的各种糖类食品，不论是天然的，还是加工精制的，在菌斑细菌的作用下，都具有很强的致龋性。实验研究显示，营养因素更为重要，新生儿营养缺乏可以增加龋病易感性。而另一方面的研究又显示通过饮食途径补充适量氟化物，又可预防和减少龋病的发生，某些非碳水化合物因素，如酪蛋白、脂肪等，以及改变食物摄入的方式和频数，尤其是含糖食品，能够调节食物的致龋性，认真做好口腔卫生也可以有助于控制龋的发生。

因此，人的营养可以从不同的水平来考虑和研究：（1）细胞或组织水平，涉及营养素的组织与细胞代谢的系列化反应；（2）机体水平主要是关于膳食，食品摄入方式，营养成分以及食物营养素的代谢包括消化，吸收，传输利用以及排泄；（3）社区水平，文化，宗教与社会经济因素，还有农业，工业与商业因素是决定社区或人群的营养状态。显然，需要多种学科，科学专家从这三个不同的途径参与研究。在预防口腔医学领域内，讨论膳食与营养问题，不仅是为了使学生了解营养状况与口腔疾病的关系，而且更重要的是为了使学生在今后的口腔临床与社区工作实践中能进行营养咨询与指导，以便预防和减少疾病的发生。

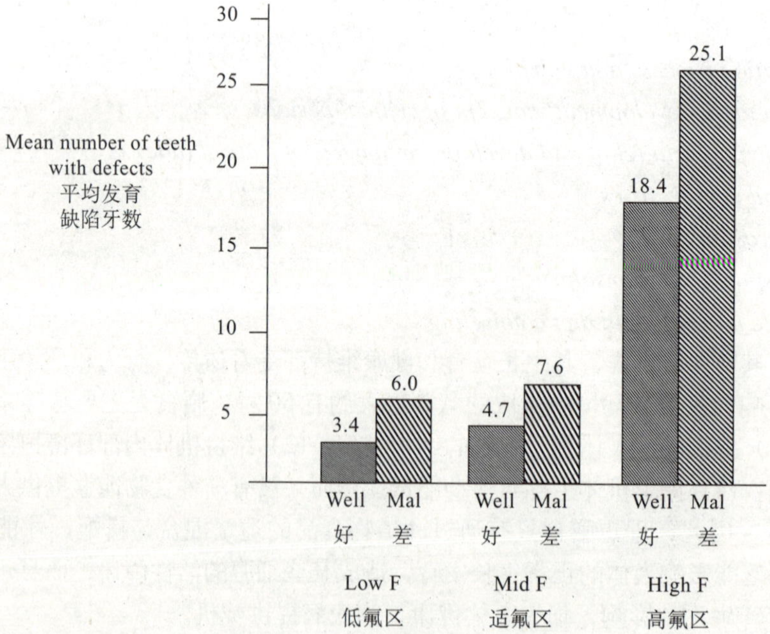

图 8-1　沙特阿拉伯三个地区营养好与差的男孩釉质发育缺陷的平均牙数（Rugg-Gunn 等 1997）

Oral tissues, like all other tissues in the human body, are dependent on their trophic environment to supply the nutrients essential for growth, development, and maintenance of health. from the moment of conception, the availability of nutrients necessary for full expression of the genetic potential of the cell determines the intensity and direction of growth and development in tissures and organs. These nutritional needs are not limited only to developmental periods but also exist at later stages when tissues have reached maturity and require nutrients to maintain the integrity of the body and to compensate for catabolic losses.,

One other aspect of nutrition that has received a great deal of attention is the concept of critical periods of human development, periods when specific nutrients are especially required by organs developing with different chronologies and rates.

Heredity, nutrition, and infection affect the development of oral tissues, just as they influence other organs and tissues. The teeth, particularly enamel and dentin, begin forming in utero and the developmental process for different teeth spans a period of 12 to 15 years. Thus, critical periods occur for specific tooth surfaces at different times. For tooth enamel, deleterious effects of malnutrition and infection become important not only because of the irreversible nature of effects imposed during critical periods of development but also because tooth enamel has no cellular mechanisms to repair tissue damage after tooth eruption. The ability of teeth to withstand a caries attack becomes impaired and susceptibility to such a disease may be markedly increased. Other organs such as salivary glandsand the immune system can also be affected by the synergistic action of nutrition and infection imposed early in development. In spite of the ability to reorganize and to repair tissue damage, once these organs have reached maturity, developmental insults may contribute to a decreased ability to protect the tooth against dental caries.

The interaction between nutrition and infection affects oral tissues early during their formative stages, but dietary patterns affect teeth after eruption through dental plaque bacteria. The quality, quantity, and intake frequency of foods included in a diet contribute to the implantation, colonization, and metabolic activity of specific bacteria in dental plaque, thus contributing to the caries virulence of these plaque bacteria. While posteruptive dietary influences on the oral environment are generally accepted, the systemic, nutritional effect on growth and development of oral tissues and the relative magnitude of these effects in humans remains unresolved and requires further investigation.

In general, investigations conducted using experimental animals and some epidemiologic studies suggest that nutrients in the diet can influence oral disease in the following ways: (1) by modifying the biochemical environment of cells responsible for formation of tissues, such as enamel, thus changing tooth structure and its composition and physicochemical properties preeruptively; (2) by altering biosynthetic reactions (proteins, proteoglycan, and lipids) and thereby modifying the nature of the calcifying organic matrix of mineralized tissues; (3) by influencing either directly, or indirectly through calcemic hormones, the cellular activity involved in imneraliaiton processes; (4) by altering the quantity and flow of saliva and its physical, chemical, or immunologic properties; (5) by enhancing or inhibiting the remineralizaiton process taking place normally on the enamel surface of erupted teeth; and (6) by influencing implantation, colonization, and metabolic activity of plaque flora on the tooth surface or in the gingival crevice. Human nutrition can be considered and studied at various levels of complexity: (1) the cellular or tissue level, which involves biochemical reactions of the tissues and cellular metabolism of nutrients; (2) the organismal level, which is mainly concerned with diets, food intake patterns, and nutrient composition, and metabolism of food nutrients including digestion, absorption, transport, utilization; (3) the community level, in which cultural, religious, and socioeconomic factors as well as agricultural, industrial, and commercial factors are considered in determining the nutritional status of the community or group. Obviously, the disciplines and scientific expertise required to contend with each of these three approaches will vary.

第一节 营养与口腔健康
Section 1 Nutrition and Oral Health

一、营养与口腔组织的生长和发育 Nutrition and oral tissue growth and development

牙，特别是釉质与牙本质，在母体子宫内形成。不同的牙发育程经历了长达12～15年的过程。营养对牙与口腔组织的影响有2个时期。一个是牙萌出之前，即人体生长发育的关键时期。许多研究显示，这一时期的牙颌，口腔与颅面，包括上下颌骨、乳恒牙、涎腺，口腔上皮，牙周结缔组织以及其他颅面组织，像唇，腭，对营养的作用特别敏感。所谓“关键时期是指大多数组织，器官或系统在一定的生长发育时期内所受到的环境因素影响，如营养不良和感染，对牙釉质可以引起决定性的不可逆转的损害—釉质发育缺陷与钙化不全，因为牙萌出之后，釉质没有细胞修复损伤的机制。受损的釉质对龋的发生易感性明显增加。人群流行病学研究提示，儿童乳牙釉质发育缺陷（Developmental Defect of Enamel, DDE）或釉质发育不全（Enamel hypoplasia, EHP）与营养不良（图8-1）和低出生体重、早产婴儿有显著关系。营养不良与感染也可对早期发育中的涎腺，免疫系统产生影响。另一个时期是牙萌出之后，膳食种类，通过牙菌斑细菌的局部口腔作用看来更为重要。其中糖与碳水化合物对牙健康的影响最为重要。

（一）蛋白质与口腔健康 Proteins and oral health

口腔的生长发育以蛋白质合成为基础。牙体与骨组织矿化以前的有机质都含蛋白质，其主要氨基酸是胶原形成的先质。在牙釉质为造釉蛋白和釉蛋白，在牙本质、牙骨质与骨组织为胶原蛋白。蛋白质，尤其是胶原蛋白对这些组织的形成与矿化有重要意义。胶原蛋白的合成比其他蛋白质更容易受营养因素的影响。

蛋白质构成牙釉质与牙本质有机质的大部分，约分别为6%与20%。蛋白质缺乏可以影响成纤维细胞、成骨细胞、成牙质细胞的活性，使成纤维细胞无力合成胶原，胶原不能由可溶性变为不可溶性以及胶原变性，口腔上皮组织与牙周结缔组织中胶原缺乏，可以使牙周组织在局部刺激因子作用下更易感炎症和变性，伤口不易愈合；可以导致乳牙迟萌，釉质发育不全，牙本质钙化不良，牙骨质沉积迟缓，以及牙拥挤与错位；还可以影响涎腺的生长发育，如颌下腺总重量。DNA，RNA 分子，唾液量以及其中的蛋白质含量均减少。因此，在孕妇妊娠与儿童生长发育期间，必需供给足够的蛋白质。

（二）脂肪与口腔健康 Fats and oral health

早期的组织学方法证实牙釉质与牙本质存有脂类成分，总脂量分别为0.51%与0.33%。在积极钙化的部位，如在前期牙本质与牙本质，还有釉质之间的邻界区存在着嗜苏丹反应（线），其中的包涵物为存在于造釉细胞与成牙质细胞中的脂肪颗粒，在长骨骨垢软骨细胞钙化区也有类似反应，表明为酸性磷脂。因此认为，在钙化过程中，在无定型磷酸钙或磷灰石开始矿质沉积期间，有磷脂参与。

细胞膜赋予高脂含量，脂类与蛋白为膜的主要成分。脂类大部分为磷脂。磷脂基本上为膜结构分子。双层磷脂为膜结构的基本特征。这种膜结构与钙化开始有关系。钙化过程，包括离子运动，特别是钙与磷酸盐通过膜进行。

脂溶性维生素E缺乏能破坏造釉器的完整。维生素A缺乏能使上皮结构变性，搅乱骨吸收与骨形成方式，使骨异常变厚。因此认为，在正常生长与骨改建中，维生素A的作用是引导破骨细胞与成骨细胞的活动。维生素A 浓度适宜可帮助稳定细胞膜功能，过多则可引起骨吸收增加。

（三）碳水化合物与口腔健康 Carbohydrates and oral health

几乎所有的研究都表明了食物中的碳水化物与龋病的发生呈明显的正相关关系。但是，关于牙的大分子碳水化物成分及其功能对牙与口腔健康的影响还了解的很少。结缔组织中的聚糖可能是营养性的，也可能是结构性的。结构聚糖有两种大分子：蛋白聚糖（Proteoglycans, PG）和葡糖蛋白（Glycoproteins），又可以把蛋白聚糖看作为葡糖蛋白家族的特殊成员，称为氨基葡糖聚糖（glyco-saminoglycans, GAG）。

人牙胚中存在着GAG，糖原和其他含碳水化物的大分子。在钙化开始之前，糖原与GAG等存在于成骨细胞，成牙骨质细胞，成牙质细胞与成釉细胞的细胞质及其周围的基质之中。在牙本质与釉牙本质界出现 GAG 之后，形成釉质的釉原，（amelogenesis）开始发生，由于利用糖原合成蛋白，因而糖原含量减少，最终在成釉细胞中完全消失。

牙乳头、前期牙本质、牙本质以及新近形成的釉质中存在着葡糖蛋白。在形成的釉质中已不存在 GAG，但在牙乳头、前期牙本质、牙本质中还可以看到。

人牙胚中的 GAG 主要是 4- 硫酸 - 软骨素（CS_4）与 6- 硫酸 - 软骨素（CS_6）。此外，人牙胚与牙乳头中还存在透明质酸（Hyaluronate, HA）。

牙周膜存在CS_4，CS_6，硫酸皮肤素（dermaton sulfate,DS），和HA等。牙髓中有葡糖蛋白、GAG 和相当量的胶原蛋白。在发育期间，牙髓中的 HA 数量有相当大的增加，而 CS（4 或 6）和DS的量则有相当多的减少。这可能与即将发生的钙化过程有关系。蛋白聚糖起到钙化抑制剂的作用。GAG等消失后，钙化即会开始。在矿化组织中，GAG总量较少。在前期牙本质中CS_6较丰富，它比CS_4有较高结合钙的能力。从前期牙本质到牙本质，CS_6/CS_4的比率减少，表示 GAG 结合钙的能力减少。随着钙的利用结果，羟基磷灰石晶体开始沉积。

因此，在钙化过程中，蛋白聚糖起到最重要的作用。由于能有效地结合钙，它可能履行几种功能：与弹性蛋白和胶原争夺钙，减少异常钙化的可能；暂时储藏钙，在适当时释放，利于基质泡有效利用；防止亚稳态磷酸钙沉淀。

（四）钙、磷、维生素 D 与口腔健康 Calcium, phosphorus, vitamin D and oral health

钙与磷是体内最丰富的矿物质，构成为骨与牙组织的大部分，占体内钙的99%（1%在血液中），磷的70%～80%（20%～30%在软组织内）。正常血清钙浓度为10mg/100ml，无机磷酸盐4～5mg/100ml。在快速生长期间，钙与磷在体内很快沉积。例如，在妊娠最后6周的胎儿快速生长期间沉积的钙为婴儿出生时总钙的一半，磷为1/3以上。出生后第一年内体内钙含量的增加比任何时候都快得多。

钙与磷的主要功能是提供骨与牙的硬度与强度，其主要化学结构为羟基磷灰石。此外，血清钙还发挥几种生命体功能：如肌收缩，血液凝固，神经应激性，心肌张缩，激活酶等。磷还作为ATP与ADP分子的一部分，在肌收缩时快速提供能量释放，还为核酸与核蛋白的基本成分，参与DNA与RNA的合成。因而与蛋白合成和遗传因素有关，还帮助碳水化物，像葡糖与糖原的吸收与代谢，又易与蛋白质、脂肪与碳水化物结合，在血液与唾液中 还有缓冲功能。

钙与磷这两种矿物质主要在小肠上部吸收（磷吸收约70%，钙20%～30%，其余由粪、尿、汗排出），主要储藏于长骨小梁内，血液与组织钙起到储藏库作用。为了保持有益于骨和牙形成的环境，钙的平衡取决于骨、肾与小肠行使的功能适当，至少有一种激素（甲状旁腺激素）和一种维生素（Vit.D）是平衡的基础。

维生素D族为固醇类，只有D_2与D_3两种有营养价值。D_2来自植物，特别是真菌与酵母菌中的前维生素。D_3由人类皮肤产生。也在鱼肝油、动物来源的食品如蛋类、奶油、肝脏等中发现。维生素D的吸收发生在有胆盐与脂肪存在的肠道内。任何肝胆疾患引起的脂肪吸收不良，都会干扰其吸收。它主要储藏于肝脏，其主要作用是与钙吸收，保持体内钙平衡与骨骼整体性有关。保证供给骨与牙矿化所需的充足的钙。

骨生长基本上分为两期：第一期是形成钙化基质或胶原，由成骨细胞产生；第二期为矿质期，在胶原纤维空间或间格内填入未定型磷酸钙。磷酸钙融合与不断再结晶的过程使晶体生长，直至整个基质变成为钙化组织。

牙生长发育期间，如果缺乏维生素D，首先改变的是釉质与牙本质发育不全，成釉细胞不能行使功能，釉质钙化不良，可引起部分缺陷，牙本质中球间牙本质形成空隙，代表未钙化的牙本质基质。急性维生素D缺乏的最早表现是牙本质出现钙损伤线，维生素D是正常骨的形成或钙化或病骨修复所必需的。可能有几种全身因素与釉质发育缺陷有关：如激素不平衡，或明显的膳食中缺乏钙、维生素A或D，或氟摄入过多。最可能的原因是在牙有效形成与钙化期间发生1～2天高烧。

釉质发育不全的临床表现为牙冠部出现水平向排列的凹沟，可扩展至釉质，直至釉牙本质界。如果在出生后第一年釉质形成受到干扰，恒中切牙、下侧切牙与第一恒磨牙出现沟凹；第二年出现干扰，则上侧切牙受到影响；第三或第四年干扰钙化，前磨牙与第二磨牙受到影响。

细胞过程深刻地受到营养因素的影响，但是有两个因素对口腔组织特别重要：蛋白质合成与钙化。蛋白质的合成在生长与保持状态期间由所有的细胞不断进行的。因此，细胞的生命是取决于大量的蛋白质合成的能力，蛋白质合成需要在细胞内存在着不同的营养素，如氨基酸，维生素作为辅助因素的形式，以及矿物质是过程的基础，必须由膳食提供。通过基本机制这些不同的氨基酸组成为蛋白质是很好理解的。在一个细胞内一种蛋白质的组合取决于从一个特殊信使RNA的DNA转移，它有一个编码表明顺序，其中氨基酸组成为一种特殊的蛋白质形成。另一组RNA分子帮助输送氨基酸到信使股，它与细胞中的核糖体有联系。每一条信使RNA分成与一种核糖体的聚合有联系，归诸于作为一种聚核糖体。在一条信使分成上核糖体的数量是反映了这种细胞器官蛋白质的合成能力。这已经显示在维持这种细胞器官完整性中氨基酸起到重要的作用。因此控制着细胞的某种高难度的蛋白质合成活动。在哺乳动物细胞中某些多核糖体依附于细胞内膜的一个系统，内形成性的网状组织，它通常与生产可输出的蛋白质有联系。在细胞质内游离的是其他聚核糖体，认为它可以使预期的蛋白质保留在细胞内。

控制蛋白质合成是这种现象的基本方面之一，在哺乳动物细胞中，它是部分地在核子内通过控制 RNA 的合成进行。RNA 的量是在可观察到的酶中 RNA 聚合酶的增加之后随之增加，还通过核苷基质可利用率的改变，或者通过改变DNA模板暴露于酶的数量。营养能够影响细胞中细胞质的蛋白质数量，通过控制组织可利用的氨基酸的数量，这样，以一种方面，通过信使控制转化。另外，其他营养素能够影响所形成的蛋白质的稳定性，因此，通过改变降解率影响蛋白质的合成。例如，含铁蛋白质，铁蛋白看来是通过铁而得以稳定的，因此，这种矿物营养素的浓度决定了铁蛋白在细胞中的分解率，因而，在任何一个时间存在着绝对量。

胶原蛋白的生物合成，由于它在骨、牙本质以及牙的支持结构的重要作用，应受到密切关注。这种蛋白的合成受到营养的影响，比其他蛋白质有更大程度的影响，胶原含有氨基酸如羟脯氨酸，羟赖氨酸，最初结合到多肽链中作为脯氨酸与赖氨酸并随后羟化。在羟化反应过程中涉及的营养素之一是抗坏血酸（维生素C）一种在组织修复与生长中起作用的维生素，已有很好的文献记述。

铜是一种营养基本元素也参与胶原的生物合成与另一种结构蛋白，弹性蛋白的合成。有几种类型的胶原分子，带有一种三为一组的螺旋形，纤维结构有三个链约 1000 种氨基酸残基组成。胶原的交叉连续（还有弹性蛋白）由通过一种依赖铜的氟化酶进行的。这方面更多的证据来自研究其中的 β- 氨丙晴，一种致山黧中毒物喂养动物，胶原的山黧豆中毒 α 链呈现是正常的。然而，lysyl 残基的 ε NH_2 组，涉及交叉连续中，不是氧化地脱氨基不发生交叉连续这样，正常的胶原成熟到缺少适量的铜之下不进行，其他矿物质，如丁酸锰对 glycosilation 反应是必要的，这些反应对蛋白聚糖的形成是基础，它是特有的骨形成所需的。

Nutritional aspects of oral tissue growth and development

Cell processes are profoundly influenced by nutritional factors, but two have special importance for oral tissues: protein synthesis and calcification. Protein synthesis is constantly being carried out by all cells during both growth and maintenance states. Cell life is therefore dependent on the ability to synthesize a large number of proteins. Protein synthesis requires the presence within cells of different nutrients such as amino acids, vitamins in the form of cofactors, and minerals that are essential to the process and have to be supplied by the diet.

Nutrition can influence the amount of protein in the cell cytoplasm by controlling the amounts of amino acids available to the tissue and thus, in a way, regulating the translation by the messenger. In addition, other nutrients can influence the stability of the protein that is formed and therefore influence protein synthesis by changing the rate of degradation. The iron-containing protein, ferritin for example, seems to be stabilized by iron; therefore, the concentration of this mineral nutrient determines the rate of breakdown of ferritin protein in the cell and hence the absolute amount present at any one time.

The biosynthesis of collagen protein, because of its important role in bone, dentin, and the supporting structures of teeth, deserves a closer look. The synthesis of this protein is influenced by nutrition to an even greater extent than other proteins. Collagen contains amino acids such as hydroxyproline and hydroxylysine, which are incorporated initially into the polypeptide chain as proline and lysine and subsequently hydroxylated. One of the nutrients involved in the hydroxylation reaction is ascorbic acid, a vitamin whose role in tissue repair and growth is well documented.

Copper is a nutritionally essential element that also participates in the biosynthesis of collagen and of another structural protein, elastin.

二、营养与钙化过程 Nutrition and calcification processes

通过一定的细胞，如成骨细胞与成牙质细胞形成的胶原经历着一个矿化过程，其中许多维生素与矿物元素必定参与完成一种结构作用或者是催化作用。

多年来已经观察到膳食系统，其中有一种低钙-高磷含量或者缺乏维生素D。通过与骨的形成不良有关，而引起佝偻病。在20世纪30年代后期当确定并合成了防治佝偻病的物质之后，直到30年代后期维生素D的代谢与功能才确立。近来，Deluca及其同事确定并描述了活性代谢产物。

今天，我们了解了维生素D在形成最终活性代谢产物之前在体内经历着几次转化。来自膳食或者皮肤内的7-脱氢胆固醇经照射形成的维生素D_3由血液输送至肝脏，在那里，维生素D_3转化成25-羟维生素D_3（25-OH-D_3），然后这种化合物由血液输送至肾脏，在那里再次羟化形成1.25-二羟维生素D_3（1.2-OH）2D_3。这种代谢物与其他代谢物如24，25-二羟维生素D_3，在佝偻病儿童中比维生素D_3或25羟维生素D_3引起钙吸收的更快增加。现时的证据提出，24，25二羟维生素D_3可能是一种失活形式的维生素。同时还发现在低于父母新的固醇浓度更有效。各种维生素D_3代谢物的存在。在肾与肝脏羟化酶系统的控制下允许在细胞外液维持体内钙的稳定性控制。来自小肠的钙吸收，来自骨的代谢，以及中钙的排泄控制着血清钙的浓度借助于甲状旁腺与维生素D内分泌系统的帮助。

许多其他营养物也参与到这一钙化过程。蛋白质，维生素A，C，K以及矿物质，如镁、锰，铜，锌与铁都参与这一过程。这些营养物中的某一些，像蛋白质维生素C及铜是胶原形成的基础。维生素A与锰影响到粘多糖的代谢。

Calcification processes and nutrition

Collagen formed by certain cells such as osteoblasts and odontoblasts undergoes a process of mineralization in which a number of vitamins and mineral elements must take part to fulfill either a structural or a catalytic role.

For many years it has been observed that dietary systems in which there is a low calcium-high phosphate content or a deficiency of vitamin D are usually associated with bone deformities referred to as rickets. While identification and synthesis of antirachitic substances were achieved in the late 1930's, it was not until 30 years later that the metabolism and function of vitamin D were established, and recently, active metabolites have been identified and described by DeLuca and coworkers.

As it is understood today, vitamin D undergoes several transformations in the body before forming the final active metabolite. Cholecalciferol from the diet or from irradiation of 7-dehydrocholesterol in the skin is transported in the blood to the liver, where cholecalciferol is transformed to 25-

hydroxycholecalciferol (25-OH-D3) . This compound is then transported by the blood to the kidneys, where it is hydroxylated again to form the 1,25-dihydroxycholecalciferol (1,25-OH) 2D3. This metabolite and others such as 24,25 (OH) 2D3 cause a more rapid enhancement of calcium absorption than either vitamin d3 or 25-oh-d3 in rachitic chicks. Current evidence suggests that 24,25 (oh2) d3 could be an inactivation form of the vitamin. It also was found to be more effective at lower concentrations than these two parent steroids. The presence of the various vitamin d3 metabolites, under the regulation of the kidney and liver hydroxylase systems, allows for the maintenance of a homeostatic control of calcium in the extracellular fluids. Absorption of calcium from the intestine, mobilization from bones, and excretion of calcium in urine regulates serum calcium concentration with the help of the parathyroid gland and the vitamin d endocrine system.

还有其他营养物，像维生素K，参与骨的特殊成分的合成如γ富羧基谷氨酸肽（γ carboxyglutamic acid-rich peplies）。这些因素的存在看来对于成功的形成与保持钙化组织，如骨与牙是必需的。在牙矿化期间这些基本元素的严重，甚至轻度缺乏都可能引起不全的釉质与牙本质沉积，转而对牙健康可能有害的作用。应该记住釉质与骨比较，只有一次正常形成的机会。在发育期间的缺陷不能由细胞修复，而构成不可逆转的病损。

Many other nutrients are involved in the process of calcification. Proteins, vitamins A, C, and K, and minerals such as Mg, Mn, Cu, Zn, and F are all involved in the process. Some of these nutrients, such as protein, vitamin C, and copper, are essential for collagen formation. Vitamin A and Mn affect glycosaminoglycan metabolism. Still others, like vitamin K, are involved in the synthesis of specific components of bones such as γ carboxyglutamic acid-rich peptides.the presence of these factors seems to be necessary for the successful formation and maintenance of calcified tissues such as bones and teeth. Severe and even mild deficiencies of these essential elements during the mineralization of teeth may cause the deposition of defective enamel and dentin, which may in turn have a deleterious effect on dental health. it should be remembered that enamel, in contrast to bone, has only one opportunity to be formed normally. Defects during development cannot be cellularly repaired and constitute irreversible lesions.

三、牙齿发育的阶段 Stages in tooth development

关键期的概念 Concept of critical periods

为了评价营养与感染的压力对牙齿发育的可能影响，有必要叙述牙齿发育的阶段。已经在子宫内乳牙在外胚叶内层，原始口腔或口凹约6周开始形成。从这时起，有区别的生长，具有快速间接核分裂的特征，引起牙板的形成（dental lamina）。通过衍化这个过程继续进入帽状期，并形成牙囊，直至达到钟状期，当细胞区分成釉质细胞与成牙质细胞。这时釉质与牙本质并列生长通过有规律的一种胞外基质的分层样沉积。第一阶段（包括，开始，增殖，形态分化，组织分化，以及最终并列的细胞活动）需要利用营养素，在乳牙列情况下通过胎盘提供，以及恒牙列通过循环液提供。第二阶段具有釉质与牙本质积极矿化的特点。有几名研究者研究了釉质矿化与其他硬组织，如骨不同。在成釉细胞的牙釉质形成过程中在牙本质形成开始后的短期内，成牙质细胞开始沿着牙本质分泌-薄层有机机质。在分泌活动开始之后很快在基质与柱间部位开始矿化。具有许多长而薄的像磷灰不样的物质晶体的外貌特征。通过第二阶段晶体厚度的增加而进行的早期矿化，釉质失去水分，以及基质蛋白浓度下降。这一过程从釉牙本质界向釉质表面扩展以及牙冠高度从颈部向釉质本质界进展，还进入到裂沟的基底部，牙齿的切缘与殆面区域，在发育过程中比滞后的颈部区域更全面的矿化。当釉质基质已完成其主要矿化，成牙质细胞停止其作为矿化细胞的功能时，第二阶段结束。这时细胞层形成一种分层上皮覆盖于釉质，保护釉质直至牙萌出之时，从几个月到几年有很大差别，取决于牙本身的状态。

第三阶段涉及萌出周围期，当釉质中的矿物质继续得到钙、磷与微量元素时，经历着向更加稳定的羟磷灰石晶体，还有氟磷灰石变化，在晶格表面部位通过氟离了取代羟基而产生。这一过程发生在萌出前，萌出期间与萌出之后，认为是釉质低矿化区（HAE）的一个成熟过程，在以前的发育阶段并没有完全矿化，这些 HAE 在这时在唾液中矿物质与蛋白质的作用下能够快速再矿化，它积极地奉献于再矿化的过程。第三阶段是明确的关键期，它能够决定牙齿对龋侵蚀的易感性。

第三阶段代表最后时期，当牙齿在功能上出现于口腔内，釉质是对口腔环境中的矿化与脱矿化作用随之而发生的目标。

从营养与膳食的观点看，这四个阶段代表着四个不同的时期，具有不同的牙齿发育活动的特点，以及不同的环境条件可以影响牙齿最终对龋的易感性。在前三个阶段，不能获得必要的营养素而可以影响到釉质与牙本质的内部结构与化学成分，还可能影响到形态与牙萌出的时间。在第三个阶段，膳食不平衡与过度主要影响到表膜与菌斑细菌，这样在的环境中修整着矿化 - 脱矿化的过程。

在最后的 15 年内，已经发展的一个重要概念是强调关键时期在发育中的重要性，当营养的危害可以有不利的和不可逆转的影响。这些研究提出大多数器官有三个主要的细胞生长期：①这个时期具有增生活动或者细胞数量增加的特点；②随后的时期是细胞数量继续增加，但体积增加也开始；③最后一个阶段，组织的增生是主要特征。这些不同的生长期主要营养的重要性是营养或全身性紊乱早期强加于这个过程，在增生开始时期，倾向于是不可逆转的，组织所产生的改变不能得到补偿。营养的危害对早期在有机机质的形成中发育的牙体组织能够在临床上引起釉质的可以看到的发育不全，具有成窝沟状，或严重病例，釉质缺失。如果这种压力在后期强加，当羟磷灰石晶体处于得到最大的体积与完善的程度的过程中，结果可能是钙化不良，围绕正常可见的釉质出现不透明或白垩色的区域。这个较后的时期也是依据原子的体积，与化学特性，各种无机离子，包括氟离子结合到品格之中或者进入到磷灰石晶体周围的水化作用层，这样供给釉质的化学成分。釉质发育不全与钙化不良也能由环境的压力引起，如发热性事件，化学中毒与遗传性缺陷。

釉质代表着牙齿就像人体的皮肤。这些组织都起源于外胚层，每一种都在全身地控制内环境与变量以及可能的病理性外环境之间起到作为一种保护性屏障的作用。像皮肤一样，釉质有细菌负载，可以成为病原体的隐匿场所，能够破坏这一组织的完整性，由于这些原因，一种健全的釉质表面是关键，因为它在一定程度上决定着牙齿是健康的还是患龋的。适当的营养能允许釉质形成发生，而营养不良与感染能阻碍正常釉质的形成，营养不良对所有的组织都是不希望出现的，但对釉质来说甚至更坏。这个组织，一旦牙萌出进入口腔，没有细胞机制来修复不论已经发生什么样的发育性损伤。因此，病损是大范围的不可逆转。釉质表面是经常不断地暴露于唾液及其成分的弥补作用之中是真的，但是这种作用能够受到菌斑破坏性活动的干扰并完全地被抵消。

重要的是注意到在釉质形成完成与萌出时间之间有一个相当长的周期（第三阶段），当人的釉质能够经历表面层矿化作用的广泛改变并获得像氟化物那样的元素时，有助于在晶体表面有选择的部位形成大量稳定的含氟羟磷灰石晶体。这些微量元素中有一些倾向于增强釉质的成熟，由此减少萌出后牙对龋的易感性。对人牙萌出之前成熟的机制有必要进一步研究。

To evaluate the possible impact of nutrition and infectious stresses upon tooth development, it is necessary to describe the stages of dental development. Deciduous teeth are known to begin forming at about 6 weeks in utero in the ectoderm-line, perimitive oral cavity or stomadeum. From this moment, differential growth, characterized by rapid mitosis, leads to formation of the dental lamina. The process continues through evolution into the cap stage and formation of the dental sac until it reaches the bell stage when cells differentiate into ameloblasts and odontoblasts. At this time, appositional growth of enamel and dentin begins by a regular, layer-like deposition of an extracellular matrix. This stage 1 (which includes initiation, proliferation, morphodifferentiation, histodifferentiation, and finally, appositional cellular activities) requires the availability of nutrients, which in the case of deciduous dentition, are provided through the placenta and, in the permanent dentition, from ciculating fluids.

Stage Ⅱ is characterized by active mineralizaiton of enamel and dentin. Enamel mineralization, which has been studied by several investigators, differs from that of other hard tissues such as bone. In amelogenesis, the ameloblasts begin to secrete the organic matrix in a thin layer along the dentin shortly after dentin formation has started. Mineralizaiton starts in the matrix and the interprismatic areas soon after secretory activity has begun. It is characterized by the appearance of numerous long, thin crystals of apatite-like material. The initial imneralization is followed by a second phase in which crystals increase in thickness, water is lost from enamel, and the matrix protein concentration is reduced. This process spreads from the dentino-enamel, and from the height of the crown it progresses cervically toward the cemento-enamel junction and also into the fundus of the fissures. The incisal and occlusal regions of the tooth are more fully mineralized than the cervical areas which lag behind during development. Stage Ⅱ ends when enamel matrix has completed its primary mineralization, and amelolasts cease functioning as mineralizing cells. At this time, a cell layer forms a stratified epithelial covering over the enamel to protect it until time of eruption, which varies from a few months to years depending on the tooth.

Stage Ⅲ involves the peri-eruptive period when the mineral in enamel continues to acquire calcium, phosphorus, and trace elements and undergoes phase changes toward more stable crystals of hydroxyapatite and also fluoroapatite, which occurs through fluoride substitution of hydroxyl ion in surface positions of crystal lattices. This process takes place before, during, and just after eruption, and can be considered a maturation process for hypomineralized areas of enamel (HAE) that were not fully mineralized during the previous developmental stage. These HAE can be remineralized quickly at this time under the action of minerals and proteins in saliva, which contribute actively to the process of remineralization. Stage Ⅲ is definitely a critical stage that could determine the susceptibility of the tooth to carious attack.

Stage Ⅳ represents the final period when the tooth is functionally present in the oral cavity, and enamel is subjected sequentially to the mineralization and demineralization action of the oral environment.

From a nutritional and dietary viewpoint, these four stages represent four different periods that are characterized by different tooth developmental activities and different environmental conditions, which may influence final tooth susceptibility to caries. Failure to obtain the necessary nutrients during the first three stages may therefore affect the internal structure and chemical composition of enamel and dentin, as well as possibly affecting the morphology and time of eruption of the tooth. Dietary imbalances and excesses during stage Ⅳ affect mainly pellicle and plaque bacteria, thus modifying the mineralization-demineralization processes in the tooth environment.

Within the last 15 years, an important concept has been developed that emphasizes the importance of critical periods in development when nutritional insults may have detrimental and irreversible effects. While working with whole rat brain, Winick and Noble observed that there is a definite pattern and sequence in the changes of DNA and total protein. These studies and others suggest that for most organs there are three major periods of cell growth: (1) a period characterized by hyperplasic activity or an increase in the number of cells; (2) a subsequent phase during which cells continue to increase in numbers but also start to increase in size; and (3) a final stage in which hypertrophic growth of the tissue is the main characteristic.

It is important to notice that there is an extended period of time between completion of enamel formation and time of eruption (stage Ⅲ) when human enamel can undergo extensive changes in mineralization of the surface layer and acquire elements such as fluoride that contribute to formation of large, stable crystals of hydroxyapatite containing fluoride in selected sites on the crystal surface. Some of these trace elements tend to enhance maturation of enamel and thus reduce caries susceptibility of the tooth after eruption. Further research is necessary to understand the mechanisms of preeruptive maturation of enamel in humans.

四、营养与牙周组织 Nutrition and the periodontium

坏血病是一种经典的营养缺乏病。柑桔类水果 - 特别是酸橙汁 - 预防坏血病。坏血病具有牙松动牙龈出血的特点。维生素 C 只是许多能够影响牙支持组织的营养素之一，这并不奇怪，因为围绕在牙周围的组织由上皮，结缔组织，包括胶原与血管和骨组成。所有这些都会受到各种营养素缺乏的影响。不仅营养素缺乏，需要讨论，而且膳食结构，食物过敏症，以及膳食成分对口腔黏膜可能的有害与保护作用也是相关的。

围绕着牙的组织有两个大标题可以考虑：第一，支持牙的结构 - 牙龈，牙周韧带，以及围绕的牙槽骨，第二，口腔黏膜 - 主要是上皮，但还有其下层的结缔组织。

Scurvy is a classical nutritional deficiency disease. As a result of Lind's clinical trial, citrus fruits-lime juice in particular-prevented scurvy and British sailors were known as "limeys" for over a century. Loose teeth and bleeding gums characterize scurvy. Vitamin C is just one of the many nutrients which can affect the supporting tissues of teeth, which is not surprising since tissues surrounding teeth consist of epithelium, connective tissue including collagen and blood vessels, and bone, all of which are known to be affected by deficiencies of various nutrients. It is not only nutrient deficiencies which need to be discussed-the texture of the diet, food allergies, and the possible harmful and protective action of dietary components on the oral mucosa are also relevant.

The tissues surrounding the teeth can be considered under two broad headings. First, the structures which support teeth-the gingivae, periodontal ligament, and the surrounding alveolar bone-and, second, the oral mucosa-principally the epithelium but also the underlying connective tissue.

牙周组织是由上皮，胶原纤维，血管，其他结缔组织元素，牙骨质与骨组成。如果营养缺乏对这些组织没有相反的影响，会很奇怪。从实验鼠，Guinea猪、狗的实验提供较强的证据，证明有相反的作用，但在人体的证据要少得多。只有在维生素C缺乏的情况下，牙周组织主要受到影响。就总体而言，当营养适当时，牙周组织将会从中获益，但是家上面普遍接受作为适当水平的膳食补充营养素看来并不会更多的改善牙周健康叶酸水平不适当似手在一定人群的牙龈组织中存在，在口腔内局部提供叶酸，这些组织能够从中受益（例如一种漱口液），到目前为止，最重要的保持人的牙周健康的方法是用一把合格的牙刷定期彻底机械地去除牙菌斑。

Periodontal tissues are comprised of epithelium, collagen fibres, blood vessels, other connective tissue elements, cementum and bone. It would be very surprising if nutritional deficiencies did not adversely affect these tissues. There is strong evidence of adverse effects from experiments on rats, guinea-pigs and dogs, but there is much less evidence in humans. Only in the case of scurvy (ascorbic acid deficiency) are the periodontal tissues primarily affected. Overall, periodontal tissues will benefit when nutrition is adequate, but dietary supplementation of nutrients above what are commonly accepted as adequate levels does not seem to improve periodontal health further. Inadequate levels of folate appear to exist in gingival tissues in defined groups of people and delivery of folate to these tissues locally in the mouth (for example in a mouthrinse) can be beneficial. By far the most important way of maintaining periodontal health in humans is regular, thorough physical removal of dental paque with a satisfactory tooth-brush. For a fuller review of this subject the reader is referred to Rugg-Gunn (1993) and to chapter 6 of this book in which periodontal conditions are considered in more detail.

（一）碳水化合物 Carbohydrates

限制或增加碳水化合物对所形成的菌斑以及牙龈炎发展的影响，在动物与人体已有了几项研究，大多数是研究糖，而不是淀粉或碳水化合物作为一个整体。几项研究，通常坚持几周，显示膳食补充糖增加菌斑量与牙龈出血。相反，限制膳食糖两年以上引起菌斑形成减少以及较弱的趋向于较少牙龈炎。

Carbohydrates

There have been several investigations in both animals and human subjects of the effect of carbohydrate restriction or additon on the quantity and quality of plaque formed and the development of gingivitis. Most of the studies have investigated sugars rather than starches, or carbohydrate as a whole. Several studies, usually lasting a few weeks, have shown that supplementing the diet with sugars increases the quantity of plaque and gingival bleeding. Conversely, restriction of dietary sugar over 2 years resulted in reduced plaque formation and a weak trend towards less gingivitis.

（二）纤维性食物 Fibrous foods

没有证据支持纤维性食物有益于牙周健康，对人来说，纤维性食物表现：不去除牙龈组织邻近部位的牙菌斑；不增加牙龈上皮的角化作用。

通过增加唾液流动增加口腔食物的清洁作用，但很少表现为与牙周病有关。

一般来说它含有的非奶外源性糖的水平是低的，因此，它是引起龋齿和增加菌斑生长的非奶外源性糖含量高的一种好的取代食品。

但是不能取代现代社会中的认真刷牙。

Fibrous foods

Evidence does not support fibrous foods beneficial to periodontal health. In summary, it would appear that in humans, fibrous foods:

do not remove plaque from areas adjacent to gingival tissues;

do not increase keratinization of the gingival epithelium;

may help to maintain the supporting tissues of teeth (bone and periodontal ligament) ;

increase clearance of foods from the mouth by increasing salivary flow, but this would appear to be of little relevance to periodontal disease;

are generally low in non-milk extrinsic sugars and are therefore a good substitute for foods high in non-milk extrinsic sugars which cause dental caries and increase plaque growth.

But they are not a substitute for careful tooth-brushing in modern societies.

The periodontal tissues are composed of epithelium, collagen fibres, blood vessels, other connective tissue elements, cementum, and bone. It would be very surprising if nutritional deficiencies did not adversely effect these tissues. There is strong evidence of adverse effects from experiments on rats, guinea pigs, and dogs, but there is much less evidence in humans. Only in the case of scurvy (ascorbic acid deficiency) are the periodontal tissues primarily affected. Overall, periodontal tissues will benefit when nutrition is adequate, but dietary supplementation of nutrientsabove what is commonly accepted as adequate levels does not seem to improve periodontal health further. Inadequate levels of folate appearto exist in gingival tissues in defined groups of people and delivery of folate to these tissues locally in the mouth (for example in a mouth-rinse) can be beneficial. By far the most important way of maintaining periodontal health in humans is regular, thorough, physical removal of dental plaque with a satisfactory toothbrush.

五、牙齿在营养中的价值 The value of teeth in nutrition

在现代社会中，人牙已丧失了其大部分最重要的功能-即食物准备-就是人牙列处于一种功能减退状态。现代人只用其一部分潜在的咀嚼力。相反，我们很关心其外观与交流，目前，在大多数人类社会中，到目前为止认为牙的最重要作用是增强外观。在决定一个人在社会中的完整性面部外观是非常重要的。

如果我们的牙齿处于功能不良状态，是否需要适当的，或者良好的营养化？生产完全的液态膳食在技术上是可能的。但有两点不同看法：第一，对大多数人来说缺牙在社会上是不能接受的；第二，液态腾食通常（不总是）缺少能量。

在我们考虑是否牙列不好相反的会影响营养之前，良好的营养很明显是重要的。有几点值得提及：

（1）增加人群的高度是良好营养的一种标志，特别是关于能量与蛋白质的摄入，另一方面，儿童肥胖在增加，所以进食健康食品与锻炼是重要的；

（2）现在经过 10 多年已经很清楚在子宫内营养影响到成人期疾病的发生（如心血管病），已经很清楚过度的消耗膳食脂肪是心血管病的一种重要危险因素，过度消耗糖引起龋齿，并且很可能是糖尿病的一种危险因素；

（3）膳食引起或预防癌症的能力 – 在几乎所有的身体系统内 – 非常强调这一点。

所有癌症的1/3是可以通过可行的膳食改变而预防的。足以得出这样的结论营养是健康与疾病的一种非常重要的决定因素。有三方面的考虑：第一，营养不良引起疾病；第二，年幼儿童缺牙或牙疼可以引起营养不良，生长迟缓；第三，老年人牙列不完整导致营养不良。然而，在我们考虑给予什么指导之前，我们需要考虑有什么样的证据，在此基础上作为提供信息的基础。

从三个水平上考虑证据的用处，每一个都重要：

（1）牙列不完整是否相反的影响到食物的选择？

（2）牙列不完整是否影响到营养的摄取或者营养状态？

（3）牙列不完整是否影响到健康？

关于食物的选择有许多证据，有些是关于营养的摄入或者营养状态，但是关于健康实际上没有证据，遗憾的是因为健康是所有这一切中最相关的结果。我们发现，食物的选择能够受到牙列不完整的影响，但是否导致营养不良？或者在临床上是否改变了营养状态？

Since teeth in modern societies have lost the major part of their most important function-namely food preparation-it has been said that the dentition is in a state of hypofunction'. Modern humans use only a fraction of their potential chewing force. Conversely, we are very concerned with appearance and communication and, in most human societies now, by far the most important role for teeth is enhancing appearance. Facial appearance is tremendously important in determining an individual's integration into society.

If our teeth are in a state of hypofunction, are they required at all for adequate or optimal nutrition? It is technically possible to produce complete diets in liquid form. There are two counter arguments: first, a lack of teeth is socially unacceptable to the majority of people and, second, liquid diets are usually (not always) poor in energy-an attribute taken advantage of by purveyors of slimming foods.

Before we consider whether a poor dentition can adversely affect nutrition, it is important to be clear that good nutrition matter. Some points are worth mentioning.

The increasing height of our population is an indication of better nutrition, particularly with regard to energy and protein intake. On the other hand, obesity in children is increasing so that eating the right foods and exercising are important.

It is now over 10 years since it became clear that nutrition in utero influences the occurrence of disease (e.g. cardiovascular disease) in adulthood. It is well known that excessive consumption of dietary fats is an important risk factor for cardiovascular disease and excessive consumption of sugars the cause of dental caries and probably a risk factor for diabetes.

In the previous seetion, the ability of the diet to cause and prevent cancer-in almost all systems of the body-was strongly emphasized. About one third of all cancers are preventable by feasible changes in diet. Chapter, but suffice to conclude that nutrition is a very important determinant of health and disease.

Thus, there are three areas of concern: first, that poor nutrition causes disease; second, that lack of teeth or painful teeth in young children may cause undernutrition and retarded growth; and, third, that an impaired dentition in elderly people results in undernutrition.

There is much evidence regarding food choice, some regarding nutrient intake or nutritional status, but virtually no evidence regarding health. this is a pity as health, after all, is the most relevant outcome. As we shall discover, food choice can be affected by an impaired dentition but does this result in malnutrition? Likewise, is a change in nutritional status clinically relevant?

（一）不完整牙列，咀嚼能力与食物选择 The impaired dentition, chewing ability and food choice

已有充分数量发表的研究得出结论牙齿数量的缺失与人们进食困难转而影响食物的选择是成比例的。直接测量咬合力与肌电图法已显示戴义齿的人咬合力大大降低（只有有牙人的 1/5 与1/6），如果义齿不舒服，咬合力会进一步降低，咀嚼能力与真牙存在的数量密切相关。表现出20～21颗牙是极限。低于这个极限，咀嚼能力下降，但在这个数字以上缺牙没有明显影响。这 20 颗牙必须有咬合关系，更准确地说，至少必须有 10 对咬合的牙。

对戴义齿的人来说，不仅是硬质食物有问题，而且带子的食品与小粒食品与粘性食品也有问题，毫无疑问，煮熟的蔬菜，碎肉增加义齿患者的可接受程度。

The impaired dentition, chewing ability, and food choice

There has been a sufficient number of studies published to conclude that the number of teeth lost is proportional to the difficulty that people have in eating foods and that this in turn affects food choice. Direct measurement of bite force and electromyographic methods have shown that people with dentures have much reduced bite force (only one fifth or one sixth that of dentate people) and that this is reduced further if dentures are uncomfortable. Chewing ability is closely correlated with the number of natural teeth present, and there appears to be a threshold of 20～21 teeth. Below this threshold, chewing ability declines, but above this figure loss of teeth has no apparent effect. These 20 teeth must occlude, so it is perhaps more accurate to say that there must be at least ten occluding pairs of teeth.

It is not only hard foods that are problem foods for denture wearers, but also foods with seeds and small particles (which get under dentures) and sticky foods. Undoubtedly boiling vegetables and mincing meat increase their acceptability to denture wearers.

（二）不完整牙列、膳食、营养摄入与营养状态 The impaired dentition, diet, nutritional intake and nutritional status

人们的营养摄入与营养状态与其牙状态的关系方面的研究太少，特别缺少有很好对照的研究；在 1967 ~ 1968 年在英国老年人中进行的研究表明，700 名受试者中 13% 确定为有咀嚼不充分的问题。不仅能量的摄入低于有充分咀嚼能力的人，而且还有肉进食少20%，土豆，绿色蔬菜与生的非柑橘类水果少 40%。三种营养素 - 能量，蛋白质，维生素 C− 与咀嚼不充分的人有关系。在瑞典进行的一项约有400名老年人的调查记录，牙列有问题的那些人蛋白质与维生素B_1摄入较低（在说明了可能的混淆因素之后，如教育，婚姻状况收入）。在芬兰的一项调查发现在无牙颌患者与有牙的比较，其血清中的半胱氨酸，维生素C与铁浓度较低。在加拿大也有报告无牙颌患者水果、蔬菜与“纤维”食品摄入较少。

“非淀粉多糖”（NSP）一词现在偏向于“膳食纤维”，因为水果与蔬菜是NSP的良好来源，但是对牙列不完整的人难以咀嚼，NSP是一种危险营养素，1994年在英国进行了首次这方面调查，无牙颌者有中等NSP摄入10.4克/天，与有牙者组15.1克/天比较。在按性别，社会阶层调整之后，56%无牙颌组摄入NSP低于现时英国的营养指导18克/天，有牙组从所有丰富的来源获取的NSP明显地多，如全麦面包，谷物，蔬菜与水果。

1995年调查营养摄入与牙状态的关系，经统计学调整了年龄、性别、社会阶层与宗教的影响之后，平均每日摄入NSP，蛋白质，钙，非血铁，烟酸，维生素C以及内源性与奶糖无牙成人明显地较低，也看到同样的趋势，当牙的状况在21颗或以上，对20颗或少于此数或咬合配对的牙数（OP）NSP的摄入对存在咬合配对的牙数特别敏感-无配对牙的人平均13克/天与有5个以上配对牙的人比较为16克/天，在口腔健康状况差的这些人中，血浆铁深度较低，缺牙者与有牙者比较，其血浆维生素A、抗坏血酸盐以及α-维生素E的水平较低。

看来十分清楚水果与蔬菜的消耗以及NSP的摄取在无牙颌的人较低。非常可能的是一种原因与结果的关系，但是还不能保证，因为现在所拥有的所有数据仅来自横断面研究。一种因果关系只能从长期的纵向研究才能确立。

The impaired dentition, diet, nutritional intake, and nutritional status

There have been far too few studies of nutrient intake and nutritional status of people in relation to their dental state and there is an especial shortage of well controlled studies. In the study of elderly people in Britain in 1967-8 already referred to, 13 per cent of the 700 subjects were judged to have "insufficient mastication". Not only did they have lower energy intake than those with "efficient mastication" but they also ate 20 per cent less meat and 40 per cent less tomatoes, green vegetables, and raw non-citrus fruits. Three nutrients-energy, protein, and vitamin C-were of concern in those with "insufficient mastication".

A survey of nearly 400 elderly people in Sweden recorded lower protein and thiamine intakes in those with poor dentitions, after taking possible confounding factors (such as education, marital status, and income) into account. A survey in Finland found lower concentrations of serum pantothenic acid, ascorbic acid, and iron in those who were edentulous compared with dentate people. Fruit, vegetables, and "fibre" intake was also reported to be lower in edentulous people in Canada.

The term "non-starch polysaccharides"(NSP) is now preferred to "dietary fibre". Since fruit and vegetables are good sources of NSP, but are difficult for those with impaired dentition to chew, NSP is a risk nutrient. One of the first investigations into this was undertake in the UK as recently as 1994. The edentulous group had a median NSP intake of 10.4 g/day, compared with a median of 15.1g/day in the dentate group (Fig) , after matching for gender and social class. NSP intakes of 56 per cent of the edentulous group were below the current UK nutritional guidelines of 18g/day. The dentate group obtained significantly more NSP from all the rich sources, such as wholemeal breads, cereals, vegetables, and fruit.

The 1995 National Diet and Nutrition Survey related nutrient intake to dental status. After statistical correction for the effects of age, gender, social class, and region, the mean daily intakes of NSP, protein, calcium, non-haem iron, niacin, vitamin C, and intrinsic and milk sugars were significantly lower in the edentate adults. The same trends were also observedwhen dental status was expressed as 21 or more versus 20 or fewer teeth, or number of occluding pairs (OP) of teeth. Intake of NSP was particularly sensitive to the number of occluding pairs of teeth present-a mean of 13g/day in those with no OP compared with 16g/day for those with over five OP. plasma iron concentration was lower in those with poor oral status, and edentate subjects had lower plasma levels of retinal, ascorbate, and α -tocopherol compared with dentate subjects.

It seems quite clear that consumption of fruit and vegetables and intake of NSP are lower in edentulous persons. It is highly likely that this is a cause-and-effect relationship, but we cannot be sure since all the data presently available are from cross-sectional studies. A cause-and-effect relationship can only be established from longitudinal studies.

（三）不完整牙列与健康 The impaired dentition and health

很少有直接证据表明一个不完整牙列引起不健康，但是很多间接证据表明可能是这样。例外的是噎塞。

间接证据表明一个不完整的牙列对健康的影响是大的，口腔状况差影响到食物的选择以及膳食的摄取－水果与蔬菜，全麦面包，NSP是特别危险－有许多证据显示水果与蔬菜消耗少，以及NSP增加许多疾病的危险－几种器官的癌症，憩室病与胆结石。

一项相当大的瑞典研究发现中年无牙颌男性与女性与有牙者比较更经常有两种或多种心血管病的危险因素，在调整了性别与年龄对数据的影响之后。这些因素包括饮食习惯-高脂与高糖的摄入以及低维生素的摄入－以及吸烟。同意这样的发现在牙不完整的人，NSP的摄入较低，一项美国人的调查发现这样的人明显地接受更多的药物治疗而引起胃肠功能紊乱。

噎塞食物不是闹着笑的。在美国每年约有3000人死于噎塞食物；这是第6种最普通的意外死亡的原因。在加拿大每年有300以上这样的死亡，同样地在英国，每年记录有300以上的人死于“咽喉异物-这些人的一半是65岁以上的人。这可能是相当低的噎塞食物死亡的报告-例如，它们常常被记录为“咖啡心脏”。因为在一项调查完成的所有尸检病例中发现在进食期间突然死亡的比例是食物窒息与闭塞性冠状动脉病为55：1。

牙齿起到什么作用呢？至少有9篇发表的文章强调牙健康差在食物窒息中的作用。这些死于食物噎塞的较高比例是无牙颌与一般人群比较。食物团的大小对死亡的责任经常是很大并且通常显示很少有咀嚼的证据。有几个作者已经提到这些人戴全口义齿口腔内缺乏感觉，作为一个原因是这些人试图吞咽大的没有咀嚼过的食物团块。

从这些相当不完全的证据，看来是噎塞食物是比通常想像的更为普遍的一种死亡原因，缺牙似乎可能是一种危险因素。口腔医生与营养学家应该告诫无牙颌老年患者需要为吞咽准备适当大小的食物。

The impaired dentition and health

There is little direct evidence that an impaired dentition causes ill health, but much indirect evidence that it is likely to do so. the exception is choking, which we will come to later.

The indirect evidence that an impaired dentition affects health is strong. Poor dental status affects food choice and dietary intake-fruit and vegetables, wholemeal bread, NSP are particularly at risk-and there is much evidence that low consumption of fruit, vegetables, and NSP increases the risk of a number of diseases-cancer of several organs, diverticular disease, and gallstones.

One fairly large Swedish study found that middle-aged edentulous men and women more often had two or more risk factors for cardiovascular disease compared with dentate persons, after the data were adjusted for the effects of gender and age. These factors included dietary habits-high fat and sugars intake and low vitamin intake-and smoking. In agreement with the finding of lower intake of NSP in dentally impaired persons, an American study found that such people took significantly more medication for gastrointestinal disturbances.

Choking on food is no joke. About 3000 people die in the USA per year from choking on food; it is the sixth most common cause of accidental death. In Canada, there are over 300 such deaths per year and, likewise in the UK, over 300 deaths per year are recorded for "foreign bodies in the pharynx and larynx" -half of these in people over 65 years of age. There is likely to be considerable under-reporting of death by choking on food-for example, they are often recorded as "café -coronary", since a survey of autopsies performed in all cases in which sudden death occurred during eating found a ratio of cases of food asphyxiation to occlusive coronary artery disease of 55 : 1.

So what has this to do with teeth? Well, quite a lot. There are at least nine publications which emphasize the role of poor dental health in food asphyxiation. A higher proportion of those choking to death on food were edentulous compared with the general population. The sizes of pieces of food responsible for death are frequently very large and usually show little evidence of mastication. Lack of intraoral sensation in those who wear full dentures has been mentioned by several authors as one reason for people attempting to swallow large unmasticated pieces of food.

From this rather fragmentary evidence, it seems that choking on food is a much more common cause of death than is usually thought, and lack of teeth seems likely to be a risk factor. Dentists and dietitians should warn edentulous elderly patients of the need to prepare food adequately for swallowing.

（四）改善牙列对营养的影响 The effect on nutrition of improving the dentition

现在我们知道，牙缺失是营养不良的一个危险因素，我们需要知道是否改善牙列状况可导致改进食物选择与改善营养。这个问题已经引起了几个国家多个研究团队的关注。研究有两种：首先，不良的全口义齿为良好的全口义齿听取代；第二，固定修复体已取代了义齿。结果显示，当全口义齿质量有改进时，咀嚼能力与食物选择有一定程度的提高与改进。在这方面，下颌义齿的适合程度比上颌义齿更加重要。然而，奇怪的是，完全提供固定修复体-骨结合的口腔种植桥（OIB）或组织结合桥（TIB）－取代可摘义齿并不改进咀嚼能力，食物选择或者营养摄入。

当解释上述结果时一个重要的观点是膳食指导，就总体而言，与义齿的改进异不同时进行。这明显是很重要的，但并没有经过适当的检验，仅改进牙列并不足够-同时给予良好的营养指导可能是基本的。正如Moynihan及其同事们指出的，并不是所有富含NSP的食物都难以咀嚼－膳食指导必须因人而异，实际而积极。

一个不完整的牙列影响食物选择，对健康不利，但证据是间接的，然而噎塞食物是重要的死因，特别是老年人。改善不完整牙列呈现出食物选择与营养很少有改善这可能是适当的膳食指导并不与修复体的改进同时进行。

The effect on nutrition of improving the dentition

Now that we know that loss of teeth is a risk factor for poor nutrition, we need to know whether improving the dentition results in improved food choice and nutrition. This has been looked at by a number of research teams in several countries. These studies are of two types-first, where poor-fitting complete dentures have been replaced by well-fitting complete dentures and, second, where fixed dental prostheses have replaced dentures. The results show that there was some improvement in chewing ability and food choice when the quality of complete dentures improved. In this respect, the fit of the lower denture was more important than the fit of the upper denture. However, it is surprising that, overall, providing fixed dental prostheses-with an osseointegrated oral implant bridge (OIB) or a tissue-integrated bridge (TIB) -in place of a removable denture did not improve chewing ability, food choice, or nutrient intake.

An impaired dentition is likely to affect health adversely, but evidence is indirect. However, choking on food is a significant cause of death, especially in the elderly.

Improving an impaired dentition appears to lead to little improvement in food choice and nutrition. This may be because adequate dietary advice has not been given at the same time as an improvement in dental prostheses is made.

六、营养，膳食与儿童口腔健康 Nutrition, diet and oral health in children

（一）儿童与青年人的口腔健康指导 advice for oral health of children and young people

1. 妊娠与新生儿期

在一般营养水平适当的国家，认为妊娠期间的营养对未出生儿童未来的牙齿健康影响很小，有文件资料陈述：

某些牙比其他牙对疾病的发生有较大的抵抗力，但从营养的观点看除了氟化物之外，没什么差异。比较普遍的认为既不是妊娠期间母亲的营养不良，也不是出生之后儿童的营养不良可能对易感龋齿的牙有任何可察觉得到的影响。在妊娠期或者哺乳期钙不能从母亲的牙齿传输给胎儿。已经显示氟化物是唯一的减少龋齿易感性的因素。氟化物的作用部分是它在萌出至口腔内之前与发育的牙齿结合，部分是在牙萌出后直接与牙接触。现在认为后者更重要。

当然上述文件强调牙萌出后膳食中糖的影响最为重要是正确的，但是有充分的数据表明即使在某些工业化国家，当牙齿正在形成期间，营养有一定的关联。

在营养不良的高发地区，在出生之前，釉质的形成受到相反的影响，釉质发育不全发生率较高，虽然其严重程度在新生儿以及出生之后较大。龋病的发生肯定与釉质发育不全与营养不良的存在有关。有理由假设，某些相反的事件，尽管很可能是一小部分，引起龋齿的易感性增加。

20世纪70年代以来，以某些发展中国家的流行病学研究显示龋病患病率增加时，同时釉质发育不全（EHP）也相当高，Sweeny 等人报告（表 1）EHP 患病率范围在 14% ~ 73%，因此提出某些营养不良可能是EHP的一个主要原因，他们进行的一些研究以及Nikiforuk的研究确认营养不良与 EHP 之间有正相关关系但其发病机制还不很清楚。

Advice for oral health of children and young people

Pregnancy and the neonatal period

Malnutrition and vitamin D

In countries with generally adequate levels of nutrition, nutrition during pregnancy is thought to have little influence on the future dental health of the unborn child. For example, the Health Education Authority in its latest policy document states:

Some teeth are more resistant to attack than others, but there is nothing from the nutritional point of view, fluoride apart, that can be done about this. Contrary to popular belief neither malnutrition in mother during pregnancy, not in the child after birth, is likely to have any appreciable effect on the susceptibility of teeth to decay. Calcium cannot be removed from the mother's teeth by the foetus during pregnancy or due to lactation. Fluoride is the only factor that has been shown, beyond doubt, to decrease susceptibility to decay. The effect of fluoride is due partly to its incorporation into the developing tooth before its eruption into the mouth and partly to its direct contact with the tooth after eruption. The latter is now thought to be the more important.

Certainly the above document is right to emphasie that the post-eruptive effect of sugars in the diet is of paramount importance, but there are sufficient data, reviewed in chapters 2 and 3, to indicate that even in some industrialized countries, nutrition while the teeth are forming is of some relevance.

In areas with high prevalence of malnutrition, enamel formed before birth is adversely affected, with a higher occurrence of hypoplasia, although the severity of hypoplasia is greater in enamel formed neonatally and postnatally () . Dental caries experience is positively related to the presence of enamel hypoplasia and malnutrition, and it is reasonable to assume that some, although probably a small proportion, of these adverse events lead to an increased susceptibility to dental caries.

Since 1970's, the epidemiological studies in some developing nations showed that the prevalence of dental caries was increasing, and at the same time, the prevalence of enamel hypoplasia (EHP) was rather high. Sweeny, Enwonwu and Infante et al reported that prevalence of EHP was ranging from 14 to 73 per cent and then suggested that chronic malnutrition may be a major cause of EHP. Some studies done by them and Nikiforuk identified the positive correlation between malnutrition and EHP but its mechanisms are not very clear.

EHP的患病率从4% ~ 73%在一些国家有很大的差异，在北京为11.4% ~ 22.2%（表2），clarkson等人（1989，1992）报告在英国EHP儿童患病率为10%，有一些发达国家有类似的结果报告，如瑞典5%，美国4%，相比之下，在发展中国家表现出患病率高（11.4%~73%）。在低出生体重儿童以及在出生第一个月有严重营养缺乏的儿童釉质发育缺陷特别普遍。早期研究釉质发育问题与低出生体重儿童，仅集中于EHP，排除了釉质混浊。近来的研究发展到各种类型的釉质发育缺陷（DDE）在正常出生体重儿童与低出生体重（LBW）以及早产儿之间进行比较。表中（3）显示在LBW与早产儿的DDE患病率（20% ~ 79.4%）比正常出生体重儿童（3% ~ 19%）要高。Seow 等（1987）进行的一项有很好对照的研究呈现 LBW 组体重越低，DDE 越高，出生体重为 1500 ~ 2000 克儿童平均 EHP 为 62.3%，而体重在 2500 克以上的对照组为12.7%。1996年郑树国的一项研究（北京）显示LBW与早产儿组（77.3%）比对照组（29.1%）高。

足够的数据证实儿童DDE与LBW之间的相关性，WHO指出出生体重是社区营养的一项重要指标。低出生体重是婴儿存活与健康地生长发育最重要的危险指标，也是个别婴儿所需要的保健水平的一项重要指南，LBW还反映出母亲的不适当的营养与不健康状况，还可能与一定的疾病有关系。

The prevalence of EHP was seen to vary considerably from 4 to 73 per cent and 11.4 to 22.2 per cent in Beijing, China.

表 8-1　Prevalence of EHP in primary dentition of preschool children in some selected countries

Age (yr)	Prev	F in drinking water (ppm)	Index	Country studies	References
2 ~ 3	31 ~ 73	NA	study-specific	Guatemala	Sweeney, et al, 1966
0.5 ~ 4	21	NA	study-specific	Nigeria	Emwonwu, 1973
1 ~ 4	9 ~	0.4	HHI	South Africa	Hargreaves, et al 1989
3	5 ~	NA	study-specific	Sweden	Holm, et al 1974
2 ~ 3	15 ~ 43	NA	study-specific	Sweden	Granhen, et al 1974
1 ~ 5	4 ~ 21	NA	study-specific	USA	Johnsen, et al 1984

表 8-2　Prevalence and distribution of DDE in primary dentition of preschool children in two studies in Beijing, China

Age (yr)	Normal	Opacity			EHP			References
	(0)	(1)	Pits (2)	Diffuse (3)	Linear (4)	Missing Enamel(5)	EHP total	
3 ~ 5	76.1	1.6	5.7	9.3	2.5	4.8	22.2	Li, et al, 1992
2 ~ 6	85.7	1.8	3.1	3.0	0.7	5.3	12.5	Rong,et al,1994

Table Prevalence and distribution of DDE in primary dentition of children in a case-control study in Beijing, China

Age（yr）normal DDE Opacity EHP combination

3-8（EG）** 22.7 77.3 38.1 15.3 23.9

（CG）** 70.9 29.1 12.7 11.4 5.1

*data from X G Zheng, 1996

**eg-experimental group: low birth weight and premature birth

Clarkson and O' Mullane (1989, 1992) reported that the prevalence of EHP among children from UK was 10 per cent, similar results have been reported for some developed countries, such as 5 per cent in Sweden, 4 per cent in USA. In contrast, the prevalence of EHP appeared to be high (11.4 to 73 per

cent) in developing countries, including China. The defects were particularly common among low-birth-weight children and children who experienced severe nutritional deficiency during the first month of life. In the early studies about the links between the prevalence of developmental problems of enamel and low-birth-weight children, it was only concentrated on EHP, excluding opacity of enamel. In recent studies after that time, it was often extended to various types of developmental defects of enamel (DDE) in low-birth-weight (LBW) and premature birth children compared with normal birth weight children. Data listed in Table 14.13 showed that (1) the prevalence of DDE in LBW and premature birth children was higher (20～79.4 per cent) than that in normal birth children (3～19 per cent) , (2) a well controlled study done by Seow et al (1987) appeared that higher DDE was identified in more LBW group, that means EHP was present in 62.3 per cent of children with birth weights of 1500～2000g and 12.7 per cent of control group with birth weights of more than 2500g had the defects.

In 1996, a study was done by XG Zheng in Beijing also showed that the prevalence of DDE was higher (77.3 per cent) in LBW and premature birth children compared with the control group (29.1 per cent) .

Enough data to confirm the correlation between DDE and LBW in children. WHO pointed out in a publication of "development of indicators for monitoring progress towards health for all by the year 2000"(1981) that birth weight can be an important indicator of community nutrition. Low birth weight is the most significant indicator for the risk to the survival of a baby and its healthy growth and development, and is thus an important guide to the level of care needed by individual babies. LBW also reflects inadequate nutrition and ill health of the mother. LBW may also be related to certain diseases.

表 8-3 The prevalence of DDE in LBW and premature birth children by investigators in different time

Investigator/year	LBW**		Very LBW	正常			缺陷
	%	N	%	N	%	N	
Stein, 1936	42	12					EHP***
Stein, 1947	50	16					EHP
Forester et al, 1955	20	34					EHP
Kreshover, 1958	77	35					DDE
Grahonen et al, 1962	21	68			2	60	EHP
Rosenzweig et al, 1962	24	21			1	80	EHP
Grahnen et al, 1974	43	82			15	39	DDE
Funakoshi et al, 1981	27	52					EHP
Mellander et al, 1982	31	91			40	48	DDE
Johnsen et al, 1984			52	67	26	46	DDE
Seow, 1986			79	63			DDE
Pimlott et al,1985			38	106			DDE
Seow et al, 1987	27	33	62	77	13	47	DDE
Fearne et al, 1990	70	50	83	60	37	93	DDE

表 8-4 Summary of strength of evidence linking diet to dental caries

Evidence	Decreased risk	No relationship	Increased risk
Convincing	Fluoride exposure (local and systematic)	Starch intake (cooked and raw starch foods, such as rice, potatoes and bread; excludes cakes, biscuits and snacks with added sugars)	Amount of free sugars Frequency of free sugars
Probable	Hard cheese Sugars-free Chewing gum Xylitol	Whole fresh fruit	
Possible	Milk Dietary Fibre		Undernutrition
Insufficient	Whole fresh fruit		Dried fruits

表 8-4 显示膳食与龋病联系的证据强度

Cockburn等在英国爱丁堡的研究显示在妊娠期间补充维生素D与婴儿低血钙症以及当儿童2～3岁乳牙釉质发育不全的患病率较低有明显的关系。伦敦的一项研究报告了低出生体重儿童与乳牙釉质发育不全的发生有紧密的联系。虽然引起低出生体重的原因并没有确定，营养不良可能是一个因素。这样，有一些证据表明营养缺乏，以及妊娠期间特别是维生素D缺乏能够引起釉质发育不全，因而乳牙列容易患龋。补充维生素 D 对所有怀孕与哺乳妇女都是值得做的。在现有证据的基础上，这看来至少有某些儿童的乳牙列可能看从获益。

The study of Cockburn and others in Edinburgh, UK, showed clear relationships between provision of vitamin D supplements during pregnancy and lower prevalence of hypocalcaemia in infants and lower prevalence of hypoplastic primary teeth when the children were 2-3 years of age. A study in London reported a strong relationship between low birthweight and occurrence of hypoplasia in primary teeth. Although causes of low birthweight were not given, poor nutrition is likely to have been a factor. Thus, there is some evidence that nutritional deficiencies, and vitamin D in particular in pregnancy, can cause enamel hypoplasia and thus predispose to caries in the primary dentition. Vitamin D supplementation remains desirable for all pregnant and lactating women. On present evidence this seems likely to benefit the primary dentition of at least some children.

2. 母亲的口腔健康 Dental health of the mother

在妊娠期间母亲的口腔健康有一些考虑。妊娠性龈炎是一件经过很好证明的事件，具有牙龈充血，水肿，刷牙甚至进食进出血的特点，通过刷牙去除牙石和很好的控制牙菌斑将会大大减少其发生与严重程度。产后会缓解。许多临床试验主要在新西兰进行的，已经报告了妇女用叶酸漱口可以减少妊娠性龈炎，这种治疗，可以称作为局部营养，并没有被广泛采用。

在妊娠期间，饮食习惯能有明显改变，但时间周期可能太短而对龋齿不会产生大的影响。同样地呕吐在妊娠期间作为牙侵蚀症的一个原因并没有看到对牙齿健康有较大的影响，劝阻限制含糖点心的消耗次数对母亲的健康是容易察觉的。

Dental health of the mother

Of some concern is the oral health of the mother during pregnancy. Pregnancy gingivitis is a well recognized event and is characterized by hyperaemia and swollen gingivae which bleed during brushing or even eating. Removal of dental calculus and good plaque control by tooth brushing will do much to reduce its occurrence and severity. Remission occurs post-partum. A number of clinical trials, conducted mainly in New Zealand, have reported reductions in pregnancy gingivitis in women using folate mouth-rinses. This treatment, which may be termed local nutrition, is not used widely.

Dietary habits can change significantly during pregnancy, but the time period is probably too short to have a great impact on dental caries. Likewise, vomiting as a cause of erosion during pregnancy has not been seen as a great threat to dental health. Advice to limit the frequency of consumption of sugar-containing snacks is sensible for the health of the mother.

3. 婴儿与断奶 Infancy and weaning

在婴儿出生后第一年的生命期间，膳食与营养与牙齿健康的关系通过两种方式。第一，牙萌出前的影响-乳牙列继续在颌骨内发育，恒牙列开始钙化。营养不良能够引起釉质发育不全的形成并增加对龋齿的易感性。因此，良好的全身营养对乳恒牙列都有某些意义。在英国推荐婴儿与年幼儿童补充维生素（通过为维生素A、C与D结合在一起）可能对某些儿童未来的口腔与牙齿健康有益；第二，在大约6个月左右，首次牙萌出以及这些新萌出的牙暴露于消耗含糖食物的次数与周期比任何牙萌出前的营养作用都要重要得多。

如果不额外加糖，奶的致龋性很低。口腔专业人员鼓励母乳喂养，因为母乳喂养的婴儿比奶瓶喂养的婴儿龋齿的发生趋势较低，很可能是因为缺少加糖喂养的机会以及用奶瓶喂养含糖的果汁饮料的机会较少。龋病的发生只与处长哺乳期（超过一年）有关，即使如此，也并不常见。

奶瓶装有含糖果汁饮料与龋齿发生之间有密切的联系。最近的一项调查报告，18%的学龄前儿童喝这样的饮料，近40%饮用甜果汁，因此，权威机构反复强调用水取代果汁饲料为儿童解渴。婴儿睡前给予含糖饮料可能特别对牙有伤害，因为睡眠期间唾液流动实际中止。

许多已经证实的人强调在生命的第一年中良好的喂养实践的重要性，在第一年饮食方式确立，这时学习到的行为方式往后很难改变。因为我们对于食物与健康的许多态度与健康是在这个初期社会化期间获得的。因此，这时应开始对孕妇与看护儿童的母亲进行健康教育是必需的。

Infancy and weaning

Diet and nutrition are relevant to dental health during the first year of life in two ways. First, the pre-eruptive effect-the deciduous dentition continues to develop within the jaws and calcification of the permanent dentition begins. Malnutrition can cause the formation of hypoplastic enamel and increase susceptibility to dental caries. Good general nutrition is therefore of some significance to both dentitions. These deficiencies are thought by most people to be only relevant to developing nations, but good data showing that they are irrelevant in developed countries are lacking. Vitamin supplementation (usually a combination of vitamins A, C, and D) is recommended for infants and young children in the UK and is likely to benefit the future oral and dental health of some children.

Second, the first teeth erupt at about 6 months (with considerable variation) and the frequency and duration of exposure of these newly erupted teeth to sugars in foods consumed is very important in determining whether or not they develop caries; this is much more important than any pre-eruptive nutritional effect.

Milk is of very low cariogenicity if extra sugar is not added. The dental profession rightly encourages breastfeeding, as breastfed babies tend to have lower dental caries experience than bottle-fed babies, probably because of the lack of opportunity to add sugar to feeds and the lower use of reservoir feeders and comforters containing sugary fruit-flavoured drinks. The development of dental caries is only associated with breastfeeding when it is prolonged (over 1 year) and on demand and even then, dental caries is uncommon.

The strong relationship between sugar-containing fruit-flavoured drinks used as a comforter in a bottle or reservoir feeder and the development of dental caries. In a recent survey, it was reported that 18 per cent of pre-school children used a dinky or reservoir feeder, from which nearly 40 per cent consumed sweetened juice. Authoritative committees have repeatedly urged that these drinks should not be used as a comforter and that thirsty children will drink water. Giving sugary drinks (or foods) just before the infant or child goes to sleep is likely to be especially damaging because the favourable flow of saliva virtually ceases during sleep. In addition, the importance of good feeding practices in the first year of life has been emphasized by many people who have demonstrated that dietary patterns are established during this first year, and that patterns of behaviour learnt at this time are very resistant to change subsequently. As many of our attitudes and habits concerning food and health are acquired during this period of primary socialization, it is essential that health education should start with pregnant and nursing mothers.

4. 学龄前儿童 The pre-school child

婴儿期的喂养实践对学龄前儿童的龋齿发生有重要影响。不过在 2、3 岁和 4 岁，龋齿会继续发生。在英国 5 岁儿童一半有龋。这个数字保持稳定约有 10 年，在中东、远东新兴的国家 5 岁学龄前儿童的龋齿发生率达 80% 以上。在阿拉伯联合酋长国之一的阿布扎比 1996 年的一项对 5 岁儿童进行的调查表明平均 dmft 为 8.3-1/3 以上的乳牙受到龋的影响。

关于学龄前儿童，糖摄入的数据很少，英国的一项调查，糖占能量摄入的22%。两餐吃点心以及大多数儿童在早晨与中午吃点心是普遍的。

The pre-school child

Feeding practices in infancy have been a major influence on dental caries experience in pre-school children, as emphasized in the previous section. Nevertheless, dental caries continues to occur at the ages of 2, 3, and 4 years. About half of 5 year olds have caries experience in the UK and this figure has remained stable for about 10 years. In the emerging nations of the Middle East and Far East, caries experience in pre-school children is very high with over 80 per cent of 5 year olds affected. In a survey of 5 year olds in Abu Dhabi in 1996, the mean dmft was 8.3-over one third of primary teeth affected by caries.

There are little data on the sugar intake of pre-school children. In one survey in the UK, sugar provided 22 per cent of energy intake. Between-meal snacking is prevalent and most pre-school children have snacks at mid-morning and mid afternoon.

重要的是要认识到学龄前儿童用含氟牙膏刷牙和控制糖消耗对预防龋齿是重要的。尽管实际上，良好的刷牙习惯与饮食习惯同时进行，许多研究显示二者都分别有助于牙齿健康，如果要想使儿童的口腔健康达到最佳，刷牙与膳食都应强调。

It is important to realize that both tooth-brushing with a fluoride-containing toothpaste and sugar control are important in caries prevention in the pre-school child. Although in reality, good tooth-brushing habits and good dietary habits go hand in hand, many studies have shown that both independently contribute to dental heath, and both tooth-brushing and diet should be emphasized if oral health of children is to be optimal.

5. 学龄儿童与青少年 The school child and adolescent

6～12岁之间为“混合牙列”期，乳牙脱落，由恒牙取代。这时膳食糖在口腔内的局部作用是最重要的，但营养的作用也不能完全不考虑。

整个儿童与青少年时期继续通过膳食形式补充氟是重要的是通过饮水。食盐、牛奶还是作为膳食补充，氟被结合到正在形成的恒牙之中，更重要的是为新萌出的恒牙，在它们最容易患龋和仍经历着萌出后的成熟过程时提供局部防龋作用。而其摄入量应是有限的，如果证明有患龋的可能，任何局部用氟均可应用（如含氟牙膏，含漱液，凝胶，涂料）。

5～10岁的学龄儿童膳食方面的资料很少，由于这个年龄阶段难以收集。关于青少年的膳食有很多信息。青少年为快速生长期，独立的食物选择与食物时尚。与成人一样，在英国的儿童与青少年消耗的饮食含脂肪太多（40%的膳食能量取代约35%），淀粉太少，非淀粉多糖（水果与蔬菜），铁与钙也太少，关于青少年的糖摄入有很多资料，所有的糖提供约21%的能量摄入，其中总糖摄入的30%来自内源性与奶糖（即约20%来自水果与蔬菜，奶约10%），其余70%的糖摄入来自非奶的外源性糖。内源性糖与奶糖对牙齿无威胁，是部分有利的食物组（水果，蔬菜与奶制品），应鼓励消耗这些食品。

1991年据英国食品政策医学方面委员会（COMA）报告关于膳食参考值分组的内源性与奶糖与淀粉，推荐这个组应提供大部分膳食能量，另一方面，反复显示非奶的外源性糖是引起龋齿的主要膳食原因，应限制消耗这些食品仅在用餐时间或者偶尔食用。

1/3非奶外源性糖来自糖果，80%以上有4种来源-糖果，餐桌用糖，软饮料以及饼干与糕点。没有一种在营养上是有利的，不仅是糖果是主要的糖来源，第二种是儿童的膳食脂肪。

美国儿童比英国儿童消耗的糖更多，但糖的来源很不一样。英国儿童36%的糖来自糖果与餐桌用糖，18%来自奶与水果，而美国儿童则相反，18%来自糖果与餐桌用糖，31%来自奶与水果。英国儿童进食的糖果为美国儿童的2倍，但来自水果的糖仅为美国儿童的一半，来自奶的则更少。

有多种因素决定我们对食品的选择，如可利用性，价钱，传统，文化，品味与情感。除了一般性减少糖的摄入之外，可以有选择的减少糖摄入包括一周只吃一次糖–“星期六甜食”思想在北欧已有相当大的进步 – 以及用非糖甜味剂取代糖。

The school child and adolescent

Between the ages of 6 and 12 years is the period of the “mixed dentition”-when primary teeth are shed and replaced by their permanent successors. The local intraoral effect of dietary sugars is of greatest importance but the role of nutrition on forming teeth cannot be dismissed completely.

Dietary fluoride continues to be important throughout the years of childhood and adolescence. Whether in drinking water, salt, milk, or as dietary supplements, fluoride is incorportated into permanent teeth which are still forming and, more importantly, provides a topical caries-preventive effect on newly erupted permanent teeth at a time when they are (1) most susceptible to dental decay, and (2) still undergoing post-eruptive maturation. While the amount of fluoride ingested should be limited (so that fluoride dietary supplements are not given in areas with an optimum level of fluoride in the drinking water, for example) , any number of topical fluoride agents (e.g. toothpaste, mouth-rinses, gels, varnishes) can be used, if the risk of dental caries warrants it.

There are little data on the diets of school children aged 5～10 years, partly due to the difficulties of collection at this age, but there is much more information on the diets of adolescents. Adolescence is the time to rapid growth, independent food choices, and food fads. As with adults, children and adolescents in the UK consume diets which contain too much fat (providing about 40 per cent of dietary energy instead of about 35 per cent) and too little starch, non-starch polysaccharides (fruit and vegetables) , iron, and calcium. Fairly comprehensive data are available for sugars intake in adolescent children. All sugars provide bout 21 per cent of energy intake. Of this, 30 per cent comes from intrinsic and milk sugars (i.e. from fruit and vegetables, providing about 20 per cent, and milk, about 10 per cent) of this total sugars intake. The remaining 70 per cent of sugars intake comes from non-milk extrinsic sugars. Intrinsic and milk sugars are not a threat to teeth and are part of desirable food groups (fruit, vegetables, and milk products) : consumption of these foods should be encouraged.

A multitude of factors govern our choice of food, such as availability, costs, traditions, culture, taste, and emotions. Apart from a general reduction in intake, options to reduce intake include eating confectionery at one time in the week only-the "Saturday sweets" idea has made considerable progress in Scandinavia-and substitution of sugars by non-sugar sweeteners.

表8-5 Comparison of the mean daily intake of dietary sugars by 11-12-year-old American and English children

Source	USA		England	
	143 g (24% energy) %		118 g (21% energy) %	
Milk	20	31	13	18
Fruit (excluding juice)	11		5	
Confectionery	8	18	19	36
Table sugar	10		17	
Soft drinks (including juice)		23		14

Not possible to separate data into fresh fruit juices and other soft drinks.

（二）营养、膳食与成人口腔健康 Nutrition, diet, and oral health of adults

现在，我们从复合碳水化合物（淀粉）得到的能量太少，而从脂肪与非奶外源性糖得到的太多。这种情况很适用于成人。1992年英国的COMA发表了老年人的营养，为保持老年人良好的营养状态，包含有21种推荐。随着年龄的增长，锻炼减少，食物能量的摄入也减少。而对营养素的需要不一定随着食物能量的需要减少，这意味着膳食中营养素的密度对老年人来说应是高的。推荐这个年龄组的非奶外源性糖不应超过食物能量的10%的部分理由是确保消耗含糖仪器不减弱膳食的营养密度。然而，报告认识到，限制非奶外源性糖消耗的主要原因是为了控制这个人群的龋齿。现在这些人比过去的人有更多的可能拥有自己的真牙。

1997年英国健康教育当局发表了健康膳食的8点指导方针：

①享受你的食物

②进食各种不同的食物

③进食适量以保持健康的体重

④进食大量富含淀粉与纤维的食物

⑤进食大量水果与蔬菜

⑥不要进食太多含脂肪多的食物

⑦不要太经常进食含糖食品和饮料

⑧如果饮酒，适度饮用

Presently, we get too little of our energy from complex carbohydrates (starches) and too much from fat and non-milk extrinsic sugars. This very much applies to adults. The results of a survey of UK adults, 16 ~ 64 years of age, are given in and indicate, how much diet must change in the UK.

Two other department of Health COMA reports are relevant to this discussion. First, the nutrition of elderly people published in 1992. this contains 21 recommendations for maintaining good nutritional status in the elderly. As exercise decreases with age, food energy intake also decreases. Requirements for nutrients do not necessarily decrease with food energy requirements, which means that the nutrient density of diets for elderly people should be high. Part of the reason for recommending that non-milk extrinsic sugars should be not more than 10 per cent of food energy in this group is to ensure that consumption of sugary foods does not blunt the nutritional density of the diet. The report recognizes, however, that the main reason for restricting consumption of non-milk extrinsic sugars is to control dental caries in this group of people, who are now much more likely to have their own teeth than was the case in the past.

Eight guidelines for a healthy diet was published by the health education authority in 1997. These eight guidelines are given as follows.

① enjoy your food; ② eat a variety of different foods; ③ eat the right amount to be a healthy weight; ④ eat plenty of foods rich in starch and fibre; ⑤ eat plenty of fruit and vegetables; ⑥ don't eat too many foods that contain a lot of fat; ⑦ don't have sugary foods and drinks too often; ⑧ if you drink alcohol, drink sensibly.

1. 成人生活中保存牙列的膳食指导 dietary advice for the preservation of the dentition in adult life

(1) 保存功能牙列的重要性 The importance of preserving a functional dentition

人们希望保留其牙齿有多种原因-美观，功能，感觉牙齿为身体一部分，以及假牙感到自卑。但是，由于牙列缺失使食物选择与营养素摄入受到损害，因此，口腔医生应该鼓励并帮助保留有功能的真牙。需要告诉病人缺少上下咬㕮配对的牙对营养有影响，如果提供固定的或者活动的修复体，这对病人进行膳食指导是很重要的。

Dietary advice for the preservation of the dentition in adult life

The importance of preserving a functional dentition

People wish to retain their teeth for a variety of reasons-aesthetics, function, the feeling that teeth are part of the body, and the perceived inferiority of the artificial substitutes. But, since quality of food choice and nutrient intake are compromised by a poor dentition, dentists should encourage and assist the retention of functional, natural teeth. You need to tell patients of the nutritional impact that loss of occluding pairs of teeth may have. If fixed or removable prostheses are provided, it is very important to give dietary advice to the patient.

（2）糖与龋病 Sugar and dental caries

龋病仍然是对成年人牙齿健康的最大威胁。龋病的膳食原因十分清楚，正如口腔健康教育的科学基础手册所说，减少含糖食品与饮料的消耗，特别是摄入的次数。这对成人与儿童都适用。根龋发生在成年人。根龋的病因十分类似于冠龋，所以预防根龋的膳食指导基本上与预防冠龋是一样的。

生活方式相当大地影响着进食习惯。人们在工作时比在家里有较少的进食小吃的机会，成人口腔健康调查的结果提示妇女的口腔疾病发生比男性要多。但这可能是很好地反映出对牙齿保存的不同态度而不是不同的进食习惯。有无对照的证据表明实际龋的发展发生在工作退休的男性，这是由于有更多空闲的时间而增加了进食小吃。对许多老人来说，在家庭中最温暖的房间经常是厨房，在寒冷的天气，鼓励经常进食。老年人的社会接触经常包括茶和点心，而这样的社会接触对提高生命质量很有利，这样的习惯的膳食含义可能需要在一小部分人群中密切观察。60 ~ 65 岁以上的成年人比 60 ~ 65 岁以下的成年人从非奶外源糖中获得更多的能量。老年家庭妇女比较年轻的家庭妇女有明显的购买较高水平的包装糖的倾向。

由于人们想要更长期地保留自己的真牙，所以与无糖甜味剂的联系增多了。对儿童来说，糖代用品的重点食品是糖果、软饮料、餐桌用糖，以及药物，这些对成人也适合，茶、咖啡与其他热饮料在成年人比软饮料更普遍。用无糖甜味剂取代这些饮料中的糖可能有相当大的益处，特别是许多老人在其生活中有把甜味剂加入到热饮料中的习惯。

Sugar and dental caries

Dental caries is still the biggest threat to teeth in the adult. The dietary cause of caries is quite clear and was discussed in. as the health education authority's booklet The Scientific Basis Of Dental Health Education says, reduce the consumption and especially the frequency of intake of sugar-containing food and drink". This is as applicable to adults as it is to children. Caries of the roots of teeth occurs in adults. The aetiology of root caries is broadly similar to coronal caries, so that dietary advice for the prevention of root caries is essentially the same as for the prevention of coronal caries.

Advice, therefore, should be directed towards reducing both the amount of sugars consumed and the frequency of consumption of sugars. In practice, amount and frequency are likely to be closely correlated so that reduction in one is likely to lead to a reduction in the other.

Lifestyle affects eating habits considerably. People at work may have less opportunity to snack than people at home. Results of surveys of adult dental health have revealed higher dental disease experience in women than men, but this may well be a reflection of different attitudes to tooth preservation rather than different eating habits. There is anecdotal evidence of substantial caries development occurring in men on retirement from work, with the suggestion that this is due to an increase in snacking caused by more spare time. For many older people, the warmest room in the house is often the kitchen, which encourages frequent eating in cold climates. Social contacts for older people often involve tea and biscuits. While such social contacts are very desirable for improving quality of life, the dietary implications of such habits may need to be examined closely in a small proportion of people. Adults over the age of 60～65 years obtain more of their energy from non-milk extrinsic sugars than do those under 60～65 years of age. There is a strong trend towards a higher level of purchase of packaged sugar by older "housewives" than by younger "housewives".

（3）膳食氟与预防牙病 Dietary fluoride and prevention of dental disease

在世界范围内已经实施了把社区水氟浓度调整到最佳水平 - 至少有39个国家的2亿4千万人口在饮用 - 是有效的降低龋的发生平均约一半。大多数研究是调查儿童的氟防龋效果，因为这比较容易在氟化区与缺氟区确定和检查长期生活在那里的年轻人。然而，已经有几项调查显示生活在饮水氟适量的社区的成人牙健康状况相当好。这同时用于预防冠龋与根面龋，观察主要集中在这两种病损的共同病因学方面。

到目前为止能够看得到的在成人中还没有其他形式的膳食氟防龋作用的报告-氟片剂，食盐或牛奶。与饮水氟化相比而言，这些途径用作为公共卫生措施还是相对近年来的事，并且不太复杂。氟化物已局部应用（在口腔局部）预防成人龋齿的发生取得了相当大的成功。

Dietary fluoride and prevention of dental disease

Adjustment of the concentration of fluoride in drinking water to the optimum for that community has been implemented world wide-in at least 39 countries reaching at least 210 million people-and is effective-reducing caries experience by about half on average. Most studies have investigated the effectiveness of fluoride in children, since it is easier to identify and examine lifelong residents of a young age in fluoridated and fluoride-deficient communities. Nevertheless, there have been several surveys which have shown that the dental health of adults is considerably better when they have lived in communities with optimum amounts of fluoride in drinking water. This applies to both coronal and root surface caries, an observation which highlights the common aetiology of these two types of lesions.

As far as can be seen, there are no reports of the caries-preventive effect of other forms of dietary fluoride-tables, salt, or milk-in adults, but it must be appreciated that these have been used on a public health basis only comparatively recently and investigated much less comprehensively, compared with water fluoridation. Fluoride has been used topically (locally in the mouth) to prevent dental caries in adults with considerable success.

（4）营养与牙周病 Nutrition and periodontal disease

营养缺乏影响到人类牙周病的发生或进展的证据很少。牙周病及其先兆，牙龈炎的最重要的病因，预防与治疗的因素是控制牙菌斑，就总体而言，当营养适当时，牙周组织将会得益，但膳食补充像上述已经接受的一般水平看来不会进一步改善牙周健康。正在出现的证据是用叶酸漱口在牙龈组织可能缺乏叶酸的情况下，可以有益于控制牙龈炎。(如妊娠期间或者苯妥英治疗癫痫)，但是广泛地开出叶酸处方用于预防和控制牙龈炎还不到时候。

坏血病是仅有的主要影响到牙周组织的疾病，现在很少见，但是病人有脆弱的口腔或者牙龈出血水肿应该有所怀疑。老年男子独自生活似乎有最大的危险。维生素C治疗可以使疾病很快恢复正常。

牙槽骨在支持牙齿方面，当牙缺失之后它们的存在，支持义齿都是重要的。在动物实验已经显示钙与维生素D缺乏可以加速牙周破坏，但是在人的证据要少得多。在存在缺乏的地方，膳食指导恢复摄入适当的水平是明智的。因为这一般对骨骼有益，包括牙槽骨。当膳食已经适当时，补充就没有正当理由。

有些研究已经报告，居住在饮水供应适当氟水平的社区的人比居住在低氟工的人牙周破坏较少。氟化物已用于治疗一般性骨质疏松症，虽然其效果并不是普遍接受的。

Nutrition and periodontal disease

The main conclusion from the review of this subject in was that there is little evidence that nutritional deficiencies affect the occurrence or progression of periodontal disease in humans. The overriding factor in the cause, prevention, and treatment of periodontal disease and its precursor, gingivitis, is control of dental plaque. Overall, periodontal tissues will benefit when nutrition is adequate but dietary supplementation above what is commonly accepted as adequate levels does not seem to improve periodontal health further. Evidence is emerging that folate mouth-rinses may be beneficial in the control of gingivitis in circumstances where the gingival tissues may be folate-deficient (e.g. in pregnancy or phenytoin therapy) but widespread prescription of folate for the prevention and control of gingivitis is premature.

Scurvy is the only deficiency disease in which the periodontal tissues are primarily affected. It is now rare, but should be suspected in patients with a tender mouth or bleeding swollen gums: elderly men living on their own seem to be at greatest risk. Regression of the disease rapidly follows vitamin C therapy.

The alveolar bone is important in supporting teeth when they are present and for supporting dentures after teeth are lost. Calcium and vitamin D deficiencies have been shown in animal experiments to accelerate periodontal destruction but there is much less evidence in humans. Where deficiencies exist, dietary advice to restore intake to adequate levels is sensible, as this will benefit the skeleton in general, including dental alveolar bone. Supplementation when the diet is already adequate is not warranted.

Some studies have reported less periodontal destruction in residents of communities with adequate levels of fluoride in drinking water supplies than in residents of low-fluoride areas. Fluoride has been used in treatment of general osteoporosis, although its effectiveness is not universally accepted.

（三）对老年人的指导 Advice for elderly people

老年人对食物的选择有许多影响因素，当对全身与口腔健康进行营养指导时必须考虑到这些因素（见表8-6）。关于牙在营养中的价值，一般的结论是缺少真牙影响到咀嚼能力与食物选择。虽然在牙列不完整的人非淀粉多糖的消耗是低的，但是营养受到影响的直接证据较少。在老年人中看到的能量摄入，铁（来自肉食），维生素C与钙的减少如同其他危险的营养素一样。不完整牙列影响全身健康的直接证据很少，但这可能是由于难以支持所需要的复杂的纵向研究，如果因为牙不好而减少了水果与蔬菜的消耗，增加了全身健康的危险，这种假设是合理的。

为了防止老年人噎塞食物的危险，需要指导在入口之前切碎食物的重要性以及在吞咽之前，花费时间咀嚼食物。

Advice for elderly people

A large number of factors influence food choice in elderly people and these must be considered when advising on nutrition for general and oral health. these are listed in Table 8-6.

About the value of teeth in nutrition, the general conclusions were that lack of natural teeth affects ability to chew and food choice. There was less direct evidence that nutrition was affected, although consumption of non-starch polysaccharides is low in those with impaired dentitions. Reduced energy intake and iron (from meats), vitamin C, and calcium were seen as other risk nutrients in elderly people. There is very little direct evidence that an impaired dentition affects general health but this could be due to the difficulty in mounting the required comprehensive longitudinal studies. It is reasonable to assume that if consumption of fruits and vegetables is reduced because of poor teeth, general health is at increased risk.

表 8-6　Some factors influencing food intake and nutrition in older people

Factor	Effect
Economic	Choice of foods Cooking facilities Transport to shops
Social	Living alone Housebound Bereavement
Psychosocial-patient behaviour	Senility Depression Psychosis Unadaptability Alcohol consumption
Psychosocial-society behaviour	Retirement and nursing homes Home helps
Physiological and pathological	Changes in gastrointestinal function Impaired taste and smell Impaired function of heart, lungs, and kidneys Arthritis and immobility Diabetes mellitus

续表

Factor	Effect
Interaction of drugs with nutrients	Poor dentition Hyposalivation Changes in absorption Changes in metabolism

In order to prevent the hazard of choking on food in the elderly people, they need to be advised of the importance of cutting up food before putting it in the mouth and for taking time to chew foods before swallowing.

唾液是口腔软硬组织的主要保护者，当唾液流动减少时，进食享受较少可能感到不舒服，吞咽食团可能会有困难，认为唾液流率随年龄减少，但这不是一种简单的关系，在健康的老人唾液流率实际上并不减少，但是健康状况不佳的人比较低，到50岁大约有20%，老年人申诉口干的有40%。

唾液分泌过少或口干症的首要征兆常常是想不到的龋齿增多，其他症状包括需要饮水，讲话，进食与吞咽困难，戴义齿困难，口角裂纹，与舌裂沟有关的烧灼感以及味觉改变。在理论上测量唾液流动容易进行，但实际上需要相当小心，因为精神因素（如忧虑，照明度）能相当大地影响到唾液的收集量，测量总体唾液流动一般有用，虽然在某些情况下记录一种腺体的流动是易行和必要的。

有多种疾病或状况引起涎腺功能不良。最重要的是药物，射线，器质性疾病，精神紊乱以及减少咀嚼。这些情况常发生于老年人，所以并不奇怪涎腺功能不良在这些年龄组是普遍的。大量的药物引起涎腺功能不良，通常这些药物并不长期损伤腺体，如果药物治疗停止，唾液流动回复到近乎正常。涎腺对射线敏感，随着明显的射线用于治疗口腔肿物就会出现严重的不过逆转的功能不良。破坏涎腺组织是许多自动免疫性疾病的一种特征，包括舍古林综合征，风湿性关节炎。抑郁症与焦虑可以促进涎腺功能不良，常常是由于使用了三环抗抑郁药物治疗这些紊乱伴随着明显的口干副作用。废弃性萎缩影响到涎腺与影响其他组织一样。

虽然疾病能够引起萎缩，但是咀嚼能够增加涎腺的体积并增加唾液流动。这样，推荐需要咀嚼的食物可能是为了增进口腔健康，不仅是当咀嚼食物时引起唾液的大量的流动而且增强了腺体对未来刺激的反应能力，这是一个重要的原因推荐咀嚼无糖口香糖。

患有涎腺功能不良或口干症的人倾向于小口吸饮液体为了减轻其不舒适的感觉，可以推荐牛奶作为一种唾液替代品，除牛奶外，人工唾液的种类可分成三组-甘油与柠檬，那些依据羧甲基纤维素以及那些依据粘液素，甘油与柠檬是最简单的一种，但是如果有真牙存在，有可能受到侵蚀，另外，甘油是收敛剂并且可以“刺激”软组织。以粘液素为基础的人工唾液有最佳的特性，并且在许多国家商业上都有这类产品，通常人的唾液取一小杯作漱口或都作喷雾。某些唾液代用品是依据猪的产品，这对素食者或某些宗教信徒使用受到限制。

老年人应用药物治疗增加，老年人用多种药品普遍，约40%的老人至少每天用一种药物治疗，据报告70岁以上的老人每年接受平均20种处方，已经提到这有两种影响：第一，许多药物抑制唾液分泌，增加口腔疾病发生的危险；第二，某些药物含糖，特别是液体口服用药，老年人更偏爱。这就指出获得完整病史的重要性，包括病人用药。没有医生同意不应改变用药，但可以有机会指导病人要求或选择无糖药品。

口腔是身体的镜子，许多系统疾病在口腔有表征，这些主要是营养缺乏性疾病。口腔医生应很好的认识这些病损，指导病人，如果必要，转诊病人接受进一步治疗。这样就指出全面检查口腔黏膜，唇及口腔周围组织的重要性。

另一个作全面系统地口腔黏膜检查的原因是口腔医生可能是首先观察，认识口腔癌或者癌前病变。关于预防口腔癌的膳食信息十分清楚-避免过多酒精消耗（与吸烟），进食新鲜水果与蔬菜。同时考虑改变的效果，减少吸烟与酒消耗比增加水果与蔬菜消耗更重要。

口腔医生作为广泛的健康的一部分，应该利用适当的机会传递这些重要的健康促进信息，然而更多的是改变成人的进食习惯，尤其是老年人，比仅给予指导更为重要。

Saliva is the principal protector of the hard and soft tissues. When salivary flow is diminished, eating is less enjoyable and can be uncomfortable; swallowing a bolus of food can be difficult. Salivary flow rate is thought to decrease with age but this is not a simple relationship. Flow rate is virtually undiminished in healthy elderly people, but is lower in those who are not in good health. About 20 per cent of people up to 50 years of age and 40 per cent of elderly people complain of a dry mouth.

The first sign of hyposalivation or xerostomia (dry mouth) is often an unexpected increase in dental caries. Other symptoms include the need to drink water; difficulty with speech, eating, and swallowing; difficulty with dentures; cracking at the corners of the mouth; a burning sensation on the tongue associated with fissuring of the tongue; and alteration of taste. Measurement of salivary flow is easy in theory but in practice needs considerable care, since psychic factors (e.g. apprehension, degree of lighting) can influence considerably the amount of saliva collected. Measurement of total salivary flow is generally useful, although recording flow from one gland is feasible and necessary in some circumstances.

Hypofunction of the salivary glands is caused by a number of diseases or conditions, the most important being drugs, irradiation, organic diseases, psychological disorders, and decreased chewing. These often occur in elderly people so it is not surprising that hyposalivation is prevalent in these age groups. A large number of drugs cause salivary hypofunction, as can be seen in box. Usually these drugs do not permanently damage the glands and salivary flow returns to near normal if the drug therapy is stopped. Salivary glands are sensitive to irradiation and severe irreversible hypofunction follows significant irradiation used to treat oral neoplasms. Destruction of the salivary gland tissues is a feature of many autoimmune diseases, including Sjogren's syndrome and rheumatoid arthritis. Depression and anxiety may contribute to hyposalivation which is often compounded by the powerful xerostomic effect of tricyclic antidepressant drugs used to treat these disorders. Disuse atrophy affects the salivary glands as it does other tissues.

While disease can cause atrophy, chewing can increase the size of salivary glands and increase salivary flow. Thus, recommending foods which require chewing is likely to improve oral health, not only by causing a strong flow of saliva while food is chewed but also improving the ability of glands to respond to future stimuli. This is an important reason for recommending chewing sugarless gum.

People suffering from hyposalivation or xerostomia tend to sip liquids to alleviate their discomfort. Milk can be recommended as a salivary substitute. Types artificial saliva, apart from milk, fall into three groups-glycerine and lemon, those based on carboxymethycellulose, and those based on mucin.

Glycerine and lemon is the simplest but, if natural teeth are present, is potentially erosive. In addition, glycerine is astringent and may 'sting' the soft tissues. Mucin-based artificial salivas have the best properties and are commercially available in many countries. Artificial saliva is usually taken from a small cup as a mouthwash or as a spray. Some saliva substitutes are based on pig products and are thus contraindicated in vegetarians and people of some religions.

第二节　营养与口腔疾病
Section 2 Nutrition and Oral Diseases

一、膳食与龋病 Diet and dental caries

（一）牙萌出前的影响

在牙正在形成与发育尚未萌出的阶段，营养对牙的影响主要是改变牙的抗龋或易感龋的化学成分，如牙内葡糖蛋白含量增加，易被有害微生物所利用，使牙结构脆弱，容易产生早期龋坏。还有因营养不良或感染而导致的釉质发育缺陷，增加了龋的易感性（图8-2），我国的一些研究显示有釉质发育缺陷的儿童，乳牙患龋率与龋均分别比无釉质发育缺陷的儿童高出 15% 及 1.5。(表 8-7)。

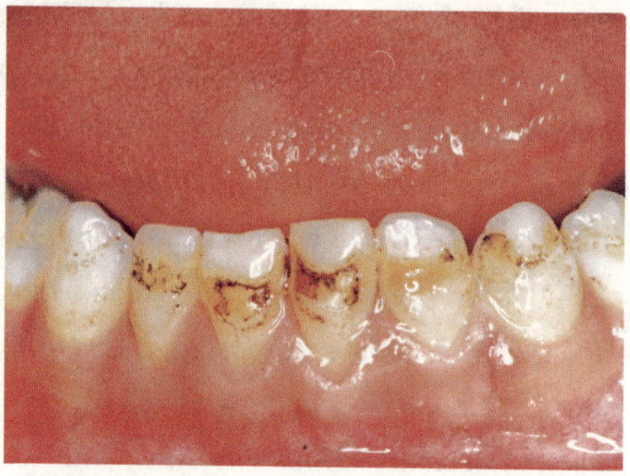

图 8-2

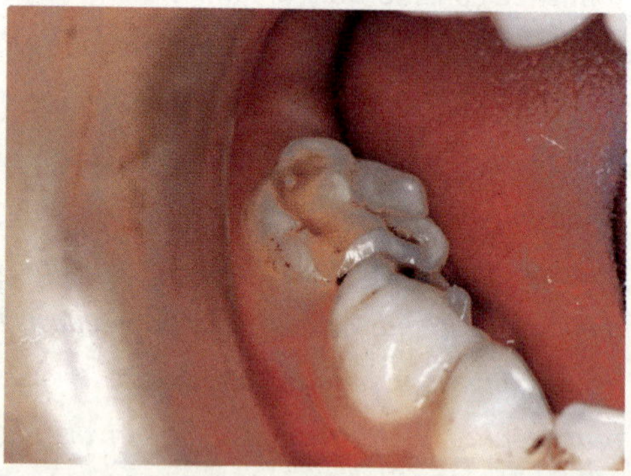

图 8-3

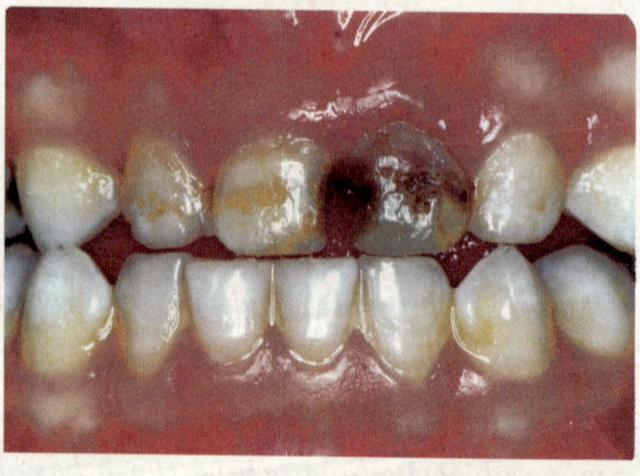

图 8-4

Enamel hypoplasia and dental caries

Caries is a multifactorial disease which cannot have one cause. Disease only occurs when the right combination of disease determinants coincides with host susceptibility and in the right environment. The anatomic characteristics of the teeth and a susceptible host, are essential factors for the initiation and progress of dental caries.

Experimental studies by animal models have demonstrated that under a chronic malnutrition status, enamel calcification will not be completed and the maturation will be delayed, as well as the time of eruption of the teeth. Until now, only a few studies have been done, and it appears that EHP is a possible predisposing factor for dental caries. A study done in rural undernourished Guatemala population showed that children with linear EHP had two to six times more dental caries than those who did not. The significantly higher prevalence of dental caries was shown even in the posterior hypolasia-

free teeth among children with EHP in the anterior teeth versus children without EHP. Distinctive tooth morphology irregularity and enamel defects may be important factor indirectly related to tooth susceptibility to dental caries.

A strong association between EHP and caries experience was observed in two Chinese studies (Table). Differences in mean decayed teeth and surfaces were seen in these studies not only between the children with or without EHP, but also among children with different enamel defect scores. The higher scores, the more caries the children experienced. It was also found in two studies that children who had EHP on their anterior teeth also had significantly more caries appearing on their posterior teeth compared with children who are EHP-free.

表 8-7 Comparison of caries prevalence and mean dmft and dmfs in chinese children with or without EHP

Concentrations of MS in saliva by categories*								
	Total		Caries		dmft		dmfs	
	n	%	n	%	mean	SD	mean	SD
Li (1992)								
DDE+	321	22.3	298	92.8	7.8	4.6	16.9	13.6
DDE-	1045	77.7	808	79.0	4.8	4.4	9.2	10.0
Rong（1994）								
DDE+	153	14.3	136	88.9	5.9	4.46	16.18	15.75
DDE-	921	79.3	703	76.3	4.54	4.22	11.96	13.58

（二）牙萌出后的影响

碳水化物食品与牙菌斑细菌在牙釉质表面的密切接触是发生龋病的先决条件。

通过膳食中糖的氧代谢，牙菌斑细菌形成的有机酸使釉质、牙本质脱矿而发生龋病。有机酸增加牙体组织羟磷灰石中钙的溶解度及脱矿化作用的发生。唾液的pH值为7时，钙、磷达到过饱和状态，促进再矿化作用。如果口腔pH值能保持充分时间的高水平。那么，可以产生釉质的完全再矿化作用。如果口腔pH值能保持充分时间的高水平。那么，可以产生釉质的完全再矿化作用；如果酸的作用太强，则脱矿化作用占优势，釉质变为更多孔状，直至最后形成龋损。龋的发生需要有糖和细菌的存在，但是受到牙易感性，细菌种类与分布，唾液的量和质的影响。

1. 细菌对龋病发病的必需性

研究证实细菌的存在是龋发生所必需的。无菌条件下喂养致龋膳食，不会发生龋坏。

2. 牙面接触食物的必要性

碳水化物必须与牙面接触才能产生龋坏，食物与牙面接触是必要条件。

3. 碳水化物对龋病发病的重要性

碳水化物是致龋膳食的基本营养成分。实验表明，蔗糖是龋病开始的必要条件。

4. 比较不同碳水化物的致龋性

动物实验与人群观察都证实，与其他碳水化物比较，如葡萄糖、果糖、麦芽糖、乳糖或淀粉、蔗糖的龋活性高，龋的发病率也较高。但是，其他糖类的致龋性也很强。因此，不能误认为其他糖类取代蔗糖就可以减少龋的发生。

膳食与营养对龋病发病的影响比较复杂，除碳水化物外，蛋白质、维生素D、钙与磷等许多营养成分还有膳食中的氟化物水平，对龋病发病都有一定的影响。

虽然牙萌出前膳食对龋病的影响比牙萌出后的影响要少得多，但维生素D、A、蛋白质-能量营养不良与釉质发育不良，涎腺肥大（即减少口腔缓冲菌斑酸的能力）使牙更易感龋。发展中国家膳食中糖缺乏，营养不足与龋无关。但营养不足与糖摄入量高，可以加重龋的危险。

Caries development

In humans is determined principally by a combination of the following factors:

1.tooth morphology and space relationships of the dentition.

2. structure and composition of enamel.

3. structure and composition of dentin.

4. fluoride status (available concentration in oral fluids, plaque, and in external layers of enamel).

5. presence of a virulent cariogenic strain of bacteria in dental plaque.

6. oral hygiene status.

7. type, amount, and frequency of exposure to fermentable dietary carbohydrates.

8. salivary (flow rate and composition, including minerals, proteins, and immunoglobulin) and gingival fluids.

Each of these factors can influence the caries susceptibility of individuals to make them either highly resistant or highly susceptible.

Diet is highly influential in caries development and can act preeruptively, as described for mineral, protein, and vitamin A malnutrition, or posteruptively by enhancing the implantation and metabolic activity of cariogenic microorganisms. This posteruptive influence of diet can be overwhelming and capable of determining rampant caries despite the beneficial effects that may have been contributed preeruptively. Additionally, some malnourished populations consume foods with high caries potential infrequently and in small quantities, in contrast to the nibbling eating pattern that is customary in some affluent countries. These underfed populations may lack adequate nutrition during tooth formation, but they also lack the cariogenic challenge that is necessary for the disease to develop. Therefore, their dental caries prevalence is low. It is only upon exposure to cariogenic conditions that their teeth seem to "melt" under such undue stress.

Types of study providing evidence for the relationship between diet and caries development

The evidence comes from a number of types of investigation. Each of these gives useful information but it would be wrong to give equal weight to each type of study. The best evidence comes from studies of the occurrence of dental caries in human populations in relation to their diet. These studies can either be observational (epidemiological) studies, in which the relationships between disease and possible causative and confounding factors are observed, or interventional studies in which diets of groups of people are purposefully altered and the effect of this intervention observed. Interventional studies are often known as clinical trials and are rightly taken as the best source of evidence. They are, however, the most difficult to undertake, as large groups of people have to adhere to strict diets for a long enough time for the effect on dental caries increment to be observed. Observational studies are the second best source of evidence and form the largest group. A problem with such studies is that the presence of confounding factors can mask the true effect.

The third source of evidence comes from animal studies. Aspects of diet, such as sugar content, frequency of feeding, and content of diet other than sugar can be controlled, and the total experimental period is short. The disadvantages of rodent experiments lie mainly in the difficulties of extrapolating the findings to humans. The fourth method has become known as enamel slab experiments. These observe the effects of diet on demineralization in slabs of enamel (cut from extracted teeth) which are held in the mouth of human volunteers in a removable plate constructed like an orthodontic appliance. The fifth type of experiment investigates the effects of foods, meals, or component of foods on the pH of dental plaque. These studies are relatively easy to do, but they measure the 'acidogenicity' of diet rather than 'cariogenicity' and, as such, are only an indication of the possible effect of diet on the development of dental caries. The sixth and final method is the simplest but weakest method: test foods are incubated with plaque or saliva (which contains plaque organisms) and the rate of acid production is recorded. In some experiments, whole enamel, powdered enamel, or calcium phosphate are added to the saliva/substrate mixture and the rate of dissolution of mineral is taken as a measure of cariogenic potential.

Evidence from all these sources will be used to indicate relevant aspects of cariogenicity of foods and the strengths and drawbacks of each type of evidence needs to borne in mind.

膳食糖与龋危险性之间关联的证据强度是多样性研究而不是单项研究的功效。通过干预性研究提供了高强度的证据。但这些研究的弱点是它们是在氟化物时代之间作出的结论。最近的研究也显示出一种关系，糖摄入与龋齿的关系虽然不如氟化物时代以前强，但是许多发展中国家还没有受益于氟化物的暴露。

暴露于氟化物（在饮水氟浓度至 0.7 ～ 1ppm，或者含氟牙膏占有市场 90% 以上的地方）提高了糖消耗的安全水平。

最好的证据表明，单糖消耗每人每年在15～20公斤以下，龋发病处于水平，即相当于每人每天摄入量为40 ～ 55克，其值相当于能量摄入的6% ～ 10%。特别重要的是在单糖消耗水平低于每人每年 15 ～ 20kg 的国家不要增加糖的消耗水平。

除了单糖的摄入量之外，其摄入频数也很重要。不论是含糖食品还是饮料的消耗频数应限制在最多每天为 4 次。

现在许多国家正经历着营养转变，而没有适当的氟化物暴露，应通过适当的载体，例如可负担得起的牙膏，饮水，食盐与牛奶，促进适当的氟化物暴露。确保实施可行的氟化物项目是国家卫生行政领导的责任。应鼓励研究可供选择的社区氟化物防龋项目。

Strength of evidence

The strength of the evidence linking dietary sugars to the risk of dental caries is in the multiplicity of the studies rather than the power of any individual study. Strong evidence is provided by the intervention studies (50, 51) but the weakness of these studies is that they were conducted in the pre-

fluoride era. More recent studies also show an association between sugars intake and dental caries albeit not as strong as in the prefluoride era. However, in many developing countries people are not yet exposed to the benefits of fluoride.

It is important to set a recommended maximum level for the consumption of free sugars; a low free sugars consumption by a population will translate into a low level of dental caries. Population goals enable the oral health risks of populations to be assessed and health promotion goals monitored.

The best available evidence indicates that the level of dental caries is low in countries where the consumption of free sugars is below 15～20 kg per person per year. This is equivalent to a daily intake of 40 ～ 55g per person and the values equate to 6% ～ 10% of energy intake. It is of particular importance that countries which currently have low consumption of free sugars (＜ 15 ～ 20kg per person per year) do not increase consumption levels. For countries with high consumption levels it is recommended that national health authorities and decision-makers formulate country-specific and community-specific goals for reduction in the amount of free sugars, aiming towards the recommended maximum of no more than 10% of energy intake.

In addition to population targets given in terms of the amount of free sugars, targets for the frequency of free sugars consumption are also important. The frequency of consumption of foods and/or drinks containing free sugars should be limited to a maximum of four times per day.

Many countries that are currently undergoing nutrition transition do not have adequate exposure to fluoride. There should be promotion of adequate fluoride exposure via appropriate vehicles, for example, affordable toothpaste, water, salt and milk. It is the responsibility of national health authorities to ensure implementation of feasible fluoride programmes for their country. Research into the outcome of alternative community fluoride programmes should be encouraged.

二、营养与牙周病 Nutrition and periodontal disease

牙周病很可能是与人的关系最为密切的疾病。50年前口腔医学家们记录了围绕无龋牙列周围支持组织的破坏，提出了营养缺乏的问题。由于观察到牙周病在营养不良的不发达国家呈现最为严重，这种看法得到了激励。于是早在50年代后期美国营养与国防部门委员会做过一次最大的流行病学调查，涉及8个国家22000人（5岁以上的人群）。所有国家的调查资料表明，牙菌斑量和年龄与牙周病的严重程度高度相关。事实上，这二个因素可以解释这些人群中90%牙周病的严重性存在的差异。只发现与牙周病严重性密切相关的营养素是血浆维生素A（不一定是维生素A缺乏的一个好指标）。这一发现与在其他国家看到的情况并不一致。几年后在世界卫生组织指导下进行了另一项重要的流行病学调查，先后在斯里兰卡与挪威调查了13岁至65岁以上5000多名男性和近3000名女性，调查牙周病与维生素A和B缺乏与否的关系。与上述第一次世界范围的调查一样，发现牙周病与口腔卫生水平（菌斑程度）密切相关。维生素A缺乏的临床表现与牙周病的严重程度无关联。相比之下，维生素B缺乏的临床表现与牙周病的分值较高有关。当口腔卫生差时，这种关联程度要强得多。

斯里兰卡人群的牙周病比挪威人群更严重，但这完全可以用斯里兰卡人群的菌斑水平较高来解释。从流行病学的观点看，菌斑量与年龄作为牙周病的决定因素似乎更重要。这些有限的流行病学资料不足以提供全面情况。有三点可以肯定，首先是牙周病发展很缓慢，在短期内任何营养评价可能是有限的，并不能反映一生的营养状况；第二，在少数人营养缺乏可能与牙周病密切相关，但这些情况很少见，在人群调查中看不到这些关系。第三，评估营养状态的有效方法难以用于流行病学的研究。

这样，是否营养不良刺激牙周破坏仍然不能肯定。但是重要的信息是围绕龈缘菌斑的特续存在，一般说来是牙周病最重要的原因。各种营养要素对牙周病的作用已经发表了许多研究文章。看来，维生素A，B，D，E或钙，不可能对人的牙周病有任何重要影响。叶酸（folic acid）通常归性维生素B族，已提出用于牙周病治疗。人类临床试验有些证据支持这一点。叶酸在DNA全成中是重要的。具有高细胞转化率的组织最可能受到叶酸缺乏的相反影响。细胞转化率在龈沟上皮特别高，使这些组织特别脆弱，易受伤害，削弱了这一上皮层作为细菌入侵的屏障功能的能力。

许多临床试验已经报告了全身与局部应用叶酸的有益效果。有一项临床试验，病人用5mg叶酸5ml每天漱口2次，与对照组比较，4周后牙龈炎显著减轻。妊娠期间，牙龈组织对菌斑能显示一种增大血管反应。提出这种反应可能是由于末端组织缺乏叶酸有关。检验这一假设，30名孕妇随机分为3组，A组接受安慰剂漱口并吸服用安慰剂片，B组用安慰剂漱口并每天吸叶酸片，C组用叶酸漱口与服用安慰剂片。补充妊娠4个月与8个月期间的最后14天，用叶酸漱口而不是服用叶酸片剂，使牙龈健康有显著改善。在第8个月期间的28天补充叶酸漱口得到类似的结果。用叶酸漱口使牙龈健康有明显改善。这些结果确信，末端组织缺乏叶酸的假设。

Periodontal disease is probably man's most prevalent disease-dental caries and periodontal disease vie for this dubious honour. Few escape the destruction of tissues surrounding their teeth. But the severity of periodontal disease varies between areas of the world seemingly quite independently of the prevalence of dental caries. In fact, it was the observations by dental scientists, 50 years ago, who recorded destruction of the supporting tissues around caries-free dentitions, which led to suggestions that nutritional deficiencies were to blame This view was encouraged by the observation that periodontal disease appeared to be most severe in underdeveloped countries where malnutrition was expected to be most prevalent.

A few years later, another important epidemiological study was undertaken under the auspices of the Would Health Organization-first in Sri Lanka and then in Norway. A total of over 5000 males and nearly 3000 females aged 13 to over 60 years were examined for both periodontal disease and the presence or absence of vitamins A and B deficiency. As in the above worldwide study, periodontal disease was found to be strongly related to levels of oral hygiene (extent of plaque) and age. Clinical signs of vitamin A deficiency were not associated with severity of periodontal disease, unlike in the extensive studies mentioned above where serum vitamin A levels were associated, but inconsistently, with periodontal disease. On the contrary, clinical signs of vitamin B deficiency were associated with higher periodontal disease scores and this association was stronger when the level of oral hygiene was poor.

These limited epidemiological data may not provide the complete picture as both these studies were of cross-sectional design. Three points are relevant. First it must be remembered that periodontal disease develops very slowly and that any nutritional evaluation is likely to have been limited to a short period and may not reflect lifetime nutritional status. Second, nutritional deficiencies could be strongly related to periodontal disease in a few individuals but these occur so rarely that these relationships are not detected in population surveys. Third, valid methods of estimating nutritional status are difficult to apply in epidemiological studies which are often carried out under difficult field conditions.

In summary, there is little evidence at present for on association between diet and periodontal disease. Current research is investigating the potential role of the antioxidant nutrients in periodontal disease. There is some evidence to suggest that periodontal disease progress more rapidly in maintaining on adequate host immune response may explain this observation. There is little evidence to indicate that the nutritional deficiencies will influence the occurrence and development of periodontal disease. Overall, periodontal tissues will benefit when nutrition is adequate, but dietary supplement of nutrients does not seem to improve periodontal health further (Table 8-8).

表 8-8　Summary of strength of evidence linking diet to periodontal disease

Evidence	Decreased risk	No relationship	Increased risk
Convincing	Good oral hygiene		Deficiency of vitamin C
Probable			undernutrition
Possible			
insufficient	Antioxidant nutrients	Vitamin E supplementation	Sucrose

Based on: McLaren D S (1992) Diet related disorders

在有些病人维生素C是明确与牙周病有关的一种营养素。维生素C缺乏导致坏血病，一种明显的牙龈肿胀，出血的症状。适当补充维生素C可用于预防和治疗。维生素C有两种代谢功能，但最重要的是它对胶原合成的关键作用。这不仅关系到组织的保持，如牙周韧带（原则上由胶原纤维组成），而且对骨基质的民保持血管壁的完整。

坏血病并不常见，只在用“面包与茶”膳食的老人可见，偶见于饮用加热牛奶的婴儿。

大多数流行病学研究试图证实抗坏血酸与牙周病之间的关系并没有成功，高于膳食标准的推荐量看来并没有与较好的牙周健康有关系。临床试验的结果并不支持大剂量应用维生素 C。

总之，现在很少有证据表明膳食与牙周病的关系，现在的研究在调查抗氧化营养素对牙周病的可能作用。有些证据提出在营养差的人口中，牙周病进展较快，营养在维持宿主免疫反应中的重要作用可以解释这一观察。很少有证据表明营养缺额影响人的牙周病的发生与发展。营养适当对牙周组织有益，但是营养补充对增进牙周健康并不明显。

三、营养与口腔黏膜病 Nutrition and the oral mucosa diseases

口腔黏膜是机体与外界接触的屏障，对外界各种反应灵敏，极易受损伤，又恢复很快。新陈代谢快，对营养缺乏反应敏感，尤其是维生素缺乏，如B族维生素（B_1、B_2、B_{12}），维生素A，叶酸，维生素C，还有缺铁性贫血，可引起许多类似的口腔表现，例如，口有炎或口角裂纹，唇炎，舌炎，牙龈炎。还伴随着许多口腔症状，如口腔黏膜充血、红肿、烧灼感、感觉过敏、疼痛、舌水肿、舌乳头肿大或萎缩，甚至出现口腔疱疹、舌溃疡、吞咽困难等。维生素B_1缺乏还可引起口腔颌面部神经炎。维生素 A 缺乏可表现为口腔白斑。

There are two major reasons for the relatively great sensitivity of the oral mucosa to physiological or anatomical changes resulting from nutritional deficiencies.

1. the oral epithelial cells probably grown and are replaced rapidly than all other cells in the body. This means that DNA, RNA and the formation of proteins which contribute to tissue synthesis and cellular turnover in the oral mucosa are extremely rapid. Therefore, intake of appropriate foods of suitable nutrient density in adequate amounts is needed daily.

2. a healthy oral epithelium can act as an effective barrier against the invasion of toxic substances into the underlying collagenous connective tissue. But this property of protection can be easily compromised by nutritional deficiency, e.g., vitamin C deficiency. In fact inadequate nourishment can cause the oral epithelium to breakdown and become infected readily which may manifest itself as an oral ulceration.

Oral tissues can undergo three major changes as reactions to a nutritional deficiency, an irritant or a change in the oral cavity. They can change functionally, anatomically and by colour.

A functional change noted in the mouth is the burning sensation caused by irritation of the nerves in the tongue or the roof of the mouth. The sensation maybe nonspecific because it may be a manifestation of a nutritional deficiency, uncontrolled diabetes or an allergy.

In contrast with the functional changes which may be reversed within a few days after the basic dietary deficiency or insufficiency has been corrected, the anatomical changes for chronic disturbances can exist for weeks or even for months. The time factor is the important difference between anatomical and functional changes.

Colour changes in the tissues can result due to several factors. The colour of the mucous membrane of the mouth is of the underlying vascular tissue which is seen through the surface epithelial tissue. The combination of the epithelial tissue and the texture and the amount of vascularity of the underlying tissues can produce variation in the light transmission and colour generaltion.

Cheilosis and angular cheilitis

The lips are readily affected by metabolic disturbances, local irritants or both. The inflammatory changes in the mucosa of the lip particularly at the commissures is the sign of some deficiency of one or more of the following nutrients riboflavin, niacin, folic acid, proteins, vitamin B_{12} *and iron.*

Glossitis

The tongue may undergo many changes in colour, size and sensitivity. The tongue is sensitive to nutritional aberrations because of the rapid growth of the epithelial cells covering the dorsum requires high amount of nutrients.

Inflammation of the oral mucosa

A patient with acute vitamin B complex deficiency as seen in alcholism will develop a markedly red and inflamed oral mucosa that sometimes has a patchy appearance as a result of isolated spots of grayish-green pseudomembrane.

Gingivitis

Gingivitis may be predisposed by certain nutritional deficiencies. Niacin deficiencies can predispose the gingival to ANUG. An acute vitamin C deficiency in the presence of local gingival irritants like plaque and calculus will cause gingivitis. Vitamin C deficiency contributes to gingivitis through defects in the capillary walls produced by the failure in collagen formation.

Iron deficiency is sometimes intimately involved with some B vitamin deficiencies and can also be suspected from the appearance of the mouth. For many of these vitamin B deficiencies, the tongue is smooth through loss of filiform or fungiform papillae (or often both types) -a red and painful tongue. While niacin deficiency is characterized by a scarlet tongue, riboflavin and biotin deficiencies are characterized by magenta-coloured tongues. If anaemiais severe, the tongue will be pale rather than red. Atrophy of the edges of the tongue in vitamin B_{12} deficiency is said to mirror the atrophy of the gastric lining in these patients.

Aphthous ulcers are very painful, often discreet ulcers and frequently in the oral mucosal sulci. Their aetiology is poorly understood, but it would appear that deficiency of folate and/or iron may be initiating factors.

Noma

Noma is a disease of the oral region strongly linked to malnutrition: it is also known as cancrum oris or orofacial gangrene. It most commonly occurs in Africa, where the prevalence is one to seven per 1000 population. It tends to occur in children aged 3-16 years and genders are equally affected.

Nutritional management of Acute Problems of the Oral Mucosa

The major consideration in the nutritional management of patients with acute problems of the oral mucosa is to provide an adequate and varied well balanced diet in a physical form and at a temperature that is not only comfortable but also soothing to sensitive oral tissues. Between eating periods, if there is an isolated painful mucosal lesions that need to be treated, a topical application of corticosteroids will be helpful.

Vitamin therapy

Supplementation of the diet with vitamin is useful when a person is unable or unwilling to consume an adequate diet. There are two major types of vitamin therapy, supportive and therapeutic. The purpose of supportive dose of vitamins is to protect the individual against the development of vitamin deficiency states during stress periods such as pregnancy or illness this supplementation is preventive.

Therapeutic vitamin preparation are indicated for the tretment of specific vitamin deficiency and for maintaining good nutritional status in patients with severe debilitating disease.

In both supportive and therapeutic vitamin supplementation it is recommended that polyvitamin preparation be used. These combinations of vitamins have complimentary functions as in energy releasing B complex vitamins, thiamin, niacin, riboflavin, pyridoxine hydrochloride and calcium pentothenate. Other combinations include:

1. vitamin B complex and vitamin C

2. combination of vitamin D with calcium and phosphate etc.

四、膳食与牙侵蚀症 Diet and dental erosion

牙侵蚀症（dental erosion）在世界许多国家已成为一个相当新的口腔健康问题，它与饮食有关。有许多证据表明在工业化国家患病率正在增加。在某些人口中，约50%的儿童受到影响。

1993 年在英国调查儿童口腔健康，首次评估牙侵蚀指数。结果发现 5 岁儿童 52% 牙腭侧面受到影响，颊侧面仅 18%。11 岁儿童的恒牙近 1/4 有牙侵蚀证据，其中 2% 的侵蚀进入到牙本质。另一项调查显示，经常饮用甜饮料与碳酸饮料的3.5～4.5岁儿童的牙侵蚀症为32%（腭侧面受到影响）。

牙侵蚀症是一种化学侵蚀与溶解。通常由于电解或化学过程引起牙体硬组织缺损是牙面受到外源性或内源性化学侵蚀的过程。外源性膳食酸，包括柠檬酸（citric acid），磷酸（phosphoric acid），抗坏血酸（ascorbic acid）苹果酸（malic acid），酒石酸（tartaric acid）和碳酸（carbomic acid）。例如，在水果与果汁，软饮料与醋中发现的。严重的侵蚀可以导致整个牙的破坏。对人的观察研究显示，牙侵蚀症与消耗多种酸性食品与饮料有关，包括经常消耗果汁软饮料（包括运动性饮料），泡菜（含醋），柠檬酸和浆果。牙侵蚀症与年龄有关，随年龄增加，软饮料摄入量最多的人更为严重。实验性临床研究显示，消耗酸性饮料或酸性含漱液使口腔唾液的 pH 值明显下降。暴露于可乐 1 小时内即可使口腔唾液的pH值明显下降。暴露于可乐1小时内即可使釉质软化，但还是可以通过暴露于牛奶或奶酪而产生逆转。动物研究显示，水果与饮料引起的牙侵蚀症，其中果汁比全果破坏性更大。因此，为了减少牙侵蚀症的发生，应该限制软饮料与果汁摄入的量与频数。

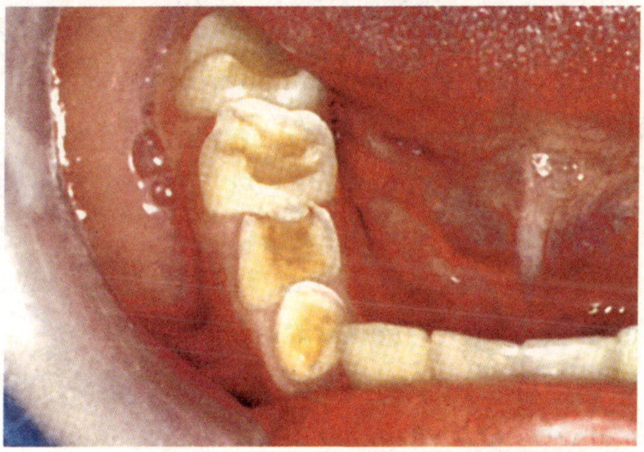

图 8-5

表 8-9　膳食与牙侵蚀症关联的证据强度

证据	减少危险性	无关联	增加危险性
相信			
很可能			软饮料与果汁
可能的	硬质奶酪		
	氟化物		
不充分			整个新鲜水果

Diet is an important and growing cause of dental erosion. There are other causes of erosion of teeth such as regurgitation o gastric fluid and exposure to some industrial acid environments but dietary acids are the significant factor. Until recently, little was known about the prevalence and severity of erosion in the population. This deficiency was corrected in the UK with the publication of the report on Children's Dental Health in United Kingdom 1993 (O'Brien, 1994) . One year later a report on the dental health of pre-school children in the UK was published (Hinds and Gregory, 1995) . Data from both these studies are given in Table . the teeth which are most affected are the maxillary incisor teeth, particularly the palatal surfaces, although the labial surface and incisal edge can be affected as well. Erosion is difficult to treat.

Dietary risk factors in dental erosion will vary between populations and between different age groups within populations. In children and adolescents, acid soft drinks are by far the biggest dietary risk factor. Sales of soft drinks have increased rapidly and the prevalence and severity of dental erosion in children seem to have increased in parallel. There has been a large increase in the UK soft drinks market with around 4000 million litres in 1992 being carbonated. The low-calorie versions have increased their share to around 26%. Overall, food consumption within the European Union (EU) of the original 12 members rose by 9.1% between 1988 and 1993. The most growth was in soft drinks, savoury snacks and frozen fruit.

What is erosion?

Erosion is defined as the 'physical result of a pathological, chronic, localized, painless (initially) loss of dental hard tissue which is chemically etched away from the tooth surface by acid and/or chelatiion without bacterial involvement'..

What causes erosion?

In broad terms, acids which cause erosion come from three sources-diet, the stomach, and the environment.

Dietary carses are listed in Table 8-12; this list includes medicaments. Not all of these are equally important, as will be discussed below.

Acids from the stomach are sometimes referred to as intrinsic acids. In broad terms, gastric acids may come to be in the mouth through vomiting or through gastro-oesophageal reflux and regurgitation.

The third source of acids which causes dental erosion is the environment. Improvements in industrial hygiene have meant that these causes are now rare in industrial countries. The addition of chlorine gas to swimming pools makes the water acid: this is usually neutralized satisfactorily but occasionally errors occur and the acidic water causes erosion to the teeth of competitive swimmers.

How to measure erosion

Our understanding of causes and prevention of dental caries and developmental defects of enamel has been helped considerably by the general use of accepted indices of measurement-the decayed, missing, or filled teeth (DMFT) and the developmental defects of enamel (DDE) indices, respectively. Erosion is more difficult to measure and a useful, easily reproducible index has yet to be established. This is further complicated by the difficulty of differentiating erosion from attrition and abrasion. The most widely used index at present is the 'tooth wear index' (TWI; table8-11) proposed by Smith and Knight.

表 8-10 The tooth wear index（TWI）

Score#	Surface	Criterion
0	B/L/Oc/I	No loss enamel surface characteristics
	C	No change of contour
1	B/L/Oc/I	Loss of enamel surface characteristics
	C	Minimal loss of contour
2	B/L/Oc/I	Loss of enamel just exposing dentine
	I	Loss of enamel just exposing dentine A defect less than 1 mm deep
	C	
3	B/L/Oc/I	Loss of enamelexposing dentine for more than one third of the surface
	I	Loss of enamel and substantial loss of dentine,but not exposing pulp or secondary dentine
	C	A defect between 1 and 2mm deep
4	B/L/Oc/I	Complete loss of enamel, or pulp exposure, or exposure of secondary dentine
	I	Pulp exposure or exposure of secondary dentine
	C	A defect more than 2 mm deep, or pulp exposure, or exposure ofsecondary dentine

in case of doubt the lower score is given.

B=buccal; L=lingual or palatal; I=incisal; Oc=occlusal; C=cervical. Missing teeth should be scored M

表 8-11 Causes of erosion

Diet	Medicaments
Acid carbonated beverages	Iron tonics
Citrus fruit juices and other acidic fruit juices	Liquid hydrochloric acid
Acidic un-carbonated beverages	Vitamin C
Wines	Acidic mouth-rinses
Cider	
Acidic herbal teas	
Citrus fruits	
Other acidic fruitsand berries	
Salad dressing	
Vinegar conserves	
Acidic fruit-flavoured candies	

Prevention of erosion

At present, prevention of erosion is based more on common sense rather than on evidence-based practice. At its most simplistic, removal of the likely causes will reduce risk. That is easier said than done. Dietary habits are subject to many powerful influences, such as advertisements and peer pressure, and are often difficult to change. Glance at figure , showing the rise in soft drink consumption, indicates the challenge.

表 8-12 Practical prevention of erosion

Inform patients of types of foods and drinks that have the greatest erosive potential
Limit the intake of acid drinks to mealtimes
Advocate consumption of a neutral food immediately after a meal（e.g milk or cheese）
Advise use of fluoride mouth-rinses or get for daily use.
Encourage the use of carbonate of soda mouth-rinses in cases of recurrent gastric reflux
Where erosion is marked, fluoride toothpaste can be placed in an occlusal guard during the night or during episodes of vomiting
Advise drinking through a straw with the straw well back in the mouth

Practical steps to take in the prevention of erosion are given in Table8-13 .

It would seem logical that the use of fluoride mouth-rinses and the topical application of fluoride varnishes or neutral gels would slow down the progression of erosion as well as reducing symptoms of sensivity.

五、营养与口腔感染、创伤 Nutrition and oral infection, trauma

（一）营养与口腔感染 Nutrition and oral infection

感染能导致营养不良，而营养不良又能使感染过程恶化。感染会减少蛋白质与其他营养素。一般来说，任何压力如创伤、疼痛或者着急都会产生负氮平衡，这样就产生分解代谢。在患严重感染性疾病期间，如伤寒，所丧失的氮相当于肌重的2～3公斤。急性期过后，需要大量蛋白质以维持必要的水平。

蛋白质缺乏性营养不良能影响抗体形成，吞噬细胞活力，组织完整性以及非特异性抵抗因素。因而可使皮肤、组织抵抗力下降，增加口腔感染的机会或加重口腔感染的严重程度。

（二）营养与口腔创伤 Nutrition and oral trauma

营养不良不仅可以降低口腔黏膜上皮的防御机能，还容易遭受物理化学性损伤和其他原因引起的创伤。另一方面，口腔颌面部创伤也影响营养物摄取。口腔颌面部中组织修复也与营养状况与营养及时补充关系密切。任何创伤或术后修复的速度与强度都需要补充和供给充分的营养。例如，补充大量维生素C可加快创伤愈合，同时供给蛋白质又有助于胶原的合成，成纤维细胞与成骨细胞的形成。蛋白质还可以纠正创伤或术中蛋白质的损失，并加速恢复，以及增加机体的免疫功能。同时提供维生素 A 和 C 有助于创伤愈合。

总之，及时补充必需的营养要素是任何创伤修复和伤口愈合以及康复的基础。

(1) Nutrition and oral infection

in considering the interactions between nutritional status and infection in the individual, two aspects should be recognized:

1. an infection usually precipitates or aggravates the malnourished state of an individual by a combination of mechanisms to be discussed later.

2.nutritional status influences host susceptibility toinfections.

(2) Nutrition and oral trauma

The nutritional requirements of a surgical patient can be determined by evaluating the following:

1. the previous nutritional state of the individual

2. the nature severity of the surgery performed

3. the amount and type of nutrients that are being lost from the body

4. the anticipated duration of the injury or disease

It is not possible to give definite recommendations for the administration of vitamins to surgical patients, but the following guidelines can be used in establishing the best levels for each case:

1. a previously healthy patient with a minor illness expected to last less than ten days, who is ambulatory and eating well and who has no history of previous inadequate nutrition, needs to be given no special consideration concerning his vitamin requirements.

2. when the foregoing qualifications are not met, the patient is given a maintenance level that is approximately twice the minimum requirement.

3. when the patient receives his nutrition by the intravenous route, he should be given a maintenance level supplemented with vitamin C.

4. when a serious illness or severe trauma exists, the requirement for the first few days should be supplied at the therapeutic level. Thereafter, the patient should receive the maintenance level until recovery is complete.

六、营养与口腔癌 Nutrition and oral cancer

（一）口腔与咽部的癌症

口咽癌是发展中国家常见癌症的2倍，接近于癌症发生病例的80%。在发达国家最近的趋势显示发病率与死亡率增加。例如，在欧洲，日本与澳大利亚。口咽癌症包括舌，龈，口底以及口咽其他部位的癌（主要受阳光与吸烟影响）在这个分类之外。到目前的认识是关于口腔癌发生的最重要的膳食影响是酒。证据是广泛而一致的。例如，有6项回顾性，与5项前瞻性队列研究报告产生的相对危险性在1.3与8.6之间。19项病例-对照研究得出的比数比（odds ratios）在 1.3 与 7.2 之间（即那些更有可能得口腔癌的人比那些没有受到膳食习惯影响的人要增加 1.3～7.2倍。对于任何水平的酒摄入与特殊的饮酒种类有关的危险性没有明确的差异。虽然在美国的一项早期研究发现饮用whisky相对危险性最大，以后的研究报告在饮不同种类的酒的人中 - 葡萄糖，啤酒，白酒与混合酒，发生口咽癌的危险性相类似。

很可能是酒的消耗与使用烟草之间有相互协同作用：高度暴露于烟酒的人与既不吸烟又不饮酒的人比较其相对危险性为 15.6 倍。

其他的膳食结构，蔬菜与水果与减少口咽癌的危险性有一致的关系。在 15 项病例对照研究中有 13 项报告至少一种蔬菜或一种水果在统计学上有显著的保护作用，其比数比不同，在 0.2 ～ 0.6 之间。

蔬菜与水果的保护性作用在校正了烟酒的消耗因素之后仍然是明显的。典型地，口咽癌的危险性在每天进食蔬菜与水果的人比不每天进食的人减少一半。进食胡萝卜，柑橘类水果与绿色蔬菜的证据最为一致。

消耗豆类，谷类，矿物质与维生素，除了维生素C之外，没有保护作用，5项病例-对照研究已经一致地报告比数比为0.3 ~ 0.6。另有一些研究也指出维生素A与E的价值。认为维生素A，C与E可以清除损伤细胞可能引起突变的游离基。

Mouth and pharynx cancers

The incidence of mouth and pharyngeal cancers is twice as common in the developing world where nearly 80 per cent of cases occur. In developed countries, recent trends show an increase in incidence and mortality-for example, in Europe, Japan, and Australia. Cancers of the mouth and pharynx include those of the tongue, gums, floor of the mouth, and other parts of the mouth and pharynx. Cancers of the lip (predominantly influenced by sunlight and smoking) and of the salivary glands are outside this classification.

Oral cancer is largely a preventable disease. The role of tobacco as the overwhelming cause of lung cancer, now the most common cancer globally, is well known. However, between 30 and 40 per cent of cancer incidence worldwide is preventable by more healthy eating, weight control, and exercise. It has been estimated that almost 87 per cent of the incidence of cancer of the mouth and pharynx can potentially be reduced by not smoking, reducing alcohol drinking, and increasing consumption of vegetables and fruits. Excluding the non-dietary risk factor of smoking, a diet high in a variety of vegetables and fruits and avoidance of alcohol may prevent between 33 and 50 per cent of cases of cancer of the mouth and pharynx.

拥有的资料对消耗咖啡或茶有增加口腔癌的危险并未提供证据。然而在南美洲一些地方把马黛茶当作茶饮用似乎是口腔癌的一种危险因素。经常饮用马黛茶者有2倍的危险性。这可能是通常高温饮用这种茶的结果。没有其他证据证实热饮是增加口咽癌的危险。

口腔癌是大部分可以预防的疾病。烟草的作用，作为肺癌的压倒一切的原因，现在是全球最常见的癌症，然而世界范围内30%与40%之间的癌症发病率是可以通过健康的进食，控制体重与锻炼来预防的。已经作出估计几乎87%的口咽癌的发病率能够通过不吸烟，减少饮酒与增加消耗蔬菜与水果可能降低。除了吸烟的非膳食性危险因素之外，膳食含蔬菜与水果量大，以及避免饮酒可以预防33%到50%之间的口咽癌病率的发生。

表 8-13　Strength of evidence relating food and nutrition to cancer of the mouth and pharynx

Evidence	Decreases risk	Increases risk
Convincing	Vegetables and fruits	Alcohol
Possible	Vitamin C	Matéa

World cancer research Fund, American Institute for Cancer Research

（二）营养预防口腔癌 Nutrition for prevention of oral cancer

1. β-胡萝卜素

是体内几种类胡萝卜素之一，是维生素A的先质。在带叶的绿色蔬菜与橘黄色水果与蔬菜中发现它的存在，也有片剂形式。在体内在一定程度上可以转化成维生素A。与维生素A缺乏综合征无关。几项研究指出，在发生消化道癌症的病人与没有发生的人比较血液中β-胡萝卜素的水平较低。这些发现引发假设β-胡萝卜素缺乏可能倾向于癌症形成。虽然给予β-胡萝卜素很少有毒性。用作一种化学预防剂是试验性的，与白斑的退化有关系，但也与癌症发生率的增加有关。作为一种化学预防剂β-胡萝卜素的作用机制可能涉及抗氧化机制还有抑制游离基的反应。

Beta carotene

Beta carotene is one of several carotenoids in the body and is a precursor of vitamin A. It is found in leafy green vegetables and yellow and orange fruits and vegetables, and it is also available in tablet form. To some extent it is converted to vitamin A in body and is not associated with hypervitaminosis A syndrome. Several studies have noted lower blood levels of beta carotene in patients who develop aerodigestive tract cancers compared to patients who do not develop cancer. These findings led to a hypothesis that beta carotene deficiency may predispose cancer formation. Although there is little toxicity associated with beta carotene administration, its use as a chemopreventive agent is experimental and has been associated with regression of leukoplakia, but also with increased cancer incidence. The mechanism of action of beta carotene as a chemopreventive agent may involve antioxidant mechanisms as well as inhibition of free radical reaction.

2. 维生素 E

在仓鼠颊囊模型中维生素E在降低口腔癌的进展方面是有效的。流行病学的研究指出，血清维生素E的水平与口咽癌的发生有相反的关系。另外，已经显示口服维生素E减少口腔黏膜的小核频数，虽然证实没有临床作用。它的作用机制被假设为一种抗氧化剂。它能够改变整个转化维生素 A 酸的某些毒性。维生素 E 与维生素 A 的联合应用，现在正在进行着化学预防的临床试验。

Vitamin E

Vitamin E has been effective in reducing oral cancer progression in a hamster buccal pouch model. Epidemiologic studies have noted an inverse relationship between serum vitamin E levels and the development of oral and oropharyngeal cancer. In addition, oral vitamin E has been shown to reduce oral mucosal micronuclei frequency, although no clinical effect was demonstrated. Its mechanism of action is postulated to be as an antioxidant agent. It can ameliorate some of the toxicities of all-trans-retinoic acid. Combinations of vitamin E and retinoids are currently being studied in chemoprevention clinical trials.

3. 姜黄素

姜黄素是姜黄的主要成分，广泛地用于咖喱粉之中。在口腔癌模型中，姜黄素抑制致癌物质诱发肿瘤发生，是无毒的，这一制剂作为一种癌症预防措施正在考虑之中。

Curcumin

Curcumin is the major component of turmeric, which is widely used in curry. Curcumin has inhibited carcinogen-induced tumorigenesis in an oral cancer model and is nontoxic. This agent is under consideration as a cancer preventive.

4. 绿茶

绿茶在世界范围内消耗，在远东地区尤为普遍。流行病学研究发现绿茶消耗与癌症，如胃与食道癌发生较低有关。儿茶素-3-茶酸（EGCG）是绿茶的主要成分，在体外口腔癌发生模型中已显示这种化合物在口腔摄入绿茶可能达到的浓度内有抑制生长的作用。临床化学预防试验正在评价这种化合物。

Green tea

Green tea is consumed worldwide and is especially popular in the Far East. Epidemiologic studies have found that consumption of green tea is associated with a lower incidence of cancers such as gastric and esophageal cancer. Epigallocatechin-3-gallate (EGCG) is the major constituent of green tea, and this compound has been shown to be growth inhibitory in an in vitro model of oral carcinogenesis, at concentrations that could be achieved by oral ingestion of green tea. This compound is being evaluated for clinical chemoprevention trials.

七、与营养不良有关的口腔表征 Oral manifestations associated with malnutrition

对一个病人的临床评价可以显示由营养不良引起的口腔组织的具体病理变化。有些与营养不良有关的口腔组织病损叙述如下：

Clinical evaluation of a patient may show specific pathologic changes in oral tissues caused by malnutrition. Some of the oral tissue lesions associated with malnutrition are discussed in the following paragraphs.

（一）唇 lips

唇的改变通常在暴露的黏膜与口角部位可以看到。核黄素烟酸与铁缺乏与这些病损有关。其他因素，如环境，暴露于极端寒冷，或干燥情况也可以产生类似病损。在一定的病例中，不良的修复体，像疱疹与梅毒，或对药物或化妆品的过敏反应也可产生类似病损。最常见的病损是：

Changes in lips are usually observed on exposed mucosa and angles of the mouth. Riboflavin, niacin, and iron deficiencies are associated with these lesions. Other factors such as environment, exposure to extreme cold, or dry conditions may also produce similar lesions. In certain cases, poorly fitting prosthetic appliances, diseases such as herpes and syphilis, or allergic reactions to drugs or cosmetics may also produce similar lesions. The most common lesions are:

1. 唇干裂 cheilosis

具有唇水肿，肿胀的特征。有些病例呈现剥脱，皲裂，垂直向皱褶增加，在萎缩性唇干裂病例，暴露的黏膜有一种羊皮纸样的外观与垂直裂沟消失。

This is characterized by edematous, swollen lips. In some cases, desquamation and chapping are present with increase in the vertical markings. In atrophic cheilosis, the exposed mucosa has a parchment-like appearance and vertical fissures disappear.

2. 口角病损 angular lesions

有时在口角部位有与念珠菌感染有关的苍白与红斑，在这个部位在半张口时，通常可以在双侧看到破碎的或浸软的上皮。在唇角部位有时可以看到口角伤痕，有时可以看到粉色或变白色的上下扩展，取决于病损最近如何形成。

Pallor and erythema are sometimes associated with monilial infections at the corner of the mouth. The broken or macerated integument in this area can usually be observed bilaterally when the mouth is held half open. Angular scars can sometimes be observed at the angle of lips, sometimes spreading up and down and with a pink or bleached color, depending on how recently the lesion was formed.

（二）牙 teeth

除了龋齿，氟牙症之外，有：

1. 线型釉质发育不全 Linear Hypoplasia

在上颌乳前牙可见此种病损，在相应的新生线部位有棕色釉质发育不全线。这与感染性疾病的发生，血清钙水平的改变以及在年龄早期的营养不良有关。

The lesions can be seen in deciduous maxillary incisors. The hypoplastic line stains brown and corresponds in position to the neonatal line. It has been associated with infectious disease attacks, changes in serum calcium levels, and malnutrition at an early age.

2. 黑色牙 Melanodontia

这种情况具有广泛的黄棕色染以及高度龋易感性的特点，流行病学资料提出，在牙齿发育的关键期间全身性营养不良是病因的一部分。

Extensive yellowishbrown staining of teeth and high caries susceptibility are characteristics of this condition. Epidemiologic data suggest overall undernutrition at critical stages during tooth development as part of its etiology

3. 错位牙 Malposition

牙齿拥挤或错位可能有营养源性，或因年幼时缺少蛋白质而干扰了颌骨发育或因乳牙过早缺失。遗传因素可能只是有影响，评价这种情况的病因时应予考虑。

Crowding nd malposition of teeth may have a nutritional origin either because of lack of protein at an early age that has interfered with jaw development or because of early loss of deciduous teeth. Genetic factors may be solely responsible and should be considered in evaluating the etiology of this condition.

（三）牙龈 Gums

牙龈组织的炎症变化普遍可见，应该鉴别以便确定其起因。

Inflammatory changes in gingival tissues are seen commonly and should be differentiated to ascertain their origin.

1. 坏血病型 Scorbutic type

这是与维生素C缺乏有关的典型症状。牙龈发红，呈海绵状，牙间乳头水肿与自发性出血，这一症状与其他征兆有关，当牙不存在时就不发生。

This is the classical symptom associated with vitamin C deficiency. Gums are red and spongy, with swollen interdental papillae and spontaneous bleeding. This syndrome is associated with other signs and does not develop when teeth are absent.

2. 牙龈炎 Gingivitis

这种情况有多种临床表现，从边缘龈组织轻度发炎到严重的牙周状况，其中有上皮附着顶端移动的牙龈剥离，骨丧失，以及形成深牙周袋。虽然维生素与蛋白质缺乏可以影响到这种组织反应，这一症状普遍是由于局部细菌的单独行动，而其他局部因素加重了这种情况，如错殆畸形，不良修复体，不良义齿或牙石，或全身性疾病，如糖尿病。

This condition has a number of stages from a mild inflammation at the marginal gum tissue to a severe periodontal condition in which there is detachment of the gingival with apical migration of the epithelial attachment, bone loss, and formation of deep periodontal pockets. Although vitamin and protein deficiencies may influence this tissue response, this syndrome commonly results from local bacterial action alone and is aggravated by other local factors such as malocculsion, poor restorations, prostheses, or calculus, or systemic diseases such as diabetes.

3. 肥大性龈炎 Hypertrophic Gingivitic

在一定的非营养性处理的过程中，如药物治疗所发生的，例如，用苯妥英，可使牙龈肿大到覆盖牙齿的程度。这种情况很可能需要一种有关的局部细菌的作用。

The gingival enlarges to such an extent that it may cover the teeth in certain non-nutritional manipulations, such as occurs with the administration of drugs, for example, phenytoin. This condition, too, probably requires an associated local bacterial action.

（四）舌 Tongue

已经发现舌是许多病理情况的一种敏感的指标，具有实质与颜色改变的特征。慢性舌炎大部分与复合维生素B，特别是烟酸，核黄素，叶酸与维生素B_{12}缺乏有关。也知道慢性铁缺乏也诱发舌炎。一定的症状，如“地图样舌”或者“犁沟样舌”存在于其他无营养缺乏的正常人之中并不可信。感染，如白色含珠菌感染，还有药物反应，晚期梅毒，肿瘤恶性变，以及某些口疮病损可以引起舌炎。

The has been found to be a sensitive indicator of many pathologic conditions characterized by changes in texture and color. Chronic glossitis has been associated with deficiency of most of the B complex vitamins, particularly niacin, riboflavin, folic acid, and B_{12}. Chronic iron deficiency is also known to induce glossitis. Certain syndromes, such as “geographic tongue” or “furrow tongue,” are known to exist in otherwise healthy individuals in whom no nutritional deficiency is suspected. Infections such as candidiasis, as well as drug reactions, late syphilis, malignancy, and some of the aphthous lesions may cause glossitis.

1. 纤维状与菌状乳头萎缩 Filiform and Fungiform papillary atrophy

这是慢性舌炎最早期的病损，并且当两种乳头同时萎缩时产生一种完全光滑性舌。它能够变成为一种红色与裂沟样外观，取决于某些乳头是否变成过度增大与融合。

This is the earliest lesion of chronic glossitis and produces a completely smooth tongue when both types of papillae atrophy. It can change to a red and fissured appearance, depending on whether or not some of the papillae become hypertrophied and fused.

2. 乳头肥大或充血 papillary hypertrophy or hyperemia

通常用压舌板可以看到舌前部的2/3，红点表明存在着充血。

This may usually be observed by running a tongue depressor over the anterior two thirds of the tongue. Red dots indicate the presence of hyperemia

3. 红紫色舌 Magenta tongue

舌呈青紫色，通常这一症状特别与核黄素缺乏有关，一般发现与口有炎与皮炎有关。

The tongue seems cyanotic, and the syndrome is usually related specifically to riboflavin deficiency. It is generally found in association with angular stomatitis and dermatitis.

4. 猩红色舌炎 Scarlet Red Glossitis

这种情况具有急性烟酸缺乏（糙皮病）与口炎性腹泻的特征。在进展阶段，口腔黏膜也变成为鲜红色。

This condition is characteristic of acute niacin deficiency (pellagra) and sprue. In advanced stages, oral mucous membranes also become bright red.

5. 牛肉样红色舌 Beefy-Red Glossitis

这种情况不同于以前那种深色的舌，而是类似深牛肉样，通常与烟酸缺乏有关，虽然其他复合维生素 B 可能对这一症状有作用。

This condition differs from the previous one in that the tongue is darker in color, resembling raw beef. It is usually associated with a niacin deficiency, although other B-complex vitamins may contribute to this syndrome.

（五）营养缺乏的其他口腔表征 Other possible oral manifestations of nutritional deficiencies

除了以上叙述的与营养缺乏有关的其他表征与症状之外，还有其他口腔表征，包括黏膜溃疡与角化病损，口腔疼痛，烧灼感，口干症，或流涎，味觉减低或消失（味觉迟钝以及有时也与锌缺乏有关的嗅觉缺失）以及口腔或舌侧黏膜的苍白。

Besides the classical signs and symptoms previously described that are associated with nutritional deficiencies, there are other oral manifestations of malnutrition that can be detected by the dentist better than by any one else. These include ulcerations and keratotic lesions on the mucosa, oral pain and burning sensations, xerostomia or sialorrhea, diminished or absent taste perception (hypogeusia and sometimes also anosmia associated with zinc deficiency) , and pallor of the oral or lingual mucosa.

Anemias, subclinical B-complex deficiencies (such as folic acid deficiency) , and vitamin A and zinc deficiencies have been found to have a part in the causation of these symptoms either directly or indirectly by diminishing the resistance or the function of the tissue. Under the influence of different stresses (for example, infection, functional stimulation, or local irritants) , a breakdown takes place and a diseased state is established.

贫血，亚临床复合维生素B缺乏（如叶酸缺乏）以及维生素A与锌缺乏已经发现是这些症状原因的一部分，直接或间接降低组织的抵抗力或功能。在不同压力的影响下（例如，感染，功能刺激，或局部刺激物），发生损坏，并确定为一种疾病状态。

第三节 口腔疾病防治中的营养指南

Section 3 Guidelines for Nutrition in the Prevention and Management of Oral Diseases

一、糖的消耗 Sugars consumption

有结论性证据表明，膳食中随意的糖消耗是致龋的。许多国家与国际专家委员会推荐：为了降低龋齿的发病率应当减少糖消耗的量与次数。然而，什么样的糖消耗水平与牙齿健康相适应？（糖的概念，英国的食品政策医学方面委员会COMA规定为非奶的外源性糖）。这个问题可以通过糖与龋之间的剂量-反应关系性质的确定来解决。然后找出在什么样的糖消耗水平龋齿发病率上升。这个水平会受到预防措施，特别是氟化物的影响，关于糖消耗水平的国际推荐必须考虑到全世界大多数人口的需要，记住在许多不发达国家氟化物一般是没有利用的。

（一）剂量反应关系 The does-response relationship

总体膳食中的蔗糖含量与作为结果而发生的龋之间的关系不一定是线性的，但是是直接的。资料提出糖与龋之间的剂量-反应关系约为S形曲线。在消耗水平低的时候，蔗糖引起的龋很少，随着糖消耗水平的增加，龋病的水平也上升。然后曲线最终变成为水平线，这时蔗糖的消耗再增加不再引起明显的龋增加。Takeuchi 发现在每人每年消耗量达到 38 公斤时 S 形剂量 - 反应达到上升之后的稳定水平。

总之，各种回顾性的研究显示当每年糖的可利用率超过10～15公斤时，龋病就增加，龋病的发病率受到糖摄入次数的影响，提出的糖消耗的“安全水平”展示在表 8-15 中。

There is conclusive evidence that free sugars in the diet are cariogenic. Numerous national and international expert committees have recommended that the amount and frequency of sugar consumption should be reduced in order to reduce the incidence of dental caries. However, what levels of sugar consumption are compatible with dental health? (“sugar”, throughout this paper, means non-milk extrinsic sugars, as defined by COMA.) This question can be approached by establishing the nature of the does-response relationship between sugar and caries, and then finding out at what level of consumption the incidence of disease increases. That level will be affected by preventive measures, particularly fluoride. International recommendations on levels of sugar consumption must consider the needs of the majority of the world’s population, bearing in mind that fluorides are not generally available in many underdeveloped countries.

The dose-response relationship.

The relationship between the sucrose content of the total diet and the resultant caries is not necessarily linear, but it is direct, as animal studies have shown. The data suggest that the does-response relationship between sucrose and caries approximates to a sigmoid (S-shaped) curve. At low consumption levels, sucrose leads to very little caries; increasing levels of sucrose are followed by increasing levels of disease. Then the curve eventually flattens out, and further increases in sucrose do not lead to appreciable increases in caries. Takeuchi found that the S-shaped does-response reached a plateau at 38 kg per person per year.

In summary, the studies reviewed show that when annual sugar availability exceeds 10-15kg per person, dental caries increases. The rate of increase in disease is affected by the frequency of sugar intake. The proposed “safe” levels of sugar are shown in table.

表 8-14 Table 8-15 Proposed “safe” levels for dietary sugar

Author	Proposed ‘safe’ levels for dietary sugar
Schulerud	
Takeuchi	30 g/person/day 10 kg/person/year if no fluoride available
Sheiham	
Sreebny	50 g/person/day 18 kg/person/year if no fluoride available
Sheiham	40 g/person/day 15 kg/person/year if fluoride available

（二）糖的摄入次数与量之间的关系 Relationship between frequency and amount of sugar intake

许多研究的证据提出，人类龋病的发病率与消耗的糖量以及两餐之间摄入含糖食品的次数是有关联的。COMA陈述：“在自由生活的人们中有三个变量，质量，浓度与频数，三者之间密切相关”。不管结论如何，大多数强调糖/龋的关系是建立在糖摄入的次数上。甚至糖与糖果工业也承认糖的摄入次数与龋病之间存在着关系。他们推荐减少次数，但不提数量。然而，在英国儿童中有结论性证据，糖摄入的次数与量之间有高度的相关性。Rugg-Gunn发现许多食物组所有的相关性都在+0.75以上，显示每天消耗含糖食品的量增加，摄入的次数也增加。含糖软饮料的相关性为+0.82。Ismail等报告北美儿童软饮料有类似的发现。这些研究表明当消耗的量越多，次数越多。这些发现对发展中国家有特殊的意义，有些国家每人每年摄入的糖低于15公斤。在这个水平以上，据联合国糖农组织（FAO）报告“消耗加工食品与饮料的次数增加”。同时显示，在不发达国家，低收入国家，糖是首要的反映收入增长的食品之一。发现 15 公斤的糖是增加次数的一个关键水平，在这个水平上。龋病发病率也明显增加。因此强烈支持WHO的推荐糖消耗应在 15 公斤以下。

Relationship between frequency and amount of sugar intake

Evidence from numerous studies suggests that caries rates in humans are related to the amount of sugar consumed and the frequency of ingesting between-meal sugary products. COMA stated: 'In free-living people these three variables, mass, concentration and frequency, are all closely and positively related to each other'. Despite that conclusion, most of the emphasis on the sugar/caries relationship has been on the frequency of sugar ingestion. Even the sugar and confectionery industries concede that there is a relationship between frequency of sugar intake and caries. They recommend a reduction in frequency but say nothing about amounts. However, there is conclusive evidence in British children of a high correlation between the frequency and the amount of sugar intake. Rugg-Gunn found that all the correlations for a number of food groups were above +0.75, showing that as the amount of sugary foods consumed per day increased, the frequency of intake also increased. The correlation for sugar-containing soft drinks was +0.82. similar findings for soft drinks were reported by Ismail et al. for North American children. These studies indicate that when more sugar is consumed, the frequency increases. That finding has particular significance in developing countries, in some of which the per person annual intake of sugar is below 15 kg. Above that level, the FAO reports that the frequency of consuming processed foods and drinks increases. They also showed that in underdeveloped, low income countries, sugar is one of the first foods to respond to a growth in income. The finding that 15 kg or sugar is a critical level for increasing frequency, and that caries rates also increase markedly at that level, is strong support for the WHO recommendation that sugar consumption should be below 15 kg.

（三）膳食糖与龋病 Dietary sugars and dental caries

从许多不同种类的研究中得到大量的证据，总起来说，这些研究资料提供了一种碳水化合物致龋可能性的全面描述。毫无疑问，在龋病发生过程中，糖是最重要的膳食因素。

世界范围的流行病学研究在国家水平之间比较了糖的消耗与龋病的发病水平。Sreebny对47个国家12岁儿童龋病患病状况（DMFT）与糖供应的数据的相关研究发现一种显著的相关性（+0.7）。52%龋病水平的变化可以用人均糖的可利用率来解释。糖的消耗水平每人每年低于18公斤的国家，龋病患病与低于3个龋均（< 3DMFT）是一致的。后来woodward等对发达国家进行的分析没有发现类似的关系。不过，糖的有效率证明龋病水平有28%的变化。在26个国家中有23个人均糖利用率低于每天50克，12岁儿童的龋均低于3（DMFT < 3）。

在世界许多国家中进行了许多横断面的流行病学研究比较糖的摄入与龋病发病的水平。在1990年代早期之前进行的研究，Rugg-Gunn已经做了总结。在21项研究中有9项比较糖的消耗量与龋病的增加发现有显著的关系，而另外的12个国家没有发现这种关系。而且，在37项研究中有23项调查糖的消耗次数与龋病水平之间的联系发现有显著的关系，而另有14项没有任何这样的联系。

在一份对纵向研究的评价中，Marthaler分析了在糖的利用率高和广泛应用氟化物的国家膳食糖与龋病活性之间的关系。他得出的结论是在采用了预防措施的现代社会中，糖消耗与龋病之间的关系仍然是明显的。

Dietary sugars and dental caries

There is a wealth of evidence from many different types of investigation, collectively, data from these studies provide an overall picture of the cariogenic potential of carbohydrates. Sugars are undoubtedly the most important dietary factor in the development of dental caries.

Worldwide epidemiological studies have compared sugar consumption and levels of dental cries at the between-country level. Sreebny correlated the dental caries experience (DMFT) of 12-year-olds with data on sugar supplies of 47 countries and found a significant correlation (+0.7) ; 52% of the variation in the level of caries was explained by the per capita availability of sugar. In countries with a consumption level of sugar <18 kg per person per year caries experience was consistently <DMFT 3. A later analysis by Woodward & Walker did not find a similar association for developed countries. Sugar availability nevertheless accounted for 28% of the variation in levels of dental caries; 23 out of 26 countries with a per capita sugar availability <50 g per day had a mean DMFT score for 12-year olds of < 3, whereas only half of the countries with sugar availability above this level had achieved a DMFT score that was < 3.

In a review of longitudinal studies, Marthaler analysed the relationship between dietary sugars and caries activity in countries where the availability of sugars is high and the use of fluoride is extensive. He concluded that in modern societies that make use of prevention, the relationship between sugars consumption and dental caries was still evident.

（四）糖的摄入减少对其他膳食成分的可能影响 Potential impact of sugars reduction on other dietary components

考虑到减少随意的糖消耗对其他膳食成分的可能影响是重要的。简单的人群膳食资料的横向分析已经显示在随意的糖摄入与脂肪摄入之间有相反的关系。因而认为减少随意的糖摄入可能引起脂肪摄入的增加。然而随着时间的推移，各种研究累积的证据显示脂肪与随意的糖摄入的变化并没有相反的关系，脂肪摄入的减少以增加淀粉的摄入而不是随意的糖摄入来抵消。Cole-Hamilton等人发现脂肪与增加的糖同时摄入的减少是因为纤维的摄入增加了。总起来说，膳食的目标是促进增加全谷物主要成分的食品，水果与蔬菜的摄入和减少随意的糖消耗不大可能引起脂肪消耗的增加。

Potential impact of sugars reduction on other dietary components. It is important to consider the potential impact of a reduction in free sugars on other components of the diet. Simple, cross-sectional analysis of dietary data from populations has shown an inverse relationship between the intake of free sugars and the intake of fat, suggesting that reducing free sugars might lead to an increase in fat intake. There is, however, a growing body of evidence from studies over time that shows that changes in intake of fat and free sugars are not inversely related, and that reductions in intake of fat are offset by increases in intakes of starch rather than free sugars. Cole-Hamilton et al. found that the intake of both fat and added sugars simultaneously decreased as fibre intake increased. Overall dietary goals that promote increased intake of wholegrain staple foods, fruits and vegetables and a reduced consumption of free sugars are thus unlikely to lead to an increased consumption of fat.

（五）氟化物与龋病 Fluoride and caries

氟化物改变着糖 / 龋剂量 - 反应曲线。在许多工业化国家龋病已经下降，在饮水氟化的地区，不考虑相对高的糖消耗水平。一种推测是当含氟牙膏广泛应用时剂量反应曲线可以向右移动并且上升不太陡峭。需要进一步研究确定氟化物对糖 / 龋的剂量 - 反应曲线的形式有什么样的影响。不论如何，研究提示的事实是在今后20年在世界大部分人口中不可能拥有含氟牙膏，因此提出作为一个国际目标，10%的能量来自糖作为一个推荐的可以接受的水平是合理的。任何其他途径都不会无视不发达国家的人们的糖消耗快速增加。每个儿童每增加一颗龋，每一百万儿童就需要额外增加300名牙医来充填牙，如果龋病在不发达国家继续按照现在的发病率增加，口腔保健的费用就需要占某些国家总体卫生预算的 1/3 以上。

Fluoride and caries

Fluoride alters the sugar/caries dose-response curve. Caries had declined in many industrialized countries and in areas with water fluoridation, in spite of relatively high sugar consumption. One could speculate that the dose-response curve may be shifted to the right and rise less steeply when fluoridated toothpaste is widespread. Research is required to establish what effect fluorides will have on the shape of the sugar/caries dose-response curve. Whatever that research reveals, the fact that fluoride toothpastes are unlikely to become available to most of the population of the world in the next 20 years suggests that 10% energy from sugar as the recommended acceptable level is justified as an international goal. Any other approach will demonstrate a blatant disregard for people in underdeveloped countries, where sugar consumption is increasing rapidly. With the increase in sugar there is an increase in caries.

An increase of one decayed tooth (DMF) per child requires an extra 300 dentists to fill the decayed teeth per million children. If cries continues to increase in underdeveloped countries at the present rate, the cost of dental care would require more than a third of some countries' total health budgets.

二、健康促进方面 Health promotion perspectives

只有在能够得到实施时，膳食推荐才有价值。为了洞察可能的改变考虑影响个人膳食摄入和了解膳食的障碍因素是有用的。表8-17构建了反映许多影响膳食摄入的因素。有些发现可以讨论。

传统的一日三餐正在减少，特别是在年轻人中间，转变简单的晚餐并增加快餐。有贫穷背景的儿童，膳食贫乏自出生开始很低的母乳喂养率，儿童经常断奶，给予不健康的膳食，脂肪含量，精制的外源性糖与钠的摄入量太高。以每天进食松脆食品，甜食与含糖汽水饮料为正餐。

较高的社会经济人群对健康的进食信息有更多的反映，并且拥有的收入可以作较好的营养选择。在较低的社会经济人群，对健康进食的反映较冷淡，由于收入制约而加剧。需要努力鼓励改变习惯与常规。

最成功地促进改变特殊食品种类的消耗是由食品生产工业界进行的。例如，早餐增加谷物，然而，在宣传健康的与不健康的食品的花费上仍有明显的不平衡。例如，1991年在英国，仅花费4.5百万英镑在宣传新鲜水果与蔬菜方面，相比之下，花费在宣传松脆食品与点心方面的有28百万英镑，巧克力方面为83百万英镑。英国人均消耗水果与蔬菜相当低。为53公斤。比西班牙或希腊少一半。欧盟平均几乎达到81公斤。美国一日5次活动强调在每日膳食中供应5次水果与蔬菜。这个目标是吸引人的。因为容易理解，依据现有的信息，像“进食你的绿色食品”和“一天一个苹果”，一种简单的措施而不是用克或者百分比；另外，信息是正面提示多吃而不是少吃。

仅靠群众性教育期望产生快速的社会性变化是不现实的。一种健康促进途径需要涉及多个政府部门的合作。然而在克服组织的惰性，各种兴趣的竞争以及消费者的误解方面都存有相当大的困难。

政府的教育政策与卫生政策比较之间的相互影响在英国是一件有意义的事情。源自一个部门的法规，如教育部门，起到削弱另一个部门，如卫生部门，法规的作用。提供学校用餐就是一个很好的说明。这个例子说明需要政府各部门之间的协调行动。

最近在美国与挪威看到的在全民水平上的成功的膳食变化。认识到达到成功的两种不同途径。在美国由美国心脏基金会发起的一项教育活动强调膳食措施与锻炼对降低血清胆固醇的重要性。这项活动是由其他志愿组织发起进行的，并且引起了广泛的态度变化。因为较多的强调个人对健康的责任，疾病直接加重了个人的经济负担，鼓励改变的作用很大，因而取得了成功。

相比之下，挪威采取的是更为经典的健康教育途径，在发展营养政策的过程中，建立了一个基础广泛的营养委员会，包括农业，食品工业，公共卫生监督，著名的医生与营养师以及公众共同参与。这二个国家在减少总脂肪摄入与吸烟同时发生看到了健康的明显改善。

Health promotion perspectives

Dietary recommendations are only of value if they can be implemented. To gain insight into likely change, it is useful to take into account influences on individual dietary intake and known dietary barriers. Figure has been constructed reflecting many factors affecting dietary intake. Some of the findings described below are discussed.

The traditional pattern of three meals per day appears to be declining, particularly among younger groups in the population.

Higher socioeconomic groups are both more responsive to healthy eating messages and possess the income to make better nutritional choices. In lower socioeconomic groups, responsiveness to healthy eating may be weaker, exacerbated by income constraints. The effort and incentive needed to change established habits, and routines that have led to longstanding dietary inadequacies, are greater in the socially deprived.

Changing consumption of specific food items has been most successfully promoted by the production industry, e.g. the growth in breakfast cereals. However, there is still an enormous imbalance between the amounts spent on advertising healthy and unhealthy foods.

It is unrealistic to expect rapid societal changes in diet based on mass education alone. A health promotion approach is needed involving cooperation between several government departments. However, there are considerable difficulties in overcoming organizational inertia, competing interests and consumer misunderstandings (WHO, 1990) .

表8-15　Factors affecting dietary intake. adapted from scottish health and home department（1993）

Individual	Food	Environment
	Taste	
Age	Appearance	Home/unemployment
Sex	Food type	Urbanization
Education	Meal/time context	Family age
Income	Cost	Season
Nutrition knowledge	Seasoning	Household size
Cooking skills	Texture	Family illness
Attitudes to health	Storage	Shift work
Attitudes to change	Preparation method	Mobility
Illness	Health connotation	Social pressures
Teeth	Symbolic content	Health pressures
	Cultural value	Role models
	Ecological value	
	Preferences-constraints	
	Food choice	
	Food consumption	

牙友甜食为成功口腔健康促进的一个范例 Tooth-friendly sweets as an example of successful dental health promotion。

牙友的想法有25年之久，始于瑞士致力于开发一项由瑞士卫生部接受的口腔内pH值的遥感勘测系统作为非致龋性食品的一项有效检测。1983 年瑞士成立了一个组织“Aktion Zahnfreundlich”作为牙科医生与工业界之间一个伙伴，为了促进牙友的思想注册了一个标识，通过 pH 值检测可以把这个标识展现在糖果包装上。

1983年以来，已有7个国家加入，现在已有4个检测中心。这些全国性牙友协会为非盈利性组织。

牙友思想并不是没有相反的意见：有争议的是这样的糖果，大部分没有能量。已知多元醇能引起腹泻。它们可能鼓励一种甜味，通常比类似的含糖食品更贵。其积极的方面是现在已相当好地接受了这一检测系统，引起龋齿与牙侵蚀症的产品不可能通过检测，糖果作为最大的膳食糖来源是目标。为消费者提供一种选择，在瑞士与芬兰均未见有肠道功能紊乱的问题。有二个理由特别重要-第一，牙友甜食是取代含糖食品而不是增加；第二，有益于口腔健康。Marthaler（1990）在他的欧洲龋病谱改变的评论中是这样说的：

In two cases, however, favourable dietary changes are thought to have occurred: the reduction of caries prevalence in Finnish and Swiss children is not likely to be fully explained exclusively in terms of fluorides and improved oral hygiene. In Finland, the widespread use of xylitol as a sweetener may have been a factor in the improvement of dental health; in Switzerland a lowered cariogenic challenge is suggested by the widespread use of nonacidogenic sweets which already in 1985 constituted 10% of the total of sweets sold.

三、合理营养与膳食指导 Adequate nutrition and diet counseling

合理营养是健康的物质基础，而平衡膳食（balanced diet）是合理营养的唯一途径。平衡膳食是指由各种食物以一定数量一定关系彼此组合而成，能够提供人体所需要的所有营养素。多年来“平衡膳食”一直是健康教育的重要内容，但是，有些人简单地认为选择所需要的食物只是为了避免蛋白质、维生素与矿物质的缺乏。泛用这个概念有可能导致另一些疾病的发生。为了避免这种误解，又提出了“合理膳食”或“审慎膳食”（prudent diet）的概念，但也有学科的言外之意和限制。为此美国国家科学院食物与营养委员会提出了“健康膳食”（healthy diet）的概念，它包含着需要各种正确信息的想法。营养不良不仅包含着营养不足，还包含着营养过剩与营养素不平衡的问题。

（一）合理营养 Adequate nutrition

人们所需要的营养素都来自于膳食。牙医学家确定了 50 种营养素分成为六大类：碳水化物、脂肪、蛋白质、维生素、矿物质与水。

1. 碳水化合物 Carbohydrates

通常每天提供总热量需要的 40% ~ 50%，包括淀粉类食物，如含量丰富的全麦面包、谷物、面粉类食品、水果与蔬菜，特别是土豆，是碳水化合物的主要来源。这些食物也含有相当量的维生素与矿物质。

糖与甜食，像糖果、蜜饯、果酱、果汁与饮料并不提供什么热量，因而不作为一般推荐的范围。考虑到牙菌斑的形成，可能引起的龋病与牙龈炎，口腔病人或易感人群应尽可能避免糖与甜食。

2. 脂肪 Lipid

脂肪是最集中的能量来源，含有的热量相当于等量碳水化物与蛋白质的2倍，同时它又是许多脂溶性维生素的载体，如维生素A、D、E、K和基本脂肪酸，特别是亚麻酸（Linoleic acid）和花生四烯酸（arachidonic acid），而且还有多种不饱和脂肪酸，能降低血脂。

乳制品是脂肪的良好来源。其他来源有肉类、人造黄油、果仁、植物油等。

3. 蛋白质 Protein

蛋白质由 22 种氨基酸组成，大多数来自食物，并可通过体内制造。但其中有 8 种不能由体内制造，必须从膳食中得到，称为基本氨基酸。这种完全蛋白质来自动物食品，如肉类、鱼类、禽类、蛋类与乳类。同样重要的还有来自面包、谷物、果仁与豆类等的不完全蛋白质。如果在同一膳食中摄入像肉、奶这样的完全蛋白质将会增加不完全蛋白质的价值。必须充分提供每一种才能构成，修复和维持所有的组织。它也是形成酶、激素用于调节机体过程，产生抗体以对抗感染所必需的。

4. 维生素 Vitamins

维生素A是生长、视力、皮肤健康、抗感染的基本需要。一般应从全奶、奶油、奶酪等乳制品中得到。也可以从蛋黄、人造黄油、肝、深色与黄色蔬菜中获得。

维生素 D 一般可以通过阳光作用于皮肤产生。如果阳光有限，应给生长发育中的儿童补充，通常强化牛奶为适当来源。

维生素C与B族维生素为水溶性，不能在体内储藏。因此，一定要通过平衡膳食每天补充人体所需之量。维生素C为牙龈与血管健康所必需。最好由新鲜水果，尤其是各种柑橘与新鲜蔬菜中得到。B 族维生素由 4 类食物（谷物、动物食物、豆类及其制品、蔬菜水果类）提供。

5. 矿物质 Minerals

18种矿物质是调节和保持机体过程的基础。钙的最佳来源是奶，奶酪与绿色蔬菜等。富含铁的食物是肉类（尤其是肝）、蛋黄、全麦面包、与谷物、干果类、干豆类以及绿叶蔬菜。碘化食盐是获得一定碘量的最佳途径。普通食盐与几乎所有食品都能提供钠。WHO 推荐每人每天食盐摄入量不超过 6 克。肉、鱼、奶和咖啡中含适量的钾，更多的来自蔬菜、柑橘类水果、甜瓜、香蕉与杏子。茶水可以经常补充氟，还有其他一些矿物质可以从平衡膳食中得到。

6. 水 Water

一般不把水看作一种食物，但它是人体所有组织所必需的。水也是氟的最普通来源，每人每天需饮水或饮料 6 ~ 7 杯才能保持身体良好的水平衡。

7. 纤维 Fibres

纤维是不能消化的食物的一部分，它不是一种营养素，但常作为平衡膳食的一部分，纤维性食物有助于口腔自洁作用，并刺激肠蠕动，因此可作为促进牙与牙龈健康的食品。

（二）膳食指导 Diet counseling

针对我国居民的营养需要和膳食中存在的主要缺陷，1997年中国营养学会常务理事会通过了“中国居民膳食指南”。现根据促进口腔健康的需要，摘要介绍如下：

1. 食物多样，谷物为主 Various foods, cereals as main food

人类的食物应该是多种多样，才能满足各种营养需要，达到合理营养，促进健康的目的，提倡人们广泛食用多种食物，包括五大类：(1) 谷物及薯类；(2) 动物性食物；(3) 豆类及其制品；(4) 蔬菜水果类；(5) 纯热能食物，包括动植物油等。

2. 多吃蔬菜，水果和薯类 More consumption of vegetables, fruits and potatoes

蔬菜与水果含有丰富的维生素、矿物质和膳食纤维。种类繁多，营养成分不尽相同，甚至悬殊很大。这些食物对维持牙龈、牙周组织与口腔黏膜健康必不可少。

3. 常吃奶类，豆类或其制品 Often consuming milk products, legumes and its products

奶类除含丰富的优质蛋白质和维生素外，含钙量也较高，且利用率也很高，是天然钙质的极好来源。我国居民膳食提供的钙质普遍偏低，平均只能达到推荐供给量的一半左右。我国婴幼儿佝偻病较多，乳牙患龋率很高，还有乳牙釉质发育不全，与膳食钙不足可能有一定联系。研究表明，给儿童青少年补钙可以提高骨密度和牙的抗龋能力。

4. 经常吃适量鱼、禽、瘦肉、少吃肥肉和荤油 Often eating appropriate fishes, fowls, eggs, lean meat, less fat and animal oil

这些动物性食物是优质蛋白，脂溶性维生素和矿物质的良好来源，更适合人体的需要，且赖氨酸含量较高，有利于补充植物蛋白中的赖氨酸不足。它对萌出前牙釉质、牙本质与牙骨质矿化、胶原合成与骨钙化，保持牙支持结构的健康，抗感染与增加口腔防御功能都是必需的。

5. 食量与体力活动要平衡，保持适当体重 The balance between the amount of foods and physical activity, to maintain healthy body weight

一日三餐之间应避免食用含糖食品，只随三餐少量食用糖类，减少龋发病的危险因素，防止肥胖，减少糖尿病、冠心病的危险因素。

6. 吃清淡少盐的膳食 Less salt in diet

7. 限量饮酒 Limiting alcohol drinks

烟酒嗜好是影响口腔健康加重牙周病的有害因素。

8. 吃清洁卫生，不变质的食物，预防感染性疾病从口腔进入 Eating clean and unchanged quality of foods and preventing infectious diseases entering in the mouth

（三）饮食习惯的形成与改变 The formation and modification of food habits

日常生活中的许多活动很少引起人们的关注。特别是饮食习惯。然而，习惯是有意识的行动。随着时间的推移，形成的一种反复固定的实践方式，具有无意识地自动地完成动作的固定倾向。

饮食习惯反映出一个人选择与摄取食物的态度与想法，喜欢与不喜欢，经验与实践。这些习惯的形成受到文化，社会，经济，情绪与生理方面的影响。养成良好的饮食习惯，能够选择对身心最有益的食品，而不良的饮食习惯则会引起膳食的质量问题。不良饮食习惯的原因是可以改变的。知识匮乏，或对适当膳食的无知，常常可以通过教育，针对不良饮食习惯造成的原因加以改进。

Many of our daily activities require little or no thought. This is especially true of eating. Habits, however, originate as a result of conscious acts. With the passage of time and as a result of constant repetition and practice, we establish a fixed tendency to perform these acts almost unconsciously and automatically. This is how we acquire a habit.

Food habits are the sum of our attitudes and ideas, our likes and dislikes, our experiences, and our practices with respect to food selection and eating. These habits grow out of cultural, social, economic, emotional and physiological influences. If we have good food habits, we choose foods that are best for the optimal functioning of mind and body. Poor food habits indicate eating practices which result in a diet of inferior quality. The cause of poor food habits could be obstinacy to change, ignorance of what constitutes an adequate diet, or poverty. Often, though, through education and reason, poor food habits can be improved.

1. 个别咨询的重要性 The importance of personal counseling

需要时养成习惯，不需要时改变习惯。成功的饮食咨询包括调整饮食习惯与实践，必须清楚选择食物的目的或理由，即饮食为了什么。

评价膳食的适当与否只是整个饮食咨询服务的一部分。同样重要的是需要明白为什么某人选择一定的食物以及饮食方式。只有在了解的基础上，才能作出现实的变更或改进，争取病人最大可能的合作。

努力帮助人们增进健康，尤其是口腔健康，只有以人为本，个性化，针对其特殊的需要与问题，才可能取得成效。为什么学校健康教育项目进行了多年，但在降低龋病或牙周病方面并没有明显效果，主要原因是提供的信息太概念化和一般化，没有直接针对个人。因此，没有为学生个别吸收或利用，以改善自身健康。直到成为病人，见到口腔医生时才讨论其个人的口腔问题，医生提供个别指导，信息才成为有价值和可能有效果。

如何为病人提供有效的咨询服务，首先，了解饮食习惯的形成，影响饮食习惯的有关因素，才能知道如何改变。

Habits are formed when there is a need to be filled and can be eliminated by doing away with the need for them. Consequently, for successful diet counseling, which involves modification of food habits and practices, we must deal with the purpose or reason for the food selection, which we call the why of the diet.

Evaluating the adequacy of what a patient ets is only one part of a total diet counseling service. It is equally important to understand why he selects certain foods and eats the way he does. On the basis of this understanding we can make realistic modifications or improvements with which he will most likely be able to cooperate. Most effects to help a person to improve his health in general, and his dental health in particular, will fail unless they are personalized to meet his particular needs and problems.

Dental health has been taught and even stressed in the elementary school classrooms for many years. Yet, in spite of these health courses, dental caries is still the most prevalent disease in the United States today. Why has this type of dental education program been so nonproductive in terms of significantly reducing dental caries or periodontal disease? One major reason is that the information taught is too conceptual and general and not directly applicable to the individual. Therefore, it is not actively absorbed or used by the learner for his own improvement. It is not until the patient goes to his own dentist to discuss his personal oral problems and the dentist provides him with personalized advice that the information becomes valuable and possibly effective.

As a preamble to a discussion on how to effectively counsel a patient with respect to the why of his diet, especially as it relates to the food habits which may have contributed to dental caries or periodontal disease, this chapter will attempt to explain the factors that influence these food habits and how they can be modified.

2. 从婴儿到老年饮食习惯的形成及其影响因素 The development of food habits from infancy to old age

（1）婴儿时期　当母亲根据婴儿需求而不是按钟点规定用母乳或奶瓶喂养婴儿时，饮食习惯开始形成。换言之，婴儿学习进食，使饥饿得到满足。母亲是主要影响婴儿对食品的态度与饮食习惯的人，这种影响十分明显。儿童是从父母那里得到喜欢的或不喜欢的食物。大多数是好的，也有不好的，包括不良的饮食习惯。

婴儿与儿童时期是对多种食物产生积极态度的最佳时期，他们相信在父母影响下，感到安全时，大多愿意尝试新的食品。

In Infants. Food habits begin to form when the mother gives the bottle of her breast to the infant on demand rather than by the clock. In other words, the infant learns that he can eat and be satisfied when he is hungry. He doesn't have to denied his milk because his hunger drive came ahead of an arbitrary "2 o'clock feeding." This gives the infant a positive, good feeling about eating and confidence in the mother as a good provider of food. When she starts to feed new foods to the toddler and says that they taste good, the child will believe her. It is quite evident that the mother is the prime influence on the child's attitudes toward food and his eating habits. In fact, the child usually acquires the food likes and dislikes of his parents. Although this, for the most part, is good, it can also be bad if they happen to have poor food habits and set a poor example. In general, infancy and childhood are the best time in which to develop a favorable attitude toward variety in food. Children are not highly adventurous about trying new foods, but they are most willing to adventure with a new food when they feel secure under the influence of parents they trust.

（2）儿童时期　随着儿童成长，伙伴，朋友，亲戚对其饮食习惯能产生负面影响。食品常作为一种奖励或爱的表示。

In children. As the child grows up, siblings, friends and relatives can exert negative influences on his food habits. In the case of peers, there is rivalry and jealousy that can dictate habitual poor food selection; for example, "I want a lollipop because Johnny has one." Or food can be used as a reward or as a means of expression of love by the grandmother who pays a weekly visit to see the grandchildren.

（3）青少年时期　倾向于从家长以外摄取更多食品，常选择碳水化合物含量高而营养价值低的食品。由于这个时期，容易饥饿，为满足饥饿之需要，常吃点心。青少年1/3以上的热量摄入来自二餐之间的点心。改变饮食习惯的关键是改变点心的种类而不是进食方式。

In adolescents. The adolescent tends to eat more and more meals away from home. He often chooses foods high in carbohydrates and low in satiety value and is therefore often hungry. To satisfy this hunger, he resorts to frequent snacks also high in starches and/or sugar. It has been postulated that as much as one third of a teenager's calorie intake comes from between-meal snacks. Since the need for acceptance by peers is great in this group, the frequent snacking is usually not so much from choice as from wanting to do what the rest of the "gang" does. Therefore, any efforts to improve these eating habits should be concerned with improving the type of snack eaten rather than the eating pattern.

(4) 青年时期　影响饮食习惯的主要因素是关于食品价值的误导性信息，缺乏知识，不成熟或受经济条件限制，使青年人容易接受不良的饮食习惯。

In young adults. As a young adult, indifference and misinformation about food values rather than food dislikes seem to influence food habits. It may be the "in" thing to be on a macrobiotic diet or a special quickie weight reduction diet even though neither of them is adequate and probably can be harmful. It is probably both lack of maturity and lack of knowledge and maybe even lack of funds that makes the young college student susceptible to poor food habits.

(5) 成年时期　饮食习惯难以改变，主要影响因素来自社交活动，宴请，送礼，以糕点甜食居多。

In adults. Food habits in adults are stubborn and more resistant to change and improvement. The adult may be guilty of acceptance-seeking. Take the case, for example, of status foods. How many people really like caviar, or pat é de fois gras? Yet we eat them at parties because they are status foods. Sweets, confections and desserts also have a very positive social connotation. Candy is frequently brought as a hostess gift; and what is a dinner party without a fancy dessert to top it off?

(6) 老年时期　因孤独影响老人的饮食习惯，缺乏热情与食欲，或者如果加入集体组织，缺少个人自主选择。

In elderly. Loneliness will influence food habits in the elderly. Some older people either have lost their enthusiasm and appetite for food or they just don't care to bother to prepare proper meals for themselves. On the other hand, if they join a group and become socially involved there may be less self-pity and less dwelling on their infirmities; instead they may exchange recipes and menus and thus develop more interest in food.

3. 其他影响饮食习惯的因素 Other basic influences on food habits

(1) 环境方面 Environmental

①地理环境　饮食受当地农产品，季节差异的影响。

Geographic. As a rule, one usually eats the foods that are indigenous to a locality because they are so readily available and therefore more economical.

②文化　地区性文化，民族，宗教差异的影响。

Cultural. Racial, national and religious groups have retained some of their food practices for generations.

③经济　家庭经济状况。

Economic. The economic status of the family influences how much of which foods are going to be bought or eaten.

(2) 心理方面 Psychological

①情感　饮食习惯受情感因素的影响很深。

Emotional. Food habits are considered difficult to modify because they can have superficial or deep emotional origins.

②以往经历　以往愉快的与不愉快的经历影响。

Associations with past experiences. There are foods which we don't eat because they are associated with former unpleasant incidents

③奖励　父母亲奖励儿童喜欢吃的食品。

Reward. Foods are also used as weapons for praise

④不喜欢　有些食品因其外形，颜色，味道而不喜欢。

Dislikes. There are some foods to which we react in a negative fashion merely because we don't like their appearance, color, consistency or odor.

(3) 生理方面　对某些食品过敏，特殊医疗条件下的特殊饮食，以及全身状况等因素影响饮食习惯。

Physiological

Allergies, special diets for specific medical conditions, and systemic conditioning factors in general influence food habits.

(4) 教育方面　改变饮食习惯是有效的一种方式是媒体交流（如广播，电视，报纸）遗憾的是信息太多而难以区分真伪。

Educational

Probably one of the most effective influences on changing eating habits is the mass communication media-television, radio, magazines, and newspapers.

4. 改变饮食习惯 modifying food habits

培养好的饮食习惯比较容易，而常常是改变不良饮食习惯困难得多。然而，改变不良的饮食习惯还是可能的。但是，需要回答以下三个方面的问题：

It is always easier to build a good food habit than it is to correct a poor one. But poor habits can be modified and even eventually changed if one stops trying to justify them. The answer to successfully modifying food habits is based on answers to these questions:

(1) 病人现时的营养状态怎样？　What is the patient's nutritional status?

开始时，评估病人是否存在主要的或次要的营养不适当的问题。通过采集有关病史，膳食史，临床观察与实验检测，如果需要可以做营养状况评价，如果营养缺乏仅为食物摄取不足，可以把实际摄入量与推荐量作比较。

It is important to begin with an assessment of whether there are primary or secondary nutritional inadequacies. Through adequate pertinent medical and diet histories, clinical observations and laboratory tests, if needed, such a nutritional assessment can be made. If the nutritional deficiency is only a food intake deficiency (determined by comparing the actual amounts of food eaten)

(2) 选择食品的原因是什么？　What are the reasons for food selection?

从环境，心理，生理影响方面广泛讨论食品选择的原因。最简单的获得信息的方式是了解病人生活方式方面的信息，掌握病人一天的常规活动是关键，健康习惯，喜欢，不喜欢的食物以及一般个性。

The environmental, psychological and physiological influences just discussed are the general broad areas where the causes for food selection are found. The simplest way of ascertaining this information is to try to elicit information on the patient's vocation, avocation, spare-time activities, health habits, food likes and dislikes and general personality traits.

(3) 如何动员病人改变饮食习惯？ How does one motivate a patient to modify his food habits?

有 4 个预先决策步骤：意识，兴趣，参与，行动，然后进入第 5 步 – 习惯改变。

There are four preliminary decision stages through which a person goes in order to arrive at a fifth and final decision to change his habit. The stages are awareness, interest, involvement, action, and habit.

①意识　认识问题的存在，但没有采取任何干预行动。

Awareness is recognition that a problem exists, but there is no inclination to do anything about it

②兴趣　进一步确认问题，尚未采取行动。

Interest is a greater recognition with no inclination to act

③参与　有兴趣明确打算采取行动。

involvement- "I have definitely had my last hard candy."

④行动　尝试开始改变习惯。

Action- "I gave up hard candies and I chew sugarless gum instead because I just have to prevent the dry feeling in my mouth."

⑤习惯　在较长时期内有规律地采取一定的行动。

habit- "I haven't chewed or sucked on a hard candy in six months."

例如：限制糖摄入量，以控制龋齿发生。

①认识：糖和甜食产生酸，导致龋齿发生。

②兴趣：可能我应放弃吃糖，因为我不想有任何牙疼之苦。

③参与：我已决定这是最后一次吃糖。

④行动：我已放弃吃糖，只吃无糖口香糖以防口干。

⑤习惯：我不吃糖已有 6 个月了。

从实际观点看，采用认识问题，参与及个性化的途径改变病人的不良饮食习惯。

From a practical standpoint, we use the problem, participation and personalization approach for modifying patient's food habits.

①问题　解释牙病问题的性质与结果以及不良饮食习惯如何影响。

Problem. We explain the nature and the consequences of the dental problem and how poor food habits have influenced it.

②参与　提供病人机会，通过实际膳食分析，简单计算不适当的方面，鼓励自行解决。

Participation. We provide the opportunity for the patient to find his own solution; we encourage self-help by guiding him into actually doing the dietary analysis and making the simple calculations that show him the areas of inadequacy

③个性化　通过提供适当的可供选择的方案，使病人容易接受和改变。

Personalization. We try to make it easy for him to make changes by suggesting suitable alternatives. We start with the patient's present diet, leaving in those familiar and well-liked foods that have no adverse effect on his dental health. using these foods as a nucleus, we try to gradually improve the quality of the diet by providing a few acceptable substitutes at the start. We encourage the patient to choose his own diet based on what he has learned is right, and letting him delete what is wrong. We reinforce his choice by approval and commendation. At a later visit, if the patient has succeeded in coping with the first group of recommendations, further modifications will be suggested.

虽然没有一种确切的方法可以帮助改变所有病人的不良饮食习惯，但从这三个方面着手进行，还是取得了一些成功。

Although there is no sure way to motivate all patients to alter their food habits, we have had some success by:

Helping patients to understand the nature of the etiology of their disease.

Helping patients to understand themselves and to determine why they have once rejected but now are willing to accept certain foods.

Allowing them to prescribe for themselves a diet with which they could cooperate without difficulty.

小结 summary

通过本节学习，主要帮助学生了解营养与口腔健康的重要关系，营养如何影响口腔健康以及在什么时期营养将会对口腔健康产生什么样的影响。营养与口腔健康疾病的关系，以及营养对口腔疾病的发生，发展以及结果的影响。熟悉糖消耗与龋病发病的关系以及膳食的健康促进方面，营养、膳食与慢性病的预防，合理营养的基本内容。掌握膳食指导的基本原则以及帮助人们改变不良饮食习惯的基本途径。

思考题 Review questions

1、 Describe two nutritional factors influencing growth and development of oral tissues?
2. What is the concept of critical periods in tooth development?
3. Are good nutrition matters important to oral health?
4. What is a major cause of enamel hypoplasia (EHP) ?
5. Based on the current evidence, what recommendations could be made in preventing dental caries
6. From the scientific basis, how to maintain periodontal health?
7. Discuss the strength of evidence in related to nutrition and diet for dental disease
8. How does one motivate a patient to modify his food habits?

参考文献 References

1. Dominick P. Depada Preventive Dentistry Section II, Chapter 7, Nutrition Conseling in a preventive practice P PSG Publishing Company, Inc, 1979, 103-146
2. Richard E. Stallard, A textbook of Preventive Dentistry, Chapter8, Nutrition in oral health and disease, W B. Saunders Company, 1982
3. Abraham E. Nizel. Nutrition in Preventive Dentistry: Science and practice, W.B. Saunders Company, 1972
4. Rugg Gunn, et al. Diet. Nutrition and oral health. Oxford, 1997
5. Promod k, Dayal, et al. textbook of oral medicine. Chapter 14. Nutrition and oral diseases. Jaypee

Brothers Medical Publishers (p) Ltd. India, 1998
6. 中国营养学会. 中国居民膳食指导. 1997
7. WHO technical Report Series 916, Diet nutrition and the prevention of Chronic Diseases, WHO, Geneva, 2003
8. Murray, JJ. The prevention of dental disease, 2nd edition. Oxford Medical publications, 1990
9. 卞金有等. 预防口腔医学. 第 4 版人民卫生出版社, 2003
10. Cynthia M. Pine Community oral health. Wright, 1998
11. Eugene P. Lazzari Dental biochemistry 2nd edition. Lea & Febiger, 1976
12. Maynihan P. Oral health, diet and other factors BDJ vol, 2000 188 No. 6: 308-312

（卞金有）

第九章　口腔癌及其预防
Chapter Ⅸ Oral Cancer and its Prevention

概述 Overview

本章主要介绍了口腔癌的流行病学，包括发病率、死亡率及口腔癌在年龄、性别、种族、患病部位等方面的差异；口腔癌有关的主要致病因素；口腔癌前病变；口腔癌的早期诊断、检查和预防。

This chapter briefly introduce the epidemiology of oral cancer, including the incidence and mortality, differences between age, sex, site and race; the causal factors related to oral cancer; the oral precancerous lesions; the diagnosis of initial stage, examination and prevention of oral cancer.

要点 Key points

- 口腔癌的定义
- 口腔癌的致病因素
- 主要的口腔癌前病变
- 口腔癌的初级预防和二级预防
- *Definition of oral cancer*
- *Causal factors related to oral cancer*
- *Oral precancerous lesions*
- *Primary and secondary prevention of oral cancer*

第一节　口腔癌流行病学及其有关致病因素
Section 1 Epidemiology of and Factors Related to Oral Cancer

一、口腔癌的流行病学 Epidemiology of oral cancer

口腔癌（oral cancer）是指涉及口腔、主要是口腔黏膜的恶性肿瘤。口腔癌狭义的概念是指口腔鳞癌。它是发生于舌、口底、腭、牙龈、颊和牙槽黏膜的一种癌症。口腔癌广义的概念是指唇癌、涎腺恶性肿瘤、口咽癌也可以包括在口腔癌之中。口腔癌是世界上第六种最常见的癌症。

1. 发病率 Incidence

衡量口腔癌的患病情况多用发病率（incidence）。发病率是指在特定时间内（通常是1年）某一特定人群新发生口腔癌的人数，常用十万分之几来表示。有关口腔癌的流行病学的资料不是很理想，很多国家没有做过这方面的调查，有些资料不是全国性的、而是某些地区的。

口腔癌在全世界都有发现，不同地区的发病率不同。表 9-1 显示的是世界上 24 个地区的口腔及咽部恶性肿瘤的发病率，可以看出口腔癌的发病率的差异很大，最低的是日本女性，估计标化发病率为1.8/10万；最高的是美拉尼西亚的男性，估计标化发病率为47/10万。我国口腔及咽部恶性肿瘤的估计标化发病率男性为8.7/10万，女性为6.0/10万。口腔癌的高发地区是印度次大陆、法国、巴西和中东欧。在地理位置相同的区域各个国家口腔癌的发病率也有显著的差异。

美拉尼西亚的口腔癌的发病率非常高的原因未详细研究过，可能与嚼烟和吸烟有关。几十年来很明确的口腔癌的最好发地区是南亚，口腔癌与鼻咽癌的最好发地区是东南亚。在印度、孟加拉国、巴基斯坦和斯里兰卡，口腔癌是最常见的癌症，占全部癌症的 1/3。

表 9-1 是来自世界卫生组织的数据，包括了唾液腺的恶性肿瘤，数据更加详细。

表 9-1 Estimated age-standardized incidence rates per 100 000 population for oral and pharyngeal cancer, in 1985, for 24 world areas (Parkin et al)

Area	Male	Female
Eastern Africa	14.2	9.5
Middle Africa	15.0	10.0
Northern Africa	15.6	8.7
Southern Africa	13.4	3.4
Western Africa	3.5	2.6
Caribbean	13.3	4.0
Central America	4.6	2.4
South America（temperate）	8.1	2.3
South America（tropical）	18.7	4.9
North America	14.2	5.1
Eastern Asia: China	8.7	6.0
Eastern Asia: Japan	4.5	1.8
Eastern Asia: Other	9.3	3.0
South-East Asia	14.5	9.8
Southern Asia	25.1	14.9
Western Asia	9.1	7.5
Eastern Europe	10.7	2.4
Northern Europe	6.5	2.8
Southern Europe	11.4	2.5
Western Europe	16.6	3.2
Australia/New Zealand	15.1	4.8
Melanesia	47.0	25.6
Micronesia/Polynesia	10.0	4.6
USSR	15.7	3.0
All areas	14.0	6.5

2. 年龄分布 Age distribution

全世界范围内口腔癌的发生都随着年龄的增加而增加。在西方，98%的口腔癌患者的年龄超过了40岁。国内统计资料显示以40～60岁为发病的最高峰，而西方国家则多发生于60岁以上，其发病的最高峰值比我国约大10岁。但从上世纪80年代以来，无论在西方国家还是我国，在患病年龄上均有逐渐增长的趋势，其主要原因可能与整个人群平均寿命的延长有关。然而，在世界上口腔癌的高发地区，许多口腔癌患者是35岁以下的，这源于大量地滥用各种形式的烟草。此外，在过去的二三十年里西方国家口腔癌的发病率有明显的上升，特别是在年轻男性中，这种趋势还将继续。

3. 性别分布 Gender distribution

男女都可以发生口腔癌，但男性比女性更容易患口腔癌，主要原因是男性更多地吸烟和大量饮酒，而吸烟和大量饮酒又是口腔癌的最重要的危险因素。工业化国家中男性口腔癌患者是女性的2～3倍。近年来口腔癌的发病在女性中有明显增加的趋势。上海第二医科大学口腔鳞癌的统计资料表明，女性患者的增长速度远大于男性患者：1960～1965年间男女患者之比为2.82：1，而1986～1990年间男女患者之比缩小至1.39：1。美国在20世纪50年代的调查显示男女患口腔癌的比率是6：1。女性发病增加的原因可能是吸烟和饮酒的人数上升了；另外口腔癌多见于65岁以上的人群，而65岁以上人群中女性比男性多20%。

口腔癌的性别差异在各地区之间有明显的不同。在口腔癌的高发地区例如印度，女性患舌癌和其他口腔内癌症的多于或等于男性，在印度妇女嚼烟草（有时吸烟）是很普遍的现象。

4. 部位差异 Site differences

在我国，以舌癌、颊黏膜癌、牙龈癌、腭癌等为常见，唇癌较少见。在美国，舌癌是最常见的口腔癌，美国1985～1996年间确诊的口腔癌中有30%发生在舌，其次是唇癌和口底癌。在其他发达国家情况也类似。但在发展中国家，因为生活习惯的差异情况有所不同，例如，在印度颊癌是最常见的口腔癌。口腔癌的好发部位与地区、气候、种族、生活习惯等均有一定关系。

5. 种族差异 Ethnic variations

已经知道种族可以影响许多类型的癌症。黑人中的癌症比白人中的多见，口咽癌在黑人中是第4位易患的癌症，而在非西班牙白人中排在第七位。亚洲人和西班牙人与白人和黑人相比，口腔癌在男性和女性中的发生都少。虽然这种结果和遗传因素有关，但更多的是生活方式和习惯的不同造成的。例如，中国人患鼻咽癌的是白人的20～30倍。

6. 死亡率 Mortality

全世界每年因为各种癌症死亡的人数超过200万。在美国每年因癌症死亡的超过55万人，其中口咽癌导致的将近1万人。黑人口腔癌的生存率低于白人，可能因为黑人的社会经济地位较低，以及黑人中吸烟饮酒的广泛流行。亚洲人和西班牙人口腔癌的发病率和死亡率都低于白人和黑人。不同的死亡率说明了口腔癌发病的不同，差异是种族、文化和环境因素共同造成的。Levi等人调查了1985年至1989年间不同国家的口腔癌和咽癌的死亡率，其中香港、新加坡、法国和匈牙利的死亡率高居前列，香港和新加坡的死亡率高居前列的原因可能是鼻咽癌在其中所占的比例大，法国和匈牙利排在前面的原因是烟草和酒的大量使用。

This chapter deals with malignant neoplasmas affecting the oral cavity, principally the oral mucosa. Table 9-2 shows the ninth vision of the International Classification of Disease (ICD) coding system of the World Health Organization. The term oral cancer in a narrow sense is most frequently taken to include squamous cell carcinoma of the tongue, cheek, gum, palate, floor of the mouth, and unspecified parts of the mouth.

表 9-2 Locations as described by the ICD-9

ICD-9 code description	
140 ~ 149	Malignant neoplasms of lip, oral cavity and pharynx
140	Lip
141	Tongue
142	Major salivary gland
143	Gum
144	Floor of mouth
145	Other and unspecified parts of mouth
146	Oropharynx
147	Nasopharynx
148	Hypopharynx
149	Other and ill-defined sites within lip, oral cavity and pharynx

The epidemiology of cancer is usually described in terms of the incidence and mortality. Incidence may be defined as the number of new cases in a specific time period (usually 1 year) for a specified population conventionally expressed as cases per 100,000.

The databases of oral cancer are far from ideal: many parts of the world produce no data at all, in others (often among the most populous), the data may come from localized, atypical regions.

The incidence of oral cancer varies with different parts of the world. Figures in Table 9-1 and Table 9-2 illustrate the marked global variability in oral cancer incidence. An age-standardized rate (ASR) is a summary measure of a rate that a population would have if it had a standard age structure. Standardization is necessary when comparing several populations that differ with respect to age because age has such a powerful influence on the risk of cancer. The most frequently used standard population is the World standard population. The calculated incidence or mortality rate is then called World Standardized incidence or mortality rate. It is also expressed per 100,000.

The incidence of oral cancer increases with age in all parts of the world. Most patients are over 40 years old. Oral cancer occurs either in females or in males, but more frequently in males. The male-to-female ratio is now 2-3:1 in the industrialized countries.

The tongue and floor of the mouth are the most common sites for primary squamous cell carcinomas in the oral cavity in the Western world. However, buccal and retromolar trigone mucosa are the most frequently encountered primary sites in those parts of the world where tobacco chewing and chewing of betel nuts are most prevalent.

Ethnic background is known to influence many types of cancer. Oral and pharyngeal cancer is the fourth leading cancer site in black men and the seventh leading site of cancer in non-Hispanic white men. Oral cancers in men and women occur less frequently in Asians and Hispanics compared to whites and blacks.

Mortality may be defined as the number of deaths from a particular disease for a given time period for a specified population conventionally expressed as deaths per 100,000. There is much geographical variation in oral cancer mortality. (Figure 9-1 plots age-standardized death certification rates for mouth and pharynx cancer (ICD-9 140-149) in various countries for the period 1985-89.) Globally, oral cancer is the sixth most common cause of cancer-related death.

二、口腔癌的行为特征 Oral cancer behavioral characteristics

口腔癌本质上分为两种—癌瘤和肉瘤，癌瘤源自上皮；肉瘤源自肌肉、神经、血管或结缔组织。

早期的口腔癌瘤有特殊的生长特征：（1）明显的表面区别—上皮角化不全；（2）肿瘤沿着小涎腺导管生长；（3）横向癌化；（4）多中心口内起源；（5）多样的口外恶性肿瘤。鳞状细胞癌在晚期癌瘤中心变硬或形成溃疡，而疼痛是晚期的症状。涎腺肿瘤生长缓慢，常为无症状的肿胀，很少溃疡。

肉瘤生长快速，最常侵犯下颌骨，破坏骨组织或造成骨硬化。肉瘤患者一般均是比较年轻的，当病人的瘤体直径超过2cm时，淋巴结常受累。肿胀、疼痛、一个或多个牙齿松动是口腔癌的常见表现。此外，口腔恶性肿瘤患者，特别是口底癌的老年患者一般都伴有口腔败血症、营养不良、体重下降、贫血、蛋白质缺乏、维生素缺乏、支气管肺炎、肺气肿、慢性气管炎、动脉硬化症等疾病。只有不到 1% 的口腔癌是从其他部位转移到口腔的。

三、口腔癌前病变 Oral precancerous lesions

虽然口腔癌在开始的时候常有外观上的变化，但在临床上也有许多可以确定的癌前病变，这些病变是可以检查出来的。提高对口腔癌前病变的认识有助于降低口腔癌的发病率和死亡率。最常见的口腔癌前病变有白斑（Leukoplakia）、红斑（Erythroplakia），扁平苔藓和口腔黏膜下纤维性变也可以发生癌变。这些病变的患病率在不同的地区和国家不同，具体数据见表9-3所示。虽然不是所有的口腔癌患者在患病前都有明显的黏膜变化，但是白斑等癌前病变还是为预防口腔癌提供了机会。

白斑可以发生在口腔内的任何部位，大多数是良性角化过度的表现。虽然烟草或急慢性刺激可以导致角化过度，但白斑的病因不清楚。

现有的调查结果显示不同地区白斑的患病情况不同。明尼苏达的一项研究发现27443名成人中有 0.1% 的人患有白斑，另一项研究是 18 万多的 17 ~ 26 岁人群中白斑的患病率是 1.5%。印度南部四个州的村民的患病率从 0.2% 到 5% 不等。而在印度西北部 Ahmedabad 调查了 57518 名 35 岁以上的纺织厂工人，白斑的患病率接近 12%。

白斑可以自行消退，也可以恶变。白斑的恶变率一般是低的，已经报道的在纵向研究中观察到的白斑的恶变率不同，从 0.1% 到 10% 左右。白斑活组织检查若有上皮异常增生，那么白斑癌变的危险性增加。虽然异常增生的严重程度有临床意义，但是轻度增生或没有增生的白斑病人也有癌变的危险。红白斑、红斑癌变的危险性比白斑高的多。不同的研究发现红白斑、红斑的癌变率是均质型白斑的 4 ～ 7 倍。

下列情况要引起高度的重视：（1）白色病变中有红斑的成分；（2）镜下有异常增生；（3）临床表现为增生的疣状白斑；（4）镜下可见伴有白色念珠菌感染的白斑；（5）不吸烟的白斑病人；（6）疼痛或有不适的感觉（白斑病人通常是没有症状的）；（7）红色病变（增生性红斑、红斑）。这些情况可能意味着上皮已经有了异常增生或癌变。

口腔扁平苔藓的病因不清，目前认为是一种免疫性疾病，主要发生在成年人，发病的平均年龄约为 50 岁，30 岁以下的人群很少见，女性多发，大约是男性的 2 倍。口腔扁平苔藓可以存在于口腔内的任何部位，但是，颊黏膜是其最常发生的部位。不同的研究显示口腔扁平苔藓的恶变率从 0.4% 到 5.6% 不等。

口腔黏膜下纤维性变的患病率很低，但是其恶变率较高，印度的大量研究显示 15 年内口腔黏膜下纤维性变的恶变率可以高达 7%。

Although in common use, the term precancerous/premalignant lesions are unsatisfactory because they imply that perhaps irreversible steps along the multistage process of genetic alterations leading to invasive carcinoma have definitely taken place. However, the risk of a lesion becoming malignant within the life span of the patient is highly unpredictable and relatively low. Furthermore, such lesions may regress. Additionally, in much of the Western world, most of these carcinomas arise without the patient or clinician being aware of a pre-existing lesion. However, in high-incidence areas of the world, notably South Asia, the reverse is the case-tobacco or areca nut chewing habits result in chronic lesions and the majority of oral cancers arise from such lesions. These carcinomas have a distinctive natural history which is much less aggressive than carcinomas arising de novo in the West.

A preferable term is potentially malignant lesions and conditions, among which there is a greater risk of malignant change. This broad group is generally classified under lesions and conditions, the latter being more generalized and widespread, with significant systemic involvement. These conditions are associated with mucosal atrophy and altered mucosal homeostasis without a discrete lesion being visible clinically. We generally consider the potentially malignant lesions to include leukoplakia and erythroplakia of various clinical presentations (such as homogeneous, verrucous, nodular or speckled) and mixed lesions. Potentially malignant conditions are usually taken to include sideropenic dysphagia (mucosal atrophy associated with chronic iron-deficiency anaemia), erosive lichen planus, oral submucous fibrosis, discoid lupus erythematosis, tertiary syphilis and actinic kerotosis.

The prevalence of potentially malignant oral lesions and conditions is different. A very wide range of figures is reported in literature. The details are shown in Table 9-3.

The causes of leukoplakia and erythroplakia are unknown. Leukoplakia that clinically has an erythematous or red component is far more likely to undergo dysplastic or malignant epithelial changes than other forms of leukoplakia. In examination, considerations of the following potential risk factors are essential: (1) an erythematous component in a white lesion, (2) microscopic dysplasia, (3) a clinical appearance of proliferative verrucous leukoplakia, (4) associated candidiasis seen microscopically,

(5) a nonsmoking patient, (6) pain or irritation (leukoplakia is usually asymptomatic) , and (7) a red lesion without a white component, which also may represent a dysplastic or malignant lesion.

Although not all oral cancers are preceded by clinically evident premalignant mucosal changes, such changes give an opportunity for preventive measures.

表 9-3 Prevalence of potentially malignant oral lesions and conditions

	Country	No. of persons examined	Prevalence (%)
Lesions			
Leukoplakia	Guam	2004	0.4
	India	4734	3.5
	Hungary	5613	3.6
	New Guinea	3996	8.1
	India	30 000	1.6 ~ 3.3
	India	2004	6.5
	India	5000	2.4
	New Guinea	1226	4.6
	India	7286	5.2
	India	50 915	0.2 ~ 4.9
	India	101 761	0.7
	India	57 518	11.7
	India	4559	1.6
	Sweden	20 333	3.6
	Germany	4000	2.2
	Burma	6000	1.7
	Cuba	749	2.1
	Saudi Arabia	674	1.9
	USA	23616	2.9
	USSR	1569	8.0
	Sweden	20333	0.7 ~ 24.8
	The Netherlands	1000	1.4
	Thailand/Malaysia	234/233	1.3
	Hungary	7820	1.3
Erythroplakia	India	50915	0.02
	Burma	6000	0.1
Condition			
Oral lichen planus	USA	23616	0.12

	Country	No. of persons examined	Prevalence (%)
	Burma	6000	0.4
	India	35 000	0.02 ~ 0.4
	India	7639	0.1 ~ 1.5
	Sweden	20 333	1.9
	Thailand	234	3.8
	Malaysia	233	2.1
	Hungary	7820	0.08
Oral submucous fibrosis			
	South Africa		
	Pretoria/Johannesburg	1000	0.5
	Durban	1200	0.6
	Capetown	---	1.3
	Durban	2058	3.4
	India		
	Bombay	10 000	0.5
	Lucknow	10 000	0.5
	Bangalore	10 000	0.18
	Trivandrum	5000	1.2
	Ernakulam	10 287	0.4
	Srikakulam	10 169	0.04
	Bhavnagar	10 071	0.2
	Darbhanga	10 340	0.07
	Singhbhum	10 048	0
	Pune	101 761	0.03
	Agra	7286	0.6
	Goa	5449	0.04
	Ernakulam	---	0.65
	Bhavnagar	---	0.06
	Burma	---	0.1

四、口腔癌有关的致病因素 Causal factors related to oral cancer

导致口腔癌的确切病因不清楚，根据长期的临床研究和实验研究，口腔癌的发生可能与下述的多种因素有关。

1. 烟草 Tobacco

烟草的烟雾中含有4000多种化合物，一支香烟燃烧产生大约500mg的气体和微粒，其中的1～35mg是焦油（芳烃），而焦油中含有最强的致癌物质。吸烟（Smoking）是全世界流行的能导致多种严重疾病的重大健康问题。

大量的流行病学研究已经证实吸烟和口腔癌有密切关系，口腔癌患者中吸烟的比例是非口腔癌人群的2倍多。美国加州大学旧金山分校对403名口腔癌和咽癌患者平均追踪观察了5.1年，发现72%的患者吸烟，而且58%的患者每天吸烟超过1包，说明吸烟者是口腔癌的高危人群。

另外，吸烟还可以加重再次发生原发口腔癌（second primary cancer）的危险性。一项研究观察了203名口腔癌和咽喉癌的病人，这些病人都是癌症根治了3年以上的，其中120名病人继续吸烟，120人中有37%发生了再发性原发癌；而81名不吸烟或已经戒烟的病人中只有6%发生了再发性原发癌。许多实验室研究显示从烟草产品中分离出的一些碳氢化合物可以导致动物的颊黏膜癌。这些致癌物质中最强的苯并芘与核蛋白结合，是致突变和致癌的。

2. 烟斗、雪茄、鼻烟和无烟烟草 Pipes, cigard, snuff and smokeless tobacco

口腔癌与使用烟草之间的关系不仅仅有纸烟，还包括雪茄、烟斗、无烟烟草等。已经从烟斗、雪茄和无烟烟草中分离出了致癌物质，虽然对这些形式的烟草与口腔癌关系的研究不如纸烟的广泛，但已有的研究显示烟斗、雪茄和无烟烟草与口腔癌有密切关系。

近年来烟斗产品的生产和消费都有所下降，而抽雪茄和小雪茄的人数上升了，在美国每年消费约500万支雪茄，过去的5年中抽雪茄的人数增加了50%。研究显示抽雪茄的人患心脏病、肺病以及口腔癌、喉癌、食道癌、肺癌的危险性升高了。部分原因是雪茄与纸烟相比，通常焦油、尼古丁、一氧化碳的含量多许多。如果雪茄是用烟叶包装，这些物质的含量和危险性更高。1支雪茄中焦油和尼古丁的含量相当于半包到1包纸烟的含量。要特别关注吸鼻烟和咀嚼烟草的致癌危险性。据估计有超过1200万的美国人使用无烟烟草，其中300万是21岁以下的。在美国的东南部，妇女常常吸鼻烟或嚼烟，她们口腔癌的发病率和死亡率都高。无烟烟草的致癌作用与长期使用有关。已经知道鼻烟和嚼烟中的不燃物亚硝胺是主要致癌的，其他致癌物质的含量少。使用无烟烟草最常引起的口腔问题是牙龈萎缩、过度角化和着色。

在撒丁岛、委内瑞拉和哥伦比亚等地区，一些人将小雪茄或卷烟叶的燃烧端放入口腔吸，叫做倒吸烟。在倒吸烟流行的地区，腭癌的发生率高。

3. 嚼槟榔 Betel chewing

印度、斯里兰卡、巴基斯坦、孟加拉国、缅甸、泰国、柬埔寨、马来西亚、新加坡、印度尼西亚、菲律宾、新几内亚、中国内地和台湾等地区有嚼槟榔的习惯，这些地区口腔癌的发病率高。在印度口腔癌占了全部癌症的15%～65%，在印度南部是最常见的癌症。不同地区槟榔的制作不同，有的地区直接咀嚼槟榔子，有的地区将槟榔子与石灰混合后再嚼，在印度是用槟榔叶包裹槟榔子、烟草、熟石灰和香料后咀嚼。

4. 饮酒 Alcohol drinking

35年前的一项研究已表明大量饮酒是发生口腔癌的重要因素，543名男性口腔癌患者中有1/3的人每天喝超过7盎司的威士忌酒，对照组的这一比例是12%。另一项调查发现，108名舌癌患者中有44%的人以及68名口底癌、腭癌、扁桃体癌患者中有59%的人有明确的肝脏酒精硬化。饮酒导致口腔癌的途径有以下几种，包括局部和全身作用：（1）酒精的脱水作用使口腔黏膜对酒精饮料中的致癌物质（亚硝胺、碳氢化合物）更敏感。（2）酒精的即刻代谢产物是乙醛，乙醛可以损害细胞，饮中等量的酒后唾液中就有相当量的乙醛形成。（3）在酒瘾很大的人群中酒精性肝病很普遍，肝病降低了肝脏对致癌物质的解毒作用。（4）酒精的能量高，大量饮酒后常常影响人的食欲，从而影响了人体对营养物质的摄取，加之酒精性肝脏的代谢能力受损，影响了营养物质的吸收。因此，长期大量饮酒导致营养缺乏，而营养缺乏显著降低了机体对癌症的抵抗力。大多数大量饮酒的人同时又吸烟，吸烟和饮酒的协同作用更增加了患口腔癌的危险性，这已被许多研究证实。

5. 营养 Nutrition

饮食和血清中维生素A含量低与口腔癌和口腔癌前病变有关，这是基于维生素A缺乏与过度角化的关系，以及在口腔癌高发的国家维生素A的摄入量低。维生素A原（类胡萝卜素）是有效的抗氧化剂，能控制细胞的自由基，而极不稳定的细胞自由基能导致变异和癌瘤的发生。

维生素C有助于阻断亚硝酸盐向亚硝胺的转化，但是没有证据表明口腔癌患者有缺乏维生素C的，或者补充维生素C有助于预防口腔癌。 维生素E也是一种抗氧化的维生素，但是缺乏维生素E或补充维生素E既不增加患口腔癌的危险性也不降低患口腔癌的危险性。缺铁性贫血是Plummer-Vinson综合征的部分表现，其他表现还包括吞咽困难、舌炎、黏膜萎缩。Plummer-Vinson综合征与增加发生舌癌的危险性有关，但是口腔癌患者并未表现缺铁。营养在口腔癌患者的治疗和恢复中起着重要作用。营养不良和非正常的体重下降与并发感染、恶病质和预后差有关，而营养丰富的饮食利于肿瘤的控制和预后。

6. 病毒 Viruses

能感染口腔组织又具有潜在致瘤作用的病毒有两种：疱疹病毒（Herpesvirus）和人乳头状瘤病毒（Human papillomavirus）。

感染人体组织的单纯疱疹病毒有 8 种：

单纯疱疹病毒 1（HSV-1），单纯疱疹病毒 2（HSV-2），带状水痘病毒（VZV；HHV-3）；EB 病毒（EBV；HHV-4）；人巨细胞病毒（CMV；HHV-5）；人疱疹病毒 6、7、8（HHV-6、HHV-7、HHV-8）。

其中的 HSV-2、HHV-3、HHV-5、HHV-7 与口腔癌没有关系。而单纯疱疹病毒 1、EB 病毒、人疱疹病毒 6 和人疱疹病毒 8 可能在口腔癌的形成中起一些作用。

目前已确定的人乳头状瘤病毒（HPVs）有90多种，感染人体的黏膜和皮肤。其中的HPV-16 和 HPV-18 可能在口腔癌前病变的恶变过程中起作用，被认为是口腔癌的危险因素。

7. 局部因素 Topical factors

长期以来，临床医生注意到不良的口腔卫生、牙列状况差（例如锐利的牙尖或边缘嵴，不良的修复体等）与口腔癌有关系。在化学物质致癌的动物实验中，黏膜有创伤及反复刺激的部位容易发生癌变。许多口腔癌患者癌瘤发生的部位有折断牙齿、义齿卡环或不合适的义齿边缘等慢性创伤刺激。有研究显示这些局部刺激本身并不是口腔癌的危险因素，在有其他危险因素存在的时候，局部刺激造成的慢性溃疡可能促进癌瘤的发生。

8. 太阳辐射 Sun radiation

户外工作者例如农民、渔民、邮递员等患唇癌的危险性较大，因为长期暴露于紫外线。证据来自许多国家，包括那些高纬度的国家例如芬兰和瑞典，因为空气洁净紫外线容易穿透；包括离赤道近的国家，因为日照的时间长，例如希腊的乡村唇癌占了口腔癌的60%。美国加利福尼亚的一项研究显示妇女患唇癌的危险与其一生中在日光下的暴露有关，而唇膏和其他遮光剂有保护作用。

The exact cause of oral cancer is unknown and may remain a mystery because of the multifactorial nature of carcinogenesis. Evidence indicates that although inherited genes do influence cancer risk, heredity alone explains only a fraction of all cancers. However, there is little evidence of a strong effect of familial and genetic predisposition to oral cancer.

Tobacco was first introduced to western civilization by the Spanish explorers of America in the early sixteenth century. At first, it was simply smoked in pipes, but, as it became more popular, it was also chewed and snuffed. Cigarettes were first made in Spain in the mid-seventeenth century, and, in the twentieth century, they became the most popular form of the tobacco habit.

There is absolutely no doubt that, on a global scale, the use and abuse of tobacco products is the major cause of oral cancer. The use of tobacco in all forms-cigarettes, cigars, pipes, chewing preparations, and snuff-increases the risk of eventually developing oral carcinoma. The association is based on the following facts:

- *Carcinogenic agents have been isolated from tobacco condensates.*
- *Tobacco can induce cellular change and tissue atypia.*
- *Patients with oral carcinoma use tobacco more than persons in control groups do.*
- *Tobacco used in various forms has been associated with an unusually high prevalence of carcinoma of specific oral sites.*
- *Continued smoking is a factor in the development of multiple oral carcinomas.*
- *The mortality ratio from oral carcinoma for smokers is greater than for nonsmokers.*

There are several ways in which alcohol is thought to contribute to oral cancer, by both local and systemic mechanisms. There is now clear evidence that ethanol increases the permeability of oral mucosa to water itself and to many water-soluble molecules, probably including important carcinogens. The immediate metabolite of ethanol is acetaldehyde. Some of this may be formed locally and damage cells. Indeed considerable amounts of acetaldehyde can be found in saliva after moderate alcohol consumption, owing to the action of bacterial alcohol dehydrogenases. Alcoholic liver disease is common in heavy drinkers and this reduces the detoxification of active carcinogens. Alcohol is high in calories, which suppresses appetite in heavy drinkers. This contributes to inadequate diet. Metabolism is further damaged by liver disease. As a result nutritional deficiencies are common, and, these contribute significantly to lowered resistance to cancer.

Both tobacco use and alcohol consumption are important independent risk factors for oral cancer and there is evidence that their combined effect is greater than the sum of the risks from exposure to either on its own.

第二节 口腔癌早期诊断、检查和预防

Section 2 Examination, Diagnosis of Oral Cancer and its Prevention

一、定期检查与早期诊断 Examination and diagnosis of initial stage

早期口腔癌的症状因肿瘤所在部位、来源、程度等的不同而不同。最常见的症状是不愈合的溃疡，伴有不同程度的疼痛，偶尔病变有出血。这样的症状通常在病人看医生之前已经存在了几个星期到几个月。无症状的病人有时候是在进行常规的口腔检查时被医生发现有可疑病变的。牙龈或牙槽骨肿瘤的很早期的症状常类似牙龈炎或牙槽窝的脓血症，发展了的牙龈恶性肿瘤可以表现为几个相邻牙齿的松动，一些牙龈癌或腭癌的病人可能会觉着所戴的义齿不合适了。

来源于口腔黏膜的原发癌的临床特征是多样的，可以表现为溃疡性、外生性、侵入性、或者表面增生的病变。溃疡性病变通常有不规则的边缘，而且溃疡基底的软组织变硬。外生性病变表现为菜花样不规则的生长，或者平坦的粉色、粉白色增生。有时候，表面侵入性癌症或原位癌的表现是红色或粉色的平坦的天鹅绒样的病变。有过多角蛋白的鳞癌、疣状癌表现为白色乳头状突起样的病变，表面有不同程度的角蛋白碎屑。侵入性病变的表层很小，但其下方波及的软组织范围大。来源于小涎腺的肿瘤以黏膜下肿块为主，最常发生在小涎腺最密集的部位硬腭，肿块增大后其表面的黏膜破溃形成溃疡，这时难以判断肿块是来源于上皮还是来源于涎腺。肉瘤也来自黏膜下的软组织，同样表现为黏膜下肿块。棕黑色病变是黏膜黑色素瘤的特征。

口腔黏膜的检查同牙列的检查一样要系统、仔细。首先用视诊，观察口腔结构和表面颜色的变化很重要，例如观察溃疡的边缘是否有凸起、萎缩的黏膜的范围、黏膜颜色的改变等等。特别需要注意口底、舌背边缘、舌根等口腔内的隐蔽部位，这些部位的病变容易逃脱检查者的视线。

视诊之后进行触诊，触诊是非常重要的检查方法。肿瘤即使是小肿瘤，其临床表现的独立性可以将其识别，也就是与周围黏膜相比肿瘤组织变硬了，即所谓的肿瘤组织所特有的癌样硬化，这种硬化使得正常的黏膜组织向肿瘤的转变很容易通过触诊感觉到。口腔癌导致的溃疡常有像围墙一样的边缘，是由活跃生长的肿瘤组织构成的，通过触诊可以感觉到溃疡基底厚而硬。触诊时不能遗漏颌下和颈部淋巴结。硬而不光滑的淋巴结，或者淋巴结区域有压痛都要高度怀疑肿瘤存在的可能。遇到有疑问的病例还可以用另一种重要的检查方法，将异常部位与对侧相对应的健康部位进行比较，即对称性比较。

检查时发现牙槽嵴有长出肉芽的不愈合的拔牙伤口，以及没有牙周病的牙列有松动的牙齿时，要注意可能有深部肿瘤的发生。在上颌的后部区域这些变化不罕见，这是破坏了牙槽骨的肿瘤长入口腔黏膜的结果。

表层溃疡和早期肿瘤经常被误诊为机械刺激导致的慢性感染性病变而采用漱口液、抗生素等来治疗。一个不能忽视的有助于诊断的问题是，因为慢性炎症细胞的浸润，长期创伤性溃疡的边缘增厚，溃疡周围的黏膜可见白斑样的变化。血管丰富的口腔黏膜再生得快，创伤性溃疡一般在去除刺激因素后的8～14天愈合。如果采用了漱口液、抗生素等治疗后溃疡仍未愈合，常考虑有恶性病变的存在，要建议病人尽快做进一步的诊断检查。

只要在检查中发现有可疑病例都需要做活组织的病理检查，诊断口腔癌的金标准就是活组织切片检查的结果。

二、口腔癌的预防 Prevention of oral cancer

1. 戒除烟草 Tobacco cessation

烟草在口腔癌的发生中起着非常重要的作用，所以停止使用烟草是预防口腔癌的基础，同时也促进了全身的健康。众所周知吸烟给人体健康带来的危害，英国卫生部统计，每 10 秒钟世界某地就有一个人死于吸烟引起的疾病。在发达国家，男性死亡者中有24%、女性死亡者中有 7% 是吸烟导致的，在发展中国家稍低，分别是 21% 和 4%。但是，发达国家烟草的消费量在下降，而发展中国家烟草的消费量却在上升。

终止烟草最简单的方法就是不吸烟，但是因为烟草中的尼古丁有成瘾性，使得戒烟很难。目前药物疗法对戒烟有一定的帮助，药物疗法有：（1）尼古丁替代疗法，是用其他途径来源的尼古丁代替烟草中的尼古丁。最普遍使用的是皮肤贴，能够稳定地释放定量的尼古丁。其他的还有鼻用喷雾剂、雾化吸入器、口香糖等方式。（2）服用药物，一些抗抑郁药有效果。应用最广泛的是 bupropion（Zyban），bupropion 具有多巴胺能和去甲肾上腺素的特性。药物治疗有许多副作用，包括口干、过敏、失眠和行为改变。

临床试验证明了药物疗法有一定的功效，治疗结束后通常有40%～60%的人停止了吸烟，1 年后随访还剩有 25% ～ 30% 的人。用药物疗法的同时，对吸烟者进行健康教育效果更好。

2. 初级预防与二级预防 Primary prevention and secondary prevention

初级预防以病因预防为主，针对致病因素采取预防措施，未病先防。口腔癌的初级预防就是不接触或者减少口腔癌的危险因素，口腔癌的主要危险因素在上节已经讨论过了。总括起来说，使用烟草、大量饮酒和不健康饮食的作用能够解释90%多的口腔癌病例。即使已经有了口腔癌前病变，如果减少对烟酒的依赖，这些癌前病变发生恶变的机会就会减少，在印度开展的一项大范围的初级干预的临床试验已经得出了关于这方面的令人鼓舞的证据。因此，除了口腔医生有责任，所有的卫生工作者都有责任和机会对公众进行健康教育和健康促进，以减少口腔癌的发生。

最有利于降低口腔癌危险的饮食是多吃进食蔬菜和水果，偶尔进食点红肉、加工过的肉类和蛋类食物。在瑞士进行了一项不同种类的食物对口咽癌危险性影响的病例对照研究，结果显示，经常进食蛋、红肉、猪肉和加工过的肉类能明显增加患口咽癌的危险。相反，减少口腔癌危险的食物有牛奶、鱼、生的蔬菜、烹调过的蔬菜、柑橘类水果和其他水果。表9-4是美国癌症协会推荐的预防癌症的饮食和行为。

表 9-4 American Cancer Society guidelines on diet, nutrition and cancer prevention

1. Choose most of the foods you eat from plant sources
Eat five or more servings of fruits and vegetables every day
Eat other foods from plant sources, such as breads, cereals, grain products, rice, pasta or beans several times each day
2. Limit your intake of high-fat foods, particularly from animal sources
Choose foods low in fat

Limit consumption of meats, especially high-fat meats

3. Be physically active: achieve and maintain a healthy weight

Be at least moderately active for 30 minutes or more on most days of the week

Stay within your healthy weight range

4. Limit consumption of alcoholic beverages, if you drink at all

5. Do not smoke

6. Avoid sexually transmitted infections

二级预防又可以称为三早预防，即早期发现、早期诊断、早期治疗。疾病处于早期阶段，及时采取适当的治疗措施，阻止病理过程的进展，尽可能达到完全康复。做好癌症的二级预防，能够延长病人的生存时间，提高他们的生活质量。

口腔癌二级预防的关键是早期筛查出口腔癌和潜在恶性病变的存在。对疾病的筛查是非常精确的科学，必须遵循已经建立的原则。口腔癌符合其中的部分而不是全部的标准。对口腔癌进行筛查的基本原理是基于这样的事实，即口腔癌在早期没有症状，局限，经常有白斑、红斑等潜在恶性病变的存在，而这些癌前病变能够通过简单的系统口腔黏膜检查发现。

现在还没有像筛查乳腺癌和宫颈癌那样适宜对所有人群进行口腔癌筛查的方法，一方面因为对口腔癌的自然病史不是充分了解，另一方面必须有足够的证据证明筛查方法的有效性和成本效益是合理的。因此，目前不推荐对所有人群进行口腔癌的筛查。但是，牙科诊所经常是发现口腔黏膜异常的第一场所，牙科医生有责任抓住机会对每一位病人（包括那些定期进行检查的人），特别是有吸烟、饮酒、嚼槟榔等习惯的病人进行口腔黏膜的检查，即使病人不是因为黏膜病就诊的。这种利用病人就诊机会进行的检查可以称为机会筛查，除了牙科医生，受过训练的初级卫生保健专业人员也可以进行口腔癌的机会筛查。

甲苯胺兰（Toluidine blue）染色检查作为诊断口腔癌和癌前病变的辅助手段目前受到很多关注。经过适当训练，甲苯胺兰染色在对高危人群进行筛查和帮助确定活组织检查部位时有重要作用。大部分研究显示甲苯胺兰染色能够检查出100%的侵袭性口腔癌，50%或低于50%的上皮异常增生能被检查出来。在黏膜健康完好的人群中甲苯胺兰染色检查的假阳性率很低。但是，有炎症、溃疡或糜烂的黏膜同样能着色，所以有些情况下单次应用甲苯胺兰染色的假阳性率可以高达48%，10～14天后普通的溃疡或创伤等病变愈合了，再染色一次，假阳性率降至11%。甲苯胺兰染色时舌背部总是着色，因为染色剂进入了舌乳头间的缝隙中，这使得该方法在舌背部的应用受到限制，除非病变发生在舌背部有萎缩的区域。在甲苯胺兰的使用中，训练、经验和好的临床判断力才能够确保这种辅助手段的合理使用。所有甲苯胺兰染色阳性的病例都需要做活组织切片检查。

3. 预防口腔癌的挑战 Challenges in oral cancer prevention

对公众教育、劝告病人、筛查等等要想取得成功，卫生保健工作者都面临着相当大的困难。口腔癌的最高危人群常是那些在接受医生邀请进行筛查、接受预防建议和行动上最不合作的，特别是那些社会经济状况较低的老年人群、戴全口义齿的以及重度吸烟饮酒的人群。另外，有的研究发现公众对口腔癌最重要的危险因素有混淆和缺乏了解，许多人误认为癌症不会发生在口腔。如果公众对口腔癌的性质、预后和常见的致病因素知道的很少，他们未必能理解一些预防措施，例如避免吸烟、减少酒精饮料的摄入和定期检查口腔黏膜。

口腔癌和癌前病变的筛查方法有其自身的特点，因为疾病的患病率低，筛查方法往往产生固有的假阳性的比例高。然而，鉴于口腔癌的严重性，必须选择高灵敏度的筛查标准，即使产生较多的假阳性病例。产生假阳性病例有两种结果：第一，发生一些不必要的费用，筛查结果出来后这些假阳性病人需要做进一步的检查以得出全面的诊断。第二，给这些被错误分类的病人带来痛苦，将他们置于一种等待最终诊断结果的不确定的状态中，另外活组织检查也会不舒服。因此，假阳性的错误分类关系到了筛查方法的成本效益和被涉及到的病人的情感状态。

在口腔癌和癌前病变的筛查中需要考虑的另一重要事项是目标人群的应答率，也就是依从性的问题，依从性包括对筛查的依从和筛查阳性者对随访的依从。按照每单位成本的收益，将筛查项目针对口腔癌的高危人群可能是最经济有效的策略，但是如果这些人群的依从性差可能会严重威胁筛查项目的经济生存能力。一些试点项目在工作场所进行，方便了人们的筛查，获得了比寄信邀请筛查更好的依从性。虽然采用了许多策略来提高依从性，但是利用人们进行常规的口腔检查或健康检查的机会进行口腔癌的筛查可能是更合适的方法。

4. 化学预防 Chemoprevention

口腔癌的化学预防是指有口腔癌前病变的人通过补充某些制剂使癌前病变消退、减少或使癌前病变的恶变率降低，从而起到预防口腔癌的作用。目前研究的比较多的制剂有维生素 A、类维生素 A 和 β- 胡萝卜素等，许多这方面的临床试验都是在印度进行的。

从动物实验的结果可以观察到维生素A可能有益于控制癌症和白斑，在动物实验中维生素A缺乏导致了上皮的过度角化。一些白斑病人服用大剂量的维生素 A 酯（每天超过 300,000 单位），角化过度的口腔白斑发生了逆转，停用维生素 A 后，白斑又重现了。作用的机理尚不清楚，可能是作用于上皮生长、抑制蛋白和细胞分化。用维生素A进行化学预防的缺点是因为肝脏的储存有限和毒性使得机体不能耐受大剂量的维生素A，最常见的副作用有皮肤干燥、皮疹和瘙痒症。类维生素 A 和 β- 胡萝卜素也可以使口腔白斑减退，但是停用后白斑很快又出现。与 β- 胡萝卜素相比，接受类维生素 A 的白斑病人发生恶变的比率低，然而合成的类维生素 A 的毒性大，限制了它的有效性和使用。

Bowman-Birk抑制剂是从大豆中提取的蛋白酶抑制剂，许多体外实验和动物实验已经证明了它有化学预防的作用。32 名白斑病人使用 Bowman-Birk 抑制剂 1 个月，31% 的病人有了积极的临床反应，其机理可能是作用于神经膜致癌基因的表达。总之，口腔癌的化学预防方法目前尚处于研究阶段。

With such well-known risk factors as tobacco and alcohol it is theoretically possible to prevent a substantial proportion of oral cancers. Stopping the habit of tobacco use is a fundamental part of prevention and treatment of oral cancers because tobacco plays such an important role in oral carcinogenesis. Many approaches for tobacco cessation have been used, with varying degrees of success. These approaches include filters, aversive conditioning, advertising regulations and legislation, counseling, pharmacotherapy. Clinical trials involving pharmacotherapy have demonstrated some limited efficacy, usually a 40% to 60% smoking cessation by individuals at the end of treatment but only 25%～30% at one-year follow-up. The best results are seen when pharmacotherapy and counseling are combined.

Primary prevention is the approach which concentrates on removing risk factors from the community with the intention of minimizing the number of cases of the disease which arise in that community, namely reducing the incidence of disease. If effective at an affordable cost, this is clearly the best approach in terms of both public and personal health gain.

The major risk factors for oral cancer are analysed in last section. Taken together, the effects of tobacco use, heavy alcohol consumption and poor diet probably explain over 90% of cases. The primary preventive approach of oral cancer is therefore clear. Even for patients who already have precancerous lesions, there is encouraging evidence from a large primary intervention trial in India that the chance of these undergoing malignant change is reduced if the patients can be persuaded to curtail their dependence on tobacco. In industrialized countries reducing smoking and alcohol consumption is a general health promotion strategy. Health promotion directed towards lowering the incidence of oral cancer is reinforced by general health policy through a common risk factor approach. Dentists and all health care professionals have an obligation and excellent opportunities to contribute.

Disease prevention or health promotion messages can be directed at whole communities, targeted at sectors of the population such as youth, prepared specifically for defined populations such as employees of a business or factory or delivered to individual 'clients' such as dental patients or those attending a health centre, antenatal clinic, physician's office, etc. There will be much common ground in the material suitable for these approaches. Dentists and doctors can obtain literature suitable for use in their offices or hospitals from many sources including, in many cases, national medical and dental associations and national health promotion and cancer prevention agencies. Much excellent material is available on the Internet.

Adequate (neither under- nor over-) nutrition is essential to host resistance against all diseases and this is strongly true of cancer. Many studies have shown that intake of protective nutrients is more effective when these are derived from natural foodstuffs rather than from synthetic food supplements. This is particularly important in smokers and drinkers.

Secondary prevention refers to the detection of cases of the disease in question at an early stage in its natural history at which intervention is likely to lead to cure, or to minimize morbidity and reduce eventual mortality. This is the category which encompasses screening. It is a complex area of science and the risks and benefits need careful evaluation in every situation.

The rationale for screening for oral cancer is based on the fact that these malignancies are asymptomatic and localized for a period of their natural history and are often preceded by potentially malignant lesions and conditions such as leukoplakia, erythroplakia and submucous fibrosis, when they can be detected by simple systematic oral examinations. However, population screening for oral cancer can not be recommended, because there is insufficient evidence for its utility or cost-effectiveness.

Logically, a stronger case can be made for targeting screening to at-risk populations-in the context of oral cancer perhaps to smokers and heavy drinkers over the age of 40.

Opportunistic screening, namely offering a screening test for an unsuspected disorder at a time when a person presents to a doctor-or a dentist or any other suitably trained primary health care professional-for another reason, is rational and cost-effective. This is the basis of the screening examination of the oral soft tissues recommended at every dental visit, perhaps also at periodic visits to a family physician. We have the manpower available-ourselves as trained specialists in what constitutes normal and abnormal tissues-and it need take only approximately 3 minutes for the month at least. This we have a duty to perform.

表 9-5 a.b.c.d.e.f., Oral Cancer Data from WHO

a.Oral Cancer - AFRO

Age - standardized Incidence Rate(100,000)*

Country		Cancer location				Year
		Salivary gland	Lip	Tongue	Mouth	
Algeria	M	2.3	0.6	0.2	0.5	
	F	0.1	0.1	-	0.2	1990 ~ 1993
French Reunion	M	0.5	5.4	0.3	6.2	
	F	0.2	0.4	0.2	0.6	1988 ~ 1992
Mali	M	0.2	0.5	-	0.3	
	F	0.3	0.3	0.4	0.3	1988 ~ 1992
Uganda	M	0.4	0.2	0.3	1.0	
	F	-	0.2	0.8	1.7	1991 ~ 1993
Zimbabwe African	M	-	1.1	0.9	0.5	
	F	-	-	0.4	0.3	1990 ~ 1992
Zimbabwe European	M	1.0	-	2.9	2.4	
	F	-	5.7	-	0.9	1990 ~ 1992

b.Oral Cancer - EURO

Age - standardized Incidence Rate（100,000）

Country		Cancer location				Year
		Salivary gland	Lip	Tongue	Mouth	
Austria	M	0.5	0.4	1.6	3.9	
	F	0.4	-	0.2	1.2	1988 ~ 1992
Belarus	M	0.8	5.8	2.6	3.6	
	F	0.3	0.8	0.2	0.4	1988 ~ 1992
Croatia	M	1.4	3.0	3.6	3.1	
	F	0.5	0.6	0.4	0.4	1988 ~ 1991
Czech Republic	M	0.9	1.6	2.1	2.2	
	F	0.5	0.3	0.4	0.4	1988 ~ 1992
Denmark	M	0.6	2.7	1.2	2.6	
	F	0.4	0.3	0.5	1.3	1988 ~ 1992
Estonia	M	0.5	2.3	2.5	4.1	
	F	0.5	0.3	0.4	0.5	1988 ~ 1992
Finland	M	0.6	3.5	1.0	1.0	
	F	0.5	0.6	0.6	0.7	1987 ~ 1992
France**	M	0.9	2.9	8.0	12.4	
	F	0.6	0.3	1.0	1.5	1988 ~ 1992
Germany East	M	0.5	1.5	1.6	1.8	
	F	0.8	1.0	4.1	5.3	1988 ~ 1992
Germany West	M	0.8	1.0	4.1	5.3	
	F	0.3	0.2	0.5	1.1	1988 ~ 1992
Iceland	M	0.8	2.0	1.1	1.7	
	F	0.4	0.2	0.5	1.3	1988 ~ 1992
Ireland	M	1.2	3.1	1.4	2.3	
	F	0.2	0.4	0.7	0.6	1988 ~ 1992
Israel Jews	M	0.7	3.3	0.8	0.8	
	F	0.5	0.9	0.6	0.6	1988 ~ 1992
Israel non Jews	M	0.1	1.5	0.2	0.5	
	F	0.2	0.9	0.4	0.5	1988 ~ 1992
Italy**	M	1.6	4.6	3.8	8.4	
	F	0.7	0.6	1.2	2.4	1988 ~ 1992
Latvia	M	0.6	2.8	2.1	2.6	
	F	0.3	0.3	0.2	0.3	1988 ~ 1992
Malta	M	0.2	2.3	0.8	1.4	
	F	1.0	-	1.2	1.1	1992 ~ 1993
Netherlands	M	0.6	1.7	1.4	2.1	
	F	0.4	0.2	0.8	1.1	1989 ~ 1992
Norway	M	0.6	2.3	1.3	1.7	
	F	0.4	0.5	0.6	0.8	1988 ~ 1992
Poland**	M	0.8	6.3	1.7	2.2	
	F	0.5	0.7	0.5	0.6	1988 ~ 1992

续表

Country		Cancer location				
		Salivary gland	Lip	Tongue	Mouth	Year
	M	0.7	3.9	5.1	5.4	
Slovakia	F	0.3	0.7	0.3	0.4	1988 ~ 1992
	M	0.5	2.0	3.5	5.0	
Slovenia	F	0.2	0.3	0.3	0.6	1988 ~ 1992
	M	0.8	12.0	5.2	4.9	
Spain**	F	0.6	0.7	0.9	1.0	1986 ~ 1992
	M	0.6	1.6	1.0	1.5	
Sweden	F	0.6	0.4	0.6	0.8	1988 ~ 1992
	M	0.9	3.0	4.8	5.3	
Switzerland**	F	0.8	0.8	1.4	1.5	1988 ~ 1992
	M	0.5	0.5	1.2	1.5	
UK, England & Wales	F	0.4	0.1	0.5	0.7	1988 ~ 1992
	M	0.7	1.2	1.9	2.8	
UK, Scotland	F	0.5	0.3	0.7	1.4	1988 ~ 1992
	M	0.6	3.9	3.0	2.3	
Yogoslavia	F	0.4	0.8	0.3	0.3	1988 ~ 1992

c.Oral Cancer - SEARO

Age - standardized Incidence Rate（100,000）*

Country		Cancer location				
		Salivary gland	Lip	Tongue	Mouth	Year
	M	0.6	1.1	6.5	10.8	1988 ~ 1992
India**	F	0.7	1.0	3.7	8.9	
Thailand**	M	0.4	0.3	2.0	2.5	1988 ~ 1993
	F	0.5	2.7	1.2	3.0	

d.Oral Cancer - AMRO

Age - standardized Incidence Rate（100,000）*

Country		Cancer location				
		Salivary gland	Lip	Tongue	Mouth	Year
Argentina	M	1.8	2.7	1.0	2.4	1990 ~ 1994
	F	0.3	0.3	0.8	0.6	
Brazil**	M	2.2	4.6	1.0	5.5	1989 ~ 1992
	F	0.5	1.7	0.6	2.0	
Canada	M	3.3	2.2	0.8	2.7	1989 ~ 1992
	F	0.5	0.8	0.5	1.2	
Colombia	M	0.3	1.2	0.6	2.3	1987 ~ 1991
	F	0.1	1.0	0.5	1.4	
Costa Rica	M	1.3	1.1	0.4	0.8	1988 ~ 1992
	F	0.5	0.6	0.5	0.6	
Ecuador	M	0.2	0.4	0.5	0.7	1988 ~ 1992
	F	-	0.2	0.3	0.2	
Peru**	M	0.3	0.7	0.6	1.3	1988 ~ 1991
	F	0.3	0.5	0.5	0.6	
Uruguay	M	0.9	2.9	1.0	2.7	1990 ~ 1992
	F	0.1	0.5	0.4	0.9	
	M	1.9	2.5	1.0	3.0	
USA-white	F	0.3	1.1	0.7	1.6	1988 ~ 1992
	M	0.0	4.5	0.9	5.4	
USA-black	F	0.0	1.1	0.7	1.9	1988 ~ 1992

e.Oral Cancer - EMRO

Age - standardized Incidence Rate（100,000）*

Country		Cancer location				
		Salivary gland	Lip	Tongue	Mouth	Year
	M	0.4	0.5	0.2	0.6	
Kuwait-kuwaitis	F	0.8	-	0.3	0.7	1988 ~ 1993
	M	0.7	0.7	0.7	0.5	
Kuwait-non kuwaitis	F	0.2	0.1	0.5	0.8	1988 ~ 1993

f.Oral Cancer - WPRO

Age - standardized Incidence Rate（100,000）*

Country		Cancer location				
		Salivary gland	Lip	Tongue	Mouth	Year
	M	1.1	13.5	2.8	2.8	
Australia**	F	0.7	3.2	1.0	1.3	1988 ~ 1992
	M	0.5	0.1	0.7	1.0	
China**	F	0.4	0.1	0.5	0.8	1988 ~ 1992

续表

Country		Cancer location Salivary gland	Lip	Tongue	Mouth	Year
French Polynesia	M	0.2	-	3.3	4.5	
	F	0.3	-	1.1	2.6	1989 ~ 1992
Hong Kong	M	0.7	0.1	2.1	1.9	
	F	0.6	0.0	1.2	0.8	1988 ~ 1992
Japan**	M	0.8	0.2	2.0	1.9	
	F	0.4	0.1	0.8	0.7	1988 ~ 1992
Korea, Republic of	M	1.6	-	0.7	0.6	
	F	-	0.2	0.3	0.7	1986 ~ 1992
New Zealand-non Maori	M	1.2	3.4	1.5	1.8	
	F	0.6	0.9	0.7	0.8	1988 ~ 1992
New Zealand-Maori	M	0.7	0.7	2.4	3.6	
	F	1.3	-	1.0	1.2	1988 ~ 1992
Philippines	M	1.2	0.1	2.6	3.1	
	F	1.0	0.1	2.1	3.2	1988 ~ 1992
Singapore-Chinese	M	0.6	0.0	0.7	0.6	
	F	0.6	-	0.7	0.6	1988 ~ 1992
Singapore-Malay	M	0.6	-	0.4	1.1	
	F	0.2	-	0.2	0.4	1988 ~ 1992
Singapore-Indian	M	0.3	-	2.8	3.7	
	F	1.3	-	0.6	3.6	1988 ~ 1992
Singapore-Viet Nam	M	0.7	0.1	0.8	1.1	
	F	0.5	0.2	1.0	1.1	1991 ~ 1993

小结 Summary

通过本章的学习，要掌握狭义的口腔癌和广义的口腔癌的内容、主要的口腔癌前病变包括什么、口腔癌的主要的致病因素以及口腔癌的预防。熟悉口腔癌的流行病学、口腔癌的行为特征、口腔癌的检查和早期诊断。

思考题 Review questions

1. 我们日常生活中的哪些方面与口腔癌的发生有关系？
2. 在临床工作中如何做好口腔癌的预防？

参考文献 References

1. 卞金有. 预防口腔医学. 人民卫生出版社, 2003
2. 邱蔚六. 口腔颌面外科学. 人民卫生出版社, 2000
3. 郑麟蕃等, 实用口腔科学. 人民卫生出版社, 2000
4. Cynthia Pine M, Community Oral Health. Wright, 1998
5. Jatin P Shah, et al. Oral Cancer. the United Kingdom, 2003
6. Murray JJ. CBE, et al. The Prevention of Oral Diseases, 4th edition, Oxford University Press, 2003
7. Richard E. Stallard, A Textbook of Preventive Dentistry, second edition, W. B. Saunders Company, 1982
8. Sol Silverman, Oral Cancer. 4th edition, the United State, 1998
9. Parkin DM, Pisani P, Ferlay J. Estimates of the worldwide incidence of eighteen major cancers in 1985. Int J Cancer, 1993; 54: 594-606
10. Linda M Martin, et al. Cancer prevention in dental practice: oral cancer screening and tobacco cessation advice. J Public Health Dent, 1996; 56: 336-340

（王文辉）

第十章　特殊人群的口腔保健

Chapter X Oral Health Care for the Special Groups

概述 Overview

本章介绍了特殊人群的主要口腔问题，阐述了他们口腔保健的需求和口腔卫生服务的策略。通过对本章的学习，应了解孕妇、学龄前儿童、学龄儿童、老年人以及残疾人等特殊人群的主要口腔问题，掌握针对不同人群的基本口腔保健策略和方法。

This chapter introduces the main oral health problems in several groups of population with special needs. The demands and strategies of oral health care among them are illustrated. Through this chapter, the main oral health problems of the pregnancy women, the preschool and school children, the elders, and the handicapped should be understood. The basic strategies and approaches of oral health care services for them should be grasped.

要点 Key points

- 婴幼儿口腔检查、家长的口腔健康咨询的内容；
- 婴幼儿口腔卫生指导的内容；
- 学校口腔保健项目；
- 老年人的主要口腔问题；

第一节　妇幼口腔保健

Section 1 Oral Health Care for the Maternal and Child

预防口腔医学的目标是帮助婴幼儿免除其罹患乳牙龋齿的危险，使儿童熟悉并乐于接受口腔检查，并且从婴儿期尽可能早地实施口腔预防保健措施以取得更好的口腔疾病预防效果。

在疾病发生之前，口腔医生应具备确定其发生潜能的评判能力，并制定有效的措施来预防其发生，这便是有效的预防性干预，而不是疾病发生之后的治疗。虽然在婴儿出生之后，儿科医生会定期为婴儿进行全身检查、生长发育评估、预防并及早发现疾病，但是儿科医生难以提供全面的口腔健康评价和口腔预防保健咨询。这些则是口腔医生的职责。

The dental profession possesses the knowledge and technology to assist parents in raising children free of dental disease. Dentistry's goal is to help infants and toddlers avoid the pain and devastation that accompanies early childhood caries, provide them with a pleasant, non-threatening introduction to dentistry, and to potential exists, the preventive process must begin early in infancy (birth to 1 year of age), to ensure a successful outcome.

As health professionals, it is necessary to identify the potential for the development of disease, and institute effective measures for preventing the initiation of the disease; it is then a sound and logical practice to intervene prior to the onset of the disease, rather than treat the effects of the disease. Examples exist in pediatric medicine with "well-baby" evaluations and immunization programs. Pediatricians recommend that the infant be evaluated five times during the first year, and three times during the second year of life. Although these visits are aimed at evaluating development, prevention, or early detection of disease, physicians are not trained to provide a thorough dental evaluation or proper preventive dental health counseling. It is the dental profession that must be proactive and assume the responsibility.

一、妊娠妇女的口腔保健 Oral health care services for pregnant women

妊娠妇女的口腔卫生保健包括两个方面，一方面是维护妊娠妇女的口腔健康，另一方面是为婴儿未来的口腔保健提供准备。为妊娠妇女提供口腔保健的目的是（1）减少妊娠期龋病、牙周病的发生或阻止已经发生的口腔疾病进一步发展；（2）增进妊娠妇女的口腔保健知识，提高自我口腔保健能力，以便能够为未来婴儿提供更好的口腔护理；（3）减少口腔内致龋微生物的数量以降低母婴传播的危险性。

The oral health care services for the pregnancy women include two aspects, one is for the expectant mother and the other is for the unborn child. The aims of providing oral health care services to the pregnancy women are (1) to reduce the possibility of onset and/or progression of caries and periodontal disease throughout the pregnancy; (2) to improve the oral health care knowledge of the expectant mother so that a greater possibility of better oral health care for the expected child would be achieved; and (3) to reduce the number of cariogenic organisms in the mother's mouth.

1. 产前口腔保健 Prenatal considerations

通常情况下，妇女一旦确诊怀孕便迫切关注自身和胎儿的健康。在这个时期，口腔医生就应参与到妊娠妇女的保健工作中。通过口腔健康咨询，口腔医生便成为母亲口腔保健知识的来源。

口腔健康咨询应尽可能早地成为到妊娠妇女保健的一部分，因为妊娠的前三个月是关键时期。牙胚在妊娠的第四到第五周形成，第九到第十二周牙齿和骨骼的早期矿化开始。这个时期的不良刺激会导致胎儿牙颌畸形。例如：唇腭裂是由于在妊娠第四到第六周时颌骨不能融合而形成的。很多因素都可能导致胎儿畸形，如基因变异、创伤、严重的病毒感染、酗酒、以及吸烟等。在胎儿的整个生长发育时期，任何过度刺激都会导致胎儿细胞生长发育短暂而不可逆的抑制。

In the short period after the diagnosis of pregnancy, an expectant mother is exposed to a barrage of information applicable to her health and that of her unborn child. Dentistry should be included in this routine. At the time of the dental counseling session, a knowledgeable dental professional should be the source of the essential information.

Dental counseling should come early, since the first trimester of pregnancy is a critical time. All organ systems are forming during this period. Tooth buds begin formation at the fourth to fifth week of gestation followed by the initial mineralization of bones and teeth from the ninth to twelfth week. Stress experiences by the unborn child at this time can produce dento-oral deformities. For example, a cleft lip or palate results when the maxillae fail to unite between the fourth to sixth weeks. These changes can result from a variety of etiologic factors affecting the mother such as genetics, stress of an injury, severe virus infection, alcohol toxicity, or smoking. An excessive stress to the fetus at any critical time in development can result in a temporary but often irreparable arrest in cellular growth.

妊娠期合理的营养是必须的。尽管妊娠妇女严重营养不良才会影响胎儿的生长发育，日常膳食还是要提供足够的蛋白质、脂肪、碳水化合物、维生素以及矿物质。虽然产科医生通常会给妊娠妇女补充各种营养素，但是适当地摄入主要营养素通常可以满足这些营养的需要。妊娠母体的骨组织会为胎儿的生长发育提供巨大的矿物质储备。

所有产科医生都应建议妊娠妇女早期接受口腔检查、口腔健康咨询、以及必要的、适当的口腔治疗。如果有可能，妊娠妇女最好选择一项灵活的、与自身的口腔健康状况相匹配的口腔保健项目，包括预防措施的应用、定期口腔检查、必要的口腔治疗等。很多妇女在妊娠期间忽视了口腔保健，最终导致严重的口腔问题。妊娠期间尽量避免X线照射，如果必须进行X线照相，最好避开妊娠期前三个月，并且对腹部进行必要的保护。所有的口腔治疗要在妊娠中期的三个月之内完成，因为妊娠后三个月随着胎儿的增大会影响母亲的体位，不便于进行口腔治疗，而且容易导致胎儿早产。除了提供所需的口腔治疗之外，口腔医生还要为妊娠妇女提供口腔预防保健方案，通过适当的措施帮助妊娠妇女维护良好的口腔卫生和健康的口腔环境。

Proper nutrition during pregnancy is essential. Although nutritional deficiencies in the mother usually must be severe to affect the unborn child, a daily balanced diet provides the necessary proteins, fats, carbohydrates, vitamins, and minerals. This requirement can usually be met by the adequate intake of the four basic food groups, although the obstetrician may desire to prescribe nutritional supplements. Bones of the maternal system form a large mineral reserve for use by the developing child.

All obstetric services should advice the expectant mothers to receive an early dental examination, preventive dentistry counseling for themselves and the future child, as well as necessary treatment. If available, the mother-to-be should be encouraged to seek a flexible dental program where prevention, monitoring, and therapy is commensurate with the severity of the dental condition. Many women who become pregnant are already long overdue for nine more months could cause severe oral problems. Dental radiographs for emergencies may be necessary, but should be avoided whenever possible during the first trimester. If radiographs are necessary, careful gonadal and abdominal shielding is required as with all dental patients. All dental treatment should be completed by the end of the second trimester, since the position of the baby by the third trimester affects the woman's posture, making long dental appointments quite uncomfortable. Once the treatment is completed, the attending dentist should supply feedback to the observation, indicating completion of the primary, secondary, and tertiary preventive dentistry treatment plans. All these emphasize on excellent maternal oral health.

2. 妊娠妇女面临的口腔问题 The mother-at-risk

通常妊娠之后，妇女罹患龋病的危险性会增加，这并不是怀孕本身造成的，而是因为饮食习惯和结构发生了改变，如食欲的增强、餐间甜食、零食的次数增加等。另外，妊娠反应的呕吐导致胃酸逆流也会引起牙齿舌面的酸蚀和脱矿。

避免饮食习惯的不良改变，减少餐间零食和甜食的次数可以最大限度地降低龋病发生的危险性。如果妊娠妇女生活在饮水氟浓度很低的地区，可以考虑适当应用氟化物。有研究表明怀孕母亲摄入氟化物可以降低婴儿出生后龋病发生的危险性。妇女在妊娠期间需要接受适当的口腔预防和治疗措施，定期进行口腔检查，由口腔医生局部应用氟化物或提供氟化物补充剂。

A pregnant woman is often at considerable risk of caries development. The mother's teeth do not lose calcium as postulated in a number of myths; instead, the risk of dental caries probably increases because of changes in eating habits. For example, the sucking of hard candy to reduce nausea, dietary cravings, and frequent between-meal snacks of refined carbohydrates can raise the caries potential of the dental plaque. In addition, the mother often experiences nausea or "moming sickness" causing vomiting with a regurgitation of stomach acid which may cause erosion and demineralization of the lingual surfaces of the teeth. Many times, only a toothbrush or a sudsy dentifrice is needed to trigger a gag reflex.

Avoidance of aberrant eating habits and snacking, and exercise of sugar discipline can greatly minimize the possibility of caries development. If the mother is living in a nonfluoridated area, fluoride supplements should be considered. There are few reports available that indicate a decrease in caries prevalence of children born to mothers taking fluoride. Since the supplement brings the level of fluoride intake to one part per million, there is no danger of excessive intake by the mother. There is the possibility of some benefit to the child. In addition, the expectant mother should be provided with appropriate treatment and recall appointments during the period of pregnancy. Professionally applied topical fluorides and systemic fluoride supplementation can benefit from the additional daily home use of fluoride dentifrices and mouth rinses. These measures will both prevent demineralization of the teeth, as well as facilitate reminearlization in the event of the development of an incipient lesion.

二、婴幼儿的口腔保健 Oral health care services for infant and toddler

1. 龋病——感染性疾病 Dental caries - an infectious disease

已有证据表明婴幼儿龋病是经由母婴传播变形链球菌而获得的感染性疾病。特异菌斑学说认为龋病是由特异性细菌引起的，纵向研究也提供证据表明变形链球菌是主要的致龋菌。因其具有以下特征：

（1）只有在牙萌出之后，口腔内才有永久变形链球菌的定植；

（2）如果口腔内已经有成熟的菌群存在，变形链球菌很难再植入；

（3）蔗糖为变形链球菌在牙面的粘附提供了便利；

（4）婴儿口腔内变形链球菌主要来源于家庭，尤其是母亲；

（5）母亲口腔内很低水平的变形链球菌就足以传播到婴儿口腔内。

Evidence suggests that dental caries is an infectious disease process initiated via the transmission of Streptococci mutans from parents to their infants. The specific plaque hypothesis suggests microbial specificity in dental caries, and longitudinal evidence supports the role of S. mutans in caries initiation. The following characteristics of S. mutans are important relative to dental caries in children,

a. Permanent S. mutans colonization of the oral cavity in infants occurs only after the eruption of teeth.

b. S. mutans has difficulty colonizing in an oral cavity already colonized by mature oral flora.

c. Sucrose facilitates the adherence of S. mutans to the tooth surface.

d. The source of infection of the infant with S. mutans is from within the family, most like the mother.

e. A minimum threshold level of maternal S. mutans is necessary for transmission of the microorganism to the infant.

母婴之间变形链球菌的传播主要发生于婴儿乳牙萌出阶段。如果婴儿食用含高糖的饮食，并且口腔内感染了变形链球菌就增加了龋病发生的危险性。婴儿早期就要实施良好的口腔清洁措施，采用低糖的饮食和良好的喂养方式。

因此，预防儿童龋齿的关键是采取各种措施减少母婴致龋菌传播的机会，母亲有必要从妊娠六个月开始一直到婴儿乳牙萌出后其口腔内建立起成熟的、稳定的、非致龋的菌群的过程中始终维持良好的口腔卫生。口腔保健服务应包括定期的口腔检查、适当的口腔预防性洁治、口腔内细菌检测、以及口腔健康监测。母亲可采用机械性和化学性菌斑控制方法，除了刷牙之外，还可采用牙齿冲洗，应用针对变形链球菌的抗牙菌斑漱口水如洗必太漱口等措施。对婴幼儿来说，最重要的就是从婴儿出生后就严格控制致龋食物的摄入，维护良好的口腔卫生。

Transmission of S. mutans to the infant most likely occurs during the first year of life, after the eruption of teeth. If the infant has a high sucrose diet in the presence of S. mutans the conditions are favorable for the initiation of caries. The early establishment of oral hygiene measures and the adoption of a low cariogenic diet and low risk feeding patterns should begin in infancy.

With the above bulleted points as a backdrop, it is possible to develop the guidelines that minimize the possibility of transmission of a cariogenic flora from the members of the family that will be most closely associated with the child. The most important goal is to reduce the bacterial challenge to the point that the potential for transmission of S. mutans is minimal. For the mother especially, this will require the continual maintenance of a high level of oral hygiene. Preferably, such a program should commence no later than the sixth month of pregnancy and continues throughout the time of the eruption of teeth and onward until a mature, stable, nonpathogenic plaque has been established (very low S. mutans count) on the child's erupted primary teeth. Such a program includes appropriately spaced professional visits for prophylaxis, bacterial counts, and monitoring oral health. For the mother, the manual and chemical plaque control procedures may include, in addition to the toothbrush, irrigation devices and use of such antiplaque rinses as chlorhexidine, which can specifically target S. mutans. For the child, the most important procedure from time of birth would be a restriction of cariogenic foods, and oral hygiene attention.

2. 早期预防干预的基本原理 Rationale for early preventive intervention

(1) 早期儿童龋 Early childhood caries

婴幼儿三岁之前就可以罹患龋病，有报道1岁婴儿的乳牙就发现了早期龋。儿童乳牙龋是婴幼儿乳牙列最主要的问题。以前的名称有喂养龋、奶瓶喂养龋、奶瓶喂养口腔疾病、奶瓶喂养综合征、婴儿奶瓶龋坏以及口腔奶瓶龋等。早期儿童龋的特点是口腔内发生猖獗性龋坏，早期累及上颌乳切牙，随后累及第一乳磨牙。主要病因是长期持续性用奶瓶喂养婴幼儿，儿童的乳牙长期暴露于奶瓶中的食物包括牛奶、婴儿配方食物、果汁、饮料或其他含蔗糖和碳水化合物的流食中。

在乳牙萌出、牙菌斑堆积的情况下，婴儿在睡觉时摄入含糖食物是导致婴儿发生龋病的一个危险因素，不应在婴儿午睡或夜晚睡觉的时候含着奶瓶（奶瓶中装着致龋性食物）或安慰奶嘴。因婴儿睡觉时口腔内唾液分泌减少，口腔内存留部分食物会形成酸性的口腔环境。这种酸性口腔环境主要累及上前牙。婴儿在哺乳或吸吮奶瓶时，舌头覆盖在下前牙上面，流质食物直接与上前牙接触，因此，在上前牙经受酸性环境反复侵袭的情况下，下前牙依然完好无损或仅轻度累及。婴儿吸吮习惯的不同，其他牙的累及程度也不同。

Dental caries can and dose occur in infants and toddles well before 3 years of age. Early infant caries has been observed in children as young as 12 months of age.

One of the first major hazards to the child's primary dentition is early childhood caries. This condition has also been referred to as "nursing caries," nursing bottle caries, nursing bottle mouth, baby-bottle syndrome, baby-bottle tooth decay (BBTD), and bottle-mouth caries. The caries pattern of this condition is highlighted by rampant dental caries initially involving the maxillary primary incisors and progressing to the first primary molars in latter stages. It is caused by continual, prolonged exposure of the primary teeth to milk, infant formula, fruit juices, soft drinks, or other sugar/carbohydrate-containing fluids placed in the nursing bottle.

Once teeth erupt, the practice of offering a child a bottle filled with cariogenic fluid as a pacifier or at naptime or bedtime should be discouraged. Once teeth erupt and plaque accumulates, the ingestion of sugar-containing fluids during bedtime or naptime places the child at considerable risk for dental caries since salivary flow decreases during sleep and the fluid pools around the teeth, creating a highly acidic environment. This permits the pooling of the oral fluids around the maxillary anterior teeth. Not all primary teeth are equally attacked. During sucking of the nipple of either the bottle or the breast, the tongue overlies the lower incisors, which directs the sweetened liquid against the maxillary incisors and to the back of the palate. The mandibular incisors often are either completely intact or only slightly affected, while the maxillary incisors bear the brunt of the repeated acid attacks. The other primary teeth are involved to various degrees, depending on the sucking habits of the infant.

乳牙龋的早期表现是牙颈部龈三分之一处出现白色釉质脱矿区，随着活动性龋的发展，病损区颜色变成褐色。最后，龋损从牙颈部继续发展导致乳牙牙冠的破坏或折断直至残存牙根。

有些母亲随意哺乳婴儿（需求喂养：24小时之内哺乳次数超过10次），这样母乳喂养的婴儿很有可能发生早期儿童龋。有时，即便没有这些不良的早期婴儿喂养习惯，婴幼儿也有可能发生早期儿童龋。早期干预措施会为婴幼儿提供预防乳牙龋发生的良好口腔环境。

乳牙龋齿导致的乳牙早失对儿童面部的发育会造成长远的影响。如果婴儿需要用奶瓶作为安慰来入睡，奶瓶中应当只装饮用水。

The caries attack begins with the appearance of white areas of demineralization around the gingival third of the teeth. With time, these incipient lesions begin to turn brown as active caries progresses. Eventually, the carious lesions that ring the cervical areas of the teeth can result in entire crowns being lost, either by fracture of the undermined enamel or by the continuous action of the caries.

In either event, only the exposed root is left in the alveolar.

Early childhood caries can also occur in some breast-fed children who are nursed every time the infant indicates a desire for feeding (demand feeding, with 10 or more nursing events over a 24-hour period). On occasion, there will be a pattern of multiple, severe caries in a toddler without a substantiated history of early nursing patterns that placed the infant at an increased risk. The caries process is certainly multifactorial and at times, a definite cause may not be identifiable. Nevertheless, sound primary preventive strategies early on will provide the appropriate environment for the prevention of dental caries.

The loss of teeth resulting from early childhood caries can have far-reaching effects on the child's eventual face growth. If a bottle is to be used as a pacifier, it should be filled with water.

（2）疾病的预防——积极的途径 Disease prevention - a proactive approach

口腔专业人员能够通过有效的方法预测龋病发生的可能性，采取有效措施来预防其发生，因此在疾病发生之前采取干预措施远比等到疾病发生之后采取治疗措施更为理想。例如：儿科的健康婴儿评估和计划免疫就是初级预防的措施。儿科医生通常建议婴儿在出生后第一年中进行5次评估，第二年中进行3次评估。尽管这些儿科检查目的在于评价儿童的生长发育、预防疾病的发生、尽早发现疾病，但儿科医生通常不能进行婴儿口腔健康检查或提供适当的口腔保健咨询。口腔专业医生必须积极主动承担这个职责。

As health professionals can identify the potential for the development of disease and have effective measures available for preventing the initiation of disease, it is a sound and logical practice to intervene prior to the onset of disease whenever possible rather than to wait and treat the effects of the disease. Examples of primary prevention exist in pediatric medicine with "well-baby" evaluations and immunization programs. Pediatricians recommend that the infant be evaluated five times during the first year and three times during the second year of life. Although these visits are aimed at evaluating development and prevention of early detection of disease, physicians are not adequately trained to provide a thorough dental evaluation or proper preventive dental health counseling. The dental profession must be proactive and assume this responsibility.

（3）公众和专业人员对口腔保健的态度 Public and professional attitude

面对乳牙龋这样的口腔问题，婴幼儿家长非常渴望其孩子能够接受早期的口腔检查和评估，并获得口腔疾病预防的知识。家长寻求婴幼儿早期口腔检查和评估的主要原因有：①渴望得到婴幼儿龋病预防的知识和信息；②渴望避免婴幼儿罹患龋齿；③渴望了解自身在婴幼儿口腔保健中的作用；④渴望得到医生的建议。

口腔健康教育最好以产科医生或儿科医生对孕妇或新产妇解释孕妇或产妇长期摄入含糖食物的危害开始。随后，作为解决的措施之一，儿科医生可以推荐含糖低的婴儿配方奶粉。最后，口腔医生必须重视学校和社区的口腔健康教育项目，使未来的父母亲认识到他们在儿童的口腔保健方面应当承担的责任。

Because of events such as early childhood caries, there is a growing desire by parents of infants and toddles to receive an early dental evaluation and obtain information on the prevention of dental diseases in their children. According to parents, the major reasons for them seeking early dental evaluations are:

a. Desire for information on preventing tooth decay for their child

b. Desire to avoid unpleasant experiences that the parents had suffered.

c. Desire to learn what their role is in their child's oral health.

d. Recommended by their pediatrician or family physician.

The education process can probably best start with the obstetrician and pediatrician explaining to the expectant or new parents the cause and consequences of continued intake of sugar fluids. The physician can further aid in reducing the problem by prescribing those bottle formulae that contain the least sugar. For instance, there is a considerable range in the amount of sugar found in the various commercially available baby foods. Finally, the dental profession should emphasize the need for high school and community dental education programs to alert would-be parents of their responsibilities in dental care for their children.

（4）婴儿的早期口腔护理 Early dental care

建立母亲每日为婴儿清洁口腔的习惯，使新生儿适应每日的口腔护理。每次进食之后，母亲应当用海绵或柔软的纱布蘸着清洁的水擦拭婴儿牙床和腭部。这样可以清除掉粘附的食物残渣。在婴幼儿期，儿童的口腔卫生都需要有家长的帮助和监督。以前，通常推荐儿童在两岁半之前要进行一次口腔健康检查。事实上，婴儿6个月大时就应该进行第一次口腔健康检查，最迟不能晚于婴儿一岁时。婴儿首次口腔健康检查的目的首先是评价婴儿口腔和颌骨的发育，其次是让婴儿熟悉口腔诊所的环境，减少未来就诊的恐惧。

The newborn should become accustomed to oral care early. After feeding, the ridges where the teeth will later appear and the palate should be gently wiped with gauze or a soft washcloth. This removes leftover food, and establishes a routine for the mother to clean inside the child's mouth. Children need directly supervised oral hygiene care throughout childhood. It was traditionally recommended that a child should visit the dental office no later than two and a half years of age. Ideally, the child's fist dental visit should occur at 6 months of age and no later that at one year of age. The purpose of this initial visit is to permit an evaluation of the mouth and jaws for proper formation and alignment of structures. A second objective of this visit is to allow the child to become familiar with the dental office and its personnel under pleasant circumstances and forestall future apprehension.

（5）婴儿早期口腔健康教育 Infant oral health education

根据联合国宪章有关“儿童的权利”章节，所有儿童应该享有同等权利，并享有健康和医疗服务的权利。乳牙龋是由生物学、行为方式、以及社会因素决定的，是与生活方式有关的疾病。婴儿在一岁左右进行早期筛查是预测和及早发现龋病危险因素以增强预防效果的最好选择。龋病危险性评估是推荐适当的预防措施的基础。

美国儿童牙科学会指出“婴儿的口腔护理首先要为婴儿提供口腔健康咨询，包括至少要在婴儿出生后 12 个月之内到口腔诊所进行一次口腔健康咨询。如果有的儿童牙齿萌出较晚，相应的初次就诊时间也可以延后，但是应当在第一颗乳牙萌出之后 6 个月之内进行初次口腔就诊。”

一项在8个月大婴儿母亲和保健人员中开展的口腔健康促进项目评价某些危险因素与乳牙

龋的关系的研究结果表明，母亲在接受了保健人员的健康指导之后，儿童的喂养方式发生了明显的改变，如改变奶瓶喂养方式，母亲用含氟牙膏给儿童刷牙，限制含糖食物和饮料的摄入，服用无糖的药物，以及预约到口腔诊所就诊等。

早期婴儿口腔保健的优点在于：

1）发现并改正不良的婴儿喂养方式，降低致龋危险性；

2）帮助婴儿家长为儿童选择低致龋性的饮食；

3）讲解并示范婴幼儿口腔清洁方法和步骤；

4）确定儿童氟化物摄入状况并推荐适当的氟化物补充措施；

5）在一种舒适、轻松的环境下，让儿童熟悉口腔诊所；

6）帮助儿童家长做好准备应对有可能遇到的儿童口腔健康问题。

According to the United Nation's Convention on "The Rights of the Child," articles 2 and 24, all children should have the same rights and have right to health and medical services. Early childhood caries is a lifestyle disease with biologic, behavioral, and social determinants. An early screening of all children at around one year of age is an excellent opportunity for early detection of risk factors and risk indicators that may increase the possibilities for its prevention. The caries risk evaluation should form the base for appropriate recommendations of prevention measures.

The American Academy of Pediatric Dentistry states:" Infant dental care begins with dental health counseling for the newborn, which should include a dental office visit for preventive oral health counseling no later than 12 months of age. However, for those children who are delayed in erupting teeth, the first visit may be postponed, but should occur within 6 months following the eruption of the first tooth."

One study evaluated an oral health promotion program involving health visitors and mothers of 8-month-old babies in order to address some of the risk factors associated with nursing caries. The oral-health promotion program significantly improved mothers recall of advice given by health visitors encouraging the use of a feeder cup, brushing their babies' teeth with fluoride toothpaste and restricting sugary foods and drinks. Significant improvements were also found in recall of advice regarding the use of sugar-free medicine and registering babies with a dentist.

The advantages of the infant oral health approach are:

a. Identifying and modifying detrimental feeding habits, reducing potential caries risk

b. Assisting parents in establishing low caries risk snacking and dietary patterns for their children

c. Explaining and demonstrating tooth cleaning procedures for infants and toddlers

d. Determining fluoride status and recommending an optimum fluoride program

e. Introducing dentistry to the child in a pleasant, nonthreatening manner

f. Preparing parents for upcoming dental events for their child (anticipatory guidance)

3. 早期儿童口腔预防干预方案 A protocol for early preventive intervention

（1）口腔健康访谈 The interview

口腔健康访谈和咨询应当简明扼要并有针对性。婴儿精力集中的时间是非常有限的，一旦婴儿产生了烦躁情绪想引起父母亲的注意时，无论婴儿家长还是婴儿对访谈内容的关注都会大大降低。经验表明口腔健康访谈和咨询最好是在口腔健康检查之前进行，这是因为：

①在口腔健康检查过程中，儿童家长的注意力和关注的心情通常会被调动起来；

②一旦婴儿在口腔检查过程中哭闹，在随后的讨论过程中，家长通常是更加直接地关注和安抚婴儿，而不能集中精力参与到讨论中来；

③口腔健康检查之前，在一个舒适、安全的环境里，儿童通常可以专注于玩具之中，这样，儿童家长便可以放心地、集中精力参与到讨论中来。

访谈应当以请儿童家长讲述就诊的原因开始。了解儿童的一般状况有助于口腔医生为儿童推荐适当的、有针对性的口腔预防措施。口腔医生需要了解的儿童一般状况包括：

①生长发育：发现婴儿生长发育的异常或怀疑有异常存在并建议进行深入的检查。同时，第一颗乳牙萌出的时间可以为牙齿的生长发育状况提供参考，解答儿童家长对于儿童生长发育情况的一些问题。

②喂养方式：婴儿时期的喂养方式是很关键的信息，医生可以通过发现不良的喂养方式来判断儿童发生早期龋齿的危险性，并帮助儿童家长改正不良的喂养方式，建议家长选择低致龋性的食物。

③疾病史：了解儿童全面的疾病史也是很重要的。在选择适当的预防措施时，应考虑任何可能对口腔健康造成不良影响的全身状况。例如：若儿童长期、多次服用含糖的药物，就要建议家长特别注重儿童的口腔清洁以减少因多次摄入糖而增加的龋齿危险性。

④预防评估：口腔医生以儿童牙齿生长发育状况、儿童家长的口腔保健态度以及儿童的口腔卫生习惯等信息为口腔健康访谈的基础，与家长一起讨论，并为儿童选择适当的口腔预防措施。家庭中其他成员牙齿龋坏情况，父母亲对儿童口腔保健的态度以及父母亲对访谈的反应等方面都要加以考虑。

⑤氟化物补充的情况：医生在给儿童开出氟化物补充剂的处方之前，必须清楚儿童饮用水中氟化物的含量，再相应开出氟化物补充剂的服用剂量。有的家庭居住在自然村庄中，饮用井水，但是儿童一天中大部分时间在幼儿园或学校中度过，而这些地方已经实施了氟化水源。因此，医生在给儿童开出氟化物补充剂处方时，一定要谨慎行事，要全面了解、准确评价儿童所有可能摄入氟化物的来源。

如果儿童每日摄入的氟化物量不足，应告诉家长儿童每日补充适量的氟化物对其牙齿是非常有益的。对婴儿来说，服用氟滴剂是最好的方法。儿童三岁左右，就可以改为吞咽氟片。随着儿童年龄的增长，儿童可以先咀嚼氟片，并使磨碎的氟片在口腔内存留一段时间再吞咽，以发挥氟化物局部和全身的防龋功效。

⑥口腔卫生习惯：评价儿童口腔清洁方法和状况有助于帮助儿童家长明确其在儿童口腔护理方面的责任。如果婴幼儿已经开始刷牙了，医生就要了解是谁、在什么时间、如何进行刷牙的，并询问儿童家长是否在帮助儿童刷牙的过程中遇到什么困难。

一项在美国进行的研究表明，大约有一半被访问的儿童家长在婴儿 12 个月时开始帮助儿童刷牙，在儿童 18 个月以前开始刷牙的有 75%。在这个时期，婴幼儿刷牙所用的含氟牙膏的量要很少，大约有豌豆粒大小即可，以避免婴幼儿吞咽过多的氟化物。儿童6岁时，可以采用每日氟水漱口的方法预防龋齿，这也可以成为终生口腔保健的方法之一。

The interview process and counseling session should be thorough and specific, yet concise. The attention span of the infant is limited and once the child becomes bored and seeks attention from the parents their attentiveness to your discussion will be limited. Experience shows that the interview and preventive counseling are best accomplished before the examination of the infant for the following reasons:

a. Specific parental concerns can be identified and addressed during the examination;

b. Should the infant fuss during the examination (normal behavior) the parents usually direct their attention toward the child during the ensuing discussion and not toward the dentist;

c. The child can be kept busy with toys, etc., before the examination in a nonthreatening environment and the parents will be better able to direct their attention toward the dentist.

The interview should begin with a discussion of the parents' reason for seeking care. Historical information gathered at the initial interview would assist the practitioner in developing the most appropriate and individualized preventive program for the family. Categories of helpful information are discussed in the following paragraphs.

Growth and development.

An abnormal pattern of development may be discovered or suspected, prompting a referral for further evaluation. Also, the date of the eruption of the first tooth will provide a baseline for determining dental development patterns and assist in answering future questions from parents regarding their child's dental development.

Feeding history

Knowledge of the feeding patterns during infancy is critical to assist the dentist in assessing the child's risk for developing early childhood caries by discovering potentially harmful feeding habits and to help form a basis for recommendations regarding proper feeding practices that minimize the potential for dental disease.

Medical history

A complete medical history is important. Knowledge of any systemic conditions that may adversely affect dental health will assist in developing appropriate preventive strategies. For example, long-term, frequent intake of sucrose-based medications may require additional recommendations for tooth cleaning to offset the increased caries risk from the sucrose intake.

Preventive assessment

Information regarding dental development, dental health attitudes, and current oral hygiene practices will serve as a starting point for counseling parents regarding an appropriate preventive program for their child. A history of tooth decay in the family will provided insight into the environmental influences as well as parental attitudes regarding dental health and serve to guide the dentist's discussion regarding preventive strategies.

Flouride supplementation

It is important to know if the child has access to fluoride in drinking water. It is not sufficient to establish that a family lives in a fluoridated community. On occasion, the family may drink bottled water, which contains an unknown quantity of fluoride. On the other hand, a family drinking well water may or may not be receiving systemic fluoride depending upon the concentration of fluoride in the water. Before any fluoride supplements are prescribed, the water should tested for fluoride concentration and supplements prescribed accordingly. Some families live in rural settings with well water, but the child spends the majority of the day in a location with fluoridated water such as a day care facility or school. Therefore, an accurate assessment of all potential sources of fluoride intake should be explored before making any recommendations regarding fluoride supplementation.

If the daily intake of fluoride is insufficient, parents should be informed that small daily dosages are beneficial to a child's teeth. This can initially be best accomplished by the use of fluoride drops. Around the age of 3, the drops can be replaced by fluoride tablets, which are swallowed. Later, as the child gains skill in chewing the tablet, the fluoride-laden saliva can be swished around the mouth and then swallowed to provide a topical application as well as systemic benefits. The practice of using a tablet a day should continue until the child is at least 12 years old, although many believe that fluoride supplementation should be considered as long as the individual - child or adult - has a fluoride-deficient intake.

Oral hygiene

An assessment of current tooth-cleaning activities is important to establish the parents' role in oral hygiene for their children. Many parents think that allowing an infant or toddler to brush their own teeth is adequate. If the infant's teeth are being brushed, it is important to establish how, when, and by whom, and inquire whether the parents experience any difficulties during the process.

In one study in the United States, almost half of the parents interviewed had stated toothbrushing programs for their infants at 12 months and 75% had done so by 18 months. With such infant and toddler toothbruhing programs, only a small amount, approximately the size of a pea, of a fluoridated dentifrice should be used in order to avoid the possibility of the child ingesting an excess of fluoride. Around the age of 6, daily fluoride mouth rinses may be initiated as part of the total lifelong oral health program.

（2）口腔健康咨询 Counseling

口腔医生通过与儿童家长进行访谈、咨询获得信息，在此基础上建议家长在儿童龋病的预防方面发挥积极的作用。家长需要在下列几个方面承担责任以维护儿童的口腔健康。

Based upon the information gathered to this point, the practitioner is ready to provide recommendations on how parents can play an active role in preventing dental disease in their child by assuming the responsibility for the following procedures.

1）口腔卫生 Oral hygiene

在儿童口腔清洁方面，家长必须意识到：儿童的父母亲或家庭中其他成员必须对婴幼儿口腔的清洁承担全部的责任。儿童在 6 ～ 8 岁之前自己很难彻底地清除牙菌斑。

①在一个舒适的环境中，婴幼儿在舒适的体位上接受口腔清洁。口腔医生要给儿童家长示范儿童接受口腔清洁时舒适的体位；

②婴儿口腔清洁不需要牙膏。很多情况下，牙膏可能会因其味道和起泡而使得婴儿拒绝接受口腔清洁措施；如果使用牙膏，牙膏的用量为豌豆粒大小以防儿童吞咽过多的氟化物；

③口腔清洁时要选择小头、软毛的儿童牙刷；

④婴幼儿每日至少要清洁一次口腔；

⑤婴幼儿晚间的口腔清洁可以在儿童进食最后一餐之后进行，而不要等到入睡之前，因为，在疲惫的情况下婴幼儿容易哭闹而不接受口腔清洁。

Parents should be educated regarding the following tooth-cleaning recommendations.

A parent, other adult or older sibling must assume total responsibility for tooth cleaning in infants and young children. Many children are unable to perform adequate plaque removal until 6 to 8 years of age.

Tooth cleaning should be done in a comfortable location and pleasant environment. Positioning will be demonstrated during the examination.

A dentifrice is not necessary for infants. In many cases, it may be a source for objection because of the taste and foaming action.

If a dentifrice is used, only a pea-sized amount should be placed on the brush to avoid ingestion of excess fluoride.

Tooth cleaning should be accomplished with a small, soft-bristled toothbrush.

Tooth cleaning should be accomplished at least once daily.

The evening tooth cleaning may be easier to accomplish following the infant's last feeding instead of waiting until just before bedtime since a tired infant can frequently be fussy during the procedure.

2）饮食控制 Diet management

婴幼儿时期，婴幼儿的饮食是由家长或托儿所控制的。因此，家长需要了解以下信息：

①婴儿 12 个月龄时就应停止用奶瓶喂养；

②婴儿睡觉时不应用奶瓶来做安慰；

③奶瓶中只能装入牛奶或配方奶；

④每日多次的母乳喂养，喂养的时间过长也是龋病的危险因素；

⑤避免夜间哺乳；

⑥婴幼儿通常每日需要多次进食；

⑦餐间零食最好选择低致龋性的食物；

⑧就龋病的危险性来说，致龋性食物总的摄入量远没有每日摄入的次数以及食物在口腔内存留的时间带来的危险性大。

Parents have control, for the most part, over their child's diet during the early years. The exceptions include time spent with babysitters and in day care settings. Parents can have some influence in those situations, however, if they make their wishes known. The following information should be shared with parents.

a. Infants should be weaned from the bottle around 12 months of age.

b. The bottle should not be used as a pacifier nor given during bedtime or naptime.

c. Only formula or milk should be offered in the bottle.

d. Frequent, prolonged episodes of breast-feeding could be a caries risk.

e. Nursing through the night should be voided.

f. Infants and young children generally will eat more frequently than three times daily.

g. Between-meal snacks should consist of foods that have a low cariogenic potential.

h. Total amount of cariogenic foods is not the issue, rather the frequency of ingestion and retentiveness of the food are the factors that contribute to the caries risk.

3）口腔检查 The examination

口腔健康访谈和咨询之后，医生开始对婴幼儿进行口腔健康检查。年龄小的儿童通常不需要牙科躺椅和照明灯。口腔检查的主要目的是让婴幼儿在安全舒适的环境下接受口腔医生的检查，3岁以下的幼儿最好是面对面地进行检查。这样的体位能够提供一个相对稳定而舒适的氛围，有利于儿童家长的参与，对于缺乏认知能力的幼儿来说，父母在场能够起到安抚的作用。如果婴幼儿需要支撑，医生可以采用坐位，用大腿的前部轻轻地稳住儿童的头和口，同时家长抓住儿童的双手，并用肘部稳定住儿童的双腿。采用这种体位大多数儿童都能够配合进行口腔检查。即便如此，如果婴幼儿哭闹，家长也要意识到这是正常的，而不要认为婴幼儿不配合。

Once the interview and counseling aspects of the visit are completed, the dentist is ready to proceed with the examination of the infant or toddler. The dental chair and overhead light are neither required nor very useful for examining children this young. Since one of the prime objectives is to provide a dental examination in a pleasant, nonthreatening manner, the procedure is best accomplished in the knee-to-knee position for children under 3 years of age. This position provides a stable, yet comfortable environment that incorporates the security of parental involvement, which may produce a calming effect on infants and toddlers who lack the cognitive ability to cooperate. Should the child offer resistance, the dentist can easily and gently stabilize the child's mouth and head cradled in the lap while the parent holds the child's hands and can stabilize the legs by cradling them with the elbows. Many of the infants and toddlers accept the examination procedures in this position without resistance. It is important in those instances where the children resist or cry that the parents be assured that the behavior is normal (and expected) for the child's age and should not be considered "bad" or "uncooperative."

口腔检查时，首先用手轻轻触摸儿童的头部和颈部，让婴幼儿熟悉医生的检查活动。在使用口腔检查器械之前，医生先用手指轻轻触摸儿童的口腔。护士或牙科助手可以用手电筒提供照明。可以将一个手指放在上颌最后一颗磨牙远中的牙龈垫上来稳定口腔。在完成口腔软组织检查之后，用一支湿润的、软毛儿童牙刷清洁牙齿（去除牙菌斑）。基本不需要橡皮杯或摩擦剂来去除牙面上的色素沉着。医生在实施口腔清洁的同时讲解并示范给家长，更重要的是要让家长有机会在医生的监督和指导下自己演示一遍儿童的口腔清洁过程。这样能够帮助家长克服自己不愿意为儿童清洁口腔的心态，尤其是在儿童哭闹拒绝的时候。有时，儿童的牙齿排列紧密，牙齿邻面堆积了大量的牙菌斑。这时要让家长学会如何用牙线和牙线支架去除这些部位的牙菌斑。要求家长每日至少要为儿童清洁一次牙齿。这个年龄的儿童无需使用牙膏，如果使用牙膏，一定要控制牙膏的用量。

要让儿童家长相信，即便有些儿童一开始时会拒绝接受家长为其进行口腔清洁，但是随着婴幼儿慢慢适应了家长每日口腔清洁程序之后，婴幼儿的口腔清洁就很容易进行了。在此情况下，即便婴幼儿哭闹拒绝接受，家长也不应该放弃。不要过多关注是否彻底地清除了牙菌斑，主要是让婴幼儿养成一个每日清洁口腔的好习惯。在儿童很配合的情况下，可以尽量彻底地清除牙菌斑。如果婴儿在出生后 12 个月内建立了每日清洁口腔的良好习惯，就可以避免儿童在两岁左右产生强烈的逆反心理和不合作行为。

The examination should begin with a soft touch, evaluating the extraoral head and neck conditions first, allowing the child to become accustomed to the dentist's actions. The examination of the oral cavity should begin by using the fingers to palpate the oral structures before introducing the dental instruments. Illumination can be provided with a penlight or flashlight held by the dental assistant. Access and stabilization of the mouth can be obtained by placing a finger on the gum pad distal to the most posterior tooth in a maxillary quadrant. Following inspection of the oral soft and hard tissues, a dental cleaning (plaque removal) is accomplished with a soft bristled, moist, child-sized toothbrush. Rarely will a rubber cup and polishing paste be required for stain removal. The tooth-cleaning process is discussed and demonstrated as you remove the plaque. At this point, it is very important that the child be repositioned with the head cradled in the parent's lap and the parent given the opportunity to practice the tooth-cleaning process with the dentist's supervision and guidance. This will help some parents get over their reluctance to clean their children's teeth, especially when the child resists. Occasionally, some infants and toddlers exhibit tight contacts between the anterior as well as the posterior teeth, which accumulate considerable plaque. The parent can be shown how to clean these areas using dental floss in a holder with relative ease. The parents are advised that they need to perform tooth cleaning for their children at least once per day. It is emphasized that toothpaste is not required and is usually objectionable to the infant. If it is used, only a minimal quantity should be placed on the brush.

It should also be emphasized early that when the child is becoming accustomed to the routine of having a parent brush the teeth, the tooth cleaning should not become an unpleasant struggle for those infants and toddlers who initially resist the procedure. On those occasions where the child struggles considerably, the procedure should not be abandoned. Rather, less attention can be placed on performing thorough plaque removal, while maintaining a consistent effort to establish a routine with the child. A more thorough tooth cleaning can be performed another day when the child is more cooperative. Parents can be reminded of other routines that are accomplished in spite of the child's objections, such as washing the child's hair. If the tooth-cleaning routine is established during the first 12 months, strong objections and resistance to the procedure during the "terrible twos" can usually be avoided.

首次就诊结束时，需要跟儿童家长总结以下内容：

①报告临床口腔检查所见；

②根据临床检查所见，提供适当的建议；

③询问并回答家长依然存在的问题；

④再次强调家长在儿童口腔护理中的作用和责任；

⑤提供一项适宜的应用氟化物的方法；

⑥依照家长的需要分发口腔健康教育材料；

⑦提供预见性的口腔卫生保健指导；

⑧确定适当的预约就诊时间。

The appointment is concluded by addressing the following areas:

a. Provide the parents with a summary of your clinical findings.

b. Make appropriate recommendations based upon the clinical findings.

c. Solicit and answer any remaining questions that the parents may have.

d. Reinforce the parents' role and responsibilities in their child's oral-health care.

e. Establish an optimal fluoride program (pending any water analysis) .

f. Distribute educational pamphlets/brochures as desired.

g. Provide anticipatory guidance information.

h. Establish an appropriate recall schedule.

4）预见性的口腔卫生保健指导 Anticipatory guidance

预见性的口腔卫生保健指导是向家长提供在下一次口腔就诊之前，儿童可能发生的生长发育方面的变化以及家长需要关注的问题。任何情况下，都应向准父母亲提供口腔预防保健的信息和预防项目。附录 10.1 ～ 10.3 中列出了相应的内容。

Anticipatory guidance is a process for preparing the parents for upcoming developmental changes and concerns that may arise before the next scheduled dental visit in order to minimize the negative effects that may arise. Wherever possible, preventive oral health information should be provided to expectant parents during prenatal education programs. Examples of such information are provided in Appendices 10.1 ～ 10.3.

5）确定预约就诊时间 Establishing a recall schedule

根据儿童的患龋危险性评价结果、临床检查所见、儿童生长发育的时期以及婴儿喂养方式和饮食习惯，确定就诊时间表，通常3，6，12 个月后再次复诊。附录 10.4 中列出了一个适宜的复诊时间表的例子。

The recall appointment may be scheduled for 3,6, or 12 months depending upon the child's potential risk for developing dental disease based upon clinical findings, stage of dental development, and feeding or diet patterns. Examples for determining appropriate recall schedules are listed in Appendix 10.4.

三、学龄前儿童的口腔保健 Oral health care services for preschool children

在我国，大部分儿童6岁上小学。在此之前，绝大多数的城市儿童和大部分的农村儿童都会在幼儿园或学前班度过一段时光。幼儿园儿童大多年龄在3 ~ 5岁间，这个时期也是乳牙龋齿快速增加的关键时期。另外，儿童5岁左右乳牙开始脱落，恒牙开始萌出，有的儿童在此过程中会感到不舒服，牙龈肿胀、疼痛。家长必须了解这方面的情况，必要时寻求口腔医生检查处理。

家长要承担起儿童口腔清洁的责任，并坚持每天至少一次在家里为儿童清洁口腔。多数儿童在 6 ～ 8 岁之前自己不能很好地清除牙菌斑。

这个时期口腔保健的重点是在幼儿园。幼儿园必须对儿童的口腔保健承担主要责任。首先幼儿园的老师需要掌握口腔保健知识和口腔护理方法。他们每年要接受口腔健康教育培训来学会如何指导儿童进行口腔护理。

幼儿园老师学会如何为儿童进行口腔健康教育和指导是幼儿园口腔保健的关键。口腔专业人员可以为幼儿园老师提供指导，采用多种形式对老师进行培训，制作口腔健康教育材料，如挂图、科普读物、录像带等，为幼儿园老师提供更多的口腔保健信息。

对幼儿园儿童进行口腔健康教育的途径与进行其他科学教育的途径是一样的——循序渐进。口腔健康教育要设计成针对不同年龄的儿童，提供需要不同灵活性、不同复杂程度的口腔护理内容。如幼儿园儿童的灵活性较差，只学会自己刷牙就可以了。另外，教育的策略可以是将口腔健康教育和口腔护理结合到儿童的日常活动中。

Normally, in China, children aged 6 years are enrolled in a primary school. Majority of the children in urban areas and some of the children in rural areas have experience of being cared in kindergartens or preschool institutions before their enrollment in a primary school. Most of children in these institutions are 3 to 5 years old children and most primary caries occurred and developed during this period. Primary teeth start to exfoliate and permanent teeth start to erupt when children are around 5 years old. Occasionally, children may experience pain and inflammation in gum, feel discomfort, parents should informed this situation and sometimes urgent dental care is needed.

Parents should assume total responsibility for tooth cleaning in young children and continue to practice tooth cleaning for their children at least once a day at home. Many children are unable to perform adequate plaque removal until 6 to 8 years of age.

Kindergartens where children spent most of daytime should assume main responsibility for oral health care of children. Oral health care should introduce to kindergarten teachers. They should received training on oral health care annually and are taught to teach children.

Teaching teacher to teach is important in oral health care in kindergarten. Dental professionals can provide teachers with guidance information, with a multimedia approach in the training sessions. In addition, oral health education materials, such as, posters, charts, and videotapes should be produced and sent to teachers and parents.

The approach to teach oral heath to children is the same with the approach to teach children other academic subjects, step-by-step. Oral health programs should be planned so that each higher-age level receives a greater diversity and complexity of subject matter and practical experience. For example, kindergarten children have least dexterity than primary school children, only toothbrushing is more easily taught and practiced. In addition, educational strategies can integrate oral health topics into daily activities.

如今，口腔医生已经拥有适当的技术和知识，拥有能力帮助家长，使得儿童在无龋的情况下健康成长。口腔医生应当积极、热心地承担其责任，并在疾病预防方面成为卫生专业人员的带头人。口腔医生不应该忽视 3 岁以下婴幼儿的口腔卫生服务需要。我们应该利用知识和技能，教育准父母和父母发挥他们做好儿童口腔护理的重要作用，从婴幼儿开始预防口腔疾病。

The potential exists today for dental-health professionals to assist parents in raising caries-free children. The knowledge and technology are available and the request for this service is growing. The dental professional has the opportunity to accept this role with enthusiasm and continue to be a leader among the health professions in disease prevention. The dental profession must not ignore the oral health needs of infants and toddlers under 3 years of age. We must instead, take advantage of our knowledge and technology and begin our disease prevention efforts with children as infants and educate parents-to-be and new parents regarding their important role in the oral health of their children. By doing so, we can provide a pleasant and logical introduction to dentistry and promote the profession in a most positive way.

第二节　中小学生口腔保健
Section 2 Oral Health Care for School Children

如今，我们有能力预防和控制学龄儿童发生的大多数口腔疾病。尽管根据世界卫生组织的龋病患病状况指标，我国学龄儿童恒牙龋病的患病状况属于很低水平，但我国学龄儿童的大部分龋齿都没有得到治疗。并且，我国学龄儿童的口腔卫生状况和牙周健康状况也不乐观。因此，学龄儿童的口腔保健仍需要加强。

Today we have the ability to prevent or control most oral diseases or conditions of school-aged children. For example, thousands of children and youths in the United States have been benefited from the use of these preventive procedures, and dental caries has been reduced dramatically among them. In fact, recent data show that nearly 55% of these children are caries-free in their permanent dentition, although the percentage decreases dramatically with age. In China, data from the Second National Oral Health Survey showed that the caries prevalence was 45.81% in 12-year-old school children, and 52.43% in 15-year-old school children. According to the standard levels of caries status recommended by the World Health Organization (WHO) , the caries status of Chinese 12-year-old children was very low. However, 88.45% of caries in the 12-year-old children and 82.84% of caries in the 15-year-old children were untreated decays. Furthermore, the oral hygiene and periodontal health status of the children was poor. Data from the Second National Oral Health Survey of China showed that only 31.01% of the 12-year-old children and 21.58% of the 15-year-old children had healthy periodontium (CPI = 0). Therefore, oral health care for the school-aged children should be improved.

一、口腔健康教育的责任者 Who is responsible for oral health education

学龄儿童主要依赖家长和以学校为基础的口腔保健项目来获得口腔保健的信息，包括口腔疾病预防和治疗的措施等。很多学校老师认为对儿童的口腔健康指导应该是家长和保健人员，而不是学校老师的责任。如果家长普遍能够作好儿童的口腔保健，老师有这样的想法也是合理的。但是，如果儿童生活在经济状况拮据的家庭，或者儿童家长的文化教育程度不高，那么儿童的口腔保健常常被家长忽视，家长只有在儿童出现牙齿疼痛时才会带儿童就诊。很多家长都很难有时间来关注儿童的口腔健康。如果社会口腔卫生服务系统不完善，他们就更难就诊了。在这些家庭中，儿童的口腔保健并不是家长首要关注的问题，他们首先要解决的是温饱问题。

School-age children, especially younger students, largely depend on parents and/or school-based programs for oral health information or for inclusion in preventive dentistry or treatment programs. Many teachers believe that oral health instruction should be the responsibility of parents and health educators - not teachers of academic subjects. This belief might be legitimate if, universally, parents were able to care for their children's oral health. A child reared in a home where the parents are subject to economic and educational disadvantages is often dentally neglected. In these homes, parental intercession in the oral health care of a child frequently begins with seeking help to relieve pain, often a difficult task because access to dental care is not easy for them. Too many working mothers and single parents find it very difficult to take time off from work to tend to their children's health, especially when there are additional barriers to access. Others may be apathetic or so overwhelmed with how to feed their family that oral health simply is not a priority in their lives.

受过高等教育的家长，他们的口腔保健知识水平通常也不高。况且，在家长的影响下，儿童行为的改变远比在学校老师的监督下难得多 。在口腔卫生保健方面，很多家长都不知道如何帮助儿童，他们需要有一个学校口腔保健项目来帮助儿童。只要有可能，家长要参与到学校儿童口腔保健项目中来。家长可以通过带头、督促等方式发挥积极的监督作用，强化学校口腔保健项目的内容，促使儿童口腔保健态度和行为的改变。如果有可能，对家长的口腔健康教育要与对儿童的口腔健康教育同步进行，这样，家长不但增进了自身的口腔保健知识，也有能力指导、帮助自己的孩子维护口腔健康。这样的口腔健康教育过程通常要纠正家长对口腔保健的不正确的观念，同时也要考虑到家长的经济接受能力。

所有的儿童都有接受教育的权利，每名儿童都应该成长为有知识、有能力的成年人。健康的儿童有更强的学习能力。学校和健康是密不可分的，因此，学校保健项目是预防儿童疾病、促进儿童身体健康的基础。

典型的学校保健项目包括三方面的内容：健康教育、保健服务以及维护有益于健康的环境。也有人将这三方面的内容扩展到八方面的内容：健康教育、体育锻炼、保健服务、营养监测、健康促进、咨询和心理服务、健康的学校环境，以及学生家长和社区参与。认为通过这些综合内容能够解决目前社区面对的复杂问题。确切地说，学校卫生保健项目同其他项目一样，必须是基于服务人群需要的综合保健项目。

Even with highly motivated and educated adults, their knowledge about oral health is often minimal. In addition, behavioral change may be more difficult to influence at home under parental guidance than under the tutelage of a teacher. In other words, many parents themselves do not know how to help their children help themselves and need to support of a school health program. Still, whenever possible, the parent must be included in a school-based oral health program. Parents can provide strong positive reinforcement, either through role-modeling or verbal messages that support the attitudinal and behavioral changes promulgated in the school setting. Ideally, parent education should parallel child education; in this way, parents can learn to improve their own oral health as well as have the guidelines to assist their children. This educational process of parents is often necessary to help overcome the barriers raised by their past adverse experiences with dental treatment and its financial hardships.

The bottom line is that all children have the right to a good education to enable them to be knowledgeable, productive adults. A healthy child is better able to learn. Schools and health are inextricably linked; thus, school health programs are the underpinnings of promoting health and preventing diseases among our children.

Typically school health programs have had three major components: health education, healthy services, and a healthful environment. More recently some have expanded this triad to an eight-component model that includes health education, physical education, health services, nutrition services, health promotion for school staff, counseling and psychological services, a healthy school environment, and parent and community involvement. Those who advocate the eight-component model believe that it is more comprehensive to help solve complex problems now faced by communities. No individual model is best. Rather, school-based programs, like other health programs, should be comprehensive and based on the needs of the population they are designed to serve.

二、创建有效的学校口腔保健项目 Creating effective, school-based oral health programs

学校口腔保健项目应该包括以下内容：知识、技能、动机、预防措施和治疗服务的利用以及安全健康的环境。更重要的是教育系统的政策支持以及学校领导和老师愿意将健康教育和健康促进的内容纳入到教学计划中。

口腔医生和口腔保健人员要承担起向公众传播基本口腔保健知识的责任，鼓励人们选择健康的口腔保健行为，促进口腔健康。在我国，完全依靠口腔专业人员来进行人群的口腔健康教育是不够的，需要学校、大众传媒以及口腔保健用品生产商的共同努力。

To involve communities, families, or individuals in assuming responsibility for their own oral health, many ingredients are necessary. These include but are not limited to: knowledge, skills, motivation, access to preventive agents and treatment services, and a safe, healthy environment. Further, decision makers and teachers must be willing to include health education and health promotion in schools. Finally, policy is important. For example, smoke-free schools are a result of a policy that bans the use of tobacco products - by all - on school campuses. Such policies help deter students and faculty from using these products.

It is impossible for the dentists and dental health workers in our country to assume the tremendous task of imparting essential oral health education to the public and encourages appropriate behaviors that are requisite to optimal oral health. Much of this education can be accomplished through schools, mass media, and industry.

1. 计划——成功的关键 Planning - key to success

成功的学校口腔保健项目需要针对不同年龄的儿童设计整体的计划、明确目的及参与人员的责任。一个项目涵盖从一年级到高中三年级的所有年龄组的学生是最理想的但也是不现实的。如果在一所学校中开展口腔保健项目，最常见的是涵盖小学一年级到六年级的学生。

好的计划会形成一个目标明确的、能够融入到整个学年教学活动中的学校口腔保健项目。计划必须包括社区需要评估、确定优先解决的问题、预算以及明确的评价内容。详尽的行动计划可以作为一个健康教育的工具来说服我们希望能够参与到项目中的个人或组织，也可以成为寻求经济资助的依据，当然，计划也是项目执行过程中的行动指南。

广泛一致的团队有利于将不同的资源、不同人群的要求以及广大的利益结合到一起。在项目计划的早期就要建立起来协调一致的儿童家长、社区领导、学校管理者和老师以及口腔专业人员的合作精神。任何一项口腔保健项目都必须有口腔专业人员的参与。

A successful school-based program does not just happen. An integrated plan of action for specified ages is essential, as is a clear delineation of program responsibilities and objectives. It should be noted that, although including all grades- grade 1 in primary school through grade 3 in high school - is desirable and ideal, it rarely occurs regarding oral health. When oral health is addressed in a school setting, it is more often confined to grade 1 through grade 6 in a primary school.

Judicious planning ultimately will result in meaningful, target-specific programs that are integrated throughout the school years. Planning must include a community needs assessment, establishing priorities, developing a budget, and a strong component of evaluation. Developing a written plan of action is necessary for a variety of reasons. The plan can serve as an educational tool to inform individuals and groups, especially those that are needed to "buy in" as a partner in the endeavor. A written plan also can be used to solicit funds to help underwrite the proposed program. And, of course, the plan serves as a guide for all who are actively involved to help maintain focus on the objectives.

A diverse and committed work group helps to ensure a greater variety of input, a representative audience, and a broad-based sense of ownership. It is essential that cooperative working relationships be established in the initial planning stages among parents, community leaders-business and political, teachers, school administrators, and oral health professionals. A dental representative should be a member involve in all school-based oral health program.

2. 健康教育的内容 Educational considerations

学校应该承担起对学生进行口腔健康教育的责任。有效的学校口腔健康教育项目的关键在于有责任心的、拥有口腔保健知识的老师。然而学校老师接受的口腔知识主要是口腔的解剖和生理功能、牙周组织以及涎腺等。这使得老师只能教授学生口腔的基本知识。应进行定期培训以保证老师拥有不断更新的口腔保健知识。教育主管部门应该为学校老师提供这样的培训计划。

学校老师和口腔专业人员有时会置疑学校口腔健康教育的意义，在学校中进行口腔健康教育会占用学生学习其他科目的时间，难道口腔保健知识比其他学科知识更为重要吗？口腔专业人员还会置疑仅仅进行口腔健康教育而不结合预防和治疗措施的效果。在学校中学到的口腔保健知识和技能对于成年之后的口腔健康有着显著的意义。

Traditionally, public schools have accepted the responsibility of teaching oral health as a part of general health. Committee, knowledgeable teachers are the cornerstones of all effective, school-based oral health education. However, the dental subject matter contained in many texts used in teachers' colleges relates mainly to the anatomy and physiology of the teeth, the supporting tissues, and salivary glands. Such a background enables schoolteachers to teach and promote basic information about the oral cavity. Teachers cannot be expected to possess expertise in a constantly changing pool of scientific knowledge relating to prevention and dental treatment options. As a result, they may be reluctant to teach what could be incorrect or obsolete information in these areas. Periodic in-service training to upgrade teacher health knowledge, including oral health, would greatly help the faculty to develop greater competence and confidence. To help attain this objective, the authorities should supply the teachers with a regular update of advances in dentistry.

Teachers and the dental profession alike have questioned the priority given to school oral health education programs. Sometimes the questions are asked by the educators because the time taken for dental education competes with the time needed for other subjects, is oral health instruction more important than, for instance, mathematics or vocational training? Health professionals also question the time devoted to school programs that feature mainly information transmittal, rather than a combination of education and preventive/treatment regimens. Education, alone, rarely suffices. For example, it is pointless to provide plaque removal instruction if toothbrushes are not provided and the instruction is not practiced in the classroom. Individuals, who are not provided assistance in shaping health attitudes, beliefs, and habits early in life, are likely to suffer the consequences of reduced productivity in later years. Health-related knowledge and skills acquired in public school may become more meaningful in adult life when the importance of good health becomes more apparent.

3. 学生的参与 Student participation

所有学生都应获得口腔保健信息，享受基本的口腔卫生服务，获得适当的口腔治疗。除口腔健康教育以外，氟水漱口、口服氟片等学校口腔保健项目都要针对最需要的人群，即高危人群。所有符合高危人群标准的学生享受同样的预防和治疗措施。

学生参与到项目中的程度是很重要的因素，个人的积极参与对于行为、态度和信念的改变会起到很大的作用。积极有效的参与有利于增强口腔疾病预防措施的效果，更好地维护口腔健康。

Philosophically, all children should be entitled to receive maximum information and primary preventive oral care. Providing maximum oral health treatment for all children, however, is not feasible. Poor children have a higher percentage of untreated decayed teeth than non-poor children. Hence, a school-based program, other than classroom education, fluoride mouth rinses, or tablet program, should be selective in targeting the children most at risk as eligible for a higher level of care. Once criteria are established defining "high risk", all students meeting the high-risk criteria should be eligible for the same preventive and treatment benefits. In a study, it was found that following a few years of participation in an intensive caries prevention program, individuals were transformed from high risk to low risk.

The extent of student involvement in program activities is an important issue. Personal involvement and participation tends to have a greater effect on behavior, attitudes, and beliefs. Active participation likely enhances interest in oral disease prevention measures and having a healthy mouth.

三、健康教育的内容 Content of health education

一个地区或学校中学生的需求，以及人、财、物的资源决定了口腔预防和治疗服务的可能性。附录 10.5 列出了口腔疾病预防和早期发现口腔疾病的一些相关内容。

The needs of students in a particular school or district coupled with available resources - human, equipment, and financial - will dictate necessary preventive and treatment services, education, and policies. Appendix 10.5 provides a list of topics that students should be taught regarding prevention and early detection of oral diseases and conditions.

1. 龋病的预防 Dental caries prevention

(1) 氟化物 Fluorides

学生应知道龋病是由多种因素引起的感染性疾病，是可以预防其发生、阻止其发展以及逆转其进展过程的，并且知道如何才能做到这些。他们应知道全身用氟和局部用氟的措施、知道氟化物在牙齿萌出之前、之后都会发挥其防龋作用，当然，氟化物最主要的作用是抑制釉质脱矿，促进再矿化。

Students need to learn that dental caries is an infectious disease with a multifactor etiology. And, they need to know that the disease can be prevented, arrested and reversed and how to do so. Students should be taught that the appropriate use of fluorides and pit-and-fissure sealants are our best defense against this disease. They also need to know about systemic fluorides, that is, fluoride intended for ingestion- community water fluoridation, school water fluoridation, and dietary fluoride supplements - as well as topical fluorides - those fluoride products that are not intended to be ingested - toothpastes, mouthrinses, and operator-applied fluorides. Everyone needs to know that fluoride works both pre-eruptively and post-eruptively, but the primary ways that fluorides work are to inhibit demineralization and facilitate remineralization.

(2) 窝沟封闭 Pit-and-fissure sealants

对于窝沟封闭，学生应知道为什么窝沟封闭能够预防龋齿，在何时进行哪颗牙齿的窝沟封闭以及需要重新封闭的可能性。更重要的是，学生和家长应知道已经封闭的牙齿不需要进行充填。

Regarding dental sealants, students need to know how sealants protect occlusal surfaces of the teeth from decay; the ages at which teeth should be sealed and the need for possible reapplication of sealant material. Further, and very important, students and parents need to know that teeth that have been sealed should not need to be restored with a filling.

(3) 饮食和营养 Diet and nutrition

美国农业部食物金字塔明确指出糖的消耗应该是中等程度的。过多甜食不仅对牙齿不利也容易造成肥胖。所有的健康教育都要包括饮食和营养指导的内容。学生应知道摄入碳水化合物，尤其是糖是龋病发生的关键因素。在进行饮食指导时，可以结合氟化物的防龋作用、窝沟封闭的应用以及口腔卫生措施等一起来阐明龋病的预防措施。对于进食甜食，最好的建议是，如果需要进食，最好选择在用餐的同时且控制摄入的量。在饮食指导方面，我们应当鼓励人们摄入不含糖的零食，减少高脂、高盐食物的摄入。

The United States Department of Agriculture's food pyramid makes it clear that sugars should be consumed only in moderation. Sweets not only are unhealthy for teeth but also are often in foods (cakes, pies, cookies, etc.) that are laden with unhealthy fats. Basic information on diet and nutrition should be a part of all health education. Students need to understand that consumption of carbohydrates, especially sugar is a key component of the caries process and that sugar must be present for caries to occur. Ideally, when discussing diet in relation to oral health, information should be taught with a parallel emphasis on the preventive benefits of fluoride and how they remineralize incipient lesions, which prevent them from becoming overt, and on the use of pit-and-fissure sealants and oral hygiene measures. In the United States, especially in recent years, more emphasis has been placed on making the tooth more resistant to decay with the use of fluorides and dental sealants. Perhaps the best message about sweets is that if you must consume sugars, do so at meals and in moderation. It is important that in our efforts to encourage consumption of non-sweet snacks that we do not encourage the use of high fat and high sodium foods.

常常是学生刚接受了限制甜食摄入的教育，又禁不住诱惑，购买了甜食。因此，学校应该是一个避免学生摄入过多甜食的场所。学校的营养师要减少学生每周摄入糖果的次数，可以选择新鲜的水果来代替。

另一项措施就是学校内禁止售卖糖果、饮料，代之以牛奶、水果、果汁等。最近的研究表明摄入水果和蔬菜能够预防口腔癌和心脏疾病。学校口腔保健项目要鼓励学生增加蔬菜和水果的摄入。学校的管理人员和营养师可以通过制定学生菜谱、限制甜食的售卖等措施肩负起维护学生口腔健康的责任。

Often, after a teacher has taught that sugar is one factor that causes tooth decay and suggests that the child avoid excessive and frequent ingestion of refine carbohydrates, the child then goes to the cafeteria. There, the child is confronted with attractive, sugar-laden deserts. The question then is "What message do students really get - the message they hear in the classroom or the message they see, smell, taste, and enjoy in the cafeteria?" Schools should provide an environment that promotes avoidance of an excessive intake of sugar consumption. One important method of meeting this objective is for the school dietitian to reduce the number of days a week in which confections are available. Instead, desserts such as fresh fruits can be offered that are nutritionally sound and limit the amount of sucrose consumed.

A second strategy for reducing student sucrose intake is for the school principal or superintendent to remove all vending machines that dispense candy and junk foods and soft drinks. Many schools have removed these kinds of machines or have substituted more nutritional snacks, including milk, fruit, and juices. Recent evidence suggests that the consumption of fruits and vegetables may provide a protective effect against oral cancers and heart disease. These school-based programs are designed to increase student consumption of fruits and vegetables to at least five-a-day. Dietitians and school administrators can act as gatekeepers to better student health by exercising control of the menu and the items in the vending machines respectively.

2. 牙龈炎的预防 Preventing gingivitis

彻底的牙菌斑控制是预防和治疗牙龈炎的基础。因此，学生要知道如何用牙刷、牙线彻底地清除牙菌斑而不损伤口腔软组织。老师要给学生讲述刷牙的技巧、牙线的使用等。

尽管没有证据表明仅靠刷牙可以预防龋齿，但是有明确的证据表明结合含氟牙膏的刷牙可以有效地预防龋齿。因此，应鼓励学生用含氟牙膏刷牙。

如果学校口腔保健项目仅讲授如何有效地清除牙菌斑而不提供牙刷和牙膏，这样的项目很难成功，尤其是经济拮据家庭的学生可能负担不起牙膏和牙刷的费用。即：如果没有牙刷，健康教育的效果将大打折扣。如果在学校进行刷牙的口腔健康教育，不仅要演示正确的刷牙方法，还有提供牙刷和牙膏以便学生能够在老师的指导下练习使用正确的方法。

Thorough mechanical plaque removal on a routine basis will essentially prevent and reverse gingivitis. Thus, it is important for children and youth to know how to remove plaque using a toothbrush and dental floss without injuring their soft tissues. For some children daily toothbrushing in the classroom may be both needed and desirable; but, in most cases, it is impractical. Despite the need for emphasis on toothbrushing, some basic problems arise. Many teachers are willing to teach the mechanics of toothbrushing so long as they do not have to demonstrate the unfamiliar details of plaque control. In fact, the issue of toothbruhing is often played down since too frequent repetition can be considered boring by students.

Other than preschool teachers, very few teachers are willing to incorporate daily toothbrushing into their classroom schedule. The daily need for hygienic storage and continued replacement of worn-out and lost brushes also poses problems for a teacher. Unless replacement toothbrushes are make available to the children without cost, dedicating classroom time for activities in which several students may not benefit due to economic or other factors is resisted. Finally, few classrooms have the water supply and the sinks necessary for conveniently scheduling daily brushing as a classroom activity.

Despite these problems, some classroom brushing programs have been a success. Although little or no evidence supports toothbrushing alone as a means of preventing caries, overwhelming evidence supports the fact that toothbrushing with a fluoride dentifrice is beneficial. Thus, one objective of toothbrush instruction is to encourage children to use a fluoride dentifrice when brushing teeth and not simply to teach toothbrushing as an exercise.

When a program just teaches plaque removal without providing toothbrushes and toothpaste for the students to practice, this approach, while well intended, may send very poor messages, especially among lower socioeconomic children who cannot afford toothbrushes and toothpaste. That is, the importance of this procedure will be lost if the child does not own a toothbrush. If toothbrushing instructions are provided in a classroom, it is critical not only to demonstrate proper procedure but also to provide brushes and toothpaste so that students can be observed practicing to help correct in appropriate methods.

四、体育运动中的口腔保护 Preventive dentistry in sports

体育运动是学生学习中的一项主要内容，许多体育运动中，口腔都容易受到伤害。不仅在踢足球中学生要佩戴口腔护套，在拳击、冰球以及曲棍球运动中都需要佩戴口腔护套。

口腔护套是在上下颌牙齿间放上软塑胶。这种装置能够缓冲来自于唇、颊、牙齿，以及上下颌间的暴力，减少颌骨骨折、颈部损伤、脑震荡、脑出血、昏迷、严重中枢系统损伤以及死亡发生的可能性。

如果没有佩戴口腔护套或护套没有起到保护作用，最常见的需要急症处理的口颌损伤就是牙齿撕脱。上颌牙齿最容易累及。一旦发生牙齿撕脱，可以抓住牙齿的牙冠部位冲洗牙齿，并轻轻放回原位。如果不容易复位，也不能让脱落的牙齿变干。在去口腔诊所就诊过程中，牛奶是很好的牙齿保存液。牙齿复位之后需要结扎固定7～10天，固位后的牙齿需要进行根管治疗。

预防口面部损伤的另外一项重要措施是乘车时系安全带，尤其是青少年。交通事故中青少年常遭受口颌部、颜面部、头颈部的损伤，然而佩戴安全带则能够减少发生这些损伤的机会。

Sports are an important morale ingredient for both student athletes and the student body. In many of the sports, the oral structures of these athletes are highly vulnerable to damage. Football is not the only school sport for which orofacial protection is needed. At the amateur level, sports that now mandate the use of mouthguards during practice sessions and in games as boxing, football, ice hockey, and field hockey.

A mouthgruard is constructed of soft plastic that is placed between the maxillary and mandibular dentition. These devices help to prevent violent contact between the lips, cheeks, and teeth, and between the upper and lower teeth. It reduces the possibility of fractured jaws as well as lessening the likelihood of neck injuries, concussion, cerebral hemorrhage, unconsciousness, serious central nerve damage, and death.

When a mouthguard is not worn or fails, one of the most frequent orofacial injuries requiring emergency treatment by the dentist is the avulsion of teeth. Maxillary teeth are the most vulnerable. When avulsion occurs, a recovered tooth should be held by the crown to rinse and then gently replaced at the site of origin. If the tooth cannot be easily reinserted, it should not be allowed to dry. Milk is a good transport solution on the way for emergency treatment at a dental office. After replacement, a minimum 7- to 10-day splinting period is advised. All avulsed teeth with fully formed roots eventually need endodontic treatment.

Equally or more important to prevent serious facial injuries is that the use of seat belts should be strongly advocated across all age groups but perhaps especially among youths who tend to believe they are not vulnerable. Car accidents involving youths frequently result in orofacial, head, and neck injuries, which could be reduced with the appropriate use of seat belts.

五、综合口腔保健项目 Comprehensive oral health programs

解决儿童口腔问题的手段是初级预防而不是治疗。从经济学的角度来说，对可以预防的疾病，应采用花费很少的预防措施来预防其发生，而不是等到疾病已经发生后，采用费用很高的治疗措施。从人文的角度来说，更应鼓励实施预防措施，而一旦预防措施失败了，再采用治疗措施。研究表明目前大部分的早期龋都可以采用窝沟封闭和再矿化的方法来控制。牙龈炎也可以通过综合性口腔卫生措施，如预防性洁治、机械和化学性菌斑控制等方法来控制。

目前，需要关注低收入家庭的儿童是否能够得到卫生服务。这种卫生服务必须是能够接受的、公正的、经济上能够承担得起的，并且是能够得到的。关键是口腔专业人员、健康教育者以及公共卫生机构要采取措施使得口腔卫生服务能够纳入到卫生服务项目计划中。决策者要发挥积极的作用使得口腔卫生服务能够共享国家的卫生资源。

Treatment is not the answer to solving children's oral health problems; rather primary prevention is the key. From an economic viewpoint, there is little rationale for treating a disease at great expense, when the disease can be prevented at a much lesser cost. From a human viewpoint, there is even less reason not to develop strong preventive programs supported with treatment programs when prevention fails. Research has shown that incipient dental caries can be largely controlled by techniques now available, such as sealant placement and remineralization therapy - techniques that are little publicized and underused by the profession. Gingivitis also can be controlled by a combination of oral hygiene practices - prophylaxis, chemical and manual plaque control.

Many communities are focusing on how millions of underprivileged children can be provided with health care. As a keystone of this effort, care must be acceptable, equitable, affordable, and accessible to all. It is critical that the dental profession, health educators, and public health agencies take the steps necessary to ensure that oral health is represented in the planning and implementation of such national efforts. Policy-maker must play a major role in ensuring that dentistry's share of funds will be available.

学校综合口腔卫生保健的优点包括（1）学生能够接受到口腔预防措施和口腔治疗；（2）学生更容易接受学校口腔治疗；（3）学校口腔保健项目增强口腔健康教育的效果；（4）口腔保健服务是学校保健的补充，从而达到学龄儿童全面保健的目的。健康教育、健康促进以及预防措施相结合的口腔保健项目大大减少了学生就诊口腔诊所接受治疗所耽误的课程时间，也减少了学生因为牙齿疼痛而耽误的课程或在接受口腔治疗之前、之后的恐惧。在学校实施综合口腔保健项目是可行的，在人员、经费和材料方面也是有成本效益的。这样的口腔保健项目已经在一些国家和地区建立起来，其他地区可以根据经济能力，采取不同水平的学校综合口腔保健措施。

There are several advantages to a comprehensive, school-based program: (1) students are available for preventive or treatment procedures; (2) school-based clinics may be less threatening than private offices; (3) school dental programs facilitate and increase the effectiveness of teaching oral health subjects; and (4) dental services supplement the school nursing services by providing total health care for schoolchildren.

A combined education, promotion, and preventive program in the school would greatly reduce the amount of classroom time lost in traveling to a treatment facility. Comprehensive school programs also would obviate the loss of study time due to pain and apprehension before and after treatment. Combined school-based educational and preventive dentistry programs for all schools could be feasible and cost-effective in terms of staffing, money, and material. Most important, with comprehensive school programs the decayed, missing, and filled teeth of students should demonstrate a substantial and steady decrease over time. A few of these kinds of programs have been established. Others could be established at different levels, depending on available funds.

1. 初级水平的学校综合口腔保健项目 Level 1

初级水平的口腔保健项目包括采用口腔健康教育课程，使学校老师和健康教育者能够组织、开展口腔健康教育。开展氟水漱口或含氟牙膏刷牙等预防措施。这两种预防措施都经济有效，容易实施。

Level 1 should include the use of a comprehensive oral health education curriculum. Providing such a curriculum minimizes the need for teachers or health educators to locate and organize lessons in an unfamiliar field. In addition, the teacher with the help of a school nurse and/or adult volunteer can conduct weekly fluoride mouth rinses or administer daily fluoride tablet regimens. The nurse might be responsible for preparing the mouth rinses or making the tablets available on a schedule approved by the teachers. Health educators, if available, help coordinate and integrate all health education activities. They have extensive training in educational principles and health, and are accustomed to working with school faculty. Fluoride mouth rinse or fluoride tablet regimens are easy to accomplish, economical, and effective. Neither of these self-applied, school-based fluoride regimens should be used if community or school water fluoridation is available.

2. 中级水平的学校综合口腔保健项目 Level 2

中级水平的学校口腔保健项目增加了口腔洁治。经过训练的口腔洁治员能够参与到学校口腔保健项目中，进行口腔预防性洁治、应用各种氟化物防龋措施、进行口腔卫生指导和饮食指导、实施窝沟封闭以及进行口腔筛查，建议学生采取必要的口腔检查、诊断和治疗。

国外很多学校和地区都有流动口腔治疗车，为学生提供预防性洁治、口腔疾病检查等服务。也有的学校安装简易的牙科设备为学生提供口腔服务。定期的口腔洁治能够预防牙龈炎的发生。另外，学生通过与口腔洁治员的接触能够更加愿意进行自我牙菌斑控制，愿意接受必要的口腔治疗。

Level 2 programs include level 1 activities plus the addition of a dental hygienist to the school health staff. The inclusion of a dental hygienist in a comprehensive school health program is critical. A dental hygienist is educated to plan and participate in school programs that include oral prophylaxes, use of variety of methods of fluoride application to foster remineralization, teaching oral hygiene procedures, counseling on diet, placement of pit-and-fissure sealants, and screening and referral for suspected oral pathology for definitive diagnosis and treatment.

Many school districts or public-health agencies have dental trailers that are used to provide prophylaxis and screening programs for students. Others use portable equipment that is set up in a room designated by school authorities. Older, teenaged students are more likely to present with gingivitis and calculus. A periodic prophylaxis by a dental hygienist during the school years may help avoid the onset of periodontitis later on. In addition, the personal contact with a dental hygienist can help motivate teenagers to develop satisfactory plaque removal techniques and to understand the need to seek professional care when needed.

3. 高级水平的学校口腔保健项目 Level 3

这一水平的口腔保健项目增加了口腔治疗，实现口腔疾病的早发现、早诊断、早治疗。为此，学生每年接受一次口腔检查，每半年接受一次高危人群筛查。

在日常的口腔预防性洁治和窝沟封闭过程中，口腔洁治员能够发现早期的口腔病损，并建议学生进行诊断和治疗。通常可以采取以下措施（1）学校给家长发通知，建议家长带领儿童寻求口腔治疗；（2）学校与某些口腔医生或医院达成协议，以一定的费用为学生提供指定的口腔治疗服务和直接的转诊服务；（3）学校将学生带到口腔医院中接受治疗或组织口腔医生为学生提供一定的免费治疗。

无论哪个水平上的学校口腔保健项目，该项目必须是经济上能够承担得起的、所有学生都能够享受到的服务，并且重点是针对高危人群。

A level 3 program consists of all of levels 1 and 2 requirements plus the addition of a treatment delivery option. This level of a comprehensive school oral health program includes the ability to identify and refer all pathology for treatment as early as possible. To achieve this level, an annual screening is indicted for all children and a semiannual screening for children classified as high risk.

During a routine prophylaxis procedures and sealant placement, a dental hygienist can identify early pathology and refer the student for expeditious definitive diagnosis and treatment.

All too often, the present method of managing schoolchildren with oral problems is for the teacher or school nurse to send home a note indicating a need for treatment and recommending that a child be taken to a dentist. This approach assumes that the parent immediately seeks a private dentist or goes to a public health clinic. In turn, it is assumed that when the dentist completes the treatment, a postcard is returned to the school hygienist or nurse indicating that the referred pathology has been treated. Theoretically, this type of system has the advantage that it uses the professional delivery systems existing in the student's community. Unfortunately, it does not always work. Not all parents respond willingly because of lack of money or insurance, apathy, or lack of available time to take the child to a dentist. This formula of "no money, no priority, no dentist, equals no care" is an elementary equation repeated countless times each year in our schools.

Another option for referral involves contracting with local practitioners to offer specific procedures for predetermined fees. In this case, the referral can be a direct transaction between the school system and dentist. The bill substitutes verification that the child received treatment. A third option often adopted is to bus children to a public health clinic. Or, in some communities dental societies have organized their dentists to volunteer to treat needy students.

The objective of whatever level of preventive care program is selected is that it be affordable, and accessible to all - with a priority for high-risk students.

六、新西兰和丹麦的学校口腔保健项目 School-based programs in New Zealand and Denmark

新西兰的学校口腔保健项目是以学校为基础、针对所有学生的、公正的、能够负担得起的、高水平的学校口腔保健项目。实际上，它是96%的学生都参加的免费口腔卫生服务，这项服务始于 1921 年。早期是年轻女性接受培训来完成牙齿充填和拔牙等工作。如今，男性和女性都接受培训成为口腔治疗员，他们只可以在公立的机构中从事口腔治疗服务，没有个人行医的执照。有上一级医生的指导和监督。他们主要是在大的学校诊所中为 5 ～ 13 岁儿童提供口腔治疗服务。

儿童每年接受一次口腔检查，高危人群每半年接受一次口腔检查。高危人群的筛选标准：

6 ～ 9 岁之间：4 颗以上乳牙有咬合面或复合面充填体，或乳、恒牙有除外唇舌面窝沟点隙的新龋损。

9 岁以上（恒牙）：第一恒磨牙咬合面充填或龋坏，9 岁之前牙齿邻面龋，或在过去 12 个月内，牙齿唇舌面窝沟点隙之外发生了新的龋齿。

预防措施主要针对高危人群采用 0.2% 的氟水漱口促进早期脱矿区再矿化，氟保护漆用于牙齿邻面龋的再矿化，新萌出的磨牙采用窝沟封闭预防咬合面龋齿。这些综合措施的开展使儿童龋齿从 1973 年的 DMFT 为 10.7 下降到 1992 年的 1.88。

The New Zealand School Dental Service likes an exemplary level-3 program. It is accessible to all, being based in the schools, equitable, with all children being able to enroll, affordable because there is no charge for service, and acceptable, with 96% of the pupils being enrolled. The service was formed in 1921 as a result of pressure on the government by the dental profession to help cope with the poor state of children's teeth. Originally, young women were trained to accomplish fillings and simple extractions. Today, both men and women are trained as dental therapists who can practice only in state institutions. They are not licensed for private practice. Supervision is provided by public health service officers and senior dental nurses. The service is based in clinics located in larger schools and takes care of all preschool, primary, and intermediate students between ages 5 and 13.

Children are examined annually, although those considered at high risk are examined semiannually. The guidelines for high risk are:

Over 6 and under 9 years of age - Four or more deciduous teeth with full occlusal or compound fillings，or new carious lesions other than buccal or lingual pits in permanent or deciduous teeth.

Over 9 years of age (permanent teeth only) - A full occlusal restoration or carious lesion on a first permanent molar, an interproximal cavity before age 9, or a new lesion in the previous 12 months other than a buccal or lingual pit.

The preventive program focuses on high-risk children. A 0.2% fluoride mouth rinse is used to prevent demineralization of "white spots," while fluoride varnish (Duraphat) is use for remineralization therapy of interproximal, enamel-limited lucencies. Finally, fissure sealants are placed on all newly erupted vulnerable permanent molars to prevent occlusal caries. This preventive emphasis and available treatment has resulted in a drop of DMFT of 10.7 in 1973 to 1.88 in 1992.

丹麦的学校综合口腔保健项目有悠久的历史。第一个学校牙科诊所在 1909 年建立。1971 年的儿童口腔保健法案是丹麦建立儿童口腔服务的基础。法案要求社会为 6 ~ 16 岁的儿童提供免费口腔卫生服务。在此服务过程中，始终贯穿着健康教育和初级预防保健。1972 ~ 1992 年间的全国口腔健康调查结果显示了丹麦学校综合口腔保健项目的效果。1986年，修改后的法案要达到的长远目标是“口腔卫生服务的目的是使人们都拥有健康的牙齿和口颌系统，并维护其终生发挥功能，这必须通过充分的自我口腔保健，综合预防措施，以及完善的治疗服务来实现。”修改后的法案包括了所有16岁以下的儿童。更加强化了氟化物的应用、窝沟封闭、每年定期检查、以及广泛的健康教育等措施。口腔疾病的治疗和错殆畸形的矫治也包含其中。新法案要求对所有的儿童、家长以及学校老师进行口腔健康教育。口腔健康教育是学校日常教学内容之一，并且设置成针对不同年龄的儿童有趣味性的健康教育内容。为孕妇提供口腔卫生指导，在新生儿的家访中为婴儿进行口腔卫生指导。对年龄稍大的儿童，教会他们如何进行口腔预约服务。提供这些服务的口腔专业人员包括牙科医生、牙科助手、以及牙科洁治员。丹麦是世界上儿童龋病患病率最低的国家之一。

Denmark also has an excellent and comprehensive school-based oral health care program. There has been a long tradition of providing oral health care to Danish children; in fact the first school dental clinic was established in 1909. The Child Oral Health Care Act of 1971 is the basis upon which the current Danish child oral health care service was established. Essentially, this legislation mandated communities to provide free dental care for children 6 to 16 years of age. The process was an incremental one with emphasis on primary prevention and oral health education of all parties.

Concomitantly, national epidemiologic data was established and maintained, which has provided the scientific evidence of the successful reduction of dental caries among Danish children between 1972 and 1992. In 1986, a new national law was introduced to replace the 1971 Act. The long-range goal of the revised national law was stated as: "The goal of the dental service is for the population to obtain healthy teeth, mouth and jaws, and to preserve them, in functional condition throughout life; this should be accomplished through a sufficient home dental care regimen, and a comprehensive preventive and curative dental health service." A major change in the 1971 Act was to include all children 16 years of age and younger. Again, the emphasis was on the use of fluorides, dental sealants, at least annual examinations and extensive educational interventions. Preventive regimens have been modified as new research has become available. The treatment of oral diseases and malocclusion also was included in the new legislation and by 1987 the system included all children. The law mandates oral health education for all children, parents, and teachers. Education in schools is a part of the regular curriculum and, thus, is adjusted for age appropriateness and at the same time to maintain interest. Oral health instruction also is provided to gravid women and oral health instruction is included in home visits for newborn and young children. Older children are taught how to make dental appointments so that they can continue their oral health care as adults. The dental teams who provide these services include dentists, dental hygienists and dental assistants. Danish school children enjoy one of the lowest caries prevalence in the world.

在我国，大部分的学龄儿童都没有享受到基本的口腔疾病预防、初级口腔保健和医疗保健服务。面对这种预防和治疗的需要，以及资源的短缺，儿童应当能够接受健康教育，获得保健信息，对于自身的健康能够有知情的选择。其次，儿童应该有机会学习如何选择正确的自我保健行为以促进自我口腔和全身的健康。最后，他们应该得到口腔疾病预防和治疗的服务。我们有能力从根本上减少儿童大部分的口腔疾病。显然也需要有政策和管理的手段使得这些经济有效的预防措施能够应用于儿童。学校口腔健康教育和促进项目给儿童青少年一个了解口腔疾病，维护口腔健康的机会。口腔医生、口腔洁治员以及各学科的学生有责任和义务促使这种综合口腔保健项目的开展。

A large proportion of our school-age children do not have access to basic preventive and primary dental and medical care. With the challenge posed by overwhelming need and limited resources, children deserve to receive information and education that enables them to make informed choices about their health. Also, they deserve the opportunity to learn skill and develop attitudes that enable them to practice appropriate behaviors to enhance their oral and general health. Finally, they deserve to receive services that prevent and/or treat oral diseases. We have the ability to essentially eliminate most oral diseases among children. Less obvious are the political and administrative means needed to make these cost-efficient measures available to the children. School-based oral health education and promotion programs give children and adolescents a chance to learn about their oral tissues in health and disease. Comprehensive, school-based oral health prevention and treatment programs provide a means not only to learn about disease, but also to maintain the health of the oral tissues and structures. Dentists, dental hygienists, and students of each discipline have an opportunity and the responsibility to help make such comprehensive programs available.

口腔健康教育与有效的口腔预防、治疗措施相结合，学校口腔保健项目就可以取得基本的成功。

事实上，采取有效口腔预防措施的学校很少。有效的口腔预防措施包括氟水漱口，口服氟片，促使釉质再矿化的措施以及含氟牙膏刷牙，所有这些措施都能够有效地降低学生龋齿的发生。只要加强自我口腔保健行为，就能取得降低龋齿的效果。员工中有口腔洁治员的学校也很少。洁治员是学校开展高水平综合口腔保健服务经济而有效的选择。洁治员可以作为学校教员来进行口腔健康教育，实施口腔预防项目，确定优先治疗人员，安排转诊服务等。

维护儿童的口腔健康需要家长、学校老师、学校管理部门以及所有卫生服务人员共同承担责任。尤其当我们国家的卫生服务目标是所有的儿童都能够享受医疗卫生服务时，更需要这些人员共同承担起责任。我们需要考虑全国性的学校口腔卫生服务政策——普及口腔健康教育知识，促进健康、采取预防措施、实施优先救护、转诊治疗服务等。

最后，如果学校开展口腔健康促进项目，它必须与整体医疗卫生服务项目相结合。

The major successes of school-based oral health program have been achieved when education has been combined with active prevention and/or treatment programs.

Unfortunately, too few schools have routinely included active preventive dentistry regimens - fluoride mouth rinses and tablet programs, sealant applications, remineralization therapy, and a strong emphasis on the use of fluoride-containing dentifrices while brushing - all of which can reduce the DMFS of a school population. This reduction can be accomplished with only a minimal change in self-behavior or compliance required of the student. A few school systems have employed dental hygienists as resources personnel to aid in the teaching programs and/or to provide primary preventive services. The availability of a dental hygienist provides an effective and economic means for schools to plan and participate in higher-level preventive programs. Hygienists can function on the school staff as oral health educators, conduct preventive programs, accomplish triage, and arrange for referral and follow up to ensure completeness of treatment.

Protecting the oral health of future generations is a commitment that must be shared by parents, teachers, school administrators, and all health professionals. This shared responsibility is especially relevant now that national health objectives for total child health care are established. Possibly the time is propitious to think in terms of a national school oral health policy - one that endorses universal access to oral health education, health promotion, preventive regimens, triage, and treatment referral capabilities for discerned pathology.

As a final note, if oral health promotion is to be accomplished through the school systems, it must be integrated with the general medical health program.

第三节　老年人口腔保健

Section 3 Oral Health Care for the Elders

从 20 世纪下半叶开始，人口的年龄构成发生了很大的变化，人均寿命的延长，老年人口的比例增大。人口统计学的变化对于医疗卫生服务，口腔卫生保健服务以及医疗工作人员都有着很大的影响。

联合国将60岁和60岁以上的人定义为老年人。但是对于老年人目前还没有一个一致的定义。一般是将到达退休年龄的人称为老年人。但是不同国家和地区的人们退休年龄不同。英国男性65岁，女性60岁。美国都是55岁。欧盟为60岁。我国男性为60岁，女性为55岁。一些学者将老年人又分为三个年龄段：65～74岁为“年轻老年人”，他们相对年轻、健康、有活力。75～84岁为“中老年人”，85岁以上为“长寿老年人”.

During the latter half of the 20th century, the age composition of the population changed dramatically, with more people living to older ages and the older population getting older. This demographic change will have a major impact on the delivery of general and oral health care, as well as on the providers of these services.

The elders are defined as those aged 60 years and over by the United Nations. Despite this, a generally agreed definition of elders is lacking. Normally, the elders are defined as people of pensionable age. However, the age of retirement varies in different countries of the world. In the United Kingdom, it is currently 65 for a man and 60 for a woman. The U.S.A. Bureau of the Census uses 55 years of age, and the European Commission uses 60. In our country, it is generally 60 for a man and 55 for a woman. Some researchers divided the elders into three categories. The "young old" or "able elderly" refers to people 65～74 years of age, who are relatively young, vigorous, fit, and healthy. People 75 years and older are called the "mid-old" or the "frail elderly" depending on their health and the thrust of the gerontologist's work. People aged 85 years and over are labeled "the oldest-old" or "the extreme aged" .

一、人口统计学分布 Demographic trends

世界人口的年龄分布发生了明显的改变。1998年世界卫生报告指出世界上有3.9亿的人口为65岁或65岁以上的老年人。估计这个数字到2025年会增加一倍。

在许多发展中国家，尤其是亚洲和拉丁美洲，预计到2025年老年人口所占的比例将会增加三倍。到2050年，全球将会有20亿人口超过60岁，其中80%的老年人口生活在发展中国家。老年人口的增加将使发展中国家面临巨大的挑战。

在我国，从建国后的四次全国人口普查结果看，60岁以上老年人口在我国人口结构中的比例从1953年的7.32%上升到1990年的8.58%。但是我国一些发达地区，60岁及60岁以上人口的比例已经超过了10%，达到了联合国规定的老年型社会的标准。

The age distribution of the world's population is changing. With advances in medicine and prolonged life expectancy, the proportion of older people will continue to rise worldwide. The 1998 World Health Report recorded 390 million people aged over 65 years. This figure, it is estimated, will double by 2025.

In many developing countries, particularly in Asia and Latin America, increases of up to 300% of the elderly population are expected by 2025. By 2050, there will be 2 billion people over the age of 60, 80% of them living in developing countries. The growth in this population is staggering, posing tremendous challenges in caring for the ageing population.

In China, data from the four national censuses showed that the proportion of people aged 60 years and over has been increasing from 7.32% in 1953 to 8.58% in 1990. In some developed areas the proportion of the elders increased to more than 10%, which is defined as an ageing population by United Nations.

二、与增龄有关的生理性变化 Physiological changes associated with ageing

生理性变化是长期的生物、心理、社会、环境的持续性变化的累积结果。许多以前认为是增龄性的变化实际上是病理过程的表现。这种变化发生于任何人群、任何机体组织、器官，只是不同的个体变化的速率不同而已。由于一些机体内部的增龄变化与疾病的表现类似，而一些正常的机体变化又能掩盖疾病过程，因此，对于老年人的护理不仅需要了解老年人正常的增龄变化，更需要区别病理性的改变和增龄变化。生理性增龄变化的四个特点是：普遍性、进展性、消耗性，以及内在性。

增龄性变化是复杂的过程，影响因素包括环境、遗传、生理和心理因素等。各种生理性增龄变化是相互作用，相互影响的。总的来说，随着身体的老化，机体的承受力逐渐降低。生理性增龄变化可以发生于机体的每一系统，影响人们的生活方式和态度，当然也包括口腔健康。

机体老化的主要结果是①生理功能减退；②自我稳定功能减弱；③免疫系统衰弱，肿瘤的发生增加，以及自体免疫能力的下降。

Physiological changes have a cumulative effect as they relate to the continuum of biological, psychological, social, and environmental processes of ageing. Many of the deficits traditionally thought to be associated with ageing are actually signs of pathologic processes. Changes occur on all people, tissues, and organs; however these changes occur with differing rates and individual variability. Variations occur at every age and in every part of the body. Since many internal changes can mimic disease manifestations, and normal changes can mask signs of disease processes, it is very important for those who care for the aged to be knowledgeable about the changes that do occur with ageing, rather than identifying changes either as pathologic or associated with the ageing process. The four characteristics of physiologic ageing are: universal, progressive, decremental, and intrinsic.

The determinants of ageing are complex, and include environmental exposures, genetics, lifestyle, and physiologic and psychological factors. Physiologic age-related changes are not mutually exclusive but rather synergistic and impact each other. In general, as the body advances in years, it tends to become less adaptive to stress. Physiologic changes associated with ageing can modify every system in the body, and impact the style and manner in which dental care is delivered.

The major results of the ageing process are: (1) a reduced physiological reserve of many body functions; (2) an impaired homeostasis mechanism by which bodily activities are kept adjusted; (3) an impaired immunologic system, as well as related increased incidence of neoplastic and age-related autoimmune conditions.

三、老年人的口腔健康问题 Oral health problems of elders

随着年龄的增长，自身免疫系统的衰弱，老年人罹患急、慢性传染病，致命性疾病的机会增加了。在老年人群中，肿瘤、心血管疾病、糖尿病以及感染性疾病很常见，老年人普遍口腔健康状况较差，主要是牙齿缺失和严重的牙周病。这些疾病不可避免地降低了老年人的生活质量。

口腔疾病通常是进行性、累积性的。增龄过程可以直接或间接地增加口腔疾病、牙齿缺失的危险性。在老年人中口腔疾病很常见，也很难得到口腔卫生服务。老年人主要的口腔问题有牙列缺损、龋病（特别是根龋）高发，而且多是未经治疗的龋齿、无牙颌，口腔功能受限、不合适的义齿、口腔癌、口干综合征、颅面部疼痛和不适等。

As people age, their susceptibility to chronic and life-threatening diseases are well as acute infections increases, exacerbated by compromised immune systems. Cancer, cardiovascular diseases, diabetes, infections and poor oral health, most notably tooth loss and severe periodontal conditions, are more prevalent in this age group. The consequences of these diseases and conditions are significant, leading to disabilities and reduced quality of life.

Oral diseases are usually progressive and cumulative. The process of ageing may directly or indirectly increase the risk of oral diseases and tooth loss, which are compounded by poor general health, illnesses or chronic diseases. Among the elders, high prevalence of co-morbidities and barriers to care are observed, together with oral health care challenges in relation to changing dentition status, caries prevalence with unmet need for care, periodontal pocketing/loss of attachment and poor oral hygiene, edentulousness and limited oral functioning, denture related conditions, ill-fitting removable dentures, oral cancer, xerostomia, and craniofacial pain and discomfort.

1. 牙齿缺失 Tooth loss

牙齿缺失是最常见的老年人口腔问题。主要是因龋病和牙周病所致。尽管在横断面研究和纵向研究中都发现随着年龄的增长，牙齿的缺失呈上升趋势，但在工业化国家，成人无牙颌的患病率从 60 年代开始却是呈现一个下降的趋势。

Tooth loss is the most common oral change associated with aging. However, no one ever lost a tooth because they celebrated a 75th birthday. Adults lose teeth because of disease, primarily dental caries or periodontal disease. Although tooth loss does increase with age in cross-sectional and longitudinal studies, the percent of adults who have lost all their teeth (i. e., are completely edentulous) has decreased from the 1960s through the 1990s in the industrialized countries.

2. 龋病 Dental caries

龋病常被认为是儿童的口腔疾病，但罹患龋病的老年人也越来越多了。龋病是成年人牙齿缺失的最主要原因。随着无牙颌的发生率越来越低，越来越多的老年人口腔内存留牙齿，龋病的危险性也增加了。根面龋是老年人常见的龋病。因此，在老年人中也要开展对儿童龋病有效的预防措施和方法。

老年人的龋病危险因素同其他成年人一样。只是，老年人常见的全身和局部疾病状况加剧了龋病的危险性。口腔卫生差延长了口腔内细菌接触食物的时间，形成口腔内的酸性环境。关节炎和中风患者自身活动性的受限影响了口腔卫生的维护。通常，日常生活活动尤其是进食方式受限的老年人，每天的口腔清洁也会受限而增加龋病的危险性。

Dental caries is often thought of as a disease of childhood. Currently, an increasing number of older adults are afflicted with this infectious condition. In fact, caries has been shown to be a major cause of tooth loss in adults. With the rate of edentulism continuing to decline, there will be an increase in the number of people with natural teeth who are at risk for caries. And root surface caries is commonly found in the elders. Thus, the preventive dental methods that have contributed to declining tooth decay rates in children will need to be applied to a growing older population.

Risk factors for caries among older adults are similar to those for all adults. Unfortunately, these risk factors are often enhanced by local and systemic diseases that are more prevalent in old age. Poor oral hygiene allows both an acidic environment and prolonged access to food sources for bacterial proliferation. Poor oral hygiene can be exacerbated by decreased dexterity, as occurs in arthritic or stroke victims. As a general rule, persons who have difficulty with their activities of daily living, particularly feeding, will have difficulty with daily oral care and are at greater risk for dental caries.

老年人食物的选择也影响他们的龋病患病状况。咀嚼能力的下降和经济状况的限制，他们常选择较软的、能够被发酵的，具有致龋性的碳水化合物作为食物。牙周病也是根面龋的一个危险因素。慢性牙周病导致牙龈退缩，牙根面暴露。牙根面或牙骨质一旦暴露于酸性的口腔环境中，很快就会发生脱矿。唾液分泌的减少也可增加龋病的危险性。接受头颈部放射性治疗的患者，涎腺受到损伤，唾液分泌量显著减少，龋病的危险性明显增加。药物治疗和原发性涎腺疾病都会引起唾液分泌量的减少，增加龋病的危险性。

Dietary choices made by older adults can greatly affect their caries activity. A decreased ability to chew and poor economic status among older adults have been shown to contribute to a diet that is higher in fermentable carbohydrates, softer, and therefore more cariogenic. Periodontal disease also acts as a risk factor specific for root caries. Chronic periodontal disease often leads to recession of gingival tissue with resulting tooth root exposure. Once the root surface or cementum of a tooth is exposed to the oral environment, it can be quickly demineralized when exposed to the acidic by-products of bacteria. Decreases in salivary flow contribute significantly to increased caries activity. Patients who have a significantly decreased flow rate secondary to radiation therapy to the head or neck, which affects the salivary glands, have demonstrated a significant increase in caries activity. Medication use and primary salivary gland disease can also cause low salivary flow, and increase the risk of caries.

3. 牙周病 Periodontal diseases

牙龈炎的主要致病因素是口腔卫生差。大多数情况下，去除牙菌斑能够减轻牙龈组织的炎症反应，牙龈炎可以治愈。研究发现尽管老年人很容易罹患牙龈炎，但是老年人牙龈组织的愈合能力没有减退。类固醇引起的牙龈炎多与绝经后的妇女采用激素替代疗法有关。一些药物治疗也能导致药物性牙龈增生，如苯妥英钠、硝苯地平等。服用这些药物时，口腔卫生差加剧了牙龈的增生。而牙龈的增生也影响了口腔卫生的自我维护。维护良好的口腔卫生、去除龈下牙菌斑和牙石能够减轻牙龈的增生。若增生的牙龈组织难以恢复，则需要采取牙周手术的方法切除增生的牙龈。

发生于老年人的牙周炎多是慢性牙周炎。慢性牙周炎目前认为是短时间的疾病活动或破坏期与长时间的疾病静止期交替进行的结果。因此，老年人的牙周组织破坏多数是长期牙周炎破坏累积的结果。研究发现老年人中急性、进展性的牙周炎不常见。急性、进展性的牙周炎常导致牙齿很早就脱落了，这说明年龄的增长并不是牙周病的危险因素。老年人衰退的免疫反应则可加剧牙周病的炎症反应。一些营养的缺乏，如维生素C，钙、锌等可能会增加老年人牙周炎的易感性，加剧牙周炎的进展。吸烟是牙周炎一个高度危险的因素。对于牙周组织的破坏，吸烟的影响与口腔微生物的影响同样重要。

The primary risk factor for gingivitis is poor oral hygiene. Removal of the plaque eliminates the inflammatory response and, in most cases, the gingivitis will heal. Some research has shown that although gingivitis forms more quickly in older adults, healing is not impaired. Medications can also alter the gingival tissue. Steroidinduced gingivitis has been associated with postmenopausal women receiving hormone replacement therapy. Gingival overgrowth can be induced by certain medications, such as cyclosporins, nifedipine, and phenytoin. Poor oral hygiene increases the risk of gingival hyperplasia when taking any of these medications. This overgrowth further decreases a person's ability to maintain good oral hygiene. To eliminate the overgrowth, oral hygiene must be improved and any plaque or calculus removed from beneath the gingival tissue. If the tissue does not satisfactorily resolve after a dental scaling, the overgrown tissue can be surgically removed.

Periodontitis is the destruction of the supporting structure of the tooth. If a sufficiently large amount of supporting bone is lost, clinically a patient may present with a chief complaint of tooth migration or movement, loose teeth, and tooth loss. Periodontal disease in older adults is commonly referred to as chronic periodontitis. Chronic periodontitis is now believed to be composed of short bursts of disease activity or destruction and longer periods of quiescence. Because periodontitis is a chronic disease, much of the ravages of the disease we see in older adults result from an accumulation of the disease over time. Research has shown that the advanced stages of periodontitis are less prevalent than the moderate stages in the elderly population. It is theorized that many of the sites of advanced periodontal disease have resulted in tooth loss earlier in life, suggesting that older age is not a risk factor for periodontal disease. As with caries, bacteria-containing plaque is the primary risk factor for periodontal disease. An altered immune response can exacerbate the inflammatory reaction in periodontal disease. Certain nutritional deficiencies, such as vitamin C, calcium, and zinc, may all play a role in the susceptibility and progression of periodontitis. People who smoke are at greater risk for periodontal disease. Smoking has been shown to be as important as bacterial destruction in the formation of this oral disease.

4. 口腔念珠菌感染 Oral candidiasis

口腔念珠菌感染分为急性和慢性感染。急性感染表现为伪膜性或萎缩性。慢性感染表现为萎缩性或增生性。老年人最常见的两种口腔念珠菌感染为急性伪膜性（急性口疮）和慢性萎缩性。急性口疮的特点是黏膜表面有凝乳状的白色伪膜。念珠菌感染后患者主诉多是口腔烧灼感。急性口疮可以发生在口咽部的任何软组织表面和舌面。临床上白色伪膜可以用纱布擦除，白色伪膜下出现红色斑块。

任何影响患者免疫系统，改变正常菌群的疾病或状态都可认为是口腔念珠菌感染的危险因素。长期服用抗生素、类固醇制剂、或进行化疗的患者容易感染念珠菌。糖尿病、艾滋病、以及头颈部放射治疗都可能是急性口疮的危险因素。与义齿有关的念珠菌感染可以是萎缩性的也可以是增生性的。上颌义齿下方可以发现与义齿覆盖的区域一致的红色斑块，不合适的上颌义齿是主要的危险因素。对于没有口腔修复体的患者，慢性萎缩性念珠菌感染常常是整个口腔广泛的发红、烧灼感。

与义齿有关的慢性萎缩性念珠菌感染常伴随着口腔和义齿的卫生状况很差。很多患者每天24小时戴着义齿，不给口腔黏膜自身恢复的机会。口干和口腔黏膜烧灼感常预示患者罹患念珠菌感染。

Oral candidiasis can be classified as acute or chronic. The acute form can present as pseudomembranous or atrophic. Chronic candidiasis can present as atrophic or hyperplastic. In older adults, the two most common types of candidiasis are acute pseudomembranous (traditionally called thrush) and chronic atrophic. Thrush is characterized by white plaques described as having a curd like appearance. Patients with Candida often complain of a burning mouth. Thrush can be found on any soft tissue in the oral cavity and pharynx, including the tongue. For diagnostic purposes, the white lesions can be wiped away with gauze, leaving an erythematous area under the white lesion.

Any condition compromising a patient's immune system or altering normal flora can be considered a risk factor for candidiasis. Oral candidiasis can occur with long-term use of medications such as antibiotics, steroid therapies, or chemotherapy. Diabetes mellitus, human immunodeficiency virus (HIV) disease, and head and neck radiation are risk factors for thrush. Candidiasis located under a denture can be either atrophic or hyperplastic. It occurs as an erythematous area under a maxillary denture that vividly outlines the tissue covered by the prosthesis. An ill-fitting upper denture is the most commonly cited risk factor. In patients without prosthesis, chronic atrophic candidiasis may present as a generalized redness or even generalized burning of the mouth.

Chronic atrophic candidiasis associated with denture use is usually accompanied by poor oral hygiene of both the oral tissue and the prosthesis. Many patients wear their prosthesis 24h per day and therefore do not allow the tissue to heal from the fungal infection. Xerostomia, or dry mouth, can also predispose a patient to this type of Candida infection, which causes a burning sensation in the oral cavity.

四、老年人口腔卫生服务 Oral health care for the elders

口腔专业人员要担负起老年人的口腔卫生服务工作。在对老年人进行口腔健康教育和健康促进时，需要强调以下内容：

(1) 每日用含氟牙膏刷牙两次；

(2) 每日用牙线清洁牙齿邻面一次；

(3) 餐后要清洁义齿；

(4) 睡觉的时要取出口腔内的义齿，并将义齿浸泡在水或义齿清洁液中；

(5) 定期进行口腔检查和洁治；

(6) 均衡饮食；

(7) 戒烟；

(8) 多饮水以防口干；

(9) 用人工唾液或含化无糖硬块糖来缓解口干；

(10) 即使所有牙齿都脱落了，也要定期接受口腔癌的筛查；

(11) 如果口腔肿胀、疼痛、麻木，要尽快寻求口腔医生或全科医生的诊治。

Dental professionals should provide oral health care for the whole population, including the elders. The following aspects should be emphasized to the elders during oral health education and promotion program.

Brush teeth twice a day with fluoridate toothpaste;

Flossing once a day;

Clean the denture after meals;

Take the denture out of the mouth when sleeping, and put it in water or a denture cleansing liquid;

Make regular dental visit for a checkup and scaling;

Eat a well-balanced diet;

Don't use tobacco products;

Drink extra water to prevent mouth dryness;

Recommend using artificial saliva or sucking sugar-free hard candy to resolve mouth dryness;

Even lost all natural teeth, the elders are recommended for oral cancer screening;

Whenever having trouble with swelling, numbness, sores, or lumps in the mouth, see a dentist or doctor as soon as possible.

氟化物对老年人和儿童的防龋功效是一样的。因此，老年人每日用含氟牙膏刷牙和应用氟水漱口可以预防龋病的发生。对于老年人中的高危人群，专业人员可以选择使用氟保护漆等防龋措施。

口腔念珠菌的感染要采取局部应用和全身抗真菌治疗。局部抗真菌治疗要连续使用 14 天以保证彻底根除真菌。如果念珠菌感染不仅局限于口腔内，或局部应用抗真菌治疗3～6周后不见好转，需要结合全身抗真菌治疗。与其他抗真菌药物比较，氟康唑是比较好的选择，因其药物反应小，每日只需服用一次，但费用略高。

For dental caries, fluoride is just as helpful for elders as it is for children. Using a fluoride toothpaste and mouth rinse can help protect teeth. Professional applied-fluoride measures, such as fluoride varnish (Duraphat), should be provided to high-risk groups.

The treatment for all types of candidiasis includes an antifungal medication. Topical (nystatin, chlortrimazole troches) or systemic (ketoconazole, fluconazole) medications are available. Topical medications should be used for at least 14 days to assure total eradication of the fungus. If the infection is more widespread than just the oral cavity or does not subside within 3 to 6 weeks of topical treatment, then systemic medication may be necessary. Fluconazole is a good drug of choice because of its once-daily dosing regimen and a minimal drug interactions compared with other systemic antifungals, but is also costly in comparison.

在未来几十年间，随着老年人口腔内存留牙齿的增多，口腔卫生服务的内容将发生巨大的变化。如今和未来的口腔医生将会诊治越来越多的老年患者。未来的老年人与今天我们所面对的老年人会有很大的不同，未来的老年人可能存留更多的牙齿，就诊口腔科的次数增加，受过较高的教育，经济状况较好，并有着非常大的口腔治疗需求。他们现在是，将来也一定是由不同社会经济状况和口腔健康状况的个体组成。口腔治疗材料和技术的提高，口腔疾病模式的改变将会对口腔医学的发展产生巨大的影响。

口腔保健人员的工作将主要是对口腔疾病和口腔异常进行诊断和治疗。口腔硬组织的疾病解决之后，将更加关注于口腔软组织疾病的诊断和治疗。口腔预防保健的措施要贯穿人们的一生。

With more older adults and more teeth per older adult, the composition of services rendered to this population will change dramatically in the next decade. The oral health professional of today and of the future will be called to treat an ever-increasing number of older adults. The future elderly will be different than the current cohort seen today. The future elderly will have more teeth, visit the dentist more often, and have a higher level of education, better finances and a dramatically different perspective of needs. They are and will continue to be a heterogeneous mix of individuals with various levels of functional, socioeconomic and oral health status. Advances in materials and technology in combination with the changing patterns of oral diseases will continue to have dramatic effects on the practice of dentistry.

The role of oral health-care professional will focus more on the diagnosis and treatment of oral diseases and disorders, using new aids and devices. As diseases of the hard tissues are resolved, more emphasis will be placed on the diagnosis and treatment of soft tissue lesions. Preventive oral health approaches need to be maintained throughout the lifespan.

第四节　残疾人口腔保健

Section 4 Oral Health Care for Compromised Individuals

残疾人是指那些因为身体、精神或情绪的问题导致日常基本生活活动受限的人。

A compromised individual is a person who has one or more physical, medical, mental, or emotional problems that result in a limitation of the ability to function normally in fulfilling the activities of daily living (ADLs).

一、辅助口腔清洁方法 Attendant care

残疾人的家庭成员或看护者、保健人员需要协助残疾人维护良好的口腔卫生。很多残疾人因为感觉、认知、或身体上的障碍而不能把握牙刷。对于这些残疾人，他们的家庭成员或看护者要学会如何帮助残疾人清洁牙齿。如果要长期坚持下去，在口腔清洁过程中，看护者和残疾人的体位就很重要。因此，推荐几种体位（图 10-1），供看护者选择应用到为残疾人进行牙齿清洁的过程中。在选择不同体位时，需要考虑残疾人的身体大小和力量强弱，看护者的身体大小和力量强弱，是否需要控制残疾人自主活动和不自主活动等因素。一个较好的

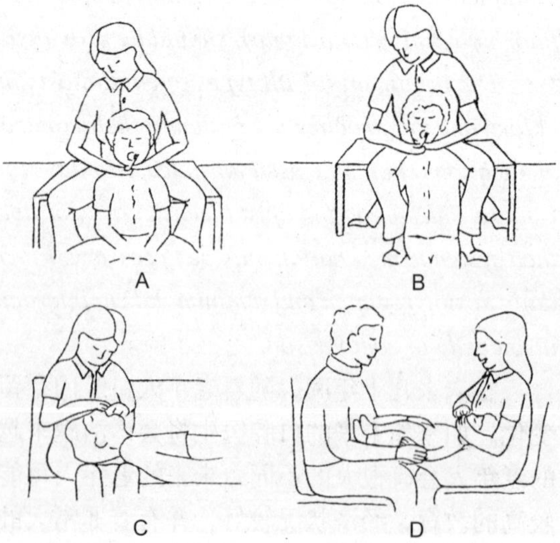

图 10-1　帮助儿童或残疾人刷牙去除牙菌斑

体位是成年残疾人坐在直背椅或轮椅上，看护者站在患者的身后。这样很容易将患者的头部固定在看护者的身体上，看护者采用清洁自己牙齿的姿势和手法帮助残疾人清洁牙齿。在他们面前放置一面镜子，看护者更容易应用给自己刷牙的方法。其他推荐的体位包括被看护者躺在床上或沙发上，或看护者坐在椅子上，被看护者坐在地板上，被看护者的头放在看护者的腿上。看护者的腿可以限制被看护者手臂的运动。看护者和被看护者必须明白，刷牙并不一定要在洗漱间进行。其实对于为残疾人清洁牙齿来说，洗漱间因为空间有限，又要与人共用，是家庭中最不适宜的地方。刷牙并不一定都需要水，因为刷牙刺激唾液分泌也能起到湿润的作用。对于极其衰弱的患者，干的牙刷很容易损伤牙龈组织，因此需要事先将牙刷湿润、变软。如果不用牙膏刷牙，就不需要漱口。不用牙膏可以有良好的视野，并且不会引起患者呕吐。如果使用牙膏和水，患者的家人或看护者最终会放弃为被看护者进行口腔清洁，或者减少口腔清洁的次数。对于正常人来说，用含氟牙膏刷牙是最基本的口腔保健内容。然而，对于残疾人来说，放弃每日应用含氟牙膏，可以选择其他形式的氟化物预防措施。

To ensure dental care and compliance with home self-care preventive programs, complete cooperation must be established among the family or caregivers, the health provider, and, to the extent possible, the patient. Many compromised individuals are unable to handle their own hygiene due to sensory, cognitive, or physical deficits. For these individuals, an attendant or family member should be instructed in the proper oral health care for the patient. If long-term compliance with instructions is the goal, the comfort of both the caregiver and the patient in performing the oral hygiene program in paramount. For this reason, a number of positions have been recommended for the caregiver to assume when providing oral hygiene care to the patient. Facts to be considered include the patient's size and strength, the attendant's size and strength, and the amount of control that needs to be exerted over the intentional or unintentional movements of the patient. One position that has proven to be successful when the patient is an adult is for the attendant to stand behind the patient, who is seated in a straight-backed chair or a wheelchair. In this position, it is easy to stabilize the patient's head by resting it against the body of the attendant. Brushing then proceeds with the attendant using the same kind of arm and brush positioning as when cleaning his or her own teeth. Performing this operation in front of a mirror takes further advantage of the attendant's own brushing habits, although a mirror is not a necessary. Other recommended positions include having the patient lie on a sofa or bed with the head in the caregiver's lap or sitting on the floor in front of a chair in which the caregiver is seated. The caregiver's legs are used as an additional restraint to the arms of the patient. Caregivers and patients should both be advised that the bathroom is not the only location in which to brush teeth. In fact, it is often the least convenient room in the house because of its space limitations and the need to share its use with other members of the family. Water is not always necessary for toothbrushing, as salivary flow is stimulated by brushing and thus provides moisture. If a patient has tender, friable gingival tissue that can easily become damaged by an initially dry toothbrush, the brush can be moistened beforehand to soften it. When no toothpaste is used, running water may not be needed. The elimination of the toothpaste increase visibility and decreases the possibility of gagging. In many cases, it has been found that when water and toothpaste were required, attendants or family members discontinued or decreased the number of toothbrushing sessions. Normally, fluoride toothpaste is an important component of an oral hygiene program in an uncompromised population. In compromised patients, however, if one must omit fluoride toothpaste from the routine, it can be compensated for by using fluorides in other forms.

如果患者希望应用牙膏，可以选择不起泡沫的牙膏。因为这种牙膏不起泡沫，且可以吞咽，因此，患者不一定要吐出来。

如果患者愿意刷牙后漱口，可以采用两个纸杯的方法。一个纸杯装用来漱口的水，另一个纸杯用来接漱口吐出的水。纸杯很轻，通常患者能够拿着两个纸杯，将需要的纸杯放到唇边。对于患有关节炎的人，不能弯腰将漱口水吐到水盆中，或者不能用口唇吐出漱口水的肌肉无力患者，这样可以防止漱口水的洒漏。

Those patients who enjoy the taste or appreciate the aesthetic value of toothpaste can use non-foaming, ingestible toothpaste. Because this toothpaste does not foam and can be swallowed, it is not necessary for the patient to be near a basin to expectorate.

If a patient likes to rinse with water or a mouthwash after brushing, a two-paper-cup technique can be used. One paper cup holds the rinse; the other is for the expectorate after the patient rinses. Because the cups are lightweight, patients can often hold both, bringing each of the cups up to their lips as needed. This two-cup technique provides a means of controlling dribbling or drooling, and it is valuable for an individual who is unable to lean over the basin, such as an arthritic patient, or for an individual who cannot purse the lips to expel the fluid, as is the case with muscular dystrophy patients.

二、维护口腔卫生的装置 Oral hygiene devices

1. 改装牙刷柄 Modifying toothbrush handles

总的来说，残疾人的刷牙原则和方法同普通人一样，但是，对于残疾人来说，维护良好的口腔卫生是很困难的。如果残疾人的灵活性足以进行刷牙时小的震颤，选择手动牙刷就能够取得较好的效果。牙刷生产商出品了大量不同结构的牙刷，加大牙刷柄的直径，可以用热水再塑形的刷柄，弯曲的刷头，多个刷头，弯曲的刷毛等，所有这些都可以满足不同需要的特殊人群（图 10-2）。一种幼儿牙刷的刷柄设计成大的椭圆形状，可以避免儿童第一次学习刷牙时，牙刷过度伸入口腔内造成口腔软组织的损伤。这样的牙刷可以给年龄较大的残疾儿童使用。即使有的儿童手指抓握力很弱或正畸夹板固定的儿童，也可以将手动牙刷的刷柄改装成需要的形状。

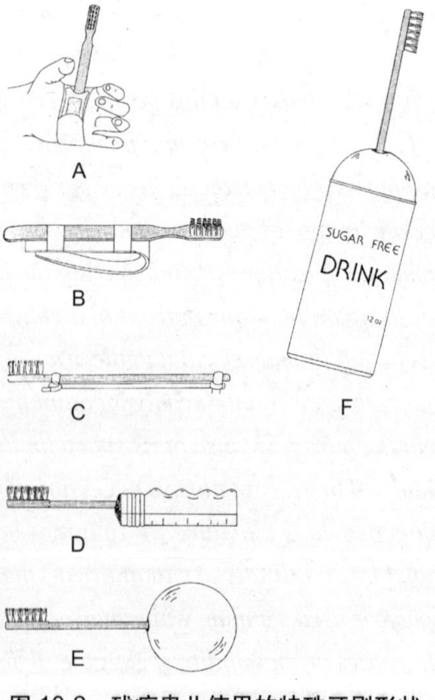

图 10-2　残疾患儿使用的特殊牙刷形状

有些残疾人因为关节受累，肘部的运动受限，可以选择刷柄加长的牙刷。有一些装置可以帮助功能受限的残疾人独立进行口腔清洁。通常情况下，用于帮助进食的装置也可用来帮助刷牙，如手掌护套，辅助日常活动的护套等。

In general, the principles and techniques of tooth brushing used for a compromised population are the same as for anyone else. In compromised individuals, however, good oral hygiene is much more difficult to achieve and maintain. If it has been determined that the patient has adequate dexterity to produce the small strokes needed to brush properly, a manual toothbrush may produce satisfactory results. Toothbrush manufacturers are now providing a variety of different configurations of brushes with increased handle dimensions, handles modifiable with hot water, angled brush heads, multiple brush head, and curved bristles, all of which can be beneficial for special needs patients. One type of brush marked for toddlers is designed with a large ovoid handle that prevents over insertion and potential intra-oral injury when a child is first learning to brush. Such a device may have application for an older compromised child. Even if the patient has a weakened hand grasp or uses orthotic splints or other adaptive appliances, a manual toothbrush can be modified to facilitate usage. There are many different methods of quickly augmenting toothbrush handles.

Patients who are unable to flex their elbows because of joint involvement can be given a toothbrush with an extended handle. Several devices have been developed to assist individuals with limited function to achieve independence. Often, products used to assist in feeding can be adapted for use in brushing the teeth, such as palmar cuffs or activities of daily living cuffs.

2. 电动牙刷 Electric toothbrushes

电动牙刷适宜于帮助残疾人维护口腔卫生。尤其适用于患者能够抓住牙刷柄，并且能够将牙刷放到口腔内，只是患者的灵活性受限，不能实施精细的刷牙动作的情况。电动牙刷的刷柄同手动牙刷一样，可以改装成便于手掌握持障碍的患者使用的形状。

对于自己能够进行口腔清洁的残疾人来说，电动牙刷清除牙菌斑的效果显著优于手动牙刷。如果看护者帮助残疾人刷牙，看护者也发现电动牙刷容易使用，残疾人乐于接受。

为特殊残疾人选择牙刷时，应该考虑残疾人的牙齿排列状况，牙弓形态，以及是否会引起呕吐反射等。

在向残疾人推荐使用电动牙刷时，需要提醒注意：过分热衷于使用电动牙刷刷牙在短时间内容易造成口腔软硬组织的损伤。

Electric toothbrushes are valuable aids in assisting compromised patients. They are especially useful when the patient has the strength to grasp the handle and place the brush in the mouth but does not have the manual dexterity needed to perform the fine movements necessary for the cleaning function. The length and diameter of the handle of an electric toothbrush approximates those of manual toothbrushes that have been modified for individuals with compromised hand function.

For patients able to perform their own oral hygiene, the effectiveness of electric toothbrushes in plaque removal has been shown to significantly improve over the manual toothbrushes. Even for caregivers, it was found to be easier and more pleasant to use.

In selecting which toothbrush is best for a particular patient, one should consider alignment of teeth in the arch, constriction of the arches, and whether an exaggerated gag reflex is present.

One additional note of caution should be considered before recommending an electric toothbrush for a compromised patient. An overzealously used electric toothbrush can cause considerable damage to the hard and soft tissues in a short time.

3. 固定牙线的装置 Floss-holding devices

牙线不适宜向所有的残疾人推荐使用。除非他已经完全掌握了刷牙的方法，否则过度强调使用复杂的牙线是没有意义的。这样做，会导致残疾人放弃所有的口腔卫生措施。不管是残疾人自我进行口腔卫生护理还是有看护者帮助进行，结果都是一样的。因此，已经掌握刷牙方法的残疾人，能够持续保持牙面上的菌斑很少的情况下，介绍他们使用牙线。

在介绍之前，对残疾人的灵活性和理解能力需要作出适当的评价。

对于一些残疾人来说，只要应用牙线柄(图10-3)，可以每日使用牙线清除牙菌斑。用一组手臂上抬受限的残疾人评价了8种牙线固定装置。其中一种得到了很高的评价，因其握持方便，容易安装牙线，并能够将牙线拉紧。尽管有些残疾人学会了自己给牙线柄装上牙线，大多数的残疾人难以完成此项工作。目前市场上有很多种可以自动安装牙线的牙线柄。但是还没有研究他们是否适合残疾人使用。因此，对于残疾人来说，不管是否用牙线柄，使用牙线清洁牙齿仍然有很大的障碍。

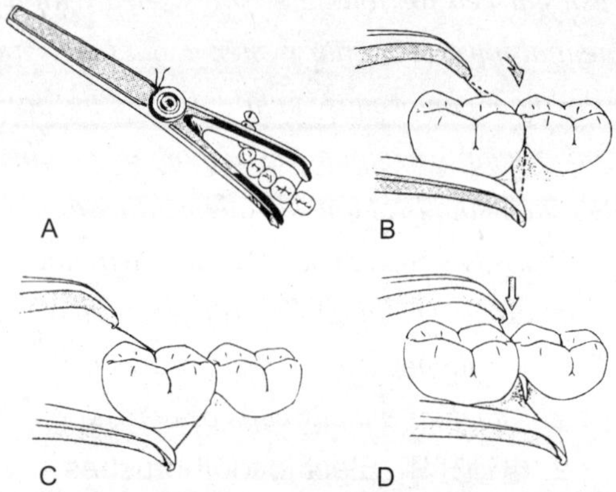

图 10-3 牙线夹持器的使用方法

Dental flossing is not recommended for all compromised patients. Unless the task of toothbrushing can be learned, it is useless to superimpose the more complex task of flossing. To do so can be so discouraging that all attempts at oral hygiene are abandoned. This is true whether the patient or the attendant is performing the program. Flossing, therefore, should be introduced on a selective basis for those patients or attendants who have mastered toothbrushing and consistently show low plaque levels on tooth surfaces.

An adequate assessment of the patient's dexterity and ability to understand the technique must be determined before flossing is introduced.

For some compromised patients, flossing can be performed regularly if a floss-holding device is used. Eight such devices were evaluated by people with upper-extremity limitations. This group rated one device significantly higher for its handle dimensions, ease of threading, and ability to keep the floss taut. Although some compromised patients have learned adaptive techniques allowing them to thread floss-holders themselves, the majority of compromised patients have great difficulty in accomplishing this procedure. There are currently on the market several brands of floss holders claiming to be self-threading. There have been no comparative studies to determine if, in fact, they offer advantages to a compromised population. Therefore, manipulating the floss with or without a floss holder continues to be a barrier for this population.

4. 牙间隙刷 Interproximal brushing

牙间隙刷可以跟刷牙一起介绍给残疾人。因为牙间隙刷的柄长而坚固，可以同牙刷柄一样进行改装。许多牙间隙刷需要将适合的牙刷头安装到刷柄上。这是一个复杂的过程，同时需要很精细的运动技巧。另外，有些残疾人的牙弓很窄，需要不同的途径和角度才能将刷头放入到牙间隙中。因此，新出现的预先安装刷头的，刷头可以弯曲的，刷头与刷柄的角度可以在90度到180度之间调节的牙间隙刷可以推荐给残疾人使用。当然，必须首先进行安装和使用的示范、练习。

Interproximal brushing may be introduced near the beginning of the preventive program. Because handles of interproximal brushes are long and sturdy, they can easily be modified in the same manner as the toothbrush. Many interproximal brushes require the assembly of the proper brush head to the handle. This is an intricate task and requires fine-motor skills. Additionally, some patients have severely constricted arches requiring unusual access and angulation of the brush head into the interproximal space. Therefore, the newer preassembled interproximal brushes, those with snap on brush heads and those where the angle of the brush to the handle can be changed from 90° to 180° are recommended for compromised patients. Demonstrations of assembly and use are definite requirements.

5. 义齿的清洁 Prosthesis hygiene

佩戴全口义齿或局部义齿的残疾人需要别人帮助清洁义齿，另外也需要取出义齿清洁口腔软组织和存留的牙齿。义齿每日都需要清洗，并且义齿每日取出的时间都要有 6 ~ 8 个小时。改装义齿清洁装置和改装义齿都有利于患者自我清洁义齿。在老人院中，口腔护士要帮助老人取出全口义齿和局部义齿，并帮助老人清洗和浸泡义齿，同时清洁老年人的口腔软组织和存留牙齿。在老人院中，老人常丢失义齿而导致消化不适，营养不良，发音困难，这些都会影响老年人的自我形象。因此，口腔专业人员应建议老人院中设置义齿鉴别程序，将老人的义齿写上名字或做上标记，这样，任何放错位置的义齿都很容易找到失主。

Compromised patients who wear full or removable partial dentures may need assistance with maintaining proper hygiene of the appliances, which must be removed for thorough cleaning or the oral soft tissues and any remaining natural teeth. The appliances also must be cleaned appropriately and should be left out of the mouth for 6 to 8 hours per day. Modifications to denture-cleaning devices as well as modifications to the dentures may aid in helping compromised patients provide their own denture hygiene. Oral hygiene care by nurses' aids in institutional settings should include removal of all full or partial dentures and scrubbing and soaking of these appliances, as well as the care of the soft tissue and teeth. Dentures are often lost in institutions by the staff, as well as by the patients themselves. As a result, residents may experience digestive complaints, inadequate nutrition, and speech difficulties, all of which can contribute to a poor self-image. Therefore, it is important for the dental consultant to set up denture-identification programs to mark prostheses with the patient's name or other means of identification. Then any misplaced appliances can be readily returned to their owner.

三、口腔预防措施 Preventive therapies

1. 饮食指导 Dietary consideration

残疾人常会因为表现好而得到甜食的奖励。这种甜食奖励的方式增加了餐间甜食的摄入次数，也增加了致龋食物的总摄入量。如果患者神经肌肉的协调能力降低，唾液分泌减少，就很难自我冲洗口腔。那么食物常存留在口腔前庭和牙齿之间，直到下次口腔清洁。为了预防龋齿，就需要（1）限制餐间甜食的次数，（2）限制高致龋性食物的摄入。如果需要进食甜食，最好在进餐的同时摄入，并且餐后立即刷牙。不鼓励睡觉前进食零食。

For many compromised patients, foods high in sugar are distributed throughout the day as a reward for having been compliant. Such a reward system encourages between-meals snacking and increases the consumption of highly cariogenic foods. With patients who have decreased neuromuscular coordination or decreased salivary flow, it may be difficult to adequately clear the mouth. Food may remain in the buccal vestibule and between the teeth until the next brushing. To reduce the cariogenic potential, it is necessary (1) to restrict between-meal snacking and (2) to limit the use of highly cariogenic foods. If sweets are to be consumed at all, they should be presented at mealtime and the teeth brushed immediately after eating. Bedtime snacks should be discouraged.

2. 窝沟封闭和应用氟化物防龋 Sealants and fluorides

残疾人的口腔健康状况常比其他人群差。龋失补中已经充填的牙齿占的比例很低，而失牙和龋坏牙所占的比例都较高。尽管一些有效的口腔预防措施越来越普遍，但残疾人受益却很少。窝沟封闭和应用氟化物应当成为残疾人龋病预防的主要措施。

在残疾人中实施窝沟封闭可能比较困难，主要是隔湿困难。脑瘫和肌肉萎缩的残疾人常可看到口腔内唾液池。由于进行窝沟封闭需时很短，通常不需要应用抑制唾液分泌的药物。可采用传统的方法进行隔湿和窝沟封闭。为了取得较好的隔湿效果，残疾人的体位通常是端坐而不是躺着。

In spite of the normalization of handicapped individuals into the mainstream of society, it appears that the non-institutionalized handicapped do not have as high as a level of oral health as the rest of the population. The F value for the DMF scores is often lower in the compromised population, whereas the D and M values are higher than in the general population. Although becoming more common, preventive strategies that would really benefit this population group are often not available on a regular basis. The use of sealants and fluorides should be considered important preventive techniques to assist in caries control for compromised patients.

Sealant application may be more difficult in compromised patients, because it may be more difficult to control moisture contamination. Salivary pooling is often seen in cerebral palsy and muscular dystrophy patients. For the short time needed to apply sealants, antisialogogue mediations are usually not indicated. Instead, the sealant may be applied in the conventional manner using the techniques to control saliva flow. To aid in moisture control the patient should be seated upright rather than in a reclining position.

口腔专业人员定期实施局部用氟防龋措施对残疾人来说很重要。一种新型的用于治疗牙本质敏感的氟保护漆现在可以用作局部用氟制剂。它有两种制剂，乳牙列用 25ml，混合牙列用 40ml。氟保护漆很容易涂布到牙面上，而且即便在湿润的环境下也有效。一些发育异常和精神障碍的残疾人常伴有吞咽困难，而不能有效地吞咽口腔内的唾液。对于残疾儿童，氟化水源和服用氟片是最基本的口腔预防保健措施。家庭自我应用的氟化物防龋措施同样重要。目前有一些可以在家庭中自我应用的氟化物防龋措施，如氟水漱口和个别托盘应用氟凝胶。对于不能将漱口水在口腔内运动的残疾人不适合应用氟水漱口。一些肌肉萎缩和中风后的残疾人不能有效地闭唇，不能将漱口水存留在口腔内，也不适合应用氟水漱口。应用氟凝胶时，需要患者将装有氟凝胶的托盘咬住4分钟，对大多数残疾人来说都是很困难的，尤其当托盘又能引起呕吐反射时。装入氟凝胶的托盘容易刺激唾液分泌，因此很难控制唾液的分泌。残疾人和看护者都难以接受大量的口水。因此，在家庭中通常很难成功应用氟凝胶。另外一种家庭用氟的方法是涂布含氟泡沫。在一项老人院中进行的研究发现，口内涂布含氟泡沫比应用氟水漱口之后唾液中维持高氟化物水平的时间长 3 个小时。

很多人发现用刷子刷氟凝胶更容易，因为这些程序与刷牙的方法一样。因此，用刷子刷氟凝胶可以应用到老年残疾人中，尤其是那些牙龈退缩的残疾人。然而，氟化物不能不加选择地分发给残疾人，让残疾人在没有监督的情况下应用，如果残疾人有理解障碍，不能遵循医生的指导就会出现问题。尽管有研究发现精神障碍的儿童独立应用含氟牙膏刷牙几乎没有氟中毒的危险，但我们在推荐残疾人使用氟化物时还应谨慎。

Regular topical fluoride applications by the dental staff are highly important for the compromised dental patient. A new fluoride-containing varnish developed for dentinal hypersensitivity is now available as a fluoride supplement. It is supplied in two doses: 25 ml for primary dentition and 40 mL for mixed dentition. Fluoride varnish can be quickly painted on and is effective even in a moist field, a particularly important characteristic for some of the developmentally disabled and mentally retarded populations who have a disordered swallowing mechanism and are therefore unable to effectively clear their mouths of saliva. For the younger patient, water fluoridation or tablets are essential. Equally important for this population is a home self-applied fluoride program. Several effective techniques are now available for home fluoride application, ranging from mouth rinses to fluoride gels applied with custom-made trays. Rinses are contraindicated for compromised patients who cannot effectively swish the solution around their mouths. Some individuals with muscular dystrophy and some post-stroke patients have an incompetent or hypotonic lip seal and cannot keep solutions in the mouth for the required period. Our experience with office-applied fluoride treatment delivered in a tray requiring the patient to keep the tray in place for a minimum of 4 minutes has demonstrated how difficult it is for many compromised patients to cooperate that long, particularly if there is an active gag reflex. A gel-filled tray also stimulates the flow of saliva, which is often difficult to confine. Neither the patient nor the caregiver likes the drooling that occurs. Therefore, home-fluoride treatments utilizing a tray-delivery method will probably not be successful. An alternative home-fluoride delivery method uses a foam applicator. In a nursing home population, it was found that the level of fluoride in saliva was higher 3 hours following delivery by an intra-oral applicator when compared to the fluoride levels in saliva after residents rinsed with a fluoride mouthrinse.

More independent populations may find brush-on fluoride gels easier to use, because their application takes advantage of an already learned toothbrushing behavior. Fluorides have been shown to reduce demineralization and enhance remineralization. Therefore, brush-on gel fluorides should be considered for use by elderly compromised patients, particularly those with gingival recession.

Fluorides should not, however, be indiscriminately given to patients for unsupervised use if some question exists as to the patient's ability to understand and follow instructions. Although it was found that little risk of toxicity when a fluoridated toothpaste was used independently by a population of mentally handicapped children, one must still exercise caution whenever recommending fluorides.

3. 化学性菌斑控制方法 Chemical plaque control

显然，我们有必要发展不依赖于残疾人自身灵活性的牙菌斑控制方法。例如用洗必太溶液擦洗残疾人的口腔。一项研究由看护者用海绵棒蘸洗必太溶液擦洗残疾人的口腔，每日一次，每周五次，与安慰剂对照组比较，试验组显示了持续的、显著的菌斑减少、牙龈炎减轻，以及牙周袋深度降低的效果。随后的研究表明每周应用两次洗必太溶液也能取得显著的效果，并且可以长期应用。

在精神障碍人群中应用缓释洗必太涂膜能减少牙菌斑、牙石，以及牙周袋的深度。在发育障碍的残疾人中，由看护者用很低浓度的（0.06%）洗必太喷雾也取得了显著的改善菌斑控制的效果。因此，对重度残疾或精神障碍的残疾人，可以由看护者应用洗必太溶液来维护残疾人的牙周健康。

It has been recognized that treatments need to be developed to manage plaque control that are less dependent on the manual dexterity of the patient. The efficacy of applying chlorhexidine by swabbing for people with disabilities has been established. In one study chlorhexidine was applied by a caregiver once daily, five times per week, for ten weeks using foam sticks. When compared with applying a placebo by swabbing, the chlorhexidine group showed consistent and significant improvement in lower plaque levels, gingivitis, and pocket depths. A subsequent study demonstrated that chlorhexidine swabbing was effective at a reduced frequency (twice per week as opposed to five times per week) and was well tolerated with prolonged use (42 weeks).

Application of sustained-release varnishes of chlorhexidine produced reductions in plaque, calculus, and pocket depths in a mentally retarded population. The effectiveness of a very low concentration (0.06%) of chlorhexidine spray delivered by caregivers was evaluated in developmentally disable patients, and resulted in significant improvement in plaque scores. Thus, for severely disabled or mentally retarded patients, a caregiver can provide chlorhexidine applications by various means and improve the periodontal condition. However, it may not be possible for these patients independently to achieve these positive results as demonstrated in a study comparing chlorhexidine and an essential oil mouth rinse.

4. 定期预防性维护 Periodic preventive maintenance

残疾人的龋病和牙周病患病率高于正常人，因此，他们需要更频繁的牙科就诊。残疾人预防性维护所需的就诊时间因人而异，因残疾人本人或看护者进行口腔清洁的能力不同而不同。通常，残疾人只有固定的收入，没有足够的经济能力支付他们所需的口腔治疗。有些残疾人口腔就诊的费用是家庭支付的，残疾人的家人意识到口腔保健的重要性，并且愿意让残疾人受益于口腔治疗措施。总的来说，残疾人没有经济能力支付他们的口腔卫生服务。对于这样的残疾人，口腔医生可以考虑采取新的收费方式来实施口腔预防措施。例如，医生可以跟残疾人达成一个每季度进行一次口腔预防性洁治的协议，如果残疾人完成了所有的治疗计划，从第一次就诊开始，随后每次就诊都可以减少一定数量的诊治费用。

Many compromised individuals have a higher incidence of caries and periodontal problems than noncompromised patients and, therefore, they should be seen more frequently. The timing of preventive maintenance appointments should be individualized and should reflect the patient's or caregiver's ability to perform oral hygiene procedures. Often, compromised patients are either on fixed incomes or have limited resources available to finance their dental care. For some, the cost of dental care is assumed by the patient's family, who realizes the importance of preventive oral care and are eager to see the patient benefit from such treatment. In general, the compromised patient has limited resources to expend on dental care. For these patients, the dental clinician may wish to consider some innovative financial arrangements to pay for preventive procedures. For example, it might be desirable if a contract could be established whereby the patient is brought in on a regular quarterly schedule for prophylaxis. Each appointment after the first one is performed for a reduced fee if the patient completes the entire series of scheduled visits.

在身体、精神、健康以及情绪方面有障碍的人通常比健康的人有更多的口腔卫生服务需要。这可能因为障碍本身有口腔的表征，但是更常见的原因是（1）残疾人本身或家庭成员对口腔卫生的了解很有限，他们不能很好地维护残疾人的口腔卫生，（2）对口腔预防措施的重要性缺乏认识，（3）难以支付口腔卫生服务费用。当残疾人到诊所就诊时，口腔医生应制定一项重点在预防的治疗计划。制定计划时要先对残疾人的感觉、认知、以及经济能力作出评价。如果残疾人自己不能进行自我口腔清洁，残疾人的家庭成员或看护者就要学会适当的口腔清洁方法和措施。

Individuals with physical, medical, mental, or emotional problems often have a greater need for dental care than their healthy counterparts. This may be because the disability itself has oral manifestations, but more commonly it is because of (1) the limited capabilities of the individual or the family members to understand and to perform important oral hygiene tasks, (2) a lack of understanding of the importance of preventive dental care, and (3) an inability to finance dental care. When a compromised patient does present to a dental office, the clinician should develop a treatment plan that emphasizes prevention. Assessments should be made of the patient's sensory, cognitive, and functional abilities and be used to customize a preventive plan. When the patient is unable to provide his or her own care, the family or an attendant needs to be taught the appropriate techniques.

特殊设计的、容易改装的传统口腔卫生工具可以用来为残疾人提供口腔清洁服务。口腔预防措施，如窝沟封闭、氟化物应用以及化学性菌斑控制方法等都应该考虑应用到残疾人的口腔疾病预防和治疗计划中。

口腔医生和口腔诊所的工作人员亲切和善地对待残疾患者，让患者感到舒适并乐于复诊。所有诊所内的工作人员都要尽力让患者感到温暖和被关怀。

大多数老年人都有很多口腔治疗需要。口腔医生可以通过与老人院的管理者交流，推荐老年人每日口腔清洁措施。口腔医生和口腔洁治员可以为老人院中的护士提供培训，由他们为老年人进行日复一日的口腔护理。

对于残疾人来说，口腔内保存健康的牙齿利于他们咀嚼和消化，也有利于保持良好的营养状况。良好的口腔健康状况带来的令人愉悦的外观使得残疾人更容易被别人所接受。良好的预防保健能够增强残疾人的自尊心。对于那些严重残疾的患者，需要特别设计的义齿来维护口腔健康。很多残疾人，因为神经肌肉功能障碍，任何义齿都难以发挥功能。自然牙列在残疾人的生活环境中发挥如此重要的作用，因此，残疾人、看护者、口腔专业人员一起采取有效的口腔卫生保健措施，维护残疾人的口腔健康极为重要。

Specialized equipment and easy-to-accomplish modifications of conventional oral hygiene devices may be employed to provide oral hygiene care. Dental preventive procedures, such as sealants, fluorides, and chemical plaque control, should be considered for each patient as part of any treatment plan.

The rapport of the compromised patient and his or her family with the dental health provider and the entire office staff is critical to the comfort and compliance of the patient. All members of the office staff need to convey a warm, receptive attitude to these special patients.

Most institutionalized individuals have great oral health needs. The dentist can play a significant role in assessing those needs by communicating recommendations for a daily oral care program to the institutional administrator. Dentists and dental hygienists can offer training to the nurses' aides who provide that day-to-day care.

For many compromised individuals, the retention of teeth in a healthy mouth improves mastication and digestion, as well as helps maintain an adequate nutritional status. The pleasing aesthetics afforded by good oral health help people with disabilities to be more welcomed by others. Good preventive care enhances one's self-esteem. For some patients who are severely compromised, specially adapted appliances may be required to maintain oral health. Many individuals, because of neuromuscular problems, have difficulty functioning with any type of oral prosthesis. Because the natural dentition assumes such an important role in the total living environment of the compromised patient, it is of utmost importance that the patient, caregivers, and the dental team work together to achieve an effective preventive oral hygiene program for such an individual.

附录 Appendices

表 10-1 Prenatal counseling (developmental age range: birth - 12 months)

Current area	Dentist's actions
Oral Development	
First primary tooth, molar eruption	Review of patterns of eruption
Formation of primary and permanent teeth	Review teething facts and myths
	Review oral anatomic landmarks
Fluoride	
Recommendation against fluoride use until 6 months of age	Discuss to assess fluoride status
Systemic fluoride management after 6 months of age	Review dentifrice use

续表

Current area	Dentist's actions
Oral Hygiene/Health	
Microflora acquisition in infants	Review of oral hygiene techniques for infants with parents emphasizing use of a soft brush and no dentifrice
Mouth cleaning techniques	
Periodicity for dental visits	
Habits	Plan for baby's first dental care visit
Pacifier use/thumbsucking	Review safe pacifier use and hygiene issues Review the mouth's exploratory role in infants Discuss effects of thumbsucking/pacifiers on oral structures
Nutrition and Diet	
Nursing caries patterns and causes	Discuss proper feeding practices Encourage weaning by 12 months of age
Role of sugars in the caries process	Discuss the role of "sugars" in dental caries initiation
Injury Prevention	
Oral trauma	Review appropriate response for parents if infant experiences oral trauma and provide emergency information/phone number

表 10-2 First dental visit（Developmental age range: 12-24 months）

Current area	Dentist's actions
Oral Development	
Completion of primary dentition/concepts of occlusion	Discuss importance of space maintenance
Spacing/space maintenance	Discuss eruption patterns and concepts of spacing
Permanent tooth formation	Emphasize oral health to protect developing permanent teeth
Fluoride	
Dietary sources of fluoride	Assess fluoride status/need for fluoride supplementation
Fluoride sources outside the home	Review dentifrice use
Toxicity and safety（dentifrices, etc.）	Discuss procedures for accidental ingestion
Oral Hygiene/Health	
Type of brush, role and amount of dentifrice	Review of oral hygiene techniques
Parent and child's role in toothbrushing/flossing	Assist parents in overcoming oral hygiene difficulties

续表

Current area	Dentist's actions
Frequency and location for oral hygiene	Plan for baby's next dental care based on risk assessment
Habits	
Pacifier use/thumbsucking	Review safe pacifier use and hygiene issues Discuss effects of thumbsucking/pacifier on oral structures
Nutrition and Diet	
The role of plaque in the caries process	Emphasize weaning if not already accomplished
Role of sugars in the caries process	Review carbohydrates and sugar intake and frequency in the caries process Review diet patterns that occur outside the home
Injury Prevention	
Primary tooth trauma and sequelae	Discuss electric cord safety and childproofing the home
Electric cord injury/childproofing home	Discuss oral trauma management for preschool and other child care situations

表 10-3 Second Dental Visit（Developmental Age Range: 2-6 years）

Current area	Dentist actions
Oral Development	
Exfoliation of primary teeth	Discuss importance of space maintenance
Eruption of mandibular permanent incisors	Discuss eruption patterns and concepts of spacing
Eruption of permanent first molars	Emphasize oral health to protect developing permanent teeth
Fluoride	
Dietary sources of fluoride	Assess fluoride status/need for fluoride supplementation
Fluoride sources outside the home	Discuss procedures for accidental ingestion
Toxicity and safety（dentifrices, etc.）	Review dentifrice use in children
Oral Hygiene/Health	
Parent and child's role in toothbrushing/flossing	Review of oral hygiene techniques and compliance
Frequency and location for oral hygiene	Child assumes more responsibility and parents supervise
Role of sealants in prevention of occlusal caries	Discuss sealants and radiographs Frequency of dental visits based upon child's level of caries risk

续表

Current area	Dentist actions
Habits	
Pacifier use/thumbsucking	Discuss effects of thumbsucking/pacifier on oral structures Discuss methods for terminating habits
Nutrition and Diet	
Snacking and sugar intake	Review carbohydrate and sugar intake and frequency in the caries process Review diet patterns that occur outside the home
Injury Prevention	
Safety during sporting activities	Discuss use of safety equipment（helmets, etc.）and mouthguards
Permanent tooth injury	Review emergency trauma management

表 10-4 Clinical findings according to child's age and expected feeding or diet patterns and dental development characteristics

	Clinical findings	Feeding or diet patterns	Dental development
3 m	Enamel decalcification Considerable plaque build-up Amelogenesis imperfecta Dentinogenesis imperfecta	Bottle used at bedtime or naptime Bottle used as a pacifier Bottle used past 12 months of age Frequent cariogenic diet or snacks	Stage of dental development has minimal influence on decision for a 3-month recall
6 m	Posterior proximal contacts No previous tooth cleaning Primary dentition crowding Moderate plaque build-up	Relatively cariogenic diet or frequent snacking on cariogenic foods	Second primary molar eruption is anticipated within 6 months
12 m	Generalized spacing present Good oral hygiene exhibited Shallow occlusal anatomy	Good dietary habits exhibiting a low cariogenic potential	Second primary molar eruption anticipated within 12 months

表 10-5 What to teach about preventing/controlling oral diseases and conditions

DENTAL CARIES	Fluoride What is fluoride What if water fluoridation How fluorides work to protect teeth from decay Effectiveness of each procedure Who needs fluoride Recommended frequency of use and duration

续表

	Pit-and Fissure Sealant What are dental sealants How they work to protect teeth from decay Who needs sealants and when reapplication of sealants Remineralization Nature's way of repairing demineralized teeth One of the most important functions of fluoride Many times, it can be used instead of fillings
Gingivitis	What is dental plaque Role of dental plaque in oral diseases How to remove plaque with toothbrush and floss Frequency of plaque removal Recommended types or toothbrushes What may happen if gingivitis goes untreated
Oral cancer	Risk factors for oral cancers Signs and symptoms of oral cancers Component of a thorough clinical oral cancer examination and recom mended frequency Who needs oral cancer examinations; when
Oral-facial injuries	Use mouthguards and headgear for sports Use seat belts at all times Use playground equipment safety

思考题 Review questions

1. 在与婴幼儿家长进行咨询和访谈过程中，访谈的内容要涵盖哪些方面的问题？
2. 简述婴幼儿口腔检查的时间、地点、方式，以及检查内容。
3. 简述不同年龄段婴幼儿口腔卫生指导的内容和方法。
4. 请设计一个学校初级口腔卫生保健项目。
5. 为什么窝沟封闭和氟化物防龋措施要针对高危人群？
6. 老年人的主要口腔健康问题有哪些，各有什么特点？

参考文献 References

1. Cynthia Pine M. , ed. Community oral health. Oxford: Wright, 1997
2. Brian Burt A., Stephen A. Eklund, ed., Dentistry, dental practice, and the community. 5th ed. Philadellphia: Saunders, 1999
3. Fejerskov Ole, Jan Ekstrand, Brian A. Burt, ed. Fluoride in dentistry. 2nd ed, Copenhagen:

Munksgaard, 1996

4. George Gluck M., Warren M. Morganstein, ed. Jong's community dental health. 5th ed, St. Louis, Mo: Mosby, 2003
5. Norman Harris O., Franklin Garcia-Godoy, ed. Primary preventive dentistry. 6th ed, Pearson Education, Inc: New Jersey, 2004
6. John MurrayJ., June H. Nunn, James G. Steele, ed. Prevention of oral disease. 4th ed, Oxford University: New York, 2003

（荣文笙）

第十一章　口腔健康促进与健康教育
Chapter Ⅺ Oral Health Promotion and Health Education

概述 Overview

本章以健康概念为基础探讨健康教育与健康促进。口腔公共卫生专业人员必须明确清楚健康促进的目的和意义在于鼓励健康的生活方式、消除健康的不平等以及赋予人们获得健康的能力。

This chapter is based on the concepts of health as turning point, to explore health education and health promotion. These who promote oral health need to be clear about their intentions and understanding the purpose of health promotion, whether it is to encourage healthy lifestyles, or it is to redress health inequalities and empower people to take control over their lives?

要点 Key points

- 各种健康的概念
- 影响健康的因素
- 健康促进与健康教育的定义
- 健康促进的策略与途径
- 口腔健康促进与健康教育的内容实践与评价
- *Concepts of health*
- *Factors influencing on health*
- *Definitions of health promotion and health education*
- *Strategies and approaches of health promotion*
- *Key issues in practice and evaluation on oral health promotion*

第一节　口腔健康促进的理论基础
Section 1 The Theoretical Basis of Oral Health Promotion

健康的概念有很多种。在理解健康的概念和影响因素的基础上，我们探讨健康促进的形成与发展。健康促进即“促使人们能够对健康作出自己的选择。”健康促进的发展经历了100多年的漫长过程，世界卫生组织在全球健康促进方面起到了巨大的推动作用，渥太华宣言规定了健康促进的基本原则。

There are a variety of views about the concepts of health. It is based on the different people with different views as turning point, to explore various factors influencing health, in order to establish a foundation of formulating and development of health promotion. “Making the healthy choice the easier choice". The development of health promotion has experienced a long period of process in more than 100 years. The World Health Organization (WHO) has played a great driving role in the global development of health promotion. The principles of health promotion are defined in the Ottaw Charter.

一、健康的概念 Concept of health

（一）健康、疾病、患病与亚健康 Definition of health, disease, illness and ill health

健康是一个内涵丰富的概念。健康一词来源于古英文的“治愈”一词，意味着“整体”，健康是一个人的完整性、健全或幸福的标志。健康观作为文化传统的一部分世代相传。在一个社会中，不同的社会组织或不同的人群有不同的健康观。

在日常生活中，健康有两方面的含义——积极的和消极的。健康的消极定义是没有病或不生病，这是西方医学科学模式中的健康含义。健康的积极定义是世界卫生组织在其宪章中所阐述的健康是个体在身体上，精神上和社会上的完好状态，而不只是没有疾病或不虚弱（WHO，1946）。

Health has two common meanings in everyday use, one negative and one positive. The negative definition of health is the absence of disease or illness. This is the meaning of health within the western scientific medical model. The positive definition of health is a state of well-being, interpreted by the world health organization in its constitution as a state of complete physical, mental and social well-being, not merely the absence of disease or infirmity (WHO, 1946).

健康是整体的，包括多个方面，而每个方面都要考虑到。整体健康意味着每方面、每方面的影响以及各方面之间的相互作用。健康的各个方面可以用图 11-1 来表示。

内圈代表健康的各个方面：

身体健康，如结实，不生病；

心理健康，如感觉良好，能适应环境；

情绪健康，能表达自我感觉，维持与发展人际关系；

社会健康，例如，有朋友可以交谈，能与他人一起参与活动；

精神健康，承认并能实践道德或宗教原则或信念；

性健康，个人的性能力能够达到双方满意。

二个外圈代表影响个人健康的宏观方面——社会健康与环境健康

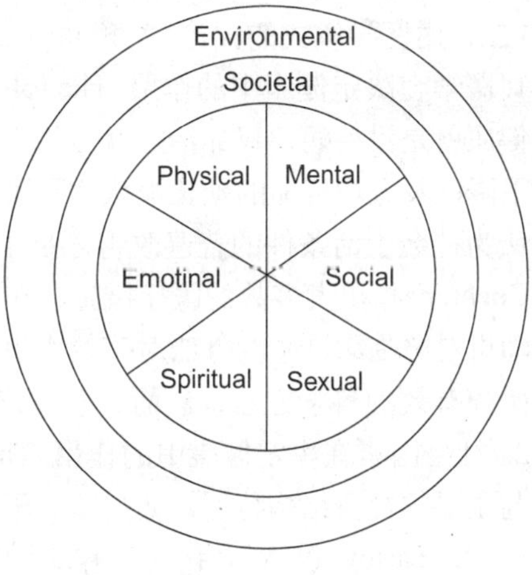

图 11-1 Dimensions of health

The inner circle represents individual dimensions of health

Physical health, e.g. fitness, not being ill

Mental health, e.g. feeling good, feeling able to cope

Emotional health concerns the ability to express feelings and to develop and sustain relationships, e.g. feeling loved

Social health, e.g. having friends to talk to being involved in activities with other people

Spiritual health is the recognition and ability to put into practice moral or religious principles or beliefs

Sexual health is the acceptance and ability to achieve a satisfactory expression of one's sexuality

疾病，患病与亚健康虽然含义不同，但常可互换应用。疾病意味着不舒服或不适，处于一种不健康的客观状态，它需要用客观的指标来测量。患病是指一种引起伤害或疼痛的状态，是主观表达的有症状的不健康的感觉。亚健康是介于健康与疾病之间的一种状态，既不完全健康，又没达到疾病的诊断标准和程度，称为第三种状态又称灰色状态或亚临床期等。亚健康有两种：一种是有不适症状存在；另一种是亚临床状态，即症状、体征已接近疾病诊断的标准或处于正常值的极限。

Disease, illness and ill health are often used interchangeably although they have very different meaning. Disease means uneasiness or discomfort. It implies an objective state of ill health which may be verified by accepted canons of proof. This abnormity may be observable and measurable. Illness indicates a condition causing harm or pain. It is the subjective experience of loss of health, and couched in terms of symptoms. Ill health is a state between health and disease. It is neither complete health, nor achieve diagnostic criteria and levels of disease, and called third state, or grey condition or subclinical stage, etc. there are two conditions in ill health: one is various uncomfortable symptoms existed, one is: subclinical condition, e.g. signs and symptoms has nearly reached the diagnostic criteria or high values of normal state.

西方医学科学持有狭隘的健康观，通常用有病或无病来表示。持有这种认识，健康是一个负面词，与是什么比较，更多地确定为不是什么。这种健康观影响巨大，不只是在专业人员范围内，而且媒体也经常引用这种观点，通过这些途径，专业定义为大部分社会所知晓与接受。

（二）对医学模式的评论 A critique of the medical model

1. 医学在决定健康中的作用 The role of medicine in determining health

健康就是没疾病，仅靠治疗就可使人恢复健康的观点已经受到了质疑。20世纪，人口死亡率的下降以及人均寿命的延长被认为是医学科学进步的结果。Mckeown等采用历史分析的方法研究认为社会生活条件的普遍改善才是主要原因，与之相比，医学的贡献很小。

Cochrane指出大多数的医疗措施，在被广泛应用之前都没有足够的证据表明其效果。因为采用随机对照临床试验的方法对疗效作出评价的医疗措施非常罕见。随机对照临床试验研究是确认医疗有效的科学方法，然而，对治疗或治愈的要求使这样的试验很难进行。

2. 社会因素在决定健康中的作用 The role of social factors in determining health

与主要的社会结构特征，如财富分配、收入、住房与雇用比较时，医学科学对健康的影响是微小的。Tarlov（1996）认为，在20世纪医疗服务对获得期望寿命的贡献只有17%。一般来说，社会资源的分配越平等，公民的健康状况就会越好、越平等。

3. 医学作为社会控制的一种手段 Medicine as a means of social control

社会学家认为医学是主要是发挥专业人员的力量。医学是有力的社会控制手段，采用疾病、患病、等分类使社会保持着稳定状态。

（三）健康如同人身自由 Health as autonomy

有人认为健康意味着人身自由，人身自由或健康受到生命医学化的搅乱。这种批评意见是医学已经得到了超过其法律经营范围的权力。生命医学化是医学的决定与技术侵入到生命周期的各个阶段，如生与死。把医生称作为生与死的决定者。

（四）外行的健康概念 Lay concepts of health

传统的医学科学将重点放在患者身上，关注疾病的治疗，忽视了对整个人群的关注，忽略了健康的积极概念。研究人员分析了公众对健康的信念或概念，发现随着年龄、性别与社会阶层的不同，人们对健康的定义、健康的差异的理解都不相同。

（五）健康文化观 Cultural views of health

健康是文化传统的一部分。不同的社会与文化对健康有不同的认识。非洲西部的阿散蒂人认为疾病是恶人或超自然力量的结果，精神抚慰仪式是治疗的一部分。关于健康与疾病的思考方式反映出社会的基本关注点和主流观点。人类学家把这种现象称为健康与疾病观念的文化特征。在多元社会中，多元文化共同影响人们对健康和疾病的理解。例如，传统的中国医学依据阴阳，男女，冷热的二元论用于症状、饮食与治疗，如针灸，中草药。

文化对健康观的影响最为明显。Crowford分析西方社会认为资本主义是西方社会的根源，资本主义是以生产力为中心的自由贸易经济体系，这种经济体系与健康观并行。健康与消费、生产有关。

（六）统一的健康观 A unified view of health

世界卫生组织试图把不同的健康观与信念协调、统一，形成了 4 种健康的理论：

1. 健康是一种理想状态

这是一种传统而积极的健康概念。它显示出健康各个方面间的相互关系，然而，具有争议的是这个概念太理想化，不能提供实际的指导意义，难以达到。

Health as an ideal state provides a holistic and positive definition of health. It is important in showing the interrelationship of different dimensions of health. However, it has been argued that this definition is too idealistic and vague to provide practical guidance for health promoters. Health in this sense is probably unattainable.

2. 健康包括精神健康与身体健康二方面

这是功能性社会学家 Talcott parsons 提出的观点。认为当人们能够完成每天的工作任务和期望发挥的作用时是健康的。这种健康功能观采用了社会准则而没有考虑到个体的差异。

Health as mental and physical fitness is a perspective developed by Talcott parsons (1951), a functional sociologist. It suggests that health is when people can fulfill the everyday tasks and roles expected of them. The functional view of health imposes social norms without regard to individual variation.

3. 健康作为一种商品

这种健康观导致对健康有不现实的期望。认为健康如同商品一样是可以购买的，而支付高额卫生费用并不能保证拥有健康。

Health as a commodity leads to unrealistic expectations of health as something which can be purchased. Health cannot be guaranteed by paying a higher price for health care.

4. 健康即为强壮

这种观点来自人类心理学，认为个人能够通过自我实现而获得健康。这一观点鼓励个人参与维护健康，而忽视了影响健康的社会环境因素。

Health as a personal strength is a view which derives from humanistic psychology and suggests that an individual can become healthy through self-actualization and discovery (Mastow, 1970). This approach encourages individuals to define their own-health but it does not address the social environment which creates health and ill health.

Seedhouse 认为这 4 种观点能够形成一种统一的健康理论。健康最终是一种手段而不是固定不变的状态。健康是能够通过人们的努力来实现的。创造以下这些条件来获得健康：

- 食物、饮水、居所、温度为基本需要；
- 获得影响健康因素的信息；
- 应用信息的技能与信念。

WHO开展了关于健康定义的讨论：健康一方面是个人或群体能够实现愿望和满足需要的程度，另一方面是改变或适应环境的程度。因此把健康看作为每日生活的资源不是目标，这是一种积极的概念。强调了社会和个人的资源以及自身能力。

Health is the extent to which an individual or group is able, on the one hand, to realize aspirations and satisfy needs; and, the other hand, to change or cope with the environment. Health is, therefore, seen as a resource for everyday life, not an object of living, it is a positive concept emphasizing social and personal resources, as well as physical capacities (WHO, 1984).

这个定义的重要性有如下几个方面：

- 确定健康是社会与个人的产物；
- 强调健康的能动而积极的性质；
- 把健康看作为基本人权和正常的社会投资。

这个观点为雅加达宣言确认健康与社会经济发展之间的联系奠定了基础。这一定义提供了多种支持健康的理由，满足了各种人群对健康的关心。对健康优先达成广泛共识，使得设计促进健康的各种活动合法化。除了初级卫生保健与发展个人技能的策略之外，WHO还在渥太华宪章中确定了更有针对性的社会参与健康的公众政策。这些策略作为健康促进的基础。然而，存在的争议是这种广泛的定义使健康促进活动难以确定重点。

健康用于不同的方面，反映生命的不同内容。由于含义的复杂性，不大可能有一个统一的定义。

因此，健康的概念无对与错之分。不同的人可能有不同的健康观，几种相互矛盾的观点可以共存。人们的社会地位、性别、种族与职业将会影响其健康观。然而，医学模式占优势的还是西方关于健康的思想。这对健康促进的价值有限，因为：

- 它依赖不为广泛接受的正常概念；
- 忽视了健康的广泛社会与环境方面；
- 忽视人们对健康的主观理解；
- 重点放在病理与功能失常方面，使医生只应对疾病，而不是主动促进健康。

健康的概念有多种含义，在具体情况下，要发现什么样的健康观起作用。对健康促进者来说，首要的是了解自己和他人对健康的理解。

二、影响健康的因素 Factors influencing on health

社会与环境因素是影响死亡率与发病率的主要因素。人群之间健康状况的不平等反映出社会结构的不平等，如社会阶层、性别与种族等。

（一）健康的决定因素 Determinants of health

20 世纪早期，感染性疾病减少，影响人们寿命的疾病主要为心血管病（近死亡的 48%）、癌症（死亡的 25%）等。

在健康的影响因素时，需要明确两个变量，一个是测量健康或亚健康变量，如死亡率或发病率；另一个是个体变量，如性别、职业等。对健康的影响可能是几种变量相互作用的结果。

Lalonde1974 年发表的报告人为对健康有影响的因素有四类：

- 遗传与生物学因素，确定一个人易患病的体质；
- 生活方式因素，如吸烟；
- 环境因素，如居住条件、污染；
- 卫生服务的范围与性质。

（二）社会阶层与健康 Social class and health

在探索健康的影响因素过程中，人们开始关注社会阶层与健康之间的关系。1980 年英国Black发表了一篇报告详细研究了死亡率与发病率和社会阶层之间的关系。自1921年以来，英国把社会阶层分为 5 级：Ⅰ级为专业人员。Ⅴ级为无技能手工工人。2001 年又修订为新 8 类。社会阶层是不同人群经历的生活方式与生活标准的一个指标，与社会地位的其他方面如收入、居住条件、教育以及工作与生活环境相关。

虽然，社会阶层与健康密切关联，但是社会阶层的指标是什么，没有一致的意见，最常用的有收入、居住环境与雇用情况等。

（三）解释健康的不平等 Explaining health inequalities

健康的不平等与社会阶层、地理位置、性别与种族有关。有4种解释：人为现象，社会选择，文化与行为以及物质主义者。

1. 人为现象的解释认为社会各阶层之间死亡率数字的差距是不真实的，而是受到测量方法的影响。因为职业分类与社会阶层结构都已经改变，不可能随着时间的过去进行比较。虽然确定社会阶层与健康的关系比较困难，相当多的研究都支持这种联系是客观的，而不是数据的人为现象。

2. 健康不平等是一种选择过程

社会选择理论认为社会阶层与健康之间的关系是健康决定了人们的社会阶层。良好的健康状况使得人们进入上层社会，而疾病或患病使得人们的社会等级下降，确实有证据表明，健康能够影响人们的社会经济状况。争论的焦点是健康是一种静态财富，不易受社会经济状况的影响。

3. 健康不平等为生活方式的结果 Health inequalities as a result of lifestyles

这一观点认为 健康与生活方式和行为有联系。不健康的生活方式与行为，如吸烟、酗酒、缺乏锻炼、高脂高糖饮食等在社会阶层低的人群中更为普遍。

4. 健康不平等与文化解释 Health inequalities and cultural explanations

有人认为，不同社会阶层的人们对待健康的态度以及对健康的保护方面存在着文化差异。

5. 健康不平等为物质缺乏的结果 Health inequalities as a result of material disadvantage

这一解释认为健康在人群中的分布反映出社会资源分配的不平等。社会阶层较低的人受教育最少、钱最少、拥有的资源也最少。

6. 卫生服务的利用 Access to health services

不同的社会人群、不同地区以及不同的种族人群之间可以利用的卫生服务资源的质量与数量有明显差异。但是，由于医疗保健对健康的影响力很轻微，健康的差异并不能完全归咎于卫生服务资源的数量和质量上的差异。

7. 解决健康不平等 Tackling inequalities in health

近 20 年来，虽然贫困对健康的影响力减弱了，健康的不平等程度却加大了。政府采取多种策略，通过媒体宣传活动、开展健康筛查以及改变个人生活方式等解决健康的不平等。Benzeval 等提出了一套解决健康不平等的政府策略。

Benzeval et al (1995) proposed a range of broad policy initiatives based on key action areas identified in the Ottawa Charter (WHO, 1986):

Strengthening individuals. This means ensuring that people have information and skills so that they are supported and enabled to make informed choices.

Strengthening communities. This means supporting people in their communities to make decisions about health issues affecting them.

Improving access to facilities and services. This involves mediating between people and service providers in order to ensure that needs are met.

Encouraging a healthy public policy. A healthy public policy underpins other areas. Wider social and economic change reduces poverty and ensures that the environment and living conditions are conducive to health.

健康促进者首先要认识到社会经济因素在决定个人与群体健康方面是至关重要的。健康促进者虽然难以改变宏观水平上的健康状况，但在制定健康促进项目时要关注健康的不平等。

三、健康促进的发展 The development of health promotion

健康促进一词被用于许多不同的方面，对健康促进的不同理解反映出其不同的来源：

- 健康的推销员（Williams）；
- 试图游说、诱使或影响个人而改变其生活方式（Gott & O'Brien 1990）；
- 结合教育、法律、财政、经济、环境与组织的干预措施，促使人们达到健康、预防疾病(Tones 1990）；
- 一种保健途径，在了解了影响健康的多因素的基础上，鼓励每个人自主选择和评价生活方式（Wilson Barnett 1993）。

WHO在健康促进方面起到了关键的作用。1977年世界卫生大会在阿拉木图向所有成员国提交了 2000 年人人享有卫生保健的原则，WHO 提出健康促进的 5 项原则。

The WHO made explicit five key principles for health promotion:

1. It involves the population as a whole in the context of their everyday life, rather than focusing on people at risk for specific diseases;

2. It is directed towards action on the causes or determinants of health to ensure that the total environment which is beyond the control of individuals is conducive to health;

3. It combines diverse, but complementary, methods or approaches including communication, education, legislation, fiscal measures, organizational change, community development and spontaneous local activities against health hazards;

4. It aims particularly at effective public participation supporting the principles of self-help movements and encourages people to find their own ways of managing the health of their community;

5. While health promotion is basically an activity in the health and social fields and not a medical service, health professionals - particularly in primary health care - have an important role in nurturing and enabling health promotion (WHO, 1977).

发展基础广泛的健康策略的背景需要依据平等、社会参与以及部门间的合作。WHO虽然强调改变生活方式、环境条件以及卫生保健，但是首先要改变基本条件。这些基本条件包括：

- 和平与自由；
- 机会均等，社会公正；
- 满足基本生存需要的条件，包括食物、收入、安全饮用水、生活环境、居住条件、安全工作环境，以及在社会中发挥自己的作用等；
- 政府承诺与公众支持。

1984年WHO开展了健康促进项目，1986年在渥太华召开了会议，1988年Adelaide，1991年 Sundsvall, 1997 年在 Jakarta 进一步概括了行动范围，在渥太华宪章中发展了健康促进的原则，概括出这些领域是重要的：

① *building a healthy public policy;*

② *creating supportive environments;*

③ *developing personal skills including information and coping strategies;*

④ *strengthening community action including social support and networks;*

⑤ *reorienting health services away from treatment and care and improving access to health services (WHO, 1986).*

WHO 认为协作、倡导与提高能力是健康促进的途径。

2005年8月曼谷会议通过的健康促进宪章提出需要策略和承诺，以便在全球通过健康促进的措施积极处理健康的决定因素。宪章指出，自渥太华宪章以来，健康促进的内容已有了明显的改变。在国家内部以及各国之间健康不平等的状况在加剧，新的消费方式、交流方式、商贸方式以及环境恶化、城市化都存在着影响健康的因素。快速而又常常不利的社会变革影响到工作条件、学习环境、家庭类型以及社区文化与社会组织结构。

健康促进是能够促使人们控制其健康及其决定因素，从而增进自身健康的过程。它是公共卫生的核心，有助于处理传染病与非传染病以及其他对健康的危害。在增进健康与人类发展中是一种有效的投资。有助于减少健康与性别的不平等。

Health promotion is the process of enabling people to increase control over their health. Health promotion is a core function of public health and contributes to tackling communicable and noncommunicable diseases and other threats to health. It is an effective investment in improving health and human development. It contributes to reducing both health and gender inequities.

WHO宪章指出，全球社会健康促进的策略需要有强有力的政治行动，广泛的参与以及连续不断的倡导。为了推动可持续性发展，所有部门与机构必须做到：宣传、投资、提高能力、制定法规与立法以及建立伙伴关系。

Advocate for health based on human rights and solidarity;

Invest in sustainable policies, actions and infrastructure to address the determinants of health;

Build capacity for policy development, leadership, health promotion practice, knowledge transfer and research, and health literacy;

Regulate and legislate to ensure a high level of protection from harm and enable equal opportunity for health and well-being for all people;

Partner and build alliances with public, private, nongovernmental organizations and civil society to create sustainable actions.

WHO宪章还指出，承诺人人享有卫生保健必须使健康促进成为全球发展议程的中心、所有政府部门的核心职能、社区与文明社会的重中之重以及良好合作的必要条件。

Commitments to health for all

Make the promotion of health central to the global development agenda;

Make the promotion of health a core responsibility for all of government;

Make the promotion of health a key focus of communities and civil society;

Make the promotion a requirement for good corporate practices.

2005年9月第八届世界预防牙医学大会通过了“利物浦宣言”——促进21世纪口腔健康的倡议行动，希望各国到2020年都应加强9个领域的口腔健康工作，包括清洁饮用水、适当的环境设施、健康饮食与良好营养、适量用氟、促进健康的生活方式、减少危险因素、利用学校平台、强调初级口腔卫生保健、增强老年人口腔健康、制定口腔健康政策、支持公共卫生研究以及建立健康信息系统。

The Liverpool Declaration: promoting oral health in the 21st century - a call for action.

四、健康促进的定义 Definition of health promotion

（一）疾病预防 Disease prevention

19世纪公共卫生措施的转变是通过健康教育提供指导和信息。20世纪后叶公共卫生措施转变为采取社会和环境措施，重点从治疗疾病转到维护健康上。不过，医学模式占优势意味着健康促进常被看作为预防疾病，并针对有高危人群。

健康教育常与初级，二级或三级预防有关。初级预防试图检查高危人群，避免亚健康开始并提供指导与咨询，二级预防则是通过早期诊断与治疗缩短病程，防止亚健康进一步发展，三级预防主要是减少机能丧失、残疾或并发症。

（二）健康教育 Health education

直到20世纪80年代中期，健康教育一词才被广泛应用于描述执业医生在促进健康方面的工作。个人能对疾病发生作出健康选择的认识形成了一种看法——有可能通过说服与传授技术，告知人们如何预防疾病，鼓励其改变行为，养成健康的生活方式。主要的途径是向人们提供有关健康与疾病的信息。

健康教育是来自以医学与教育为基础的一种专家权威的模式——由健康教育者决定是否有健康需要，倡导个人生活方式干预的性质，以及最有效的交流方式等。

当我们着眼于健康教育实践时，我们相信健康教育是提供促进健康的信息。当人们依从 健康教育的指导时，促进健康的措施就容易取得成功。

Health education may be defined as planned opportunities for people to learn about health and make changes in their behavior. It includes:

Raising awareness of health issues and factors contributing to ill health

Providing information

Motivating and persuading people to make changes in their lifestyle for their health

Equipping people with the skills and confidence to make those changes

健康教育的历史发展有两条线索，教育家与社会学家通过争论健康教育的假设，挑战预防医学的主流，是否可能，或者应该通过提供信息与说服方法促使行为改变。这样就形成了增强自我能力的原则，是许多争论的中心。增强能力是一种途径，使人们有能力对他们的生活负责，如果愿意，包括改变其行为。这不可避免地涉及专业人员的优势与控制的减少。

健康教育的途径，医学模式重点在于健康监督与达到行为改变，而教育模式依赖探索态度与价值。这些途径与健康促进更密切有联系。如社区发展，强调需要采取集体有益于健康的行动，社会模式重点在于需要影响地方和国家水平的决策者。

（三）健康促进 Health promotion

WHO把健康促进的定义从预防疾病或发现高危人群转向关注全民健康。取代了由专家与专业人员诊断问题，改为在社区由人们自己确定与其有关的健康内容。所有的人，包括教师，初级卫生保健工作者，工作场所经理，以及社会福利工作者都能参与促进健康。取代了只把健康看作为个人的责任。重视决定健康的社会因素，把健康看作为是社会集体的责任，需要组织和政府在决策中优先考虑。健康教育与健康促进的词汇常交互使用，而把健康促进看作为一把伞，健康教育可以纳入健康促进之中，其概念更加广泛。

健康促进结合各种措施，以便促进健康和控制疾病，毫无疑问，健康促进的一个主要特征是“健康的公众政策”的重要性，它可能通过立法，财政，经济与其他环境工程形式达到社会变化。

Milio第一个提出把健康促进概述为“使选择健康更加容易”，便于执业医生发挥健康促进的作用，提供信息，指导如何采纳健康的生活方式。

A phrase first coined by Milio (1986) has come to encapsulate health promotion- “making the healthy choice the easier choice”

区别健康促进与健康教育的关键特征是它涉及环境与政治行动。健康教育以自治与自愿为中心，健康教育的原则包括促进自尊与非强迫性。

（四）健康促进的整合定义 An integrated definition of health promotion

在实践中，健康促进包含不同的政治倾向性，与结构途径相对，具有个人途径的特征。

WHO 确定三种促进健康的途径：倡导，提高能力与协作。

- 倡导 Advocacy　意味着代表弱势群体的兴趣以及代表其说话或游说来影响政策；

- 提高能力 Enablement　健康促进的目的应是减少现时健康状况的差异确保有平等的机会，使所有的人都能达到最大可能的健康；
- 协作Mediation　健康促进需要多种机构，多个部门的协调与合作。在健康促进的定义中，把它解释为一个增进个人或社区健康的过程。WHO 把这些确定为提高能力，平等，合作和参与。应该把这些价值结合到所有健康与福利工作之中，它就是健康促进。

健康促进是一种确定和开展卫生工作的整合途径。中心的问题并不是健康促进的范围是什么，而是是否以一种健康促进的途径在进行。

接受这样一个定义意味着健康促进可以没有边界，因为任何情况或事件在医患之间都有健康促进的可能。

健康促进包括增加个人关于身体功能，预防疾病的方法、知识，增加利用卫生保健系统的能力、增强关于政治与环境因素影响健康的意识。

Health promotion includes increasing individual knowledge about the functions of the body and ways of preventing illness, raising competence in using the health care system, and raising awareness about the political and environmental factors that influence health.

五、健康促进的模式与途径 Models and approaches of health promotion

（一）健康促进的途径 Approaches of health promotion

健康促进有 5 种不同的途径：

- 医疗或预防　medical or preventive
- 行为改变　behaviour change
- 教育　educational
- 提高能力　empowerment
- 社会改变　social change

这些途径有不同的目的、方法与评价手段，不同的目标：

- 预防疾病；
- 确保人们知情并能作出健康的选择；
- 帮助人们获得技能与自信，以便更好地控制其健康；
- 为促进健康的选择而改变政策与环境。

所有这些途径都反映出不同的工作方法。

1. 医学途径 The medical approach

（1）目的 Aims　活动重点在于降低发病率与过早死亡率，活动目标针对全人口或高危人群，这种健康促进在于寻求增加医疗干预，预防亚健康与过早死亡，通常分为三级干预水平：初级，二级与三级。医疗途径对健康促进是普遍的。

（2）方法 Methods　预防服务的原则，如饮水氟化，是针对特殊情况的高危人群。筛查对于疾病或情况是有效的。

（3）评价 Evaluation　评价预防措施的最终依据发病率或死亡率的降低，这是一个长期过程，短期评价较有效的措施是筛查目标人群的百分比。

2. 行为改变 Behaviour Change

（1）目的 Aims 鼓励人们采纳健康的行为，是增进健康的关键。这一途径很普遍，因为它把健康看作为个人财富。很明显个人行为与社会环境因素之间存在着复杂的关系。

（2）方法 Methods 采用群众性交流方式，专家指导，自上而下的途径，提供信息，面对面咨询等。

（3）评价 Evaluation 行为改变是一种简单的测试。干预之后健康行为是否有改变？有两个问题：经过一个长周期，改变才能变得明显，难以与其他任何因素引起的改变分开。

3. 教育途径 The educational approach

（1）目的 Aims 提供知识与信息，发展必要的技能，人们能够对健康行为作出知情选择。

（2）方法 Methods 教育的内容包括三个方面：

- 认知（信息与理解）；
- 信念（态度与感觉）；
- 行为（技能）。

（3）评价 Evaluation 知识的增加相对容易测量。通过媒体活动、一对一教育、班级活动进行健康教育。用信息量的增加或疾病危险因素的意识增强来评价效果。然而，只提供信息不足以改变行为，即使向往并有能力改变的人也不能保证会去做。

4. 提高能力 Empowerment

（1）目的 Aims 使人们有能力控制其生活。这一途径帮助人们确定其自身关注的问题，并获得对其采取行动的技能与自信。提高人们的能力，需要：

- 认识和理解其能力的有限；
- 产生改变现状的迫切感；
- 意识到通过提供的信息，知识与生活技能能够改变现状。

（2）方法 Methods 这一途径称为以客户为中心，或用倡导或自我保健的词汇。社区发展是类似的工作方法，使人群能够确定他们所关心的问题并参与制定行动计划。

（3）评价 Evaluation 评价这样的活动比较困难，原因是提高能力是长期的过程。这使得评价难以确定检查出的任何改变是由于干预而不是其他因素的作用结果。

评价包括达到目的的程度（结果评价）以及人群获得能力的程度作为干预的一种结果（过程评价）。

5. 社会改变 Social Change

（1）目的 Aims 改变自然，社会与经济环境使人们易于做出健康的选择

（2）Methods 社会改变或者称为根本的途径是针对人群或全体人口自上而下的一种工作方法。虽然可以是广泛的咨询，一般在组织内部寻求改变，并且需要最高领导层的承诺。这一途径需要必要的工作技能，如游说，制定政策计划，协商与实施等。

（3）评价 Evaluation 社会改变途径的评价包括结果，如促进健康的立法，组织或规则改变。有时，其结果是长期而复杂的过程，难以证明结果与特殊的健康促进干预措施的联系。

（二）健康促进模式 Models of health promotion

健康促进模式有不同的目的而并非行动指南，但有助于鼓励思考，形成新的策略与工作方式，也有助于确定重点和设计干预的类型。

Models of health promotion serve different purposes-they are not a guide to action but may help to:

- *Conceptualize or map the field of health promotion.*
- *Interrogate and analyze existing practice.*
- *Plan and chart the possibilities for interventions (Naidoo & Wills, 1998).*

Using a model can be helpful because it encourages you to think theoretically, and come up with a new strategies and ways of working. It can also help you to prioritize and locate more or less desirable types of interventions.

有两种模式是从社会学与社会政策构架演化而来的，它们采用一种结构分析法提示关注物质与社会对健康的影响以及形成健康不平等的社会结构。显示出健康促进途径怎样受到政治理念以及关于权力，职责与自治不同价值定位的影响。

The following two models derive from sociological and social policy frameworks. They adopt a structural analysis which draws attention to the material and social influences on health and the social structures which contribute to inequalities in health. They show how health promotion approaches are influenced by political ideology and different value positions about power, responsibility and autonomy.

1. Caplan & Holland（1990）

Caplan & Holland 提出的健康促进模式有两种形式，一种与知识有关。知识被看作为从主观途径通过理解达到客观途径的一种连续性基础。客观解释来自科学（例如，健康就是没有病）仅为总体的一部分。也可以强调外行的说法和人们自身独立的解释健康意味着什么。

另一种与设想的社会性质有关。其范围从基本变化的理论到社会规范的理论。当把这两方面放在一起时就提出了健康促进的4种观点。每一种都代表着理解健康与健康促进实践的一种主要途径，具体表现出有关社会，健康概念与健康问题的主要来源的不同的理论与哲理假设。

（1）传统的观点 The traditional perspective　与医学和行为改变途径有关。知识属于专家所有，强调提供信息和促使行为改变。

（2）人类学家的观点 The humanist perspective　与教育途径有关。促使个人能够利用个人资源与技能，以最大的机会发展他们所认为的健康生活方式。

（3）偏激的人类学家观点 The radical humanist perspective　与增强能力途径有关。健康促进与增强意识有关。强调探索个人对健康内容的反映。按照这个思路，鼓励个人组成社会，组织与经济网络。

（4）偏激的结构学家观点 The radical structuralist perspective　持有结构的不平等的看法是许多健康问题的原因。健康促进的作用是处理健康与社会不平等之间的关系。

2. Beattie（1991）

Beattie提出健康促进途径所有组成部分的结构分析。指出健康促进有4种落伍。这些产生于干预方式的量纲，其范围从权威（自上而下与专家领导）到协商（自下而上与尊重个人自治）。

Beattie 的类型学产生健康促进的策略。

（1）健康说服 Health persuasion　干预针对个人并有专业人员指导。

（2）立法行动 Legislative action　由专业人员指导干预，但有意识的保护社区。

（3）个人咨询 Personal counseling　这些干预是引导客户，重点在个人发展。

（4）社区发展 Community development　这些干预类似于个人咨询，寻求增强能力或增强一个人群或当地社区的技能。

上述每一种策略对应一种不同的政治观点。这样，保守的改良主义者的观点把健康促进看作为试图纠正或恢复所看到的不足。偏激的观点是寻求动员和解放社区。

3. Tannahill（Downie et al 1996）

这种健康促进模式广为卫生保健工作者所接受。他包括三个相互包含的活动内容——健康教育、健康保护以及预防。

This model of health promotion is widely accepted by health care workers. Tannahill talks of three overlapping spheres of activity: health education, health protection and prevention.

Health education - communication to enhance well-being and prevent ill health through influencing knowledge and attitudes.

Prevention - reducing or avoiding the risk of diseases and ill health primarily through medical interventions.

Health protection - safeguarding population health through legislative, fiscal or social measures.

Tannahill's diagrammatic representation shows how these different approaches relate to each other in an all-inclusive process termed health promotion.

4. Tones（1994）

提高能力是其主要原则。目的是使人们能够得到控制自身健康的能力，重点是提高个人自我维护健康的能力。

Tones认为教育是通过增强对健康问题的意识，从而达到提高普通人与专业人员能力。这样人们更能作出选择，并对健康的公众政策造成压力。我们看到提高自我能力与社区能力之间是有区别的，二者之间是相互作用的关系。

只有当我们关注健康促进的不同方式时，才能作出判断。认识到两种方式并不总是同义的，在短期内可能感到灰心，但必须长期坚持才能见到健康促进的效果与效率。

第二节　健康促进的策略与方法

Section 2 Strategies and Methods in Health Promotion

无论采纳何种策略与方法，健康促进的难点在于怎样与社区一起工作，社区发展途径的优点与限度，什么影响到健康的行为，怎样才能帮助人们改变行为？利用媒体是否有效？以及在健康促进工作中怎样采纳人们的观点？

一、健康合作伙伴——一起工作 Partnerships for health-working together

健康促进向着健康包含着社会与环境因素的广义健康观转化。因此，促进健康不只是卫生部门的责任。为了达到更好的健康必须有三方合作：政府、社区以及个人。合作伙伴包括政府部门，如卫生局，地方局，商业机构，志愿团体与个人。WHO把这个过程称作为部门之间的合作。

Health promotion shifted towards a broad view of health encompassing social and environmental factors. Improving health cannot, therefore, be the sole responsibility of the health sectors. For 'a three-

way partnership for better health, the government, local communities and individuals will join in partnership to improve people's health.' partners include the government, health authorities, local authorities, business, voluntary bodies and individuals. WHO calls this process intersectional collaboration.

（一）定义 Definition

人们在一起为促进健康而工作有多种形式，使用许多不同的词汇：

（1）伙伴 Partnership　涉及合作者之间联合行动（国家与地方机构以及公众）。意味着权力同享。

（2）服务协议与合同 Service agreements and contracts　为增进健康，伙伴之间确定各自的职责。

（3）多种机构 Multiagency　社会服务，或教育服务，都是公共服务的法定提供者。

（4）部门之间 Intersectoral　超过任何一个部门以上，可以包括公共，私人（生意与商业）与志愿团体。

学科间或多学科工作 Inter-or multidisciplineary working，在同一组织或跨部门机构内发挥各自不同作用或功能的人们联合工作。

联合计划 Joint planning　部门内或跨部门的各种组织统一的目标，定期开会制定并实施一个联合计划。

团队 Team　通常有共同的任务，并由经过选择的人员组成，因为他们有相关的专长。

（二）政策背景 Policy background

合作在健康促进中是一个常用的词，很久以来，就已经认识到，健康促进需要各个水平上的广泛参与。WHO做出结论认为医疗服务对促进健康的贡献是有限的，因此，部门之间的合作非常重要："人人享有卫生保健需要所有相关部门的协调工作。卫生当局只能处理所要解决的部分问题。多部门合作是唯一有效的确保健康，促进健康的政策，减少自然、经济与社会环境的危险的前提。WHO21世纪的新目标包括一个具体的动员健康伙伴的目标。

"Health For All requires the co-ordinated action of all sectors concerned. The health authorities can only deal with part of the problems to be solved and multisectoral co-operation is the only way of effectively ensuring the prerequisites for health, promoting health policies and reducing the risks in the physical, economic and social environment (WHO, 1985). The WHO's new targets for the 21st century contain a specific target on mobilizing partners for health.

（三）合作的优点 Advantages of working together

合作是一种挑战，但它创造了"附加性"。有优点也有缺点。优点在于：

1. 把通常并没有看到自身能够发挥健康促进作用的组织和群体组织在一起。这意味着把健康看作为是一个整体，而不仅仅在以治疗为主题的医疗机构内。

2. 增加这些组织的知识和彼此了解，帮助澄清作用，消除对抗。

3. 合作服务计划是依据当地需要的总体情况，这将会帮助弥补缺陷。

4. 依据广泛的咨询确保正确有针对性的提供服务以及汇集社区需要的知识和意识。

5. 伙伴工作可导致更有效地利用资源，也能避免重复管理。

6. 确保给予公众同样的、没有矛盾的信息。

7. 可以解决不健康的根源，不只是症状，能够加强对不健康决定因素的意识。

影响合作的许多因素与专业人员之间的工作有关，其中最重要的两点：

- 关于工作的价值与方式，专业人员间有不同的观点；
- 人际关系，如伙伴的私生活，是以友谊与诚信为基础。

（四）合作成功的特点 Characteristics of successful joint working

健康促进需要良好的团队工作与各方的协调，理想的团队有下列基本特点：

- 共同的任务或目的；
- 成员经过选择，因为他们具有特殊的能力（专长）；
- 成员知道自己的作用以及他人的作用；
- 在工作中彼此支持；
- 成员在技能与修改方面相互补充；
- 有领导负责协调；
- 团队有一个基地。

促进健康伙伴形成的因素有（Thompson 等，1994）：

- 一个伙伴建立的过程；
- 激励支持改变的网络；
- 支持过程的物质资源；
- 一个致力于中央协调的机构或人员；
- 一个交流计划。

（五）关键合作者 Key stakeholders

健康促进的关键合作者如下：

- 政府各部门；
- 卫生当局与卫生托管机构；
- 健康教育当局与国家领导机构；
- 初级卫生保健团队；
- 医学专业机构与人员；
- 地方当局；
- 社区团体与志愿组织；
- 商业部门与雇主；
- 媒体。

WHO概括的主要原则之一是部门间的合作。合作伙伴一起工作也是健康策略的关键。然而，仅此不足以减少不平等或重新定向卫生服务或促进与说服社区积极参与自身的卫生决策。如果有一个以当地健康为方向的项目，社区发展途径对健康促进与咨询、培训、支持与资源都是必要的。渥太华宪章认为健康促进的关键过程与方法是提高能力、协调与倡导，促进健康合作者一起工作，特别是提高执业医生的协调能力。

Intersectoral collaboration is one of the key principles outlined by the WHO, if 'Health For All' is to be achieved. Partnership working is also a key to the health strategies. It is not sufficient alone, however, to reduce inequalities or reorient health services, or catalyze and persuade communities to actively participate in their own health decisions. Community development approaches are necessary to health promotion and the consultation, training, support and resources, if there is to be a local health-oriented programme. The Ottawa Charter described the key processes and methods for health promotion as enablement, mediation and advocacy. Working together in partnership for health calls, in particular, upon practitioner's mediation skills.

二、公共卫生工作 Public health work

公共卫生——促进全民健康取决于多种因素，其中许多问题需要提交给政府来解决，如交通、住房、收入、环境质量、食物、空气和水等。因此，公共卫生领域比医学更为宽广。公共卫生有以下几个特点：

- 关系到国民的健康；
- 关系到预防疾病；
- 认识到许多社会因素对健康有影响。

显然，“公共卫生”与“健康促进”概念之间有相当大的重叠。公共卫生最近的发展标志着它与健康促进的关系。

Public health-the promotion of the health of the population-depends on many factors which are the remit of government, such as transport, housing, income, the quality of the environment, food, air and water. Public health is therefore much broader than medicine. Public health is characterized by several factors:

Several factors:

A concern for the health of the whole population；

A concern for prevention of illness and disease；

A recognition of the many social factors which contribute to health.

It is apparent that there is considerable overlap between the concepts "public health" and "health promotion". The recent developments in public health flags up its relationship to health promotion.

（一）确定公共卫生工作 Defining public health work

为公众健康而工作意味着各级部门都要奉献于使人们健康和环境健康的任务。如空气或水的污染程度，地方活动能够影响到当地环境。

Taylor等（1998）提出，公共卫生被确定为是一种资源和一项活动。作为一种资源包括获取健康信息与统计资料（流行病学）以便支持影响健康状态的决策和干预。流行病学有长期的、高度的可信性，现在有一种考虑扩展流行病学的基础，以便包括外行的观点与重点，并公认社会因素对健康的影响（Naidoo 等 1998）。公共卫生行动涉及各种机构、组织、专业人员、社区、家庭与个人促进健康的活动。

（二）旧公共卫生 The old public health

现在已非常清楚，近代健康状况的改善更多地归功于公共卫生措施而不是临床医学。

It is now will known that improvements in health in recent times owe more to public health measures than clinical medicine (McKeown, 1979).

19世纪，保护和促进公共卫生是作为地方政府的任务，重点在改善提供清洁用水，废物处理，食品卫生与居住条件。19世纪后叶，环境的改善被环境科学所取代，把疾病的病因归咎于个人而不是他们的生活状况。公共卫生的重点是预防措施，如免疫注射，以及医生的防护。

20世纪中叶，随着感染性疾病的减少、与生活方式有关新的疾病增多（如冠心病与癌症），出现了公共卫生的低谷阶段。20世纪的大部分时间，公共卫生继续是地方政府解决的问题。到70年代，公共卫生变成为一门医学专业。处于边缘经费支持很少。公共卫生逐渐被认定为控制传染病。虽然，研究报告已指出社会不平等是不健康产生的原因。广泛的公共卫生观点在政治上不被重视，但一直没有消失。

（三）新公共卫生 The new public health

80年代中期，公共卫生的概念重新被人们关注，其范围也得到了扩展。新的公共卫生是从WHO欧洲地区项目目标“人人享有卫生保健”中设定健康的环境为目标而引出。渥太华宪章中把健康的公众政策作为健康促进的中心政策要点。健康促进的目的之一是关注公共卫生内容，如污染、职业危害、居住与新建定居点等。

The 1980s saw a revival of interest in the concept of public health and a reframing and broadening of its boundaries. The new public health drew on the World Health Organization (WHO) programme which set targets for healthy environments in its "Health for All" European Region targets (WHO, 1985). The Ottawa Charter identified healthy public policy as a central plank for health promotion. One of the aims of health promotion is to "focus attention on public health issues, such as pollution, occupational hazards, housing and settlements"(WHO, 1986).

渥太华宪章确定了以下基本健康资源：和平、安全居住、场所、教育、食品、收入、稳定的生态系统、可持续的资源以及社会公正与平等。Adelaide会议确定健康的公众政策其主要目的是创建一个支持环境使人们都能健康地生活着，或使人们易于作出健康的选择。Sundvall会议集中于全球的环境改变与促进健康之间的关系（WHO，1992）。雅加达宣言（WHO，1997）集中于社会、经济与政治发展与健康之间的联系。

19世纪占优势的公共卫生观点是自然环境对健康的作用，新的公共卫生是生态学观点。认为经济，环境与社会因素是相互联系的，当它们彼此之间达到适当同等的平衡时，全民都是健康的。新的公共卫生政策还意味着法定的与志愿的机构一起工作，评估所有涉及健康的公共卫生政策的实质——农业、能源、交通、防御、经济发展、雇用、居住、教育与休闲。

通过全球化和可维持发展的概念，环境运动与绿色政治的出现已影响到公共卫生的形象。经济活动的全球化意味着各国政府不再能控制那些影响到自然与社会环境的活动。例如，西方工业化国家的污染导致世界范围的气候变化，以及国际货币市场影响到全球的雇用方式，世界银行与国际货币基金，通过他们对发展国家的债务管理，已经受到抑制这些国家社会经济与卫生发展的指控。

The rise of the environmental movement and Green Politics has been influential in raising the profile of public health, through the concepts of globalization and sustainability. The globalization of economic activities means that nation states no longer control those activities which affect physical and social environments. For example, pollution from the industrialized western countries leads to worldwide climate change, and the international money market affects employment patterns worldwide.

More directly, the World Bank and international Monetary Fund, through their management of developing countries debts, has been accused of shifting social, economic and health development in these countries (Townsend, 1997).

可持续发展已经被规定为“满足现时需要的发展而不是让步于未来一代满足他们需要的能力（全球环境与发展任务，1987）”。联合国1992年政府首脑关于环境与发展会议开始的第21项议程，建立一个21世纪可以负担得起的行动项目，提出环境、社会与经济方面的发展。Rio宣言陈述：“人类是可负担得起的发展考虑的中心。在与自然协调中，他们是有权利拥有一个健康而有价值的生命”。

Agenda 21 commits governments to the following objectives on health:

Meeting the basic essential for health, e.g. safe food and water, sanitation and housing;

Controlling communicable diseases;

Protecting vulnerable groups, such as children;

Reducing the health risks caused by pollution, excessive energy consumption and waste;

Local Agenda 21, which developed as a result of the Rio Summit, is a comprehensive action plan for local development which aims to bring together local government, business, voluntary and community sectors to assess and meet local needs in a way which is sustainable. It was called “Think globally, act locally.”

（四）公共卫生与健康促进 Public health and health promotion

新的公共卫生与健康促进分享许多原则与策略。现代健康促进的原则与内容与新公共卫生的原则与内容是一致的。

The following have been identified as public health principles:

- *Health for All - equality for all citizens;*
- *A strategy for health;*
- *Involvement of the public and patients;*
- *Intelligence and surveillance;*
- *Need for strong evidence base;*
- *Importance of education, research and ethical considerations (Calman, 1998).*

The following have been identified as health for all principles：

- *Empowerment；*
- *Participation；*
- *Equity.*

Collaboration (WHO, 1985)

公共卫生原则与WHO人人享有卫生保健项目的原则为参与、平等与合作。

- 参与：公众有权利考虑并参与决策过程；
- 公平：大量证据表明健康的不公平反映出社会经济的不公平。与富足和优势的群体比较，较落后与弱势群体遭遇较高水平的不健康与早亡。还有证据表明，所有生活在较大不公平社会的人比生活在更为平等社会的人经受较差的健康状况。这提供了有利的论点，倡导较大的社会与经济公平为健康促进的一种手段。公平或公正与平等不相同。公平是公正的状况而平等将不可能达到。为同样需要的人提供同样的服务以及为减少已知的健康不平等而工作是现实的目标。

- 合作：合作或工作伙伴是第三个公共卫生原则。合作意味着与他人一起分担项目的工作。由于许多不同的因素影响到公共卫生，所以合作很有必要。这意味着任何一个部门或组织机构对健康只有有限的影响，通过一起工作，才能产生更多的改变，才有较大的促进健康的可能。

Public health is currently a high-profile issue. A key principle is replacing the medical model of health with a social model. International and national agencies that are responsible for providing the broad agenda for public health have produced a variety of supportive declarations, charters and legislation. For many, public health means the broad government functions of healthy public policy, and is a political agenda which is thought of as an activity removed from everyday practice. It is important to have a supportive public agenda, but the real challenge is to translate such lofty ideals into everyday practice, which requires a range of activities at many different levels. Central to this task are activities aimed at promoting participation, equity and collaboration.

三、与社区合作和发展社区 Working with communities and community development

社区发展是一种策略，目的在于提高人们的能力，使他们得到控制影响健康的危险因素。与社区合作以便增加他们参与影响健康的决策是健康促进的一个基本方面。

（一）社区发展 Community development

社区发展被确定为一个过程，通过它确定社区的需要或目标，满足这些需要或目标，发展自信，并愿意为这些需要或目标而工作，寻找资源（内部或外部）以便满足这些需要或实现这些目标，采取行动，在社区进行扩展，发展合作的态度并在社区实践。

（二）社区发展的关键特征 Key features of community development

发展社区健康是一个过程，通过这个过程，一个社区确定其自身的健康需要，考虑如何满足这些需要，并集体决定行动的重点。社区发展是一种理论又是一种方法，作为一种理论，其关键特征是：

- 承诺平等，破除等级制度及权力关系；
- 强调参与，并使所有社区都能赞同；
- 强调通俗知识，并重视人们的自身经验；
- 汇集经验并看到问题，共同分享；
- 通过教育，发展技能，分担与联合行动，增强个人与社区能力。

社区发展过程概括为：

- 反映社区现实的各个方面；
- 寻找并集体确定社区现实状况的根源；
- 审查问题的实质含意；
- 发展行动计划以便改变现实。

（三）社区发展与健康促进 Community development and health promotion

在健康促进中，社区发展是一种反复出现的主题。社区发展被看作为确定健康促进策略的中心。

"The people have right and a duty to participate individually and collectively in the planning and implementation of their health care"(WHO, 1978).

"Health for All will be achieved by people themselves. A well-informed, well-motivated, and actively participating community is a key element for the attainment of the common goal"(WHO, 1985).

"Health promotion works through concrete and effective community action in setting priorities, making decisions, planning strategies and implementing them to achieve better health. At the heart of this process is the empowerment of communities, their ownership and control of their own endeavours and destinies"(WHO, 1986).

"Community action is central to the fostering of health public policy"(WHO Adelaide, 1988).

"Health promotion is carried out by and with people, not on or to people. It improves the ability of individuals to take action, and the capacity of groups, organizations or communities to influence the determinants of healt,. improving the capacity of communities for health promotion requires practical education, leadership training and access to resources"(WHO, 1997).

通过社会支持、社区参与取得促进健康的作用的证据支持这些发展途径。因此，赞同社区发展作为一种根本的健康促进策略，它挑战不平等，目的在于促进参与。然而，社区发展不一定能针对根本原因。

（四）利用社区发展途径开展工作 Working with a community development approach

社区发展的方式可以不一样，但都含有三个基本要素：

1. 用户在先 User led

社区发展始于与社区人群共同确定发展的重点。即从社区人群的健康概念出发，比卫生工作者确定更有广泛的群众基础。Caulter发现工作的人认定社会、经济与环境因素，如失业、污染、居住与收入、对他们的健康的影响最重要。

社区发展工作的一个重要方面是使人们关于健康与疾病的知识正当合理，并给予发言权，不只是对医学的主要问题提出挑战。

2. 重点在于过程 Focus on Process

使社区有能力促进健康的过程被看作为是其自身权利的一项积极活动，社区发展需要更多地参与，这个过程将会增强自身的自信、自尊、感到能够控制自身的健康促进因素。这项活动是否具体针对某个健康问题并不重要，得到技能可以转化成不同的内容。

3. 重点放在易感与弱势人群的需要上 Focus on the needs of disadvantaged and vulnerable groups

社区发展的第三个特点是承认健康的不平等以及与弱势人群一起确定重点活动。取代重点放在个人的生活方式上，社区发展的重点放在健康的社会决定因素上。目的是针对影响他们健康的社会、经济与环境问题，增强人们一起行动的能力。这就意味着：

- *Working to promote the health of disadvantaged groups;*
- *Increasing the accessibility of services;*
- *Influencing the commissioning of services;*
- *Acting as an advocate and representing the interests of disadvantaged groups;*

- *Building a social profile of the community, high lighting the relationship to health status.*

社区发展途径面临着挑战。它提供了改善健康的前景，但是有许多实际困难需要克服，例如，时间花费、经费获得、责任与义务、可接受性以及专业人员的作用与评价等。

Smithies 等（1990）提出 5 种不同的社区健康行动：

- 正式参与决策机制；
- 社区行动；
- 促使社区增强能力的过程；
- 专业人员与社区人群面对面交流；
- 策略支持。

Community development does appear to address many of problems. However, it has been endorsed both at the international level, by various WHO declarations, and at the local level, by project workers.

四、帮助人们改变 Helping people to Change

人们的行为与生活方式被认为是许多现代疾病的原因。因此，健康促进的重点是改变已知对健康有影响的那些行为。除非认识到人们的行为会对自身生活环境起作用，否则这一途径不可能取得效果。

有几个理论，如健康信念模式（Becker, 1974），合理行动理论（Ajzen 等, 1980），阶段改变模式（Prochaska 等, 1984）等试图解释不同变量对个人健康行为的影响。

按照行为改变的社会心理学理论，人们的行为部分取决于自身的态度。个人对具体行动的态度（attitude）并打算采纳它是受到信念（beliefs）、动机（motivation），来自个人的价值（values）、态度（attitude）与驱动力（drives）或本能（instincts）的影响，以及社会准则（social norms）的影响。

（一）健康信念模式 The health belief model

这个模式（Rosenstock, 1966, Becker, 1974）是强调信念在决策中的功能，已用于预测保护性健康行为，如筛查对免疫注射的依从性。它认为不论人们是否改变其行为，都会受到评价其可行性与衡量成本效果的影响。换句话说，人们考虑改变其行为都要进行成本效益或利用的分析。这可以包括他们对于疼痛或创伤发生可能性（易感性）的相信程度；疾病或创伤的严重性；以及行动的效果，是否会有某些个人效益或怎样才能保护个人免受疾病或创伤的相信程度。

对于行为改变的发生，个人：

- 必须有改变的动机；
- 感到现时行为的威胁；
- 感到以某种方式改变会有好处，以及有些相反的结果；
- 必须感到有能力进行改变。

The model suggested that whether or not people change their behaviour will be influenced by an evaluation of its feasibility and its benefits weighed against its costs. In other words, people considering changing their behaviour engage in a cost-benefit or utility analysis.

For a behaviour change to take place, individuals:

- *Must have an incentive to change*

- *Feel threatened by their current behaviour*
- *Feel a change would be beneficial in some way and have few adverse consequences*
- *Must feel competent to carry out the change*

结果是指导人们行为的前提。如果是正面的或可能是正面的结果，那么个人很可能采纳这种行为。这种把行为看作为对结果的简单反应的解释并不能解释坚持有明显负面结果的行为，如吸烟或饮酒与驾车，短暂的满足可能比长期的伤害有更大的诱惑。

Becker认为个人是否能意识到自身对疾病、伤害或危险的易感性和严重程度会影响到他的行为。人们对危险的理解与评估是这个模式的中心。因此，人们的行为改变与否受到三个因素的影响：个人经历，控制能力以及对疾病危害性的认识。然而，在许多情况下，人们会有“这可能不会发生在我身上”的不现实的想法。

健康信念模式认为人们需要有某种提示以便采取行动改变行为或作出与健康有关的决定。这种提示内容需要变得引人注目或相关。提示可能是关注一个人的内部状况或外貌的改变。

The Health Belief Model suggested that people need to have some kind of cue to take action to change a behaviour or make a health-related decision. The issue needs to become salient or relevant. The cue could be noticing a change in one's internal state or appearance.

这一模式已受到广泛批评。有些批评是关于缺少不同因素的加权，试图用假设总体不大于各组成部分解释复杂行为，通过分析一套相互隔裂的概念成分而采取知情行动，并作出选择。没有考虑到相互交织，整合不同意见以及交流想法与媒体信息组合成的事由。

在预测行为或确定影响人们改变的因素方面，这一模式并没有特别帮助，但是它特别强调范围以及涉及因素的复杂性。

（二）合理行动理论与计划行为理论 Theory to the reasoned action and theory of planned behaviour

按照合理行动理论（Ajzen 等，1980），行为依据两个变量：

- 态度 attitude：相信行为的结果并做出改变的正反两个方面；
- 主观准则 subjective norms：一个人要顺从和如其他有影响的人那样所做，所指望以及达到的程度。

这两方面的影响组成为一种意向。

Ajzen等认为人们不一定与他们的意向有一致的行为表现。预测行为的能力受到一个人信念稳定性的影响，而稳定性由信念的强度决定。社会压力可以通过社会准则、社区准则、同事群体以及有影响的其他人的信念施加影响。健康促进中模仿的作用特别重要。表示关心，间接模仿行为可以来自媒体。WHO已确认为了健康，正式与非正式的社会网络支持个人与给人们以帮助的重要性。

Bandura（1977)的社会学习理论（social learning theory）提出作出健康选择的人与期望的结果（一种行动是否会导致一种特别的结果）；自我效力（人们是否相信他们能够改变）有关。自我效力的理解是依据人们对自己的评估——是否有知识和技能作出行为改变，是否外部因素，如时间与金钱，允许改变。

The Theory of Reasoned Action differ from the Health Belief Model in that it places importance on social norms as a major influence on behaviour.

The development of self-concept and self-esteem has been at the centre of work in health education and promotion. It is assumed that people with high self-esteem are likely to feel confident about themselves and have social and life skills which will enhance their feelings of personal efficacy. Because of these feelings of personal effectiveness, the person's self-esteem is enhanced.

Ajzen（1991）进一步发展了合理行动理论形成为有计划的行为理论。这一模式纳入了另一个变量——人们的行为是其认识到的控制的结果，人们想改变其生活的程度不一样。社会学习理论认为人们解释事情发生的方式是其童年经历的产物。

Control in the context of health can be understood in terms of:

Internal locus of control (the extent to which individuals believe that they are responsible for their own health).

External locus of control (people who believe that their actions are influenced by powerful others, chance, fate or luck).

（三）阶段改变模式 The stages of change model

人们行为的改变可能是一个长期而复杂的过程，而不是简单的快速决定的结果。

Prochaska等（1984，1986）提出行为获得的阶段模式，认为人们作出的任何改变都不是最终的，而是正在进行中的改变循环中的一部分。他们的工作集中在鼓励改变上瘾行为，虽然这一模式能够用于显示，当尝试改变或获得行为时，大多数人要经历许多阶段。这一过程包括下列阶段：

1. 预先打算 Precontemplation

预先打算的人不考虑改变他们的生活方式或没有意识到其行为有任何潜在危险，只有当他们认识到这一问题时，才可能发展到下一阶段。

2. 打算 Contemplation

虽然人们认识到改变的益处，但尚未准备好，可能在寻找信息或帮助，以作做出决定。

3. 准备改变 Preparing to change

当认识到效益超过成本，当改变看来可能而且值得去做时，个人可能准备去改变，寻找某些额外的支持。

4. 作出改变 Making the change

早期改变需要个人积极的决定以便进行不同的事情。明确的目标、现实的计划、支持与鼓励是这个阶段的特点。

5. 保持 Maintenance

新的行为持续不变，人们转向一种健康的生活方式。

The stages of change model differs from the other models of behaviour change, because it is principally about how people change and not why people do not change.

（四）改变的前提条件 The prerequisites of change

从人们改变其健康行为的证据提出，产生行为改变需要一定的最低条件：

1. 改变必须是从我开始 The change must be self-initiated；

2. 行为必须是明显的 The behaviour must become salient；

3. 行为显著性必须持续一段时间 The salience of the behoviour must appear over a period of

time；

4. 行为不是个人应对策略的一部分 The behaviour is not part of the individual's coping strategies；

5. 个人生活不能有问题或不确定 The individual's life should not be problematic or uncertain；

6. 有可以利用的社会支持 Social support is available。

用于健康促进中的社会心理学已受到批评，认为行为不是健康最重要的决定因素。然而，行为改变仍然是许多健康促进途径的一个特点。它必须伴随着项目进行，试图提供环境条件，使健康的选择易于变为现实。

The role of health education and promotion is neatly summarized by whitehead & Tones:

One level involves primarily influencing beliefs (assuming that attempts to directly "plug into" motivation by creating fear or otherwise generate emotional responses are of dubious value both ethically and in terms of effectiveness).

The other level is concerned with providing the understanding and skills needed to translate intention into practice. Health education is also concerned to foster healthy public policy in order to encourage the development of a health-promoting environment that both will facilitate intentions to make healthy choices and will signal the unacceptability of unhealthy practices.

健康教育也是为了鼓励健康的公众政策以便鼓励发展促进健康的环境。

行为改变的心理学概貌是清楚的，没有一个能提供一个全面的解释。然而，这些模式确定的变量呈现在人们健康行为的说明之中：

- 意识到危险性与易感性；
- 意识到疾病的严重性；
- 意识到到有助于良好健康的行为效果；
- 意识到自身作出改变的可能性；
- 意识到有影响的人如何评价行为。

Whilst these models may not help to predict who will adopt preventive health practice, they can help to plan programmes of education by making clear those factors which influence decisions.

五、媒体在健康促进中的作用 Using the mass media in health promotion

媒体是进行交流，达到大多数人的有效传播者，80%以上的人把媒体看作为最重要的信息来源。它也是说服我们购买大量产品，造成不健康生活方式的手段。媒体被用于健康促进有长期的历史。

（一）媒体影响的性质 The nature of media effects

关于媒体影响的观点，已从早期相信媒体可以产生态度与行为方面的巨大变化转化到相反的观点，那就是媒体也有负面影响。Gatherer等（1979）对49种媒体活动的评价研究认为媒体对个人的影响并不很大。目前，另一种观点认为在一定的环境条件和具体方式之下媒体是有影响力的。Tones（1994）得到结论，在健康教育中，媒体活动能达到一种很有用的目的，但也有内在的限度。媒体如何影响公众有 4 种主要模式：

1. 直接影响 Direct effects

这一模式把媒体比作为一种皮下注射，对公众能有一种立竿见影的效果。它假设一个被动的公众能通过媒体的控制而动摇。这一观点促进了发展政治广播打算转变选举的意向。这一观点被看作为一种喷雾式的大众交流。

2. 二步模式 Two-step model

这一模式认为大众交流影响权威人物，权威人物是媒体公众的积极成员。权威人物通过人际交流手段，把想法传播给其他人。这一模式提出媒体在增强意识与交流基本信息方面是重要的，但人力资源，如朋友或有名"专家"，在说服人们作出改变方面是最有影响力的

3. 使用与满足 Uses and gratifications

这一模式认为公众在选择与解释信息方面是更积极的。它认为人们利用媒体满足自身需要——强化现有的信念，或反对，或当不符合他们现有的价值与信念出现时，重新解释信息。

4. 文化影响 Cultural effects

这一模式认为媒体在创立关于健康、医药、疾病、患病的信念与价值方面起关键作用。信息交流是把消息从发送者传递到接收者。媒体是一种间接的文化交流，为不同的解释或者阅读同样的内容留有余地。

消息在特殊编码中编成为有含义的符号与标识。消息通过发送者编码再通过接收者解码。意图是应该解码信息，并按照发送者的意图理解，但是信息有充分的机会以不同的方式进行解码。

（二）媒体的作用 The role of mass media

大众交流已用于健康促进，其作用在于通过提供信息、提醒人们不健康行为的影响以及采纳健康行为、生活方式的益处来增强公众意识；通过突出一个问题，并确保经过考虑，创造一种评价气氛有助于政策改变；通过揭示损害健康的行为，强调其对疾病的影响，以及改变行为的好处，敦促人们转变态度并促进人们行为的改变。

通常，媒体采用两种主要的方式：

1. 计划广泛的活动 Planned campaigns and advertising

优点是快速到达社会各阶层的大多数人与各个人群，能够发送有针对性的信息，以适合具体的目标。

2. 不收报酬的公开宣传与媒体倡导 Unpaid publicity and media advocacy

优点是成本低，可信度较大，因为信息并不被看作是卫生组织直接促进的。

（三）社会营销 Social marketing

正如商业公司让人们购买产品一样（即使那些人实际上可能并不需要），健康促进者应能让人们选择健康的行为。现在许多营销技术已广泛用于健康促进以便影响人们对健康生活方式的接受能力。这样，使健康的生活方式看来是值得向往和易于采纳的。

媒体活动的限制之一是它们是一种单向交流过程，往往是采纳一种统一的大众信息。健康促进者正逐渐增加利用社会营销技术，以便针对特殊人群。营销按人们的态度、行为还有粗略的社会经济与人口统计学资料把人群分成不同的群体。

商业营销是依据"交换"的理念——营销员试图满足消费者的要求，以可接受的价格提供商品，而健康促进者也开始认识到影响研究的重要性，那就是仔细确定人们所能看得到的特殊健康行为的效益，并把这些结合到活动信息中去。在某种意义上，这只是应用健康信念模式，建议人们做出健康行为的改变，需要让他们看到效益超过成本，如时间与努力。

营销一种商品与销售健康很不一样。广告典型地鼓励现时的倾向，而健康促进典型地尝试与其相反。广告是与人们向往某些产品有联系，而健康促进信息是不纵容，通过暗示，没有乐趣。广告是现时销售东西，即刻消费与享受。相比之下，健康促进信息经常是未来效益超过现时享受。

（四）媒体在健康促进中的作用 what the mass media can and cannot do

在健康促进中媒体能够做到：

- 增强健康问题的意识，如戒烟；
- 帮助把健康放到公众的议事日程之中，如反复强调；
- 传达简单信息与单一信息，如婴儿放在背上睡觉；
- 如果存在其他能促使改变的因素，则改变行为，如鼓励已承诺的不吸烟者放弃吸烟。

媒体做不到：

- 传达复杂信息，如膳食中不同脂肪的相对危险性；
- 传授技能；
- 转变人们的态度或信念，如果提出的消息是对基本信念的挑战，消息更可能被疏忽，不理解或解释为其他意义；
- 在缺少其他促成因素时，改变行为。

2005年，曼谷宪章提出了更完善的便于全球化的健康促进策略。为了向着更加健康的世界迈进，需要强有力的政治行动、广泛的参与以及不断的倡导。健康促进已经建立了一套完整的已经证实有效的并且需要充分利用的策略。为了取得更大的发展，所有的部门与机构都必须采取行动：

提倡以人权与团结一致为基础的健康；

投资于可行的政策、行动与基本设施以便致力于应对健康的决定因素；

增强政策发展、领导、健康促进实践、知识转化与研究以及健康识别能力；

遵守规章与法律，确保高水平防护免受伤害；

使所有的人都能同等享有健康与幸福的机会；

与公共、私人、非政府组织以及民间团体建立伙伴关系与联盟，以便采取可行的行动。

Strategies for health promotion in a globalized world progress towards a healthier world require strong political action, broad participation and sustained advocacy. Health promotion has an established repertoire of proven effective strategies which need to be fully utilized. To make further advances all sectors and settings must act to:

Advocate for health based on human rights and solidarity;

Invest in sustainable policies, actions and infrastructure to address the determinants of health;

Build capacity for policy development, leadership, health promotion practice, knowledge transfer and research, and health literacy;

Regulate and legislate to ensure a high level of protection from harm and enable equal opportunity for health and well being for all people;

Partner and build alliances with public, private, nongovernment organizations and civil society to create sustainable actions.

The mass media are significant partners for health, but ones that need to be understood and used according to their own priorities. To expect a mass media campaign to produce large shifts in behaviour and contribute directly to reduce mobility and mortality is unrealistic. But the media can work for health by supporting individual and social change.

On an individual level, the mass media can supplement, but not substitute for, one to one education and advice. Eum with sophisticated marketing and audience research, the mass media remain a fairly blunt instrument with little opportunity for feedback or clarification. However, the media can rise awareness, provide information and motivate people to change if their environment is supportive. The media can also be used to advocate for the public health by shifting public opinion and encouraging the formation of healthy public policies.

第三节　口腔健康教育
Section 3 Oral Health Education

一、口腔健康教育的重要性 Oral health education is still important

从第二次全国口腔健康流行病学调查的结果看，44.4%的人至少每天刷牙两次，这意味着还有50%以上的人不经常刷牙或不刷牙；只有17%的人应用含氟牙膏刷牙，大部分人特别是儿童，没有用含氟牙膏刷牙；有近一半的人（47.2%）没有接受过任何口腔卫生保健指导。近三分之一（29%）的12岁儿童，三分之一以上（40.5%）的18岁青少年只有在龋齿出现症状或疼痛时才去就诊，城市人口比农村人口更为经常有定期口腔保健习惯。有些省份由于开展了口腔健康项目，龋齿出现了下降趋势，而其他很少开展活动的省份则出现了上升趋势。从口腔健康情况看，5岁儿童患龋率很高，达到76.6%，龋均为4.5，12岁及18岁儿童龋患率及龋均虽然很低（45.81%与1.03，和55.32%与1.6），但是治疗率很低（7.11%与17.52%），并且牙龈炎与牙石在所有年龄组都很常见。这些资料提供的信息说明，无论在知识、态度还是在行为习惯方面，口腔健康教育与促进仍然很重要。

二、口腔健康教育的定义与基本概念 Definition and basic concepts of oral health education

口腔健康教育是一个告知、动员与帮助人们采纳与保持保健实践与生活方式的过程，倡导所需要的环境改变以便推动这一目标的实现，指导专业人员培训与研究也是为了这个目标。健康教育是利用任何设计的学习机会，促进自愿采纳有益于健康的行为。

Oral health education is a process that informs, motivates and helps persons to adopt and maintain health practices and lifestyles; advocates environmental changes as needed to facilitate this goal; and conducts professional training and research to the same end. Health education is any combination of learning opportunities designed to facilitate voluntary adaptations of behaviour that are conducive to health.

1984年WHO提出：健康教育的目的在于达到与健康目标有关而开展的任何教育活动。这种活动能够直接针对个人、群体甚至全体人口。主要涉及三个学习领域：

- 知识，cognitive：了解实际知识，如吃甜点与产生龋齿有关联的知识；
- 信念，affective：与健康有关的情绪、感觉与信念，如相信乳牙不重要；
- 行为，behavioural：技能发展，如用牙线洁牙所需要掌握的技能。

在多数情况下，对大多数人来说，知识、态度与行为彼此的关系是复杂、能动而又针对个人的。换句话说，人类在其思想、感觉与行动方面并不是完全理性的。例如，大多数吸烟者完全认识到吸烟是肺癌的主要危险因素，然而，这种知识并没有使其停止吸烟。当知识与行为发生矛盾时，就会出现认知的不一致，许多吸烟者相信这种习惯不好，在社会上会令人讨厌，但这样的态度也并未能使其停止吸烟。知识，态度与行为之间的这种复杂而能动的关系，就是健康教育所包含的三个主要方面。

Definition of health education

Health education is defined as any educational activity which aims to achieve a health-related goal (WHO, 1984). Activity can be directed at individuals, groups, or even populations. There are three main domains of leading:

Cognitive: understanding factual knowledge, for example, knowledge that eating sugary snacks is linked to the development of dental decay.

Affective: emotions, feelings, and beliefs associated with health, for example, belief that baby teeth are not important.

Behavioural: skills development for example, skills required to effectively floss teeth.

With a complex and dynamic relationship existing between knowledge, attitudes and behaviour, it is essential that all three elements are appropriately covered in health education.

健康教育项目不能与事件分开，但它是任何治疗、预防或促进健康活动的一个方面。口腔疾病多因素变量的综合及其相互作用现在已经日益强调教育过程将有助于达到期望的健康结果。

在口腔医学以及其他卫生领域都已有很好的资料证明仅有正确的健康信息或知识并不一定能导致期望的健康行为。然而，获得知识可以起到一个工具的作用，增强人们获取准确的健康信息、卫生保健技术的能力使他们能够采取保护其健康的行动。内外变量都影响着一个人或者一个社区依从所推荐的疾病预防、健康保持或者健康促进措施，健康促进是任何结合教育、组织、经济、政治与环境支持有益于健康的行为。健康促进提出采取行动，打算改变个人的生活环境以促进健康（如社区饮水氟化）或使个人增强能力，采取预防措施的好处，或者减少或排除进入服务的障碍。

健康教育的方法与内容由医学与公共卫生领域，还有自然、生物、社会与环境科学衍变而来。在这一领域产生的概念与理论影响到健康教育者的努力与实践。在口腔健康教育领域内，那些已经为行为学家证实的许多理论常被忽略、遗忘或不能接受。口腔健康教育的目标是预防和控制口腔疾病，目的为达到这一目标的有组织的努力，应该遵循已被证明的健康教育活动的理论与相关概念。研究已经证实有效的现代健康教育理论，经过评论能够结合到未来的健康教育努力之中。

研究已经表明在许多口腔健康教育活动中，一个根本错误是假设增加人们的知识将有助于改变口腔保健行为。这一途径，依据唯一的认知模式，假设以下的顺序：

知识→态度→行为改变

如果这一关系是真实的，那么每个人提高了口腔知识水平就能导致行为改变，经过一个长时间，改善其口腔健康状况。然而，直至今天，没有一个口腔健康教育项目产生了这样的结果。

一个人的行为是内外力量作用的结果，信念、态度、兴趣、价值、需要、动机、个性、期望、理解与生物学因素、以及家庭、同事的影响、宏观经济因素如职业、教育、媒体都塑造和影响着行动。社会人口学因素，如年龄、种族或文化、性别、职业、教育与收入也对口腔健康教育实践有重要影响。当设计和实施健康教育策略时应予以考虑。这些力量的相互作用在Kressin发展的模式中已作出说明。

Kressin's model (2001)

Factors influencing the eental education process aspects of the learner (s) to consider when designing dental health education programmes:

- *Sociodemographic factors (e.g. age, sex, race/culture, income);*
- *Values, attitudes, beliefs；*
- *Readiness to change behaviours；*
- *Education.*

Aspects of the social environment to consider when designing dental health education programmes:

- *Cultural norms (e.g., how much of the population smokes, how many people floss their teeth);*
- *Cultural values/expectations (e.g., expectation that children's teeth will have brown spots/caries);*
- *How supportive the environment is for behavioural change；*
- *Possible ways in which education/information can be offered.*

很显然，教育者的努力与学习者的行为之间的直线关系通常是不存在的。为了发展一个有效的口腔健康教育项目，教育者必须认识到所有这些力量对学习者相互作用，教育者必须首先评估学习者，开发与实施一个合理的教育项目才可能导致一种持续的行为改变。由于公众的安全与保护意识增强，逐渐增加了对健康信息所持有的怀疑态度，因此非常重要的是提供给公众的健康教育信息必须是一致的，并且在科学上是正确的，证据是充分的。

三、计划口腔健康教育项目 Planning oral health education programmes

口腔健康教育项目的关键作用是养成或改变与健康以及口腔健康有关的行为习惯。个人与社会的健康与口腔健康受到社会环境的影响。个人生活方式也对健康起到重要作用。生活方式包含各种行为方式，它受价值观念、传统观念、交流与相互作用的典型方式以及语言、文化、经济、地理、年龄、性别、种族、个性、时间等影响。因此，一个好的口腔健康教育项目将依据人类生态学知识，考虑生物学与环境因素（自然与社会）之间的相互作用影响协调发展。这样的项目应灵活地适合于在不同背景之下不同人的不同需要。计划是一个工具，它以一定的技巧、资源和支持把希望达到的情况变得比较好。使用标准作为目标，指导实践。计划也是解决问题的过程。

计划口腔健康教育项目是从提供者到接受者口腔健康问题解决的过程，提供者从事传播活动，接受者做出反应。

Planning is a tool that, with a given amount of skill, resources, and support, can transform an undesirable state into a better one, using the norms as a target to guide the effort. Planning also is a process of problem solving.

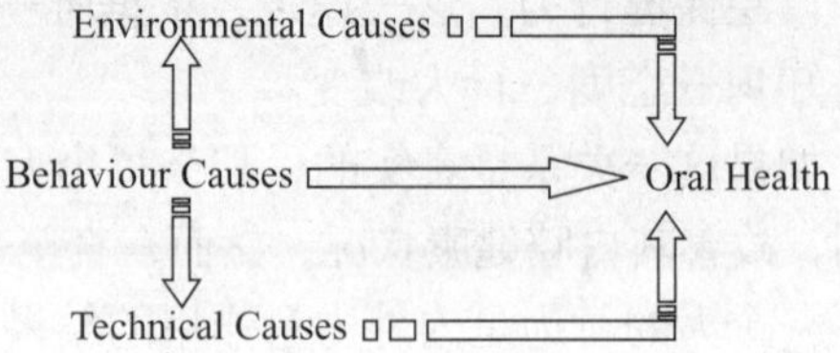

图 11-2 Three ways behaviour can influence oral health

Planning oral health education programme is a process of oral health problem solving from provider to receiver. The provider engages in diffusion activities and the receiver in adoption reactions. These relationship could be shown in Figure (图 11-2) .

口腔健康教育导致行为改变的过程有以下六个基本步骤：

1. 确定并具体规定与口腔健康有关的问题

我们没能看到问题的解决，只是因为我们没能看到问题所在。确定问题的性质是基础，我们至少可从五个方面发现问题：

（1）调查与口腔健康有关的社会问题，如个人收入、文化教育率与教育水平、安全用水、食物供应、家庭大小、社会性服务等。

（2）从流行病学调查、文献、医院病案、文件、年度报告如发病率和患病率、有关口腔健康问题的分布、问题的描述、确定范围等方面发现口腔健康的问题。

（3）确定与口腔健康有关的文化、行为方面的问题：

- 目标人群的人口普查资料；
- 关于一定的自我保健措施与疾病症状的知识、态度与实践；
- 有关个人使用牙科服务的知识、态度与实践；
- 现时口腔健康水平造成的影响。

（4）确定口腔健康教育的问题。

（5）确定有关口腔健康的管理问题。

在一个社区或一定的目标人群中发现和分析上述问题是口腔健康教育计划中必要的一步，在有限的健康教育资源下，确定哪一个口腔健康问题应成为重点，在什么基础之上，以及通过什么过程进行健康教育等。

2. 制定可以达到并可以测量的目标

在确定问题形成重点需要之后，对于已经发生的情况有了一个清楚的印象。通过口腔健康教育与促进项目，制定目标，改变这种状况就成为下一个必要的步骤。口腔健康教育项目总是针对我们要求改变什么，我们最终的工作目标是通过共同努力来达到。口腔健康教育应该有它自己可以达到的目标。在短期内，总目标不容易达到，而具体目标则比较实际，可以达到。

从一个目标到另一个目标，通过一步一步的进展，与一步达到最终目标相比是较为缓慢的，但常可能取得满意的结果。

一般来说，口腔健康教育可以分为 6 个目标：

（1）发展概念

（2）发展技能

(3) 获得信息

(4) 认识价值

(5) 交流

(6) 发展解决问题或决定问题的策略

其中每一个目标都是独立的，不同的目标需要不同的课程结构，针对不同的听众做不同的事情。这样，不同的目标需要不同的策略。

3. 确定口腔健康教育的策略

在口腔健康教育中可以使用下列 6 种策略

(1) 获得信息的策略——得到有关口腔健康的信息　主要强调通过口腔健康教育从口腔健康教育提供者那里得到一些信息，例如，口腔与牙齿结构及其功能，影响个人与社区口腔健康的因素，口腔疾病，特别是龋齿与牙周病的特点，口腔疾病预防的科学基础等。

(2) 发展概念的策略——发展有关口腔健康的概念　主要强调帮助接受者发展他们对口腔健康概念或普遍原理的理解，如涉及牙与牙龈，牙菌斑细菌，饮食与时间的相互关系。

(3) 发展技能的策略——发展有关口腔健康的技巧　主要强调掌握技巧。

(4) 认识价值的策略——发展有关口腔健康的认识价值　主要是帮助接受者认识所阐述的问题的价值以及发展他们自身阐明这些价值的能力等。

(5) 发展质询的策略——发展有关口腔健康问题的质询策略　主要强调发展接受者质询问题解决策略的各种技能以及作为问题解决者的积极自我概念，例如提出诸如“为什么近 30 年内工业化国家龋齿发病率激剧下降，而发展中国家则情况相反？”等问题。

(6) 开展结尾性讨论的策略——发表与口腔健康有关的想法与意见　主要强调发展接受者表达与讨论问题有关的想法和意见的能力。

这6种策略为一个整体可以分成2组。第一组集中学习基本知识，提供信息，概念与技能。第二组发展个人意图，提供内在的表达信息，概念与技能的思维方式。使接受者能用于讨论口腔健康的问题，解决口腔健康的问题并作出有关口腔健康的决定。

在选择口腔健康教育的适当策略中应遵循三个步骤：

(1) 确定目标　因为一种策略的基本目的是促进接受者达到具体的目标。在目标确定之后，将选择最适当的策略。在任何情况下，信息是清楚的——学习什么。

(2) 选择适当的策略　在决定学习什么之后，下一步是使用什么样的策略方法来推动学习。

(3) 建设策略　决定接受者的适当活动，确定教学技术，教学行为以及需要的详细资料，提供者与学习者一起通过做来学习。

4. 健康与口腔健康教育方法学

一般来说，有七种方法可以用于健康与口腔健康教育：

(1) 媒体活动

目标人群：普通群众，专门小组，如孕妇，青年人等。

题目：任何健康与口腔健康问题。

方法：提供一般性信息。

目的：改变行为（较小程度的行为与态度的改变）。

(2) 社区方法

目标人群：从少数人到一个村或几个村。

题目：社区的健康与口腔健康问题。

方法：提供本社区的具体信息与推荐意见。

目的：促进社区参加口腔卫生保健活动。

活动内容：每次项目的活动类似，每件事都要有社区参与-每个村或地区建立委员会，确定当地领导（经过培训），在每个阶段的计划与实施活动中与卫生官员或卫生工作者合作。社区也参与其他健康问题。这些案例主要来自发展中国家，如印度，斯里兰卡，菲律宾，泰国，中国等。

(3) 健康教育辅助法

目标人群：普通群众，不同年龄组或特殊人群或高危人群。

题目：具体的口腔健康问题。

方法：提供具体信息，包括知识，技能与态度。

目的：促使人们采取积极行动，改变某些有害行为习惯。

活动内容：内容：手册，折页，视听材料等。

(4) 成人小组讨论

目标人群：特殊或高危人群。

题目：具体的口腔健康问题，如吸烟与口腔癌，营养与口腔健康等。

方法：提供具体信息，知识，技能与方法。

目的：说服人们改变其行为习惯。

(5) 儿童小组讨论

目标人群：学校儿童。

题目：牙健康，吸烟，药物。

方法：提供知识，技能与方法。

目的：形成与修正儿童的行为与习惯。

(6) 个别交流

目标人群：病人，特殊个人，或残疾人。

题目，预防技术。

方法：通过个人交谈与示范提供知识，技能。

目的：说服个人采取具体行动，通过口腔专业人员增进或保持口腔健康状态。

(7) 规章制度

目标人群：普通群众，制造商或销售员。

题目：牙健康，吸烟，嚼烟，滥用药物，饮酒。

方法：提供信息与劝阻。

目的：说服人们改变有害行为习惯。

5. 实施与监督口腔健康教育

为影响人们与社区，获得最大多数的参加和社区参与，使其能制定出自身的口腔卫生保健目标。在这种情况下，口腔健康教育提供者必须：

（1）提供每个人学习机会，学会如何确定和分析口腔健康及其相关问题，如何设定自身的目标，例如，目标人群中至少有95%的人应该参与口腔健康教育项目，特别关注那些龋齿与牙龈炎的高危人群。应用从目标人群中得到的新资料显示他们中间存在的问题，分析其与生活方式，环境状况有关的机制，并依据其社会文化，价值，个人与社会资源，可能采取的解决办法。

（2）使口腔健康信息容易达到每个人和社区，如利用当地广播站，参与社区会议或活动。这可以为健康与口腔健康教育提供时间与空间。同时，提供者可以容易接近了解群众，从群众与社区那里学习一些东西，并从他们那里得到反馈信息。

（3）向人们表明某些可供选择的解决办法。这些办法适合于那些已经经过提供者与接受者/社区，共同努力确定的口腔健康及其有关问题。

（4）提高对提供者与接受者之间进行有效交流重要性的认识，双向交流比单向交流效果更好。

（5）把目标变成简单，可以理解，实现和可以接受的口号或海报，使社区能监督，例如，为改善牙周健康状况，要求每人每天刷牙2次，可以制作简单记录卡，发给每个人，每次刷牙后作记录，然后社区卫生工作者定期搜集分析比较。

（6）当几个口腔健康问题同时存在时，帮助人们学会如何确定重点，例如，当人们同时有急诊需要，治疗需要和预防需要时，通常只考虑去看急诊，总是忽略了每天的自我保健，这时提供者应给予一些指导和帮助。

（7）为各种年龄组或特殊人群，特别是高危人群准备手册或讲稿。

（8）模拟或示范个人与家庭保健的预防技术。

（9）建立个人与社区参与监督过程的标准与方法。

（10）在口腔健康教育项目与发送社区口腔健康中监督口腔健康教育内容取得的进展。

（11）在口腔卫生保健项目中建立与其他单位的合作。

（12）口腔健康教育项目几乎总是社区卫生发展项目的一部分。

（13）随访与复查。

6. 最后分析与评价，并报告和重新制定计划

There are six fundamental steps in the process of oral health education leading to behaviour change as follows:

(1) Identifying and specifically defining the problems related to oral health. we can not see the solution, just because we can not see the problem. Determining the nature of the problem is essential. We can find out the problems in five arrears at least:

①Identify social problems related to oral health, such as personal income, literacy rate and level of education. Safe water supply, food supply, size of family, social services, etc.

②Identify oral health problems from epidemiological survey, literature, hospital medical (dental) records, documents, annual reports, etc.

③ Identify cultural, behavioural problems related to oral health,

demographic data of target population

knowledge, attitudes and practices about certain self-care procedures and disease symptoms

knowledge, attitudes and practices concerning the use of personal dental services

impact of current oral health levels

④ Identify oral health education problems

⑤ Identify administrative problems related to oral health

(2) Setting achievable and measurable goals and objectives

In general, six goals could be classified in oral health education, these are:

① Concept development

② Skill development

③ Information acquisition

④ Values awareness

⑤ Communication

⑥ The development of problem solving and/or decision-making strategies

Each of them is unique, and different goals require a different structure for the respective lessons, and doing different things with different receivers. Thus, different goals require different strategies.

(3)Strategies defined for oral health education six strategies could be used in oral health education as follows:

① Information acquisition strategy is to acquire information about oral health

② Concept development strategy is to develop concept about oral health

③ Skill development strategy is to develop skills about oral health

④ Values awareness strategy is to develop awareness of values relative to oral health

⑤Inquiry development strategy is to express ideas and discuss opinions and ideas relative to oral health

⑥ Open-ended discussion strategy is to express ideas and discuss opinions and ideas relative to oral health

(4) Methodology in health and oral health education

In generally, seven methods usually be used in health and oral health education:

① Mass media campaigns

② Community methods

③ Health education aids

④ Group methods for adults

⑤ Group methods for children

⑥ Individual counseling

⑦ Legislation

(5) Implementation and monitoring of oral health education

To get maximum individual participation and community involvement, in order to influence people and community, and to enable them to formulate their own oral health care objectives. In this case, the oral health education providers will have to:

① Provide opportunities for everyone to learn how to identify and analyze oral health and its related problems, and how to set up their own targets

② Making oral health information easily accessible to the people and the community

③ Indicate to the people some alternative solutions for suiting the oral health and its related problems which have been identified by jointed efforts both from providers and receivers/communities

④Create awareness of the importance of effective communication between receivers and providers

⑤Translate the targets into simple, understandable, realistic and acceptable slogans or posters which the communities can then monitor

⑥Help people to learn how to set up priority among several oral health problems existed, based on their economic ability and availability of oral health services

⑦Prepare manuals or contents of lecture for various age groups and special groups, especially for high risk groups

⑧ Model or demonstrate preventive techniques for self-care and family care

⑨Set up criteria and methods for individual and community involvement in the monitoring process

⑩ Monitor the progress of oral health education components in oral health programme and improvement of the community health

(11) Set up intersectoral collaboration in oral health care programme with other institutions and agencies

(12)Oral health education programme as a part almost always joins to community health development project

(13) Follow up and reexamination

(6) Final analysis and evaluation, reporting and replanning

四、评价口腔健康教育 Evaluation of oral health education

评价是口腔健康教育的一部分，是证明信息已得到有效传送、接受和理解，并已采取了某些行动，结果是肯定的、成功的。

评价基本上是一个主观过程，凭借采用不同措施的结果达到价值判断。评价是为了估价：

（1）口腔健康需要（个人，人群，社区）

（2）口腔健康知识、态度与行为的改变

（3）口腔健康教育项目的优点和缺点

（4）口腔健康具体目标达到的程度

1. 评价的内容 What to evaluate（contents or components)

（1）价值Values　评价有关口腔健康、口腔健康教育以及口腔健康项目在一个人一生之中的价值，如生产力、社会、身体与精神方面的以及发展有效的口腔健康教育项目方面。

（2）总目标和具体目标Goals and objectives　明确陈述的、准确的、可测量的、可达到的、实际或可行的、与其他目标和观点一致的目标，包括口腔卫生实践与认知技能的范围，依据具体内容和学员所学到的具体行为。

（3）策略与方法 Strategies and methods：所陈述的与总目标和具体目标的一致性，知识、态度与行为改变所起的作用，成本——效果，可利用，可达到，可接受的程度，利用与可行性，以及一整化与结合程度。

(4) 内容（有意义的，现实的，科学的）Contents（meaningful, realistic, and scientific）：直至今日最新的、有效的、与口腔健康及口腔健康教育的观点保持一致的、依据学员的口腔健康需要与兴趣、与学员成熟的水平保持一致的一个口腔健康领域的内容以及与其他领域有关的内容。

(5) 学习机会 Learning opportunities　确定帮助学员达到目标的程度，提供学员应用或实践目标里规定的行为的机会，适合于学员成熟的水平，激发或奖励，鼓励多方面提高认识，允许与有关的经验形成一个整体，允许学员有个人差异及能力大小的不同。

(6) 其他方面 Others 环境（自然的，情感的）：评价过程本身（仪器与技术）。

2. 评价谁（人员 / 对象）Whom to evaluate（persons)?

需要直接或间接评价与口腔健康教育项目有关的任何人，如学员（不同年龄组的人），提供者 / 教师，管理人员，以及作为一个整体的社区。

(1) 学员 / 接受者 Learners/receivers

学员的口腔健康状况（项目开始前后），口腔健康需要（个人、群体与社区），口腔健康兴趣，价值，态度，行为与实践还有自我保健的认知技能。

(2) 教员 / 提供者 Teachers/providers

口腔健康教育技术/方法的效果，教员与学员和其他人员的关系，教员自身自我评价（教学行为，知识，应用的技术，个人之间的关系）由指导人员作评价，以及学员已经达到具体目标的程度。

(3) 管理人员 Administrators

口腔健康教育政策，程序以及口腔健康教育项目与口腔卫生项目管理。

(4) 社区人群 People in the community

社区人群的口腔健康需要与兴趣，社区参与的程度，社区口腔卫生服务的利用，环境状况的改善（水，食品，口腔保健品的供应等），以及口腔卫生资源的利用状况（人力，钱，时间，措施等）。

3. 评价的时间 When to evaluate（time)

评价应该在：

①口腔健康教育之前（Before oral health education）　个人与社区的口腔健康需要与兴趣，以及口腔健康状况；

②教育期间（During oral health education）　目标取得的进展，教学策略与方法，项目内容，学习机会及其他以及获取反馈信息作适当调整；

③教育之后（After oral health education）　达到提出的目标的程度，重新发展和改进现在的口腔健康教育项目。

4. 如何评价（方法 / 技术）How to evaluate（methods or techniques)

可以应用 5 种评价技术：

①书面测试 Paper tests　这是最普通的确定学员学到了什么的方法。这种方法用来评估知识最容易，但价值有限。

②自我评价 Self assessment　一般性估计（认识，自我兴趣，态度，信念与行动），具体估计（进餐次数，糖消耗量，餐间甜食，饮料，刷牙，牙线洁牙，氟水漱口，专业保健等），

结果评价（满意不满意）包括营养，糖与含糖食品消耗，口腔卫生实践，氟化物使用，以及行为习惯改变。

③个别交谈 Interviews 在口腔健康教育项目开始前后由教员与学员个别交谈是评估口腔健康知识，态度与实践改进的必要步骤之一。

一种简单的核查表会有帮助

肯定 否定 不一定

认识

自我兴趣

态度

信念

许诺

行动

④临床技术 Clinical technique 观察（由教员或学员）与简单记录，由专业人员作口腔检查，填写记录表，做出个人结论（需要重新教育，加强自我保健，专业保健，随诊）。

⑤统计技术 Statistic technique 收集目标人群资料，分组分类，制表分析，并对目标人群作出总结报告。

⑥最后结论 Conclusion

五、评价口腔健康教育方法 Methodologies used in evaluating oral health education

1. 媒体活动法 Mass media campaign

评价：通常依据项目前后对一般群众进行的横断面调查的发现：在发达国家知识的增加不超过6%，在发展中国家增加的幅度相对要大得多。态度与行为方面的改变——长期的行为改变不超过10%。许多媒体活动报告行为没有改变。

优点：对生活有影响力，但并不很大，尤其对个人。

缺点：信息不能直接指导那些感兴趣或需要的人，各种媒体效果的比较：事实上，传播信息最有效的方法完全不是通过媒体方式，而是通过口头讲述或个人接触，电台或广播车还有海报在文化程度较低的国家 / 地区非常有用。在文化水平较高的国家 / 地区。虽然电台广播也有效，但印刷材料效果排在前列。影片与电视节目，没有明显的结论。

Comparison of the effectiveness of various media.

The most effective method of spreading information infect appears to be not through the media at all, but by word of mouth and personal contact. Radio and louder-speak trucks are most useful in countries where the literacy is low, as also are posters. In a literate country, the printed word ranks high, though radio is also effective.

Films and TV-no definite conclusion.

2. 社区教育方法 Community methods

研究结果主要来自印度，斯里兰卡，主要印象并不惊人，不过有些地方作用很大。

3. 健康教育辅助资料法 Health education aids

包括各种小册子，视听仪器及其他资料。书面资料并不十分有效。两页纸的宣传品比什么也不给对增加病人的知识方面没有明显好处，打算引发某些特殊行为的传单或信件能起一定的作用。为推动儿童口腔保健给家长的信件有些作用。然而，想通过这些改变人们已经养成的习惯非常困难，看来信件与手册不是解决这类问题的好办法。影片与录像带可能对增加人们的知识和促使改变态度方面比小册子的影响要大。在候诊室内使用录音信息没有效果，因为病人不听，但在某些情况下，有些效果。

Including booklets, pamphlets, audiovisual aids and other materials, written materials are not very effective. Two page information handout was not significantly better than nothing at all in improving patient's knowledge. Leaflets and letters intended to elicit some particular behaviour can work. Letters to parents urging dental care for their children has some effect. However, it is far more difficult to get people to change well-established habits, and letters and pamphlets do not seem to be an effective method of doing so.

Films or video tapes probably have more impact than pamphlets in improving knowledge and changing attitudes.

Tape-recorded messages is ineffective in a doctor's waiting room, because they were not listened to, but in some cases, it could have some effectiveness.

4. 成人组教育方法 Group methods for adult

对小组教育方法的评价研究已经发表了许多不同的文章。直接给成人讲课，很少或者没有人积极参加。但在某些情况下，如课程内容包括营养指导与示范在改变饮食习惯方面是有效果的。还有指导刷牙减少牙菌斑是有效果的，虽然其他因素可能对这个结果也有作用。讨论可以帮助提高效果。健康教育研讨会能改进预约看病和自我保健。小组的作用：特别是很小的组，可以建立友谊关系，这可以影响到结果。但是小组压力并不总是有效的。

其他研究发现，各种形式的小组活动在知识与态度的改变方面没有明显的差异。包括有实践的小组方法，但没有讨论——有一项研究发现受训人员使用牙线的能力有明显提高，但其他方面效果不佳。

Evaluation studies of group methods have been published for many different subjects. Straight forward lectures to adults with little or no active participation. But in some cases, such as a course which included nutrition advice and demonstrations was effective in changing dietary habits, and instruction on tooth-brushing reduced plaque though other factors may have contributed to this results. Many groups including discussion may help to increase the effectiveness. Health education workshop were also found to improve appointment-keeping and self care.

5. 儿童组教育方法 Group methods for children

对儿童的健康教育大多集中在三个课题：药物，吸烟与口腔健康。课程长短与结果有关。对儿童健康教育课程的最佳时间长度并没有作过研究。短期随访的各种尝试报告表明，儿童知识稍有增加，态度也略有改变。长期研究儿童的态度与行为显示，随着年龄增加，同学之间的影响比教育项目本身更重要。

在积极参与之后的测量表明，口腔健康教育比其他教育的结果更能得到证实，因为可以对这些结果作客观测量而不是取决于主观陈述或自我报告。口腔健康教育还可以包括理想的实际示范以及对部分儿童的指导活动，因此，更便于记忆。而且，某些研究试图包括家长，包括个人有机会发现并深入到其他科目的革新项目中去，有时组织班级比赛，似乎有最佳的效果。

教学方法：传统的讲课加上较多非正式的小组讨论相当满意。直观教具辅助比书本好，两种方法结合似能增加效果，口头讲解以直观教具作辅助并且开展一些活动的方法是其中最好的。

Teaching methods; traditional lectures are contrasted with more informal group discussions are relatively satisfactory. Visual aids are better than a written text. A combination of methods seems to have an enhancing effect and that teaching by word of mouth supplemented both by visual aids and by activity methods are the best of all.

6. 个别教育方法 Individual methods

可以用个别咨询作为对还没有患病的人的一种预防技术，或者也可以在临床情况下作为治疗过程的一部分。

口腔健康研究在防治结合或者只与预防方法有关的方面，把改变行为的技术个别教给家长用于儿童身上。这些研究几乎肯定可以产生能客观检查的行为改变，如菌斑，或牙龈炎指数。

一种个人示范和教学技术，几乎用于大多数牙科研究。有时这些方面可以在模型上或者在儿童身上做比较都是非常有效的。

大多数个别健康教育方法的研究都是报告可以测量的行为改变。比较数字的改变，成功率在10%～36%。这些研究结果通过一年后的随访报告表明，有持续而满意的行为改变。个别咨询没有提到有什么负面影响。

心理对动机的影响——一项儿童口腔健康实践的研究提出责任感和领袖感有助于行为改变。

The majority of these studies of individual methods of health education report measurable behaviour changes. Where comparable figures are given, the success rates vary from 10 to 36%. Those studies which were followed up after one year report a persistent and satisfactory behaviour change. No mention is made of any negative effects resulting from individual counseling.

7. 规章制度法 Legislation

登广告或销售目的在于不鼓励吸烟的规定而不是禁止，看来对一般群众的吸烟习惯很少有作用。提供给个人遵循的规定，常被个人所回避，特别是如果力度差的时候。用于对厂商的有关规定，不能不考虑，结果最为满意。

Legislation about advertising or sale aimed at the discouragement of smoking, rather than its banning, seems to have little effect on the general public's smoking habits.

Laws which refer to individual action are frequently evaded especially if enforcement is weak. Laws apply to manufacturers and so cannot be disregarded, the outcome is the most satisfactory

8. 讨论所有发现 Discussion of overall findings

（1）成功率 Success rate　一般认为增加群众的实际知识比说服他们改变其态度要容易得多。在62项以增加知识为目的的研究中85%确实有改进。在36项以改变态度为目的的研究中只有约65%有改变的希望。一般认为行为改变比态度改变要困难得多。但在123项尝试改变行为的研究报告中有75%获得一定的成功，但这并不意味着在健康与口腔健康教育项目的研究报告中有85%的成功率。即使在统计学上有显著性差异，但实际的重要性可能太小，即使是最成功的项目，可能对少数人是无效的。由于这些原因，估价健康教育项目的成功不要把数字看得太重。虽然能说它们一点作用也没有。

(2) 评价技术 Techniques of evaluation

♦ 在评价一项实际教育项目时，在方法学上存在着困难，但实际上，在许多研究中有合理的标准；

♦ 缺少对照组，或与实验组没有可比性。前后对比的试验设计，如果不用对照组的话，可能得出错误的结果；

♦ 一般知识可以通过某种书面测验来衡量，但对把知识用于实践的能力或意愿，并不是很好的指标。而态度只有通过带有很多偏见的自我报告去衡量。通过客观方法测量行为非常满意，但其他方面也并不满意。

(3) 口腔健康教育方法的比较 Comparisons of methods in oral health education

♦ 一般认为个别教育是最好的教育方式；

♦ 小组随访，一般性指导，效果最小，这一观点可从表 11-1 中看出来：

表 11-1 口腔健康教育方法的比较

			研究的比例（括号内为%）报告肯定有改变的方面
	知识	态度	行为
媒体	7/11（64）	8/8（100）	20/30（67）
小组方法	25/28（89）	14/24（58）	35/51（69）
个别方法	10/10（100）	1/2（50）	30/33（91）

♦ 多种方法可能比一种方法好。越是个别的方法效果越好。虽然并一定是效益越大；

♦ 在增进口腔健康方面，修正行为的技术比各种小组的方法好。个别指导刷牙比在模型上示范好。但个别咨询并不比知自我教育或小组方法，或影片或有计划的学习好。个别的方式不一定要面对面；个别指导与通过录音带教育比较并未发现什么差别。与教具的相互作用和个别讲述指导比较，前者更有效。

♦ 小组方法从完全不针对个人的讲座到有很多人的小组，很可能会走向两个极端。可能在两个不同的小组之间出现很大的差别。

学校里的小组讨论看来并不有用。但各种小且方法在增加口腔健康知识方面比海报或分发牙刷，牙膏，菌斑显示片与传单更为有效。

♦ 通常书面教育指导方式的效果看一比其他方式都差。书面指导比口头指导，或与教具相互作用的效果要差。但录音带，书面资料与影片又比正规指导要好，如果联合使用多种方法，甚至效果更好。

♦ 比较研究媒体与其他方法的效果还进行的很少。

♦ 开展社区活动成功的报告表明，以社区为基础的方法很有价值，不发达国家所有的研究报告，几乎都与公共卫生措施有关。但在发达国家还没有过尝试或报告，发达国家的健康教育者几乎总是集中于直接影响个人，很少注意到社区。

社区途径可能比其他方法需要更多的资源，特别是那些非针对个人的方法，如媒体，但它可能更有效果。

在比较了各种方法之后，不应该认为一种方法总是比其他方法好。在一种特殊情况下，最好的健康教育方法将取决于3种因素。具体的场合与情况，和健康教育所倡导的，以及个人有关的因素。

- 场合与情况因素：健康教育在遇到社会压力与要求的情况下，不得不采取的行动；
- 由健康教育提出的行动：需要什么、提供什么；
- 个人因素：影响个人对健康教育做出反应的个人特点。

最后，通过10～15年期间发表的250篇参考资料的分析比较，Dr. A. Gatherer等人指出，大多数研究报告似乎设计不当，其结果是混乱而含糊或者缺乏充分对照。在理念与方法学上很少拿得出证据来。因此，作为健康教育服务的基本组成部分，应该进行更多的评价，应该付出代价，提供更多的资源，包括经费与时间，以便有批判性地做出评价，应仔细地计划与对照，小范围、更深入的研究比范围大而不准确的研究，对健康教育工作者更有帮助。质量比数量更有价值。

Finally, Dr. A. Gatherer et al., point out through 250 reference under 10-15 years, a majority of the reported studies appear to be inadequately planed and their findings too confused, vague or insufficiently controlled. There is very little evidence in ideas and methodology. More evaluation should be carried out its cost should be accepted as an essential part of the health education service. More resources, both in money and time, should be devoted to the critical appraisal of the health education services, should be carefully planed and controlled. Small and more intensive studies are likely to be of more help to the average health educator than large-scale or imprecise studies. Quality is of more value than quantity.

评价应该是任何卫生服务活动中的一个核心内容，不论是治疗，还是健康促进活动。评价是为了评估达到什么目标以及怎样达到的。因此，对任何活动的批判性评价都是为了评估什么是好，什么是坏的特征，以及改进未来活动的方法。能够做出评估的，是对结果与过程的评价测量。

设计的结果评价是评估已经达到了什么，以及是否设定的目标已经达到。在健康促进评价中能够用整个范围的结果测量，取决于所采取的活动的性质。例如，结果测量可以包括评估健康意识，知识或态度，或政策的改变（Nutbean, 1998）。在某些情况下，健康状态的改变能够用作为一定的健康教育干预的结果测量。然而，这只是适合于长期干预的项目才能达到这样的改变（Watt等，2001），能够用一整套方面来测量健康教育的结果。这些包括问卷调查，个别访谈，政策评论或健康调查，取决于评估什么样的结果。

在健康教育中，除了测量结果之外，重要的是评估包括发展与实施一种干预的过程。因此，过程评价的目的是评估实施的质量。是否应用了最适当的方法与资料？时间范围是否适当？资源是否充分？

口腔健康教育是口腔健康促进的重要组成部分，应该成为所有口腔专业人员临床职责的一个重要部分。在临床实践中，有效的口腔健康教育大部分取决于详细的计划与团队工作。重要的是所有的健康教育指导与支持都要在科学上依据正确的证据。

Oral health education is an important part of oral health promotion and should be an important part of all dental professionals' clinical duties. Effective oral health education within dental practices is largely dependent upon detailed planning and teamwork. It is important that all health education advice and support is based upon scientifically sound evidence.

Effective dental health education should ultimately provide positive values toward dental health and affect behaviour changes. Therefore, it is necessary to fully understand the knowledge level of the population and have some background to be aware of the values that population and individuals within the population have. In addition, the educator must be aware of personal values and make sure to work in a positive manner to improve the dental health of the population.

小结 Summary

通过本章学习，使学员们认识到健康促进的目的是为了改变环境，营造有益于健康和口腔健康的整个环境，而健康教育的目的是为了改变人们的行为与生活方式。

WHO早在1977年就提出了健康促进的五大原则。渥太华宪章（1989）又发展了健康促进的原则。2005 年曼谷会议通过的健康促进宪章提出了便于全球化的健康促进策略。

健康促进的整合定义包括倡导、提高能力和协作三个方面。健康促进的途径有医学或预防、行为改变、教育、增强能力和社会改变。这些途径有不同的目的、目标、方法和评价手段。健康促进途径为叙述性，而健康促进模式更具有分析性。健康促进的策略与方法涉及 5 个方面，都有特别的难点。口腔健康教育包含知识、态度与行为3个方面。口腔健康教育的关键作用是培养和改变人们的行为习惯。在健康教育中，除了测量结果之外，重要的是评价干预的过程。口腔健康教育是口腔健康促进的重要组成部分，应该成为所有口腔专业人员职责的重要组成部分。

After learning this chapter, the students should be able to understand the purpose of health promotion is intending to change the total environment which is conducive to health and oral health and health education aims to made changes in people's behaviour and lifestyle.

As early as in 1977, the WHO made explicit five key principles for health promotion. The principles of health promotion are further developed in the Ottawa Charter (1989). In 2005, the Bangkok Charter identifies the strategies for health promotion in a globalized world.

The integrated definition of health promotion includes advocacy, enablement and mediation. There are five different approaches to health promotion: medical or preventive, behaviour change, educational, empowerment and social change. These approaches will have different aims, methods and means of evaluation. The approaches are primarily descriptive, and the models of health promotion are primarily analytic. The strategies and methods adopted pose particular dilemmas. on the other hand, knowledge, attitude and behaviour are appropriately covered in health education. The key role of oral health education is to form or change human behaviour related to health and oral health. in addition to measure the outcomes of interventions, evaluation which includes developing and implementing a process of interventions is important in health education. Oral health education is an important part of oral health promotion and should be an important part of all dental professional's duties.

思考题 Review questions

1. 健康促进与健康教育的目的有什么不同？
2. 为什么说健康教育是健康促进的一个组成部分？
3. 如何评价口腔健康教育的效果？
4. WHO（1977 年）提出的健康促进五项原则是什么？
5. 健康促进的五种途径是什么？

参考文献 References

1. Technical Report Series No. 449, WHO,"Dental Health Education", 1970
2. Technical Report Series No. 690, WHO,"New approaches to Health Education in primary Health Care", 1983
3. Green, Laurence W. et al. Health Education planning- A Diagnostic Approach, 1980
4. Philip Weinstein et al. changing Human Behaviour-Strategies for preventive Dentistry, 1978
5. Parfit, A Gatherer, J. et al. Is Health Educaiton Effective, 1979
6. Kay, L. and Locker, D. Is dental health education effective? A systemic review of current evidence. Community Dentistry and Oral Epidemiology, 1996, 24: 231-5
7. Sheiham, A. The role of the dental team in promoting dental health and general health through oral health. International Dental Journal, 1992, 42: 223-8
8. Watt, R. and Fuller, S. Oral health promotion: opportunity knocks! British Dental Journal. 1999, 186: 3-6
9. Ewles, L. and Simnett I. Promoting health: a practical guide. Edinburgh. Bailliere Tindall, 1999
10. Jennie Naidoo, Jane Wills Health promotion-Foundations for practice, 2nd Edition. Bailliere Tindall, 2000

（卞金有）

第十二章　社区口腔保健
Chapter Ⅻ Community Oral Health Care

概述 Overview

本章第一节主要叙述初级卫生保健途径，初级卫生保健的五大基本原则，初级口腔卫生保健包括概念，水平作用及其限度。第二节介绍社区口腔卫生保健，包括口腔公共卫生的定义。社区口腔卫生保健模式构架，实践与评价。社区口腔健康状态及其干预，贫困社区口腔卫生保健以及综合基本口腔卫生保健。

This chapter firstly describe primary health care approach. There are five basic principles of primary health care, primary oral health care, including concept, levels, role and its limitation. The second section introduces community oral health care, including the definition of oral public health, an essential structure practices and evaluation of community oral health care models, community oral health status and its intervention. oral health care in deprived communities and integrated package of basic oral care.

要点 Key points

- *Primary health care approach*
- *Primary oral health care*
- *Community oral health care*
- *Community oral health care models*
- *Status intervention index*
- *Integrated package of basic oral care*

第一节　初级卫生保健途径
Section 1 The Primary Health Care Approach

一、人人享有卫生保健的含义 The meaning of "health for all"

"2000 年人人享有卫生保健"（health for all by the year 2000）是 1977 年第 30 届世界卫生大会通过的决议，是全球的社会战略目标。1978年在前苏联阿拉木图召开的国际初级卫生保健会议上提出了初级卫生保健（primary health care, PHC）是实现这一战略目标的基本途径和策略。这一全球性社会目标产生的背景可以追溯到上个世纪的 50 年代。

早在上个世纪 50 至 70 年代期间，通过对中国等 9 个国家的考察，对当时的世界卫生状况和卫生服务进行了全面分析，提示了四大问题：⑴健康状况存在着明显差异；⑵卫生资源分配不平衡；(3)贫穷病、富裕病和社会病对人群健康和生命带来了极大的威胁；(4)卫生计划和管理不足，为全球的卫生变革提供了重要依据。因此，2000年人人享有卫生保健的战略思想开始形成。

人人享有卫生保健意味着在一个国家内健康可以带给每个人。健康意味着一个人的幸福状态，不只是拥有健康服务——使一个人能够达到社会经济生活富有成效的那种健康状态。人人享有卫生保健含有消除对健康有害的障碍的含义——那就是说，消除营养不良、无知、污染饮水、不卫生的居住环境——十分常见的是解决单纯的医疗问题如缺少医生、医院床位、药品与疫苗。

人人享有卫生保健意味着应该把健康作为经济发展的一个目标，不仅是达到目标的一种手段。

人人享有卫生保健最终要求所有人受教育，直到变成为现实，至少开始懂得健康对每个人意味着什么。

In 1977, the thirtieth world Health assembly decided that the main social goal of governments and WHO in the coming decades should be the attainment by all the people of the world by the year 2000 of a level of health that would permit them to lead a socially and economically productive life, popularly known as "health for all by the year 2000".

In 1978, an International Conference or primary health care, held in Alma-Ata, former user, stated that primary health care is the key to attaining this target.

"Health for all" means that health is to be brought within reach of everyone in a given country. And by "health" is meant a personal state of well being, not just the availability of health services-a state of health that enables a person to lead a socially and economically productive life. "Health for all" implies the removal of the obstacles to health-that is to say, the elimination of malnutrition, ignorance, contaminated drinking-water, and unhygienic housing-quite as much as it does the solution of purely medical problems such as a lack of doctors, hospital beds, drugs and vaccines.

"Health for all" means that health should be regarded as an objective of economic development and not merely as one of the means of attaining it.

"Health for all" demands, ultimately, literacy for all. Until this becomes reality it demands at least the beginning of an understanding of what health means for every individual.

“人人享有卫生保健”取决于医疗保健与公共卫生的不断进步。通过初级卫生保健，所有的人必定能够得到卫生服务，在每一个村庄，都拥有基本医疗帮助，通过转诊服务，可以得到更加专业化的保健。免疫注射也必定能达到普遍的覆盖。

因此，“人人享有卫生保健”是一个整体概念，要求农业、工业、教育、住宅、通讯系统共同努力，正像医学与公共卫生的许多事情那样，只靠医疗保健是不可能把健康带给生活在简陋小屋中的饥民的。对于这些人的健康需要一种完全新的生活方式与新的机遇为他们提供一种较高的生活标准。

"Health for all" depends on continued progress in medical care and public health. The health services must be accessible to all through primary health care, in which basic medical help is available in every village, backed up by referral services to more specialized care. Immunization must similarly

achieve universal coverage.

"Health for all" is thus a holistic concept calling for efforts in agriculture, industry, education, housing, and communications, just as much as in medicine and public health. Health for such people requires a whole new way of life and fresh opportunities to provide themselves with a higher standard of living.

一个政府采纳“人人享有卫生保健”意味着一种承诺在广泛发展的前沿上促进所有公民健康的改善并坚持鼓励每个公民达到一种较高的生命质量。

The adoption of "health for all" by a government implies a commitment to promote the advancement of all citizens on a broad front of development, and a resolution to encourage the individual citizen to achieve a higher quality of life.

这一目标的真正含义，正如世界卫生组织所指出的：⑴人人享有卫生保健或称人人健康，不是指到2000年医护人员将为世界上每一个人治疗其全部已患疾病，也不是指到2000年不再有人生病或成为残疾；⑵健康是从家庭、学校与工厂开始，在人们生活与工作的地方保持健康；⑶人们将运用比现在更好的办法预防疾病，减轻不可避免的疾病和伤残的痛苦，并且通过更好的途径进入成年、老年并安然地告别人世；⑷所有个人和家庭在能接受和提供的范围内通过充分参与，享受到基本卫生服务；⑸在居民中平均分配一切卫生资源；⑹人们会懂得自己有力量摆脱可以避免的疾病桎梏，创造自己及其家庭生活，并明白疾病不是不可避免的。

The meaning of health for all, it is just pointed out by WHO that: (1) health for all does not mean that in the year 2000 doctors and nurses will provide medical care for everybody in the world for all their existing ailments and that nobody will be sick or disabled; (2) it does mean that health begins and is fostered or endangered at home, in schools and in factories, where people live and work; (3) people will use better approaches than they do now for preventing disease and alleviating unavoidable illness and disability, and have better ways of growing up, growing old and dying in dignity; (4) essential health care will be accessible to all individuals and families, in an acceptable and affordable way, and with their full involvement; (5) there will be an even distribution among the population of whatever resources for health care available , and (6) people will realize that they themselves have the power to shape their lives and the lives of their families, free from the available burden of disease, and aware that ill-health is not inevitable.

1981 年，WHO 又提出了到 2000 年全球应能达到的十项具体目标：

⑴每个国家所有的人至少已经能够利用基本卫生保健和一级转诊设施；

⑵所有的人在其可能的范围内积极参加针对他们自己与家庭的保健工作，并且积极参加社区的保健活动；

⑶全世界的所有社区都能与政府共同承担社区成员的卫生保健责任；

⑷所有的政府将会负担起人民健康的全部责任；

⑸全体人民都可利用安全饮用水和卫生设施；

⑹全体人民都能得到足够的营养；

⑺所有的儿童都会接受针对儿童主要感染性疾病的免疫接种；

⑻发展中国家的传染病在公共卫生方面的重要程度不会超过发达国家 1980 年的水平；

(9)应用一切可能的办法，通过影响生活方式和控制自然与社会心理环境因素预防和控制非传染病，促进精神健康；

(10)所有的人都能得到基本药物。

In 1981, WHO also proposed the following 10 global targets for the year 2000:

(1) All people in every country will have at least ready access to essential health care and to first-level referral facilities.

(2) All people will be activity involved in caring for themselves and their families as far as they can and in community action for health.

(3) Communities throughout the would will share with governments responsibility for the health care of their members.

(4) All governments will have assumed overall responsibility for the health of their people.

(5) Safe drinking-water and sanitation will be available to all people.

(6) All people will be adequately nourished.

(7) All children will be immunized against the major infectious diseases of childhood.

(8) Communicable diseases in the developing countries will be of no greater public health significance in the year 2000 than they are in developed countries in the year 1980.

(9) All possible ways will be applied to prevent and control non-communicable diseases and promote mental health through influencing life-styles and controlling the physical and psychosocial environment.

(10) Essential drugs will be available to all.

面对21世纪新的挑战，回顾“2000年人人享有卫生保健”的目标，虽然仍是一个梦想，但是其目标与策略途径的完整性、科学性、可靠性与可行性、仍然是一个值得追求的，有可能实现的目标。

二、初级卫生保健 Primary health care

初级卫生保健并不是一个全新的概念，它是经过总结过去的各种卫生保健方法，并吸收了一些新的经验而逐渐形成的。中国农村卫生工作的实践经验对发展初级卫生保健概念起到了重要影响。“人人享有卫生保健”策略的基础是初级卫生保健。著名的“阿拉木图宣言”对初级卫生保健的概念作了精辟的阐述。它明确指出“初级卫生保健是建立在实际可行，科学上正确可靠，社会上能接受的方法与技术的基础之上的一种基本卫生保健。是在自力更生，与自决精神的指导之下，通过人们的全面参与，使社区，个人与家庭都能普遍得到，其费用又能为社区和国家所承担，并能维持其不断发展的一种卫生保健。它是国家卫生系统整体的一个组成部分，行使其中心职能并成为主要重点的一部分，同时也是整个社会经济发展的一部分，它是个人家庭、社区与国家卫生系统联系的第一个环节，使卫生保健尽可能接近人们居住和工作的场所，它还构成一个连续不断的卫生保健过程的第一要素。

The basis of the “health for all” strategy is primary health care. The Alma-at conference described primary health care as: essential health care based on practical scientifically sound and socially acceptable methods and technology made universally accessible to individuals and families in the community through their full participation and at a cost that the community and country can afford to maintain at every stage of their development in the spirit of self-reliance and self-determination. It forms an integral part both of the country's health system, of which it is the control function and main focus, and of the overall social and economic development of the community. It is the first level of contact of individuals, the family and community with the national health system bringing health care as close as possible to where people live and work, and constitutes the first element of a continuing health care process.

初级卫生保健集中体现了五项基本原则，它们是：

1. 平等分配 Equitable distribution

卫生保健应能服务于社会各阶层，而初级卫生保健可以使全民享有，具有可进入、可接受、可利用、可努力达到等特点。

Primary health care is to make the health care services accessible, available, acceptable, and affordable to the target group in order to have an even distribution of health care services among different strata in the society.

2. 社会参与 Community involvement

要求社区在确定其需要，寻找解决方法，动员当地资源，以及建立必要的地方组织方面承担较大的责任。决定开展一系列的活动，并不意味着都是医疗性质的，目的是为了满足个人，家庭与社区的基本健康需要和提高生命质量。

这种社区参与比当地的卫生保健机构有更大的影响。它可以把社区领导支持所需要的卫生事业改革的承诺变为现实，并通过他们转变成政府对卫生事业改革的政治承诺。

Such involvement requires communities to assume greater responsibilities in defining their needs, identifying solutions, mobilizing local resources, and developing the necessary local organizations. It is defined as a series of simple activities, by no means all of a medical nature, aimed at meeting the essential health requirements of individuals, families, and the community, and at improving the quality of life.

Such community involvement can have a broader influence than the local organization of health care. It can be instrumental in bringing about the commitment of community leaders to support the health reforms required, and through them it can stimulate the political commitment of the government to introduce and sustain these reforms.

3. 多方合作 The multi-sectoral approach

健康不能单独存在，它受到环境，社会与经济因素的复杂的，最终是彼此相关的影响。健康只是整个生命关怀的一部分（教育，住所，营养）其改善应涉及农业，食品加工，经济与人事各部门参与计划。2000年人人达到可以接受的健康水平，仅靠卫生部门不可能实现。只有通过国家的政治决定，与卫生部门及其他相关的社会经济发展部门的协同努力才有可能达到。

Health does not exist in isolation. It is influenced by a complex of environmental, social, and economic factors ultimately related to each other. Health is only a part of total care (education, shelter, nutrition) and should be improved by involving the agricultural, food manufacturing, economic and employment sectors in planning. An acceptable level of health for all by the year 2000 cannot be achieved by the health sector alone. It can only be attained through national political will and the coordinated efforts of the health sector and relevant activities of other social and economic development sectors.

4. 适宜技术 Appropriate technology

适宜技术或者称适宜的健康技术是指在科学上是有效的，适合于当地的需要，使用这些技术的人是可以接受的，并且保持和利用这些技术所需要的资源是社区或国家能够负担得起的各种方法，操作程序，技术与设备。

初级卫生保健需要发展，适应与应用适宜的健康技术，人们能够应用和负担得起，这些包括低价值物品的充分供应，优质基本药品，疫苗，生物制品，及其他供应与设备，还有功能上有效的支持性卫生保健设施，如健康中心与医院，应当重新定向这些设施以满足初级卫生保健的需要和适应社会经济环境。

Appropriate technology or appropriate health technology, that is, methods, procedures, techniques, and equipment that are scientifically valid, adopted to local needs, and acceptable to those who use them and to those for whom they are used, and that can be maintained and utilized with resources the community or the country can afford.

Primary health care requires the development, adaptation, and application of appropriate health technology that the people can use and afford, including an adequate supply of low-cost, good-quality essential drugs, vaccines, biologicals, and other supplies and equipment, as well as functionally efficient supportive health care facilities, such as health centres and hospitals. These facilities should be reoriented to the needs of primary health care and adapted to the socioeconomic environment.

5. 重点预防 Focus on prevention

有些疾病是完全可以预防和控制的。主要是教育群众，自我保护，预防疾病的发生。一般来说，预防性花费要少于治疗性花费。

Some diseases are highly preventable and controlled. It is of extreme importance to educate the people to take care of themselves to prevent the onset of diseases.

The cost involved in prevention is generally much less than the cost used to cure diseases.

根据“阿拉木图宣言”的基本原则，初级卫生保健应致力于解决全民的基本卫生问题。其具体内容则可因不同国家，不同地区与不同人群而有所不同，但至少应包括八项最低限内容：

针对普遍存在的问题及其预防和控制方法进行的健康教育；

- 促进食品供应与适当的营养；
- 适当供给安全用水；
- 提供基本的清洁卫生环境；
- 开展妇幼保健，包括计划生育；
- 对主要感染性疾病的预防接种；
- 对地方病的预防和控制；
- 提供基本药品。

Based on Five principles of “Declaration of Alma-Ata”, primary health care should focus on the main health problems in the community, but recognizing that these problems and the ways of solving them will vary from one country and community to another. Primary health care should include at least eight elements:

Education concerning prevailing health problems and the methods of identifying, preventing, and controlling them;

- *Promotion of food supply and proper nutrition;*
- *An adequate supply of safe water, and basic sanitation;*
- *maternal and child health care, including family planning;*
- *immunization against the major infectious diseases;*
- *prevention and control of locally endemic diseases;*
- *appropriate treatment of common diseases and injuries;*
- *the provision of essential drugs.*

全面理解初级卫生保健的含义：

(1) 从居民角度看，它是必不可少的，人人享有和参与，并且是负担得起的；(2) 从技术方法角度看，它是切实可行的，科学上证明可靠的，是社区，个人和家庭都乐于接受的；(3) 从卫生角度看，它是最基本的卫生保健服务，体现卫生方针，以为群众服务为宗旨，是国家卫生体制的基础与组成部分；(4) 从政府角度看，它是各级政府的职责，是基层政权的重要组成部分，组织动员群众充分参与，和各部门协调行动；(5) 从社会经济发展角度看，它是社会经济发展的重要组成部分与原动力，是社会进步与经济发展的目标之一。

Completely understanding the meaning of primary health care:

(1) From the residents points of view, it must be necessary, and everyone have access for their participation and involvement and everyone can afford; (2) from the technical point of view, it is practical and feasible, and scientifically sound and reliable, and the community, individual and families are willing to accept; (3) from health system point of view, it is the most basic health services, which demonstrate health policies, and serve for people as its goal and as a basis of a country's health system and an integral part of it; (4) from government point of view, it is the responsibilities of governments at different levels and is an important part of local political power and organizing and motivating sufficient participation of the public; (5) from social economic development point of view, it is an important part of socio-economic development and motive power, and one goal of social progression and economic development.

三、初级口腔卫生保健 Primary oral health care

（一）基本概念 The basic concept

一个明确的初级口腔卫生保健的概念是不同水平的社区开展项目计划的前提。初级口腔卫生保健是在实际可行，科学上证明可靠，为社会和群众所要求和接受，在个人积极参加和社区参与的基础上，以自我保健贯穿于其发展的各个阶段，通过社区卫生工作者或口腔卫生工作者的实践，提供最基本的口腔卫生保健服务早期中止口腔疾病的自然发展，晚期及时治疗组织改变与症状处理，使全体社区成员都能享有的一种基本口腔卫生保健。

A clear concept of primary oral health care is a prerequisite for proper planning at different levels of the community. Primary oral health care is essential oral health care for all community members, based on the methods that are practical, scientifically sound, and socially acceptable and the public demanded, and individual participation and community involvement, and self-care throughout every phase of its development, and the provision of very basic oral health services by community health workers or oral health workers from their practice to intercept the natural history of oral diseases at an early stage. Prompt treatment of tissue changes and the management of symptoms at a later stage.

（二）基本内容 The essential components

大部分初级口腔卫生保健的最基本内容与初级卫生保健的基本内容是密切相关的，在具体做法上是可以结合为一体的：

1. 口腔健康教育与促进：针对社区群众普遍存在的口腔卫生问题，如龋病，牙周病，以及预防与控制这些疾病的知识，方法与实践，进行教育与具体指导，并且广泛动员全社区以及社区每个成员积极关注与投入。

Oral health education and promotion: focus on the common existed oral health problems of the community population, such as dental caries, and periodontal diseases, and the knowledge, skills and practice in prevention and control of these diseases, to carry out health education and hygiene instruction, and widely motivating the whole community and its members for their full attention and involvement.

2. 食品选择与营养指导：正确指导并适当限制糖类食品消耗，选择有益于牙齿与口腔健康的食物。

Food selection and nutritional counseling: correctly advising and properly limiting sugar-containing food consumption, and selecting appropriate foods which are beneficial to teeth and oral health.

3. 倡导有益于口腔健康的行为习惯与生活方式，如戒除烟酒嗜好，纠正不良习惯等。

Initiating behaviour, habits and lifestyle which are beneficial to oral health, such as cessation of tobacco and alcohol use, and change of poor habits, etc.

4. 适当调节饮水含氟量（加氟或除氟）有利于牙齿健康。

Appropriate adjustment of fluoride level in drinking water (fluoridation or defluoridation) for dental health

5. 妇幼口腔保健。

Maternal and child oral health care

6. 常见口腔病伤的适当处理。

Appropriate treatment of common oral diseases and injuries

7. 提供基本口腔保健用品。

Provision of essential oral care products

8. 在工作与生活场所防止环境受污染以利于牙齿健康。

Preventing environmental pollution at the places where the people are working and living in order to protect teeth.

9. 建立口腔保健卡，定期为群众进行口腔健康检查，并安排就近就医，及时治疗。

Formulating oral health passport, and regularly taking oral examination for the public, and referral to nearest oral health centre for treatment promptly.

（三）不同水平的初级口腔卫生保健 Primary oral health care at different levels

虽然初级口腔卫生保健有其最基本的内容，但不一定都在同一水平上，而是可以根据不同国家和地区的不同社会经济发展水平，不同的资源状况与疾病发病状况，以及群众的需求程度而变通的。根据目前我国各地区的不同情况，大致可以把初级口腔卫生保健分为三个水平或层次：

1. 一级水平——口腔健康教育，促进与防护 Oral Health education, promotion and specific protection as first level

（1）提供口腔卫生与保健信息及口腔卫生指导，包括知识，技能与实践；

（2）自我口腔保健技术示范；

（3）个人营养，饮食习惯与食品选择咨询与指导；

（4）个人口腔卫生实践，卫生习惯与生活方式；

（5）适当补充氟化物；

（6）糖消耗量，次数与消耗方式指导；

（7）提供基本口腔保健用品；

（8）监测口腔疾病发病状况。

To provide oral health and care information and oral hygiene instruction, including knowledge, skills and practice

Technical demonstration of oral self-care

Counseling and conducting individual nutrition, diet habits and foods selection

Individual oral hygiene practice, hygiene habits and lifestyle

Appropriate supplement of fluorides

The amount of sugar consumption, frequency and mode of its consumption

Provision of basic oral care products

Monitoring the trend of oral diseases status

2. 二级水平——口腔检查，早期诊断与即刻处理 Oral examination, early diagnosis and prompt treatment as second level, in addition to level 1

（9）龋齿，牙周病定期检查，记录与报告；

Regularly examine, recording and reporting about dental caries and periodontal diseases

（10）去除牙石；

Scaling（super and subgingival）

（11）窝沟封闭预防殆面龋；

Pit and fissure sealants for preventing occlusal caries

（12）预防性充填；

Preventive fillings

（13）早期龋简单处理（充填等）；

Simple treatment for early caries（fillings, etc）

(14）局部应用氟化物（涂氟，氟胶等）；

Topical use of fluorides（varnish, fluoride gel, etc）

3. 三级水平——症状保健 Symptomatic care as 3rd level in addition to level 1 and level 2

(15）缓解疼痛（机械或药物方法）；

Pain release（mechanical or drug methods）

(16）简单急诊保健；

Simple emergency care（injuries, infection and accident management）

(17）拔除松动牙；

Extraction of loosening teeth

(18）安排转诊治疗。

Appointment of referral to further treatment

上述三个不同层次的内容一般都属于初级口腔卫生保健的范畴。

These three levels are flexible and changeable; depend on changing pattern of oral diseases, community needs and individual demands, technical level of community health workers in primary oral health care.

四、初级口腔卫生保健的作用及其限度 The role of primary oral health care and its limitation

初级口腔卫生保健的目的是向社区全体成员提供必不可少的口腔卫生保健，以增进和保持人群的口腔健康水平。

初级口腔卫生保健是初级卫生保健的一个重要组成部分，与初级卫生保健的基本内容有密切的内在联系。因此，世界上许多国家制定了本国或本地区未来的口腔卫生保健目标，如2005年，2010年或2020年的目标。现在，不论是工业化国家还是发展中国家，都试图以初级卫生保健为途径，把口腔卫生的最基本内容纳入初级卫生保健之轨道，并通过培训现有的各种基层卫生工作者甚至非医务工作者来承担初级口腔卫生保健的工作任务（表12-1）。

The aim of primary oral health care is to provide the whole population with essential oral health care, in order to strengthen and maintain the people's oral health.

Primary oral health care is an important part of primary health care, and there is a close relationship in the basic content between them. Therefore, many countries in the world have formulated the national or regional goals for oral health by the year 2010 or 2020. at present time, both industrialized and developing countries are attempting to integrate oral health as one element into the contents of primary health care and to train a variety of community health workers and even non-health professionals to provide first-contact services for their community members 表 12-1)

表 12-1 Primary oral health care in some selected countries or regions

Country/Region	Organizational Mode	Type of personnel	Work range
India	Village health station	Multi-health workers	Health education preventive measures
Thailand	Village health post	Examiner, communicator, scaler	Health education, preventive measures scaling
Indonesia	Village health station	Health workers	Health education, preventive measure
Syria	School health clinic	Teachers	Health education preventive measures
Philippines	Village health station	Midwife	Health education
Hong Kong	Outside dental clinic	Dental therapist	Health education preventive measures treatment
Singapore	School dental clinic	Dental nurse	Ditto
New Zealand	School dental clinic	Dental nurse	Ditto
Sweden	School dental clinic	Dental hygienist	Health education, regular examination preventive measures treatment

初级口腔卫生保健是整个国家或地区口腔卫生保健系统与个人，家庭和社区直接接触与广泛联系的前沿阵地，也是能最大限度地深入到社区群众生活与工作的场所，因而是群众最容易得到的一种基本口腔卫生保健。它面向社区，面向全民，具有最大的人口覆盖面。这种保健应该是有组织有计划地，连续不断地向整个社区群众提供，而不受到地理，经费，文化与职能方面的限制。

Primary oral health care is the first level of contact of individuals, the family, and the community with national or regional health system, and widely link with them, bring oral health care as close as possible to where people live and work, and it is essential oral health care that most easily accessible to the people. Accessibility implies the continuing and organized supply of care that is geographically, financially, culturally and functionally within easy reach of the whole community with the maximum coverage of the population.

尽管如此，初级口腔卫生保健的限度是显而易见的。因为它不能独立存在，或者说不能孤立地开展活动，它只能是整个国家卫生与社区系统中的一部分。初级口腔卫生保健的成功与否，不仅要看它是否已建立，是否已存在，或者是否已在行使它的职能，还要看整个卫生系统其他机构，包括口腔卫生保健系统，也就是上级行政与技术部门对它的支持是否充分和足够，是否能较好地解决初级口腔卫生保健所无力解决的较为复杂的问题。因为至少有一部分群众的口腔健康状况恶化，疾病比较严重，需要比较复杂的口腔医疗和康复保健。较高水平的口腔保健机构，如二级，三级水平，应当在人员培训，技术指导，器械材料与药品供应，后勤维修，资料搜集与统计分析以及科学管理诸方面提供支持，促进与协调，不仅当地机构需要这样做，而且中间各级机构与中央一级机构也要这样做。只有这样，初级口腔卫生保健才能巩固并得到发展。

But, even this strategy can lead to success; the limitation of primary oral health care is evident. Because it cannot exist independently, or saying to make any activity separately, and it can only be a part of the whole national or community health systems, whether it is success or not, not only to see, it set up or exists, or carrying out its functions, but also to see, other sectors of health systems including oral health care system, e.g., the top administrative and technical institutions for their sufficient and adequate support of primary oral health care and assisting them to solve more sophisticated problems which can not be deal by itself. At least, oral health status is getting worse and oral diseases are more serious in some people and those require more comprehensive oral care and rehabilitative care. Oral health care institutions at higher levels, such as the second level or the third level of referrals, should provide manpower training, technical advice, dental supplies, such as equipment and materials, drugs and repairing for maintenance, data collection, and statistical analysis and scientific management, as a support, promotion, and coordination, not only the local institutes are requested to doing so, but also the mid-level and top level of institutes in doing too. Only by this way, the primary oral health care can be salivated and further developed.

五、初级口腔卫生保健人员的充分发展与利用 Sufficient development and utilization of primary oral health workers

初级口腔卫生保健与初级卫生保健一样，必须充分利用一切可以利用的资源条件，包括可以调动整个社区可能使用的人力资源。初级口腔卫生保健是由经过适当培训的社区卫生工作者提供服务的，他们所需要和所能掌握的技能以及所接受的培训取决于所提供的初级口腔卫生保健的具体服务内容与形式。口腔卫生保健的基本知识与技能完全可以根据社区群众的需求以及他们和社区所能接受的能力来决定。不论他们掌握什么样的技能和达到何种水平，重要的是他们了解社区群众真正的口腔保健需要，并真心情愿地为群众服务，得到群众的信任。他们是由社区挑选出来的，并生活在他们所服务的社区之中。所以社区卫生工作者的含义十分广泛，可以由社区多方面的人员加入，在卫生保健人员严重短缺的地区可以选择群众经过短期培训来担任，在口腔医师已经过剩的发达国家和地区可以用口腔医师来担任，例如，在瑞典，由口腔医师担任初级口腔卫生保健工作；在泰国清迈地区，是从农村青年中选择志愿者经过培训或者由牙科护士来担任；在我国农村，有100多万乡村医生，其中一部分可以经过培训担任此项工作；还有学校校医，保健老师，普通老师，工厂厂医，车间卫生员，红十字会员等，经过培训都可以参加初级口腔卫生保健工作。随着初级卫生保健人员的深入发展，还可以更广泛深入地开发利用这方面的人力，比如学生中的班组卫生员，家庭主妇，退休老人等。专业口腔卫生人员在我国的数量十分有限，而且每年增加数量不多，应该充分发挥他们的专长，其主要责任应该是指导、教育、监督基层初级和中级口腔保健人员，并负责解决比较复杂的口腔医疗保健问题。

To achieve the goal of health and oral health for all in a country or a community, it is essential to have an adequate number of properly trained health workers. The development of primary oral health care depends on the attitude and capabilities of all health workers and also on a health system that is designed to support and complement the frontline workers. To carry out primary oral health care community health workers are needed, that is to say, trained health workers who live within the community and work with other health and development workers as a team. They provide the first contact between the individual and the health system. The types of community health worker vary between countries and communities according to their needs and the resources available for meeting them. In many societies these workers come from and are chosen by the community in which they work. In some countries, they work as volunteers; or they work as auxiliary workers with special training and skills in others, even primary oral health care are delivered by the dentists in Sweden. The governments should give high priority to the sufficient development of health manpower and full utilization of human resources by defining the technical role, supportive skills, and attitudes required for each category of health worker according to the functions that need to be carried out to ensure effective primary oral health care.

六、实施初级口腔卫生保健的若干问题 Operational aspects of primary oral health care

1. 核心问题 Key problems

在一个国家或地区的口腔保健系统中，应该以哪一级为核心，是初级口腔卫生保健还是中央一级（三级）？在一般情况下，初级口腔卫生保健所提供的服务内容有健康教育与口腔卫生指导，以及一些切实可行的预防措施，至于对疼痛的缓解，可以由初级卫生保健人员提供有效药物临时止痛，或作应急处理，又可以由二级或三级医疗保健机构提供急诊保健与彻底治疗。当然复杂的治疗与康复性保健提供。虽然初级口腔卫生保健的工作范围可因不同的国家和不同的社区而有所不同，但至少其基本内容是相类似的。因此，初级口腔卫生保健应是整个口腔保健系统的核心。其他各级都围绕着这个核心，它们的工作者集中在支持初级口腔卫生保健工作，使其能连续不断地提供基本口腔卫生保健。中间一级（即二级）能够解决比较复杂的问题，能够开展技术较高，比较专业性的口腔保健工作，并且在后勤供应方面给以支持。这一级由经过较高培训的人员通过培训和指导解决实际问题支持初级口腔卫生保健各方面的工作，中央一级（三级）负责制订计划和提供管理方面的专门知识，开展专业保健，培训专家，提供如中央实验室这一类机构的专业知识以及由中央给予的后勤与经费方面的支持。

Primary oral health care is the hub of the oral health system. Around it are arranged the other levels of the system whose actions converge on primary oral health care in order to support it and to permit it to provide essential oral health care in order to support it and to permit it to provide essential oral health care on a continuing basis. At the intermediate level more complex problems can be dealt with, and more skilled and specialized care as well as logistic support provided. At this level, more highly trained staff provide support through training and through guidance on practical problems that arise in connexion with all aspects of primary oral health care. The central level provides planning and managerial expertise, highly specialized care, teaching for specialist staff, the expertise of such institutions as central health laboratories, and central logistic and financial support.

2. 制定计划 Planning

制定初级口腔卫生保健计划既须在社区水平进行，也须在中级与中央一级进行。卫生部或类似机构负责制定包括初级口腔卫生保健的国家卫生政策。初级口腔卫生保健一旦被确定为重点，就必须制定和实施这一重点项目的具体策略。这种策略必须贯彻到全国范围各级水平的初级口腔卫生保健项目中去，例如，要提高无龋儿童的百分比，就必须把口腔健康教育与适当应用氟防龋以及鼓励有益于口腔健康的饮食习惯作为基本策略。在发展策略和制订项目的过程中，必须充分考虑准备采用的技术方法，动用的资源，所需要其他各级部门的支持以及整合成一体的方法。制定中央一级计划的目的是使各个社区能计划其自身的初级口腔卫生保健活动。

Planning for primary oral health care has to be carried out in communities as well as at intermediate and central levels. The ministry of health, or its equivalent is responsible for formulating national policy, including primary oral health care policy.

Wherever primary oral health care has been identified as a priority, a specific strategy is needed for its formulation and implementation. The strategy has to be translated into a nationwide primary oral health care programme embracing all levels, supportive and referral as well as community. For example, if we intend to increase the percentage of children with caries-free, the basic strategy in oral health education, appropriate use of fluoride and encouraging dietary habits beneficial to oral health should be recommended.

In developing the strategy and formulating the programme, full account has to be taken of the technologies to be used, the resources to be employed, the support needed at other levels, and the way to organize all this into a coherent system.

3. 制定社区初级口腔卫生保健计划和组织初级口腔卫生保健活动 Planning and organization of primary oral health care in a community

制定社区初级口腔卫生保健计划和组织这样的活动方式是因社区的类型、大小，以及社区组织形式而各不相同。适合于农村的解决办法可能与适合于城市社区的解决办法大不相同。然而，必须考虑到各类社区的某些共同特点。

首先，需要确定的是最适合于社区初级口腔卫生保健项目的计划，实施与控制的机制。这些机制要根据当地的政治，行政与社会状况来决定。一个共同点是有必要就职责问题达成共识，谁对项目负责，是个人还是一个委员会，如何与其他部门协调？

在确定重点项目时，哪种方法是能保证听到整个社区居民的意见？重点一旦确定，是全部付诸实施，还是分期实施？主要取决于可以利用的资源。重点项目确定之后，必须决定应用的方法与技术，使用者与获益者都能接受。决定培训人员，掌握方法，以及所需要的设备与供应等。为了控制社区项目的实施，有必要确定指导与监督的机制。

在社区初级口腔卫生保健计划与实施过程中，必须回答这些问题。

Ways of planning and organizing primary oral health care in communities will vary with the type and size of community and with its pattern of social organization. Thus, solutions applicable to small villages may be vastly different from those appropriate for large urban communities.

At first, it is necessary to decide on the most suitable mechanisms for planning, operating and controlling the community primary oral health care programme. Local political, administrative and social patterns will help to determine these mechanisms. In all cases, it is necessary to reach agreement on responsibilities, to decide who carries ultimate responsibility for the programme and whether the same individual, or committee as the case may be. How will coordination with other sectors best be ensured?

In determining priorities, what are the best ways of ensuring that the voice of the whole community is heard? And once priorities have been determined, are they to be given effect all at once or in stages? This last question will depend on the resources available. Once priorities are decided on, decisions have to be taken concerning the methods and techniques to be employed. These have to be acceptable both to those who use them and to those on whom they are used. The decisions have been taken on the methods to be employed by the workers to be trained, and to decide on the equipment and supplies required. To control the implementation of the community programme, it is necessary to decide on the mechanisms for guidance and supervision. There are some questions have to be answered in planning and operating a community primary oral health care programme.

4. 普及程度与面向社区 Coverage and accessibility

初级口腔卫生保健的目的是向全体居民提供必不可少的口腔卫生保健。人口的覆盖程度经常用计划提供的口腔保健服务与已经提供的服务之间的比例数来表示的。这样的比例经常会引起误解。因此，必须把口腔保健项目中的具体内容与需要提供的人作比较，例如，提供儿童口腔卫生指导的人数与整个社区的儿童人数比较，以便确认实际上每个儿童都可以得到这样的指导。

面向社区是指连续不断地有组织地提供全社区容易得到的口腔卫生保健而不受到地理，经费，文化与功能方面的影响。地理上面向指距离，路上花费时间与交通工具人们可以接受，经费上社区与国家均可负担得起，文化上指采用的技术与管理方式与社区文化类型一致，功能上人们需要，随时可以得到，并且由相应的卫生团队提供。衡量初级口腔卫生保健是否面向社区，不仅要看社区一级的工作，还要看口腔保健系统的其他各级机构解决较为复杂的问题的程度，因为人们需要比较复杂的医疗保健。因此，初级口腔卫生保健的全面普及是确保整个口腔卫生保健系统合理利用的一种手段。

在不同的社区以及同一个社区的不同发展阶段，面向社区显然有不同的方式，社区的每一个发展阶段都必须根据上述因素制定面向社区的衡量标准。

Primary oral health care aims at providing the whole population with essential oral health care. Population coverage has often been expressed in terms of a numerical ratio between oral health services for providing and the population to be served. Such ratios are often misleading. Therefore, it is necessary to relate the specific components of oral health care being provided to those who require them. For example, to relate the provision of children's oral hygiene instruction to the total number of children in the community, in order to make sure that such care is in farct available to all children.

Accessibility implies the continuing and organized supply of oral health care that is geographically, financially, culturally and functionally within easy reach of the whole community. Geographical accessibility means that the distance, travel time, and means of transportation are acceptable to the people. Financial accessibility means the services can be afforded by the community and the country. Cultural accessibility means that technical and managerial methods used are in keeping with the cultural patterns of the community. Functional accessibility means that the right kind of care is available on a continuing basis to those who need it, whenever they need it, and that it is provided by the oral health team required for its proper delivery.

The accessibility of primary oral health care has to be measured not only by its use at community level but also by the degree to which more complex problems can be solved, and people requiring more complex care treated, at the other levels of the oral health system. Primary oral health care that is fully and universally accessible is thus a means to ensure that the whole oral health system is used in a rational way.

It is evident that accessibility will be defined in different ways in different societies and at different degrees of development of the same society. Each society at each stage will have to define criteria for measuring accessibility in the light of the factors mentioned above.

5. 适宜卫生技术学 Appropriate health technology

初级口腔卫生保健成功的一个重要因素是应用适宜的卫生技术。"技术学"一词与方法，技术与设备有关，还有应用这些技术方法的人能够明显地有助于解决一个口腔健康问题。"适宜性"除了科学上证据可靠之外，这种技术还是使用者与获益者都是可以接受的。这种技术学应具有与当地文化保持一致的含义。如果有必要，一定能够作适当的调整以便进一步发展。这样的技术更容易为社区卫生工作者所理解和掌握。在某些情况下，甚至可以为社区个人掌握使用。虽然不同的技术适合于不同的发展阶段，但是总希望简单易行。最富有成效的途径是确保适宜技术在问题一开始就可以利用，然后去探索，是否有必要发展一种适合于当地条件与资源的技术。

口腔保健用品，以及预防技术，材料与方法，还有简单易行的治疗技术都是适宜卫生技术的重要内容。这些技术在社区为社区卫生工作者所应用应该是简单、标记与使用说明都清楚以及确保安全。

确定与发展适宜技术，必须在国家已经制订初级口腔卫生保健的目标与策略之后加以考虑，其原则是不仅适合于社区的初级口腔卫生保健，而且也适合于各级支持机构，特别是最接近社区的健康中心或区、县医院。它是国家初级口腔卫生保健政策的一部分，坚持技术适宜，鼓励地方发展，传播信息，促进广泛应用。

An important factor for the success of primary oral health care is the use of appropriate health technology. The word "technology" means an association of methods, techniques and equipment which, together with the people using them, can contribute significantly to solving a oral health problem. "appropriate" means that besides being scientifically sound the technology is also acceptable to those who apply it and to those for whom it is used. This implies that technology should be in keeping with the local culture. It must be capable of being adapted and further developed if necessary. In addition, it should preferably be easily understood and applied by community health workers, and in some instances even by individuals in the community: although different forms of technology are appropriate at different stage of development, their simplicity is always desirable. The most productive approach for ensuring that appropriate technology is available is to start with the problem and then to seek, or if necessary develop, a technology which is relevant to local conditions and resources.

Oral care products, preventive techniques, materials and methods, and simple curative techniques, are important components or oral health technology. Technology for use in the community should be simply and clearly labeled, carry clear instructions, and be safe for community health workers to use.

The identification or development of appropriate technology has to be considered when the national goal and strategy for primary oral health care is being formulated. The principle that technology should be appropriate in the sense described above applies not only to primary oral health care in the community, but also to all the supportive levels, and especially to those closest to the community, such as oral health centres or district/county dental hospitals. It is part of national primary oral health policy, to insist on technology that is appropriate, to encourage its local development, to disseminate information about it and to promote its widespread use.

6. 人力资源与培训 Human resources and training

人是任何国家和社区最重要的资源，但这种资源却往往没有得到开发。然而初级口腔卫生保健必须充分利用一切可以利用的资源，因此，必须动员整个社区可能的人力。如果个人和家庭对他们的口腔健康承担更大的责任，则这一点是可能办得到的。他们密切关心并积极参与解决他们自己的口腔健康问题，不仅是社会意识和自力更生精神的突出表现，而且也是保证初级口腔卫生保健成功的一个重要因素。由于他们个人的参与，成为口腔卫生团队的成员，他们的联合行动对初级口腔卫生保健必须开展的主要工作是必不可少的。

除了社区卫生工作者和其成员本身之外，口腔卫生团队还包括各级支持部门的人员。团队的组成将根据人群各年龄组的不同需要而有所不同，如果说初级口腔卫生保健是口腔保健系统的核心，那么，需要得到这种保健的人就是初级口腔卫生保健的核心。

在个人与卫生系统之间接触的一级水平上，初级口腔卫生保健是由社区卫生工作者组成的团队提供的。卫生工作者的类型将根据各国或各社区的需要和满足这些需要而可以利用的资源而各不相同。这样，在不同的社会，他们可能包括一些受教育水平有限，在口腔卫生保健方面只经过初步培训的人，乡村医生、护士、医士、全科医生、校医、学校老师、厂医等。

对许多发展中国家来说，要作为向全民普及必不可少的口腔卫生保健最现实的办法是使用经过短期培训而能完成具体规定的任务的社区卫生工作者。

社区卫生工作者必须经过有计划有组织的培训和定期再教育，以便使他们在开展初级口腔卫生保健工作中发挥日益重要的作用。他们的培训与复训应该根据他们面临的确切问题，预定要完成的任务以及准备采用的方法，技术与设备来进行。

经过较高培训的口腔专业人员必须用他们的技术解决根据社会需要提出的口腔卫生问题，必须对社区卫生工作者的工作进行指导、教育、与监督，并就社区的一切有关口腔卫生的问题开展宣传与教育，除了临床技能之外，他们的社会职能与教育职能增加了。

People are the most important resource of any country and community, but all too often this resource remain untapped. Primary oral health care, however, has to make full use of all available resources, and therefore has to mobilize the human potential of the entire community. This is possible on condition that individuals and families accept greater responsibility for their oral health. their active interest and participation in solving their own oral health problems are not only a clear manifestation of social awareness and self-reliance but are also an important factor in ensuring the success of primary oral health care. By their involvement, individuals become full members of the oral health team, whose joint action is essential to make the most of what primary oral health care has to offer.

In addition to community health workers and members of the community themselves, the oral health team will include personnel in establishments at the supporting levels. The composition of the team will vary according to the varying needs of groups of the population, for if primary oral health care is the hub of the oral health system, people in need care are the hub of primary oral health care.

At the first level of contact between individuals and the oral health care system, primary oral health care is provided by community health workers acting as a team. The types of health worker will vary by country and community according to needs and the resources available for satisfying them. Thus, they may include in different societies people with limited education who have been given elementary training in oral health care, village doctors, nurses, assistant doctors, or general medical practitioners, school doctors and teachers, and manufactory doctors, etc.

For many developing countries, the most realistic solution for attaining total population coverage with essential oral health care is to employ community health workers who can be trained in a short time to perform specific tasks.

Community health workers have to be trained and retrained in a planning and organized programme, so that they can play a progressively more important role in providing primary oral health care. Their training and retraining should be based on a clear definition of the problems involved, the tasks to be performed, and the methods, techniques and equipment to be used.

The responsibilities of more highly trained oral health professionals are to apply their technical skills to solve oral health problems determined in the light of social needs, to guide, teach and supervise community health workers, and to educate communities on all matters pertaining to their oral health. They are therefore given social and educational functions in addition to their technical functions.

7. 其他方面的问题 Other relevant aspects

（1）转诊系统 Referral system

社区内的初级口腔卫生保健活动应得到逐级转诊系统的支持。对转诊单位，特别是口腔卫生系统中初级口腔卫生保健的上一级单位必须给予更多的考虑。尤其有必要评价口腔保健中心和县／区级口腔医院的职能，人员编制，制定计划，设计项目，设备，组织与管理，以便扩大其职能范围，支持初级口腔卫生保健。这些包括继续教育，指导和监督社区卫生工作者并对社区进行口腔健康教育。

Primary oral health care activities in the community should be supported by successive levels of referral facilities. Additional thought will have to be given to referral facilities, and especially to the establishments that constitute the link next to primary oral health care in the oral health system chain. In particular, there is a need to review the functions, staffing, planning, design, equipment, organization and management of oral health centres and county or district dental hospitals, in order to prepare them for their wider function in support of primary oral health care. They will include the continuing training, guidance, and supervision of community health workers as well as the education of the community in oral health matters.

（2）后勤供应 Logistics of supply

一旦决定采纳初级口腔卫生保健，就必须按轻重缓急的原则向社区供应物资。物资供应的逻辑程序包括制定计划、编制预算、采购或生产、储存、发放与控制。

初级卫生保健所需要的物质条件可以很简单，但必须十分清洁。

Once the decision has been taken to adopt primary oral health care, it is necessary to make supplies available to communities on a priority basis. The logistics of supplies include planning, and budgeting for the supplies required, procumbent or manufacture, storage, distribution and control.

The physical facilities required for primary oral health care may be very simple, but they must be very clean.

(3) 管理程序 Management process

为了确保初级口腔卫生保健的原则能够付诸实施，需要制定一个管理程序。这个程序包括制定计划和项目、编制预算、筹措资金、控制实施、评价、研究、必要时重新制定计划。

To make sure that the principles of primary oral health care translated into practice, a managerial process is required. This includes planning, programming, budgeting, financing, control of implementation, evaluation, research, re-planning if necessary.

(4) 编制预算 Budgeting

编制预算是一个关键性步骤，因为预算要对所需要的资源做出估计并调拨那些可以利用的资源，以便将某种意图变成为口腔卫生系统各级机构实现项目的具体行动。因而，编制预算必须确保把资源优先调拨给初级口腔卫生保健，从社区开始，逐步到各级机构。

按预算调拨资源，必须同时交代任务和授予职权。

Budgeting is a key step because it estimates required resources and allocates those available in such a way as to transform an intention into concrete realization of the programme at the various levels of the oral health system. Thus, budgeting has to ensure the preferential allocation of resources to primary oral health care, starting from communities and progressing through the other levels.

Budgetary allocations need to be accompanied by simultaneous delegation of responsibility and authority.

8. 评价 Evaluation

为了确保初级口腔卫生保健正常开展，并在实践过程中吸取教训，用以改进初级口腔卫生保健项目，必须建立一个评价过程。

评价有几个方面。首先需要评价的是所开展的活动与项目的社会指导思想一致性的相关程度。然后，对按计划开展的活动所取得的进展进行分析以便促进对项目运作的控制。评估项目进展的效率，目的在于通过对所花费人力，时间，经费与技术做出的努力与所得到的结果作比较以改进项目的实施。评价项目的效果，目的在于测量某些严重状况减轻的程度或者社区口腔健康状况改善的程度，包括评价社区参与项目的程度，以及对项目满意的程度。影响是指项目对社区全面社会经济发展所起的作用。

In order to ensure that primary oral health care is functioning properly and that lessons learned in the course of its operation are used to improve the programme, a process of evaluation has to build in.

Evaluation has several components. It is first necessary to review the relevance of the activities being carried out in terms of their consistency with the social philosophy of the programme. Then, an analysis is made of progress in carrying out activities as planned in order to facilitate operational control. Assessment of the efficiency with which the programme is being carried out aims at improving implementation by comparing the results obtained with the efforts expended, the latter being expressed in terms of people, time, money, and health technologies. It includes the measure of the extent to which facilities are actually being used. Review of the effectiveness of the programme aims at measuring the extent to which it appears to be reducing the severity of specific conditions or improving the oral health situation in the community. It could also include an assessment of the degree of community participation in the programme and satisfaction with it. Impact is an expression of the effect the programme is having on the overall socioeconomic development of the community.

需要选择测量变化的一些指标和针对采取的行动之后可以进行比较的各种标准。例如，必须规定评价社区儿童应用含氟牙膏每天早晚刷牙2次覆盖率增加的指标或者改善儿童口腔健康状况的指标。另一个例子是初级口腔卫生保健的目的之一是普遍享有基本口腔卫生保健，必须制订标准来评估普及的程度，可以根据前面提到的影响因素来制订评价指标与标准。如果没有，还可以设计简单的问卷调查，例如“氟水含漱方法是否儿童实际上可以接受？”或者“社区所有的群众都可以利用社区的口腔保健设施以及是否利用适当？”

There is a need for certain indicators to measure change, and various criteria against which actions can be compared. For example, indicators have to be defined to asses any increase in the coverage of community children with fluoridated toothpaste to be used, or improvement in the oral health statues of children. As another example, since one of the aims of primary oral health care is universal accessibility of essential oral health care, criteria have to be developed to assess accessibility, based for example on the factors mentioned above. When formal indicators or criteria are not available, asking simple questions can often be useful, such as “are the methods of mouth-rinsing being used really acceptable to children?” or “do all people in fact have access to the facilities and are they using them properly?”

总之，对初级口腔卫生保健工作定期进行评价可以围绕以下几个方面的问题：

（1）项目或活动是否达到了群众公认的需求？

（2）所通过的保健内容是否是群众所要求和可以接受的？

（3）项目或活动是否对提高群众的口腔健康水平有帮助，或者已经有了提高或改善？

（4）社区是否能经过努力，可以长期提供这样的保健或者还可以增加哪些新的服务内容？

In summary, for assessment of the progress in primary oral health care in a certain period of time, there are several questions which may be answered as follows:

(1) whether the programmes or activities have met the public recognized needs or demand?

(2) whether the content of primary oral health care is required by the people and being acceptable or not?

(3) whether the programmes or activities can help the people to being improve their oral health status, or has raised, or improved oral health levels?

(4) whether the community could provide such care for a long term by their efforts or which new issues of services could also be added?

第二节　社区口腔卫生保健

Section 2 Community Oral Health Care

1991年WHO的一个专家委员会的报告中指出“口腔卫生保健最主要的进展之一是逐渐强调它的科学基础，并且还指出口腔医学已经变成为口腔卫生保健”。1994年世界口腔卫生日期间，WHO又一次召开了专家委员会会议，发表了21世纪的口腔健康文件，指出“新世纪的挑战是保持和加强我们的成功之处，并且采取更加有效的机制使所有的社区，不论贫富，工业化还是发展之中，快速还是缓慢老龄化的社区，都能从我们终生保持最佳口腔健康的能力中获益。”2003年WHO的世界口腔健康报告文件中又进一步指出“不断增进21世纪的口腔健康”，并提出通过“共同危险因素途径”这一新策略预防和控制口腔疾病。那么，在社区水平上，把口腔卫生纳入到整个社区卫生服务之中可能是一个最佳的试验场所，或称为社区模式。

A report of a WHO Expert Committee addressed that “one of the most fundamental advances in oral health care has been the increasing emphasis on its scientific basis, and as a result “dentistry” has become “oral health care” in 1991. During the World Oral Health Day in 1994, a document on oral health for the 21st Century presented by a WHO expert committee's meeting, also pointed out that the challenge for the new century is to maintain and even to intensify our success and to install more efficient mechanisms to also all communities rich and poor, industrialized and developing, aging rapidly or slowly to benefit from our capabilities to maintain excellent oral health throughout life. A World oral health report for 2003 on the title of continuous improvement of oral health in the 21st century by a new strategy of the common risk factor approach for managing prevention and control of oral diseases. Therefore, at the community level, oral health integrated into community health services may be on optimal demonstration field, or called as a community model.

一、口腔公共卫生 Oral public health

口腔专业的目标是保护和保持公众的口腔健康。口腔公共卫生在美国是口腔医学8大专业之一。美国口腔公共卫生委员会采取了Winslow的公共卫生定义，并提出了口腔公共卫生的定义。口腔公共卫生是整个公共卫生的一部组成部分，直接受到公共卫生项目与政策的影响，美国疾病控制中心列出的20世纪十大公共卫生事件中，其中自1945年开始的饮水氟化就是10大事件之一。因为它在降低美国儿童的龋病（40%～70%）减少成人失牙（40%～60%）方面发挥了重要的作用。其他九大事件中免疫注射、汽车安全、工作场所安全、控制感染性疾病、降低冠心病与中风的死亡率、安全与健康的食品、母保健婴、计划生育、以及认识烟草为健康的危险因素。

早在1920年Winslow提出一个被广泛应用的公共卫生定义：公共卫生是一门科学和艺术，它从环境卫生，传染病控制，健康教育，医疗与护理服务机构对疾病的早期诊断，预防和治疗，发展社区机构，保证每个人适当的生活标准诸方面，通过有组织的全社区努力，达到预防疾病，延年益寿，促进健康与提高工作效率，并且以这样一种方式组织社会福利事业，使每个公民都能享有生来就有的健康长寿的权利。

The goal of the dental profession is to protect and preserve the oral health of the public. Dental or dental public health is one of the eight specialists of dentistry in the united states. The American Board of Dental Public Health adapted Winslow's definition to develop one definition of dental public health. Dental public health is an integral component of public health and is directly affected by public health programme and polices. The centres for Disease Control and prevention (CDC) selected a public health "top 10 list" for the twentieth century. Fluoridation of drinking water, which was initiated in 1945 is on the list because it has played an important role in the reduction of tooth decay in children (40% to 70%) and of tooth loss in adults (40% to 60%) in the united states. The other nine are vaccinations, motor-vehicle safety, safe work places, control of infectious diseases, decline in deaths from coronary heart disease and stroke, safer and healthier foods, healthier mothers and babies, family planning, and recognition of tobacco use as a health hazard.

As early as in 1920 Winslow developed a widely used definition of public health: the science and art of preventing disease, prolonging life, and promoting physical and mental efficiency through organized community effort for the sanitation of the environment, the control of communicable infections, the education of the individual in personal hygiene, the organization of medical and nursing services for the early diagnosis and preventive treatment of disease, and the development of the social machinery to insure everyone a standard of living adequate for the maintenance of health, so organizing these benefits as to enable every citizen to realize his birthright of health and longevity.

这个定义对 Winslow 认识到的社会，教育与经济因素对健康的影响有更深的理解。最近 20 年来公共卫生的重点已经在改变。在整个世界范围内，一个值得注意的倾向之一是在一国之内和国家之间在经济与社会条件方面增加了贫富之间的差距。因此公共卫生的重点之一是通过机构内的工作如城市或学校推动建立健康的环境。目的是增强社区行动，发展个人健康保护的技能。

在发展中国家，公共卫生被看作为一个复杂的领域，其中社会条件，如贫困，对未来失望，一个以自我为中心的社会，以及经济影响正日益变得重要。同时现代医学已经更多地退回到它自身的专业范畴之内。不只是生存，而是生命质量已经变成为公共卫生的核心内容；另一方面，传统的公共卫生概念已经扩展到不仅包括全体人口的健康，而且包括人群中个人的健康。

This definition shows great understanding in that Winslow recognized the impact of social, education and economic factors on health. over the last 20 years the focus of public health has been changing. One of the notable trends, common across the world, has been the increasing difference between the rich and poor economic and social conditions both within and between countries. Therefore, one of the focuses in public health is to promote the establishment of healthy environments by working in settings such as cities and schools. The aim is to strengthen community action and develop personal skills for health protection.

In developing countries, public health is seen as a complex area in which social conditions such as poverty, the absence of hope for the future, a self-centered society and economic influences are increasingly important. At the same time, modern medicine has retreated more and more into its own professional domain. Quality of life and not just survival has become a core issue for public health. on the other hand, traditional concept of public health is expanded to include, "the health of the individual in addition to the health of populations".

口腔公共卫生的定义规定为：通过有组织的社区努力，预防和控制口腔疾病，促进口腔健康的科学与艺术。这就是口腔实践的形式把社区作为一个病人服务于社区而不是个人。它关系到群众的口腔健康教育，研究与应用研究的发展，人群的口腔保健项目管理，通过社区途径预防和控制口腔疾病。

近年来，口腔公共卫生已经把它的重点扩大到包括口腔保健供给系统以及它对口腔健康状况的影响。

The definition of dental public health is defined as the science and art of preventing and controlling dental disease and promoting dental health through organized community efforts. It is that form of dental practice that serves the community as a patient rather than the individual. It is concerned with the dental health education of the public, with research and the application of the findings of research, with the administration of programmes of dental care for groups, and with the prevention and control of dental disease through a community approach.

Dental public health recently has expanded its focus to include the dental care delivery system and its impact on oral health status.

从上述情况看口腔公共卫生与社区口腔卫生二个词汇经常交互使用存在着口腔的差异。但是社区与公众意味着一群人，一个人群或一组人，有些事是共同的。从这个观点考虑，公共卫生与社区卫生可以认为是同等的。然而，现在的使用趋于“公众”意味着整个一群人而并没有考虑他们生活的具体地理区域。而“社区”则认为是生活在一个特定地理区域之内的一个人群中一群人，有一定的范围。所以，口腔公共卫生与社区口腔卫生保健实际需要解决的都是人群的口腔保健问题，其目标策略，途径，过程与结果都是一样的，所不同的仅仅是一个区域的限定或不限定而已。

The concepts and the explanations indicated that both terms of dental public health and community oral health often are used interchangeably, a distinct difference exists between them. Both community and public mean a collection of people, a population, or a group of people having something in common. From that perspective the terms public health and community health can be considered equivalent. Current usage, however, tends to define "public" to mean a general collection of people without regard to a specific geographic area in which they live. Community is used to indicate a collection of people who are located in a defined geographic area. Therefore, dental public health and community oral health care is actually required to deal with oral health problems of the population, in which the objective, strategy, approach, process and results are all the same, only one difference is within a defined area or without such a limitation.

二、社区与社区口腔保健 Community and community oral health care

（一）社区 Community

社区是西方社会学、政治学、人类学等许多学科常用的一个术语。有的学者曾对社区的90个定义进行了对比分析，发现其中唯一的共同要素是“人”。有人把社区大至一个完整的社会系统，小至一个社会组织，社会团体甚至某些具体的单位相提并论。有的则明确指出社区与社会或社会体系完全同义。有些学者完全按生物学的观点定义社区把生物分布，生存条件和自然环境作为划分社区的基本要素。有人从文化发展的角度把不同的文化传统，生活方式，价值观念以及社会风俗等作为社区规定的主要成分。也有人把生物学观点与文化要素结合起来，从两个方面来确定社区的定义。目前比较普遍的定义是社区是一个功能相互联系在一起的人类群体，他们在某一特定时期生活于某个特定地区处于相同的社会结构中，具有基本上一致的文化传统和价值观念，共同感觉到自己是一个具有相对独立性和一定自治性的社会群体。

Community as a special term is often used by many disciplines such as sociology, politics, and anthropology in the western societies. About the definitions of the community, some scholar made a comparative analysis on 90 definitions of it, and only one common element of "human being" was identified from them. Someone mentioned in the same breath that it could be a complete social system as maximum, and it could also be a social organization, social groups, and even some special units as minimum. Other one point out clearly that it is in same meaning whether or not community, society, or social systems. Following the biological perspective, some researchers defined the community by the biological distribution, survival conditions and natural environments as the essential elements of it. From the cultural development point of view, some defined the community by different cultural traditions, lifestyle, values, and social customs as the essential components of it. Moreover, other researchers defined the definition of the community from two dimensions of biological perspective combined with cultural elements. At present, the relative common definition of the community is the functional interrelationship among human groups, they are living in a special areas of the same social structure at a certain period of time, with a fundamental consistency in cultural tradition and values, and commonly feeling themselves as a relative in dependent and a certain autonomous social group.

社区的划分可能比较容易也可能比较难以确定。如果就是为了一个具体的邻近居民（不论它是否在社会学意义上组成一个实际的社区）。在工厂工作的工人，在学校里学习的儿童，或者还有其他人群，提供口腔卫生保健服务，这样的社区定义最容易，登记的人作为附近的口腔保健或者口腔保健中心提供服务的对象也可以看作为一个社区。如果对一个具体的人群没有规定职责。那么，定义一个社区就非常困难，在这种情况下，为了开展社区口腔卫生保健的目的，就可以把需要口腔保健的人，最近已经看过牙的人，或者需要继续保健的人，还有某些规定的人群可以看作为一个服务社区。总之，从实现情况出发，社区的定义应该是灵活的。

The community may be easy or hard to define. Its definition is easiest if the oral health care services for the residents of a specific neighbourhood (whether or not they constitute a true community in the sociological sense) , workers in specific places of employment, children in specific schools, or other specific groups. People registered as potential users of the services of a given dental group practice, or neighbourhood oral health centre may also be regarded as a "community" for whose oral care the practice is responsible. Definition is most difficult where there is no defined responsibility for a specific population; in such instances the aggregate of people who seek oral care, or those who have sought care recently, or those who seek care repeatedly, or some defined group of them, may be regarded as the "community" for oral health are purposes. In general, from real situation to define, the definition of community should be a certain flexible.

（二）社区口腔医学 Community dentistry

社区口腔医学或称社会口腔医学是现代口腔医学发展的一个分支，它以口腔医学为基础，采用社会调查与社会实践的途径研究口腔医学与社会学的相互关系，研究社会环境与社会因素与人群口腔健康的关系以及相互制约，相互作用规律的学科，它是在预防口腔医学的基础上发展起来的，是口腔医学社会化的重要标志，其研究对象和重点是人群口腔健康状况的变化，影响口腔健康与口腔患病的社会因素，以群体预防与健康教育为主，包括适当的治疗，修复与康复性保健。口腔医学社会化的一个基本点是把口腔卫生保健事业纳入整个社会发展的总体系统之内。社区口腔医学是为研究和制订社会口腔卫生保健发展总体规划，目标，策略，措施与方法的选择，更新观念提供理论依据，为培养 21 世纪的新型口腔专业人员提供基本理论，知识和方法。因此，在许多国家的大学牙学院内社会口腔医学作为一门独立的学科建制而被命名为教研室的名称，取代了预防牙医学这个较为传统的名称。当然，也有不少院校仍然保持着这门学科的名称，但显然，在其内容上也向社区领域扩展了。开设这门课程的主要目的是增强新一代口腔专业人员为社区群体服务的意识，以及为社区群体工作的技能。

社区口腔医学是确定、研究和解决有关社会人群口腔健康问题的一门科学和艺术，它可以立足于任何一个具体的社区全体人群或各个年龄组，通常采用社会调查，口腔健康流行病学调查和社会流行病学调查以及统计学方法等对社区人群的口腔健康状况及其相关问题作出社会分析，社会诊断并通过预防策略与措施的选择和确定以及有效的科学管理程序，发展口腔保健项目，开展社区口腔保健活动，提供社会口腔保健服务，满足社区人群的口腔保健需求，保持并进而改善一个社区的总体口腔健康状况。

Community dentistry is a developing brand of modern dentistry, it is based on traditional dentistry, and by using social survey and social practical approach to study the interrelationship between dentistry and sociology, and to study the relationship between social environment and social factors, and oral health of social groups, and to explore the inter, and interaction between them. It is developed on the basis of preventive dentistry, and an important indication of dental socialization and the subject and priority to be studied is the change of oral health in the population and influencing factors in oral health and diseases, it mainly focuses on group prevention and health education, including appropriate treatment, restorative and rehabilitative care. A basic principle of dental socialization is to integrate oral health into the whole community development system. Community dentistry is to provide theoretical basis for study, and formulization of general goals, objectives, strategies, measures, and methods by selection and renew the ideas in order to provide basic theory, knowledge and skills of new type of oral health professionals for the new century. Therefore, in many dental schools in the world, community dentistry as an independent discipline named department of community dentistry, instead of preventive dentistry as a traditional terms which still exist in other dental schools in some countries, but the content has been extended forward community sector. The main purpose of offering this subject is to produce these new types of oral health professionals with awareness of community group services and community working skills.

Community dentistry is a science and art that identifying, studying and solving oral health problems in related to the whole community members, or age groups usually community surveys, oral health epidemiological survey and social epidemiological survey and statistical methods are used to make a community situation analysis and community diagnosis through oral health status and their relevant problems of the community population, and by selecting and identifying preventive strategies and measures and effective scientific managerial procedures for the development of oral health care programmes and oral health activities and providing community oral health services for meeting the needs of oral care of the whole community members in order to maintain and to improve all their oral health status in the whole community.

（三）社区口腔卫生保健 Community oral health care

它是以一定人群的口腔健康状况改善与提高为目标，以生物心理社会三维结构的医学模式概念为基础，以社区的社会经济文化为背景，以三级医疗保健网为依托，以初级卫生保健为基本途径，以社区群体防治为主要策略，建立并逐步发展农村县、乡、村或城市的市、区、街道或者与之相应的三级口腔保健网，并通过社区试点研究，建立，发展与完善一定的口腔卫生保健服务提供系统，实现社区人人享有最基本的口腔卫生保健目标。

It is targeted on the improvement and strength of oral health status of a certain population, and based on the conceptual model in three dimensions of biological psychological and social structure, within the social, economic and cultural background of the community, and rely on three levels of medical care network, and basic approach of primary health care, and prevention and appropriate treatment for the community groups as the main strategies, to setting up, gradually developing a relevant three levels of oral health care network subsystem at the county, township and village in the rural areas or the city, district, and neighbourhood in the urban areas, and through a study on the community demonstration, to establish, to further develop, and to consummate an appropriate oral health care delivery system for achieving goal of essential oral health care for all members in the community.

三、社区口腔保健模式构架 An essential model structure for community oral health care

模式（model）是对所研究的某个实体或系统进行抽象说明，模仿与表达的一种手段。社区口腔保健模式就是通过社区试点研究，对某个社区的口腔保健服务提供系统作概括说明，并阐述这一系统的基本特征。因此，作为一种模式，既有许多共性问题，又有多样性，从而形成了多种可供选择的模式。

每一种模式都以健康概念作指导，形成一定的社区与个人健康目标：以自我口腔保健为基础，初级卫生保健为途径，以及以其支持系统为后盾，以口腔健康干预指数为标准，形成社区口腔健康目标管理，以模拟培训为基本手段，形成合理的培训系统，培训各种人员，为社区所有的人提供预防性口腔保健服务，并对已患病者提供适当治疗，使疾病停止在早期阶段，防止丧失口腔功能改变传统的口腔医学基本方法，尽可能提供非侵入性保健，必须能达到影响人们的生活方式，促进并保持口腔健康，预防和控制口腔疾病。因此，在任何情况下，预防项目必须成为重点。只有在预防项目不成功时，才采用修复与治疗性保健措施，尽可能防止功能丧失。

Each model is guided by the concept of health, and formulating a specific health objectives for both community and individuals: based on oral self-care, primary health care as approach, and its supportive systems as backup force, oral health status intervention index as a criteria, setting up the management by objective of community oral health, and simulated training as the basic methods, to forming a logistic training system for training a variety of health workers to provide preventive oral care services for all members of the community, and appropriate treatment for the ill persons to suspend the process of disease at the early stage and to prevent loss of oral function, and to change the traditional treatment methods and provide noninvasive care if possible and it must be able to influence the people's lifestyle, promoting and maintaining oral health, preventing and controlling oral diseases. Therefore, in any case, preventive programme must be at the priority, and the restorative and rehabilitative care could be provided, only when the preventive programme is fail, as possible as it can prevent loss of function.

口腔卫生保健模式的形成是依据初级卫生保健的概念，以及实现人人享有卫生保健的战略目标。这一模式的基本结构分为三个水平——初级卫生保健（含一级预防），二级卫生保健（含二级预防），三级卫生保健（含三级预防）。虽然在不同地区，不同情况下，他们之间的差别可能较大，但至少这三个水平的活动是互相补充的。这一模式的基本构成要素，亦是按这三个水平的顺序组成的。

Elements of the essential oral health care model

① Promotion oral health through lifestyles that are conducive to health

② Priority for prevention through health protection

③Community involvement and leadership; attention to social acceptability and economic feasibility

④ Integration of oral and general health

⑤ Access by all people to primary oral health care

⑥ Maximum self-care, promoting self-sufficiency

⑦ Regular public interaction through

(a) Information from the people (examination and survey)

(b) Information to the people (including quality of life messages and the promotion of health awareness)

(c) Education and instruction to the community and individuals

*⑧ Minimal intervention focused upon surface care**

⑨ Referral as appropriate and feasible

⑩ Employment of appropriate personnel and technology

⑪ First referral level

(a) General restorative and rehabilitative care

(b) Actions complementary to each of the primary health care level services, as required

(c) Specialized services not feasible at the first referral level

**Surface care is taken here to mean non-invasive preventive and/or treatment measures that are applied to the surfaces of oral structures (as opposed to surgical procedures)*

The oral health care model is based on the primary health care concept and achieving the strategic goal of health for all. Three levels of care model can be identified-primary health care (including primary prevention) , first referral (second level, including secondary prevention) and second, or final referral (third level, including 3rd level prevention) . Although distinctions between them will vary in different situations and in different communities or regions. Activities at the three levels should be complementary. Elements of the essential oral health cares model are in sequence of events rather than in order of priority.

（一）初级口腔卫生保健水平 First level of oral health care

初级口腔卫生保健的目标应该是帮助人们保持良好的健康状态而不是等待疾病发生后才不得不采取行动。最理想的是全体人口都能定期得到检查，为了完成此项工作任务，可以在社区人群集居场所建立联络点-如学校，工作地点与社区中心或卫生中心。如不可行，应该找其他的条件和机会。总的目的是建立的联络点应为社区提供最大的方便。

在项目开始阶段很可能重点要放在社区的目标人群或重点人群（学校儿童、孕妇、青少年，或者其他社区慈善机构的人们），政策应该是每户至少检查一人，确保“定期联系以保持健康”的概念传播到整个社区。

The objective at the primary oral health care level should be to assist in maintaining good oral health rather than to wait until problems of ill health necessitate action. Ideally, the whole population should be examined regularly; the contacts necessary to achieve this can be established at the usual community gathering places-schools, workplaces and health or community centres. Where this is not possible, other situations and opportunities should be sought. Overall aim should be to provide contact points of maximum convenience to the community.

初级阶段包括有一定标准的内容如下：

1. 检查

通过检查可以提供有关监测个人与社会的信息，并且可以记录和解释个人的健康状况。通过检查也可以发现少见而又严重的病情以及某些社区的高危人群，如学龄前或学龄儿童，老人，或在慈善机构里的那些人。

In the initial phase of the programme, which will probably concentrate on target or priority groups in the community (school children, pregnant women, adolescents or institutionalized people) , the policy should be to examine at least one person in every household. This will ensure that the concept of "regular contact to keep healthy" is disseminated to the whole community. The initial phase comprises certain standard elements as follows.

Examination provides monitoring information about individuals and about the community, and allows the health status of individuals to be recorded and explained. It also allows the identification of rare, but serious, conditions and in some communities, of high risk groups such as preschool or school children, the elderly, or those in institutions.

2. 自我保健

为了保持个人健康，适当的自我保健活动，有时结合表面保健（非侵入性）或转诊保健是需要的。这些活动包括：

- 针对龋病与牙周病的正确的口腔卫生方法；
- 适当应用氟化物（例如，含氟牙膏或含氟漱口液）增强口内的硬体组织；
- 注意饮食，以减少龋病的发生率以及降低龋病的严重程度。

Self-care. Appropriate self-care activities, sometimes together with surface (non-invasive) or referral care, are needed to maintain individual health. such activities include:

- *Correct mouth-cleaning to combat caries and periodontal diseases;*
- *Appropriate use of fluorides (for example in toothpaste or in rinses) to reinforce the hard tissues in the mouth;*
- *Dietary prudence to reduce the frequency and severity of caries attack.*

3. 信息

用检查的简要数据通过大众化语言向社区领导与管理人员说明社区口腔健康状况及医疗需要。采取实际而又适当的社区措施预防疾病和促进健康-如，饮水或食盐氟化或必要时饮水除氟-可以讨论。以便这些措施能在政治上得到支持并使项目能够实施。数据也应该涉及维持一个健康社区所采取的各种途径的成本问题。

Information. Summarized data from examinations can be used in explaining the oral health status and treatment needs of the community in non-professional language to community leaders and administrators. Realistic and appropriate community measures for disease prevention and health promotion-such as water or salt fluoridation or water defluoridation as necessary-maybe discussed, so that political support for such measures can be mobilized and programmes implemented. Data should also deal with the cost implications of various approaches for maintaining a healthy community.

4. 高危与特危人群

应该为发生常见的或严重的口腔疾病的个人提供有关的预防措施和由于对疾病的不重视可能产生的后果方面的信息，也应该得到必要的保持口腔健康进行自我保健的指导。还应制定转诊治疗与定期检查的计划，适当的次数与疾病发病的水平相一致。

High and special risk. Individuals at high or special risk of developing common or serious oral diseases should be given information about preventive measures and about the likely consequences of neglect; they should also receive instruction in the self-care necessary to maintain the health of their oral fissures. Referral schedules and "check up" examinations should be programmed for such individuals, with a frequency appropriate to prevailing disease levels.

5. 表面保健

表面（非侵入性）口腔卫生保健包括一系列规程，如应用窝沟封闭，与局部用氟，预防或停止龋病发展。洁治有助于控制牙周病，组织基本服务的责任应该由社区负责，以便能最大限度地适合于当地的情况与生活方式。

Surface care. Surface (or non-invasive) oral health care includes a range of procedures, such as use of sealants and topical fluorides, to prevent or arrest caries, and scaling to assist in controlling periodontal disease. The responsibility for organizing basic services should rest at community level, so that there is maximum adaptation to local conditions and lifestyles.

6. 人员

在已经有口腔保健人员的地方，口腔检查，指导自我保健，以及最基本的保健任务可以由牙科辅助人员（卫生士，治疗员）或口腔医师来完成。还有，其他卫生工作者如乡村医生，社区护士，学校卫生人员以及慈善机构的护理人员等也能作为他们现有任务的扩展，提供这类服务。

Personnel. Where there are already oral care personnel, examinations, self-care instruction and minimal-care tasks may be performed by dental auxiliaries (hygienists, therapists) or dentists. Otherwise, health workers such as village doctors, community nurses, school health personnel and institutional nursing staff could provide these services as an extension of their existing tasks.

7. 结果

在头两年提供最低限度的干预性保健，在社区需要这类服务的人数百分比可能很高，然而，随着项目的进展，这个比例应该有较大的减少，这样项目就可以逐渐集中到高危人群。预期可以得到很好的结果。因此，在初级卫生保健取得成功的地方，需要一级转诊保健干预的人数预期会减少。其余的保健需要，应该划入所有社区的经济资源来考虑。

Effect. During the first two years or so of the provision of minimal interventive care, a high percentage of the community is likely to need the service. With a successful programme, however, this proportion should reduce considerably, so that the programme can then concentrate increasingly on high-risk individuals. A progressive effect can be expected. Thus, where primary health care activities are successfully introduced, the need for interventive care at the first referral level can be expected to decline. Residual care needs at the both primary health and first referral levels should then be brought within the economic resources of all communities.

（二）二级口腔卫生保健水平或称一级转诊水平 Second level of oral health care

在一级转诊水平上，修复与康复性保健，是在适当的自我保健已经进行，初级卫生保健已经提供了检查与最基本的干预活动之后，作为一种补充。应该在有固定的，多种操作设施的场所组织，这样可以进行常规质量控制，达到合理使用各种不同技能的团队成员，正确使用并保养设备。在当地情况需要的时候，如农村人口分散，公共交通很不方便，流动服务成为一种可以考虑的选择。应该在明确的指导下选择推荐的保健，应该设计服务内容，确保人群不依赖昂贵的保健-否则反复往来可能会对口腔健康产生负面影响，由经过很好培训的人员进行修复与康复性保健，经过严格的质量控制。一旦任何初期积压下来的没有治疗的情况得到了处理之后，应该能把口腔保健需要减至最少。

Second level of oral health care (or first referral level)

At the referral level, restorative and rehabilitative care that is complementary to the examination and minimal interventive activities at the primary health care level may be provided when adequate self-care has been demonstrated. This should be organized in fixed, multi-operator facilities, so as to permit routine quality control, and ideally, achieve rational use of the different specific skills of the team members and the correct use and maintenance of equipment. Where warranted by local conditions, such as a scattered rural population with little public transport available, mobile services become an option to consider.

Recommended care options should be the subject of clear guidelines and should be designed to ensure that the population does not become dependent on an expensive care repair cycle that may have negative effects on oral health. restorative and rehabilitative care, provided by well trained teams of personnel and with strict quality control, should succeed in progressively reducing oral care needs to a minimum once any initial backlog of untreated conditions has been care for.

（三）三级口腔卫生保健水平（二级转诊水平）Third level of oral health care

依据可以利用的资源，可能只能由二级转诊水平提供的保健种类，包括肿瘤，创伤处理，遗传性缺陷，错殆畸形，以及复杂的修复问题，牙髓病以及康复。

Third level of oral health care (second referral level)

Depending on the available resources, types of care that might be provided only at the second referral level include treatment of neoplasm, and management of trauma, congenital defects, malocclusions and complex problems in prosthetics, endodontics and rehabilitation.

四、社区口腔保健模式的评价 Evaluation of community oral health care models

口腔保健项目的组织可以用一种结构 - 过程 - 结果模式进行分析，采用这个模式，可以开发，管理和评价所有的卫生系统研究，教育与服务方面，如果不提出这三个要素的任何一个，那么，要了解一个项目的成功是困难的。

The organization of oral health care programmes may be analysed in terms of a structure-process-outcome model. Health systems, research, education, and services may all be developed, managed and evaluated using this model. It is difficult to understand a programme successfully if any of the three elements is not addressed.

1. 结构 Structure

在一个社会系统内结构的种类可以确定为包括，或者可以叙述为权力结构，交流结构，政治结构或者经济结构，如政府组织，卫生组织，口腔卫生项目组织，以及社区组织，这样，它们可以以国家、省、或社区水平而存在。

Types of structure that may be identified within a social system include, or may be described as, authority structures, communication structures, political structures or economic structures, such as government organizations, health organizations, oral health programme organizations. Thus, they may exist at national, provincial or community level.

2. 过程 Process

在口腔（与一般）卫生保健服务组织中包含中 5 个基本过程：

- 获得信息，即来自单独研究与系统调查（科学研究）的监测资料；
- 传播信息，例如，通过教学，示范，写作，公布渠道；
- 应用知识与技能，即提供卫生保健与相关服务，像环境控制（例如，调节氟水平，控制有害物质等）以及保健品生产；
- 通过专业人员的道德，法律，规章，政策，指南，准则与标准的应用作出判断或评价；
- 管理，即人员，设施，材料，经费与其他促进上述 4 个过程的资源的管理。

Five fundamental processes are involved in the organization of oral (and) general health care services:

① Acquisition of information, i.e. monitoring data, from independent study and systematic inquiry (scientific research)

② Dissemination of information, e,g. by teaching, demonstrating, writing, publicizing

③ Application of knowledge and skills, i.e. provision of health care and related services such as environmental control (e.g. fluoride adjustment, regulation of harmful substances, etc.) and manufac-

ture of health products.

④ Judgment or evaluation by the application of professional ethics, laws, regulations, policies, guidelines, criteria and standards

⑤ Administration, i.e. the management of personnel, facilities, materials, funds and other resources to facilitate the four processes outlined above.

3. 结果 Outcome

在分析一个口腔公共卫生项目的结果中，公众的期望是一个明显的因素，可以在四个不同的水平上作出评价：

♦ 顺从：这里主要的要求是急诊保健，与提供者没有联系，绝对超出了基本的要求

♦ 取代或替换：主要的要求是拔牙与义齿修复。口腔医学可以帮助口腔保健人员在提供了控制疼痛的服务之后，恢复功能与外观。

♦ 修复：主要的要求是口腔修复学，包括固定修复，正畸与牙周治疗。因为牙齿有价，希望口腔保健人员保存它们。然而，应该指出的是必须通过个人的继续努力来维持治疗的结果。

♦ 预防：主要的要求是教育和帮助维持口腔健康和预防疾病。希望口腔保健人员提供必要的信息与治疗以便减少疾病，不适与成本。要使公众理解维持口腔健康的主要责任在个人而不是口腔保健人员。很清楚任何一个口腔保健项目的重要目标把短暂的，康复性与修复性保健的要求转变成期望预防为主的服务，以及培养预防为主的态度与行为。

♦ 为了符合这一目标，描述口腔健康状态及其相关因素，用于证明口腔保健的结果必须选择反映各种不同人群的理解，兴趣与需要。这样：

♦ –公众，包括的个人与公共政策制订者，特别应考虑到他们对卫生保健的可进入性和可负担程度

♦ – 卫生与口腔卫生管理者应特别考虑到卫生问题的各个方面以及可供选择的策略

♦ –临床医生，流行病学家与研究人员应该表明他们对改进诊断与治疗质量方面表现出来的掌握必要信息的兴趣。

Public expectation is a significant factor in the analysis of the outcome of an oral health programme and may be assessed at four distinct levels:

♦ *Resignation. The predominant demand here is for emergency care, and no contact with providers beyond what is absolutely essential is desired. A fatalistic attitude to health may prevail.*

♦ *Replacement. The predominant demand is for extractions and dentures. It is appreciated that dentistry may be helpful, but the onus is placed on the provider to furnish pain-free treatment to restore function and appearance.*

♦ *Repair. The predominant demand is for restorative dentistry, including fixed prostheses, orthodontics, and periodontal treatment. Teeth are valued and providers are expected to preserve them. It should be noted, however, that continuing efforts must be made by the individual to maintain the results of treatment.*

♦ *Prevention. The predominant demand is for education and assistance in maintaining oral health and preventing disease. The provider is expected to supply the necessary information and treatment to minimize disease, discomfort and costs. Primary responsibility for maintaining oral health is understood to rest with the individual rather than with the provider.*

Clearly an important objective of any oral health programme should be to convert a demand for episodic, rehabilitative, and restorative treatment to an expectation of predominantly preventive services, and to cultivate prevention-oriented attitudes and behaviour.

In line with this objective, the description of oral heath status and associated factors used to document the outcome of care must be selected to respond to the perceptions, interests and needs of various constituencies. Thus:

- *The public including individuals and public policy-makers, should be especially concerned with the accessibility and affordability of health care;*
- *Health and oral health administrators should be especially concerned with the dimensions of health problems and of alternative strategies;*
- *Clinicians, epidemiologists and researchers should express interest in the information necessary to improve the quality of their diagnoses and treatment.*

4. 主要评价模式 The underlying evaluation model

重要的是要认识到任何项目总是要以某种方法作出评价。包括在项目中的人，项目服务的对象以及较高层的决策者总是会有某些意见，即使意见是非正式的以及常常是主观的，项目管理者的目的是促进一种正式的，合理的，系统的评价过程的概念应该结合到任何项目中去。

任何卫生保健项目系统评价的基础是明确的定义项目的目标，没有很好规定的标准的正式评价是不可能的。还有，任何一个促进健康与减少疾病的项目体现出这样的概念，在还没有开展项目的情况下，会存在着更大的健康问题。从逻辑上考虑，一个项目只能在对发现的健康问题作出反映的情况下才存在。因而项目的计划和评价只应该依据对那个问题的解决的预期效果上。

然而，许多卫生项目的共同不足之处是与他们打算要解决的基本问题之间缺乏紧密的联系，没有这种明确的联系，项目评价只能限于评价项目活动的本身，而不论这些活动是否已经产生了相关的结果。因此，在进行项目评价时，分别考虑以下几点是重要的：

- 设想主要的健康问题是什么；
- 直接与问题有关联的项目目标；
- 针对项目的目标，计划开展的活动；
- 开展计划的活动所需要的资源。

因此，合乎逻辑的评价过程变成为与达到项目目标有关的资源的利用，活动的开展，以及活动所产生的效果。

It is important to recognize that any programme will always be evaluated in some way. People involved in the programme, those served by it and higher-level policy-makers will always have some opinion of it, even if that opinion is informal and often subjective. An aim for programme administrators is to foster the concept that a formal, rational and systematic process of evaluation should be integral to any programme.

Fundamental to the systematic evaluation of any health care programme is a clear definition of the programme objectives formal evaluation without well defined standards is impossible. Moreover, any programme for promotion of health and reduction of disease embodies the concept that a health problem of greater magnitude would exist in the absence of the programme. Logically, a programme can exist only as a response to a perceived health problem: it's planning and evaluation should therefore e based on its anticipated effect on that problem.

Nevertheless, a common inadequacy of health programmes is loss of the linkage to the fundamental problems they were designed to affect. Without this clear linkage, programme evaluation may well be limited to evaluation of the activities of the programme, regardless of whether these activities are producing relevant results. It is therefore important, when evaluating to consider separately:

- *The assumed underlying health problem;*
- *The objectives of the programme in direct relationship to the problem;*
- *The activities that have been planned to achieve the objectives;*
- *The resources that are required to undertake the planned activities in relation to the objectives of the programme.*

五、社区口腔保健模式的实践 Community care models for oral health in practice

（一）中国的实践 Practice in China

中国农村现有9亿多农民，约占总人口78%，有县城2137个。按我国农村社会的组织形式，每个县都是一个相对独立的行政管区。又是一个社会功能，组织结构相当完备的社区。

农村医疗卫生保健系统是以县为单位组成的县，乡，村三级网络。初级卫生保健示范县以县为基础，称为PHC示范县，在这方面中国已经积累了相当丰富的经验。

在实现2000年以及2010年人人享有卫生保健目标的进程中，以县为单位的社区模式试点研究与逐步推广都具有十分重要的示范和促进作用。口腔保健是这一目标的组成部分之一。近年来已引起各级政府的重视和社会群众的关注。作为县社区口腔保健模式的试点工作由此而引起。最早在1984年由山西运城地区的农村开始。在卫生部领导，有关专家的帮助与指导下，吸取了WHO推荐的社区口腔保健模式经验，经过几年实践取得了一定进展成为中国第一个农村社区口腔保健模式，并曾获得1989年由WHO颁发的世界初级卫生保健奖。

1989年以来，又相继创建了几种不同的模式，农村地区有黑龙江省林口县，浙江武义县及内蒙古哲里木盟模式，在城市地区，有上海与沈阳市的学校口腔保健模式，以及河南周口地区的一种新模式。资料表明，通过这些模式试点提供了三个水平的口腔保健服务，基本上可以满足目标地区群众的基本口腔保健需求，并为进一步研究发展提供了社会实践基地。为2010年人人享有初级口腔卫生保健目标的实现，提供了实践经验。其实践的逻辑程序如下：

1. Community models practice in China

there are more than 900 millions of farmers are living in the rural areas of China and it is about 78% of the total population within 2137 counties, according to the organizational pattern of Chinese rural society, each county is a relative autonomous administrative area, and also a quite complete social functional and organization structured community.

A health care delivery system within a county is composed of county level, township level and village level as an integrated network. Primary health care project is demonstrated on a county basis called

PHC demonstration county, China has accumulated a wealth of experience in this respect.

In the progressing process of achieving the goal of health for all by the year 2000, and by the year 2010, testing the community models will play an important role in demonstration and promotion through its studying and gradually expanding at a county basis. Oral health is an integral part of the goal. In recent years, the governments have emphasized on its development and the social groups have paid more attention for it. Therefore, the community models for oral health has been initiated. As early as in 1984, it has been firstly tested in Yuncheng region of the Shanxi province, under the leadership of the Ministry of Health, and conducted by some Chinese experts and following the recommendation made by WHO. The progress is there after practice for several years and then it has become a first community model for oral health in rural area of China and awarded a SASAKAWA price for primary health care by WHO in 1989. since then, there are several community models for oral health developed in succession, such as Linkou county of Heilongjiang province, Wuyi county of Zhejiang province, and Zhelimo League in the rural area, and school models for oral health in Shanghai and Shenyang in the urban area, and another new community model for oral health developed recently in Zhoukou prefecture. The data indicated that by these models tested, it provides oral health services at three levels, and meeting the basic needs of oral health care for the local population and also provides a social basis for the further development. The experiences learned from practices will be beneficial to achieve,the national goal of primary oral health for all by the year 2010.

The logical procedures for practice is proposed as follows:

1. Identify the main problems existed

(1) Oral health awareness

(2) Oral health status

(3) Oral health resources

2. Formulating the basic objectives of the model

3. Selecting strategies

4. Approaches for manpower training

5. Development of infrastructure

(1) County level

(2) Township level

(3) Village level

6. Financial sources

7. Basic equipment

8. Content and patterns of services

9. Evaluation of results

(1) Questionnaire survey

(2) Coverage of oral health services

(3) Funds collection and utilization

(4) Continuing education of oral health workers and controlling of quality of services

(5) Oral health survey

10. Main problems existed

1. 确定存在的主要问题 Indentify the main problems existed

（1）口腔健康意识：农村社区居民普遍对口腔健康的重要价值缺乏足够的认识，缺乏基础口腔保健常识，受传统观念的影响很深。据调查农村的刷牙率远低于城市，口腔卫生普遍，一般通过问卷调查可以获取有关资料。

（2）口腔疾病流行现状：主要查询近5年内的资料，农民患龋率很低，约为40%～50%，不论是患龋率还是龋均，都比城市人群低。但大多数人的龋病很少有治疗的机会，儿童的龋充填率几乎为零。由于口腔卫生差，牙周病，尤其牙龈炎与牙石比龋病严重，农村儿童的牙周健康状况比城市差。一般通过流行学调查获取相关资料。

（3）口腔保健资源严重匮乏：包括人力，经费与机构设备方面。在县，乡，村三级机构中，县级尚有不少未建立独立口腔科，乡镇一级大多数没有建立，村一级更少。县，乡二级主要为助理口腔医师提供服务，经费严重不足，几乎没有任何口腔预防保健措施。口腔保健用品的质量、数量与价值都满足不了农民的需求。一般可以通过社会调查获取相关信息。

2. 设定模式的基本目标 Formulating the basic objectives of the model

一般以人人享有最基本的口腔卫生保健为目标，以初级卫生保健为途径，把口腔卫生保健的最低限内容纳入PHC之范畴，以原三级医疗保健网为依托，建立相应的服务机构，提供三个层面的服务内容，形成一个以初级口腔卫生保健为主体的模式，其基本任务是通过健康教育与促进，逐步改变人们的传统生活方式，并采纳一些适合于当地实际情况的预防措施，逐步改善并保持社区人群的健康，减少口腔疾病的发生，对已经受到疾病影响的人提供适当治疗，防止疾病的恶化和可能的功能丧失。因此，在任何情况下，预防应成为重点。有的模式有明确的目标——人人享有初级口腔卫生保健，有的模式以PHC为基础，以儿童为重点人群，建立三级牙病防治网，重点培养初级与中级口腔保健人才，逐步扩展网点的人群覆盖面。

3. 策略选择 Selecting stratiges

在策略选择中要考虑到几个基本原则：

（1）用相对少量而简便的物资供应和器材设备，因陋就简，即可以见到效果；

（2）口腔专业人员的职能可以由其他经过培训的医务人员，卫生工作者来替换，或者其职能范围可以适当扩大；

（3）社会性干预措施与个人预防方法，在科学上要通过试验，证明有效、安全与价廉；

（4）不论人群所在社会的经济水平，文化教育，收入与职业状况如何，都有可能从中得到好处；

（5）价格合理，无论国家，还是集体与个人都能负担得起；

（6）技术方法不复杂，易于学会和掌握易于接受和利用。

4. 人员培训的途径 Approaches for manpower training

在人员培训方面，这些模式有一个共同特点，就是因地制宜，依靠本地师资力量与培训基地，定向招生，着重招生，着重选拔和培养当地的初中级口腔保健人员。培训方式有两类：一类是主要依靠当地卫校培训中初级人才，周期为2～4年，另一类为选择中级医务人员经过约1年的培训，培训由当地大学或上级专业机构负责。人力短缺状况大有改变，以运城为例，口腔医务人员与人口之比从 1∶12 万到 1∶5000。

5. 牙病防治机构建设 一般有县，乡，村三级机构 Development of infrastructure

（1）县级：设立牙病防治机构，如县牙防所或县医院口腔科，主要职能为预防技术指导，人员培训以及独立解决临床疑难复杂病症，县牙防指导机构主要负责社区项目开发与管理，监督与评价以及协调各有关部门。

（2）乡镇级：一般由乡镇卫生院设立口腔科，或设立独立牙科诊所，其主要职能负责本乡镇群众常见牙病的防治，健康教育，乡村医生培训及口腔疾病状况的统计报告。

（3）村级：一般设立村卫生室，一般由乡村医生负责村民口腔卫生指导，小伤小病与急诊的简单处理，安排转诊治疗，少数中心村单设牙科诊室，有一名助理口腔医师负责常见牙病防治，如洁治、预防性充填、松动牙拔除等。

6. 经费来源 Financial souras

一般由当地政府，社区与个人三部分经费来源组成三方投资。口腔基本保健纳入合作医疗，仍在探索之中，另有在学校儿童中实行口腔健康保险或统筹口腔保健的方式，设法解决儿童的基本口腔保健问题。

7. 基本装备 Basic equipment

必须根据农村地区的承受能力，购置最基本的牙科设备，例如简式牙椅、台式或立式或便携式电钻、国产手用器械、材料等。

8. 服务内容与服务方式 Content and patterns of services

一般服务对象为社区人群，重点对象大部分为儿童，主要服务内容包括口腔健康状况调查，口腔健康教育与口腔卫生指导，配合切实可行的预防措施如推广应用含氟牙膏刷牙、局部用氟、氟水含漱、高危儿童的窝沟封闭，以及应用非创伤修复治疗（ART）技术充填治疗早期龋以及急诊保健。条件较好的乡镇牙防机构可以提供修复性保健等。

服务方式一般为村卫生室主要提供初级口腔卫生保健服务，如健康教育，口腔卫生指导，推荐口腔保健用品，简便口腔检查，记录与报告，安排病人接受治疗等，乡镇卫生院可以开展简单充填与治疗，口腔洁治，拔除松动牙，接受转诊治疗和安排复杂治疗，指导和培训乡村医生，定期进行口腔健康调查和基本数据的统计与分析。县级牙防机构一般应独立开展较高水平的临床医疗保健协助制定县牙防发展计划并负责组织实施与评价，负责对乡镇口腔保健人员的培训与技术指导，定期组织全县的口腔健康状况调查与统计分析报告，以及全县的口腔健康教育与促进活动。

9. 结果评价 Evaluation of resuets

社区口腔保健模式试点的效果应定期组织评价。

评价内容与方法：

（1）问卷调查：评价口腔保健意识，态度，知识与行为的改变，如刷牙率；

（2）口腔保健服务的人群覆盖率：以学校儿童为重点评价人群；

（3）资金筹集与利用状况评价；

（4）口腔保健人员的定期培训与服务质量的监控；

（5）口腔健康状况的变化，以儿童人群为评价重点，涉及龋病，牙周病与口腔卫生状况的变化，每年进行一次调查，每 2 年进行一次评价。

10. 存在的主要问题 Main problems existid

（1）缺乏必要的基本信息资料，搜集资料的方法不统一，原始资料的统计分析不规范，利用不充分；

（2）有效的群体预防措施采纳的较少或覆盖面很有限；

（3）乡镇与村级机构设置与群众的需求不匹配；

（4）人员的定期培训缺少计划和组织、考核；

（5）规章制度不健全，有些政策不落实。

（二）泰国的实践 Practice in Thailand

20多年前（1984），世界卫生组织（WHO）与泰国卫生部合作在清迈发展了社区口腔保健模式为社区群众提供口腔保健服务。这个模式以初级卫生保健原则为基础，在村级水平上强调自助与自力更生为主，基本设想是通过现有的村级医疗保健机构，提供口腔健康检查，预防性指导与预防措施，急诊保健与疼痛，在开展了这些初级卫生保健的基础上，提供一级转诊保健。以此证实初级口腔卫生保健是可能的，可接受的，现实的和经济上是可行的。

发展社区口腔保健模式是对卫生保健体制进行的一项研究，其目的是在人员与资源都缺乏的发展中国家和地区，寻找适当的方式提供口腔卫生保健服务，包括对多种培训与多种提供服务方式的可行性与适当性进行评价。

泰国清迈的社区口腔保健模式在经历了10年实践探索的基础上，于1994年由WHO组织了国际专家会议进行了评价。

20 years ago, in cooperation between the World Health Organization (WHO) and the Thai Ministry of Health, a community care model for oral health has been initiated in Chiang Mai, Thailand, in order to provide oral health services for the community members. This model is based on the principles of primary health care, and emphasized on the self-sufficiency and self-reliance. The basic assumption is that oral health examination, preventive advice and preventive measures, emergency care and pain release could be provided by the current village health care units. Based on these activities within primary health care carried out, then the first referral care could be provided. The model demonstrated that primary oral health care is possible, acceptable, practical and economically feasible.

The development of community care model for oral health is a study on the health care system; its aim is to seek an appropriate way to provide oral health care services in the developing countries and regions, including the evaluation of feasibility and appropriateness in different ways to train health workers and to provide services.

In 1994, in cooperation with the WHO, the Intercountry centre for oral health organized an international experts meeting for evaluating of community oral health care model tested in Chiang Mai after implemented for 10 years.

结论：社区口腔保健模式在短期试点研究的过程中，取得了较为明显的效果，但是在长期可持续发展的过程中，也暴露出不少需要进一步探索，研究和解决的问题.

Conclusion: in the process of short-term testing, the community care model for oral health has reached the significant effectiveness. However, in the long-term continuing developing process, it revealed many problems which needs to be further explored, studied and to be solved.

六、社区口腔健康状态及其干预 Community oral health status and its intervention

为了有组织有计划地在一个社区范围内根据社区群众的基本口腔卫生保健需求提供相应的服务，并且评价这一社区的口腔保健服务系统在促进社区人群口腔健康方面的效果与效率，监测与评价社区人群口腔健康与疾病的变化状况，而且还可以在地区，国家甚至国际水平上作分析比较，帮助确定可能出现的其他口腔健康问题，并适时采取适当的干预措施以及进一步调查研究，在日本人体功能研究所的指导下，以“零点”概念为基础，设计了一个口腔健康状态干预指数系统，并在泰国清迈的社区口腔保健模式的试点研究中，经过了10几年的实际应用，取得了比较成功的经验，证明对社区口腔卫生保健的计划，实施与评价有一定的参考价值，尤其对发展中国家的社区。

In order to provide relevant services, based on the essential needs of oral health care of the community population within a well organized and planned community, and to evaluate the effectiveness and efficiency of promoting oral health of the community groups served by the community oral care service system, and to monitor and evaluate the change of oral health and oral diseases. Moreover, to analyse and to compare it among regions, countries and even at the global level and assisting to identify the possible occurrence of other oral health problems and taking an appropriate intervention promptly and making a further investigation, the Human performance Institute, Atami, Japan devised a system for oral health status intervention index based on the Zero concept which has been tested in the community care model for oral health in Chiang Mai, Thailand for more than 10 years, and a quite lot of successful experiences has been obtained. It demonstrated that the system has a certain values in planning implementing and evaluating of the community oral health care programme, especially in the communities of developing countries.

1. 零的概念（concept zero）

问题的解决是基于一种科学原理及其有关范围，目标及其有关指数之间的关系。解决问题的途径是评价与目标的关系。卫生保健目标为“O”，意味着健康或无需保健，提供的信息量最少。这一目标是通过自我保健并应用适当的措施，而达到人群的口腔及其周围组织健康。这一套数字术语的逻辑性安排的基础是目标及其确定的有关范围作为“O”，对于“O”的应用，我们可以联系目标来规定并评估与既定目标有关的机构与活动。因此，对任何一次对既定目标有关的社会活动的完成情况进行定量评价，用数字的形式反映出有送的信息是很好的指征。

“O”在空间规格中代表实体，当一个问题在其实体中被觉察到，寻求一种解决的办法一般波及到测量。测量需要有一个起点，测量就是以这一起点为依据进行的。这一点也以“O”来表示。因此，选择数字术语使信息内容的安排系统化，采用“O”的概念，便于问题的解决。这些问题包括健康状态人体测量，人类遭遇，保健机构规格，操作规格，学习训练以及可靠的数据收集。

The orientation, planning and implementation of the community care model are geared to the concept of “health” or absence of need for care (“concept zero”) and use of the status and Intervention (SI) Index.

In addition to identifying the goal of health care, “concept zero” provides the basis for a logical numeric scale for use in classification and recording and in relating the goal and the scope of concern in a given health area. For this project, the goal for community oral health is "O"(i.e, absence of the need for oral health care) and as regards the health of the oral cavity and associated and surrounding tissues in the individual the goal is also "O".

With the use of 0 and the numbers 1 to 9, the meanings of which are defined in the SI index in relation to 0, care specifications, settings, and activities can be related to the goal of oral health. the "concept zero" approach means that the need for any activity, setting component, or intervention must be justified in the context of an approach to the goal.

2. 状态干预指数 The status intervention index（SI index）

状态干预指数是对健康与卫生保健来说是一种清楚而不庞大，普遍有关的分类方法。表明健康状态的指数是以 0 至 -1 的范围形式来表示。0 代表健康状态或无需保健，而 0.9 为保健的上限。-1 表明残疾状态或处于保健范围之外的依赖状态。因此，负数越大表明健康状况越糟，情况也越复杂，需要侵入性口腔卫生保健。

The status intervention index is a clear, unambiguous, and universally relevant classification to health and health care. The index which represent the health status is in the form of a scale range from 0 to-1。The scale zero represents the healthy status or the absence of need for care and -0.9 the upper limit of care. The scale -1 represents the state of being handicapped or dependence status which lies outside the realm of health care. Therefore, the higher negative numbers on the scale represent progressive worse health status and also increasing complex and invasive oral health care.

而且，干预变得越来越复杂，治疗费用上升，并且还存在着治疗失败与错误的危险在治疗期间与治疗后还有更多的疼痛与不适。所有这些因素都要包括在指数设计之中。

健康状态的种类为个人口腔健康状况的诊断分类提供了基础，随后数字诊断系统能用来保持流行病学记录。而且，历为每一种状态有相应的干预表，SI指数也能用于特殊状态／干预各类所需要的器材的分类以及不同干预所需要的不同种类的提供人员。

SI指数的另一个优点是当与显示口腔疼痛与典型的干预结果的适当的口腔组织模型一起应用时，还能起到一种口腔健康教育与促进的简单工具的作用，这样的教育也可以使人们对所需要的口腔卫生保健种类作出知情决策。这种能力在发展中国家的社区水平特别需要，因为那里的口腔保健服务与资源常常是有限的。

因此，口腔健康状态干预指数（OSI）已经为国际标准组织（ISO），FDI与WHO正式采纳。

"1" 表示最大的信息量，需要最大限度的干预措施，如外科手术，颌面修复等。介于0～1 之间的状态划分为 12 步干预程序，简述如下：

前3项指数（0.0～0.2）为监测，自我保健，健康教育与卫生指导，以及初级预防性保健（牙面保健），作为促进与保持口腔健康程序；后4项指数（0.3～0.6）为经过临床治疗，恢复健康程度；最后 4 项指数（0.7 ～ 1）为经过临床修复，达到康复程序。

这套 SI 指数与上述的所有口腔健康指数，如 DMFT，DMFS，CPI 等均有关联。

"1" expresses the maximal information and needs maximal intervention, such as surgical operation, maxillo-facial prosthesis etc. the status between 0 ～ 1 were divided into 12 steps for intervention procedures, which are summarized as follows:

The first 3 indexes (0.0 ~ 0.2) including monitoring, self-care, health education and hygiene instruction and primary preventive care (surface care) as the procedures of promoting and maintaining oral health; the next 4 indexes (0.3 ~ 0.6) as the procedures of clinical treatment and restorative health; the last 4 indexes (0.7 ~ 1) as procedures of clinical restoration and rehabilitation.

This set of SI index and all oral health index described above, such as DMFT, DMFS, CPI, etc is interrelated.

Moreover, as the interventions become more and more complex, the cost of treatment also rises, and so does the risk of treatment failure and error in treatment. There is also more pain and discomfort during and after the treatment, as there is in the absence of it. all these factors have been carefully included in the design of the index.

The health status categories provide a basis for classifying the diagnoses of oral health conditions for individuals, and subsequently the numerical system of diagnosis can be used for keeping epidemiological records. Furthermore, since for each status category there is a corresponding list of interventions, the SI Index can also be used for classifying materials and instruments needed for specific status / Intervention categories, and manpower categories.

Another advantage of the SI index is that, when used together with appropriate models of oral tissues showing oral diseases and results of typical interventions, it can serve as a simple tool for oral health education and promotion. Such education will enable people to make informed decisions about the kind of oral health care needed. This ability is particularly needed at the community level in developing countries, where oral health services and resources for them are often limited.

Therefore, the Oral Status and Intervention Index (OSI) has been formally adopted by the International Organization for Standardization (ISO) , FDI and WHO.

表 12-11 The status and Intervention（SI）Index for classifying health status and procedures

Concept 0	Health and health care										Concept-1
Health	–.0	–0.1	–0.2	–0.3	–0.4	–0.5	–0.6	–0.7	–0.8	–0.9	D
	Collection of information	Self-care	Maintenance of surface support, or structure	Position anatomy dimension	Loss of support, structure, function	Partial		Full	Replacement Fixed	Removable	e p e n h
Absence	Oral health status and care needed										d a
of need	0	1	2	3	4	5	6	7	8	9	e n
for care	Recording	Self-care mouth	Maintenance	Maintenance-restoration Gingival-tooth		Tooth		Surgery	Replacement		n d c c
	status	Monitor explanation exercise	Surface by performer	Position	support	dentine named	Pulp	Access removal	Fixed	removable	e a p

表 12-12 Classification of oral health status and intevention categories by means of the SI Index

scale	Oral health status	Type of intervention
0	Perfect oral health	No need for any care
−0.0	Unknown	Periodic examination
−0.1	Presence of plaque, gingival bleeding	Self-care after instruction by qualified health personnel
−0.2	Early (reversible) stage of caries, calculus, stain	Surface care, (e,g. scaling and fluoride application)
−0.3	Positional and cosmetic defects and dentofacial anomalies	Orthodontic care, tooth straightening and repositioning
−0.4	Affections of tooth-supporting tissues, periodontal pockets, loose teeth	Tooth root cleaning and smoothing, care of periodontal pockets to restore tooth stability
−0.5	Dental caries, decay of enamel and dentine	Filling of teeth and placement of crowns
−0.6	Affections of pulp and pulp chamber	Pulp care
−0.7	Teeth decayed beyond restoration, dental impaction dental fracture trauma and swelling	Surgical care of oral tissues: extraction of teeth, removal of oral lesions, repair of trauma
−0.8	Absence of 1-3 consecutive teeth requiring replacement in order to improve chewing ability or appearance	Fixed tooth replacements, enamel-bonded crown abutter or implanted
−0.9	Few to many teeth missing or completely edentulous	Fitting of partial and full dentures

表 12-13 Oral health and oral health care and oral health manpower categories

scale	Manpower categories
0	No need manpower
−0.0	Parents, individuals, teachers, dental assistants, dental hygienists, dental therapists, pediatric dentists, dentists
−0.1	Parents, school nurses, factory hygienists, dental therapists, local physicians, dentists
−0.2	Dental hygienists, dental therapists, and dentists
−0.3	Dental hygienists, dental therapists, technicians and dentists
−0.4	Dental therapists, dentists
−0.5	Dental technicians, dentists
−0.6	Dentists
−0.7	Dentists
−0.8	Dental technicians, dentists
−0.9	Dental technicians, prosthetic dentists and oral surgeon
−1	Oral maxillo facial surgeon and prosthetic dentists

3. 结论

SI指数是一个多种健康，保健图表与记录方式的输入信息系统，并且是个人与社区健康状态的指标，以及干预种类的指标，指数的数字就可以用来编排健康状态与所需保健。

建立在“0”概念与SI指数基础上的一种管理监督信息系统广泛采用数字编码记号和编排口腔卫生保健所需要的信息，并且作为开展和试验社区口腔保健模式项目的一个组成部分。

Conclusion

The SI Index is (a) a system for entering information in a numerical form onto health can care charts and records, and (b) an indicator of personal or community health status and of types of intervention. The digits in the index become the first digits of numerical terms used for coding health status and the care needed.

A management, monitoring, and information system based on “concept zero” and the SI index, that makes extensive use of numerical codes for recording and arranging the information needed for oral health and care, is also being developed and tested as part of the project of community care model.

七、贫困社区口腔卫生保健 Oral health care in the deprived communities

1978年发表阿拉木图初级卫生保健宣言时，有两件事当时并未预见到：一个是80年代全球的经济危机，另一个是艾滋病流行及其预防控制问题。在许多发展中国家出现的经济，社会，还有政治危机对人群健康也有负面影响，如健康状况，服务提供，能得到的卫生保健及其覆盖面，服务费用与服务质量。在大多数贫穷国家，人均收入低，人口增长快（约3%），口腔卫生保健服务差，龋病患病普遍，严重性增加，贫困人群中的未治龋或拔除的龋牙比例高，加上贫困直接引起的失业，低收入，低教育水平，膳食不当，居住条件差，拥挤，不洁饮水与不良环境，感染性疾病，污染，事政，压力，不稳定与不安全等。而个人，家庭与社区的健康需要应建立在公正，尊重与平等的基础上之。

在健康方面的平等意味着每个人都应有平等的机会发挥其潜力。不平等意味着不公正，在许多贫穷国家和社区，尽管也作出了许多努力，但人们的健康状况与卫生保健仍趋于恶化。

健康是基本人权，口腔健康是全身健康的重要组成部分。是公共卫生的重要问题，但并未引起足够的重视。

口腔疾病的重要特点是可以利用简单，廉价而有效的预防方法，存在的主要问题是在许多情况下并没有得到适当的应用。若能开展社区口腔卫生保健项目，将能提供较好的机会，改善服务状况，并最终增进社区的口腔健康。这些以社区为基础的项目，更有可能建立在自力更生，自我管理的基础之上。因正为如此，1992年柏林宣言为项目计划人员在计划，实施与评价贫困社区的口腔卫生保健项目方面提供了指导，目的在于改善贫困社区的口腔健康与口腔保健服务。

When the Alma-Ata Declaration was formulated in 1978. There were two developments which were not foreseen or anticipated. These are the rapid global economic crists of the 1980s and the AIDS pandemic with the current problems of its prevention and control. The economic, social, as well as political crises in most developing countries have adversely affected health in terms of: provision of services, access and coverage, financing of services, quality of services, and status of health. Many of these poorest nations have low per capita incomes and increases in their populations of around 3% per annum. Their oral health services are grossly moldistributed. Dental caries is common in most poor countries and the severity is rising. The deprived have a high proportion of their decayed teeth unfilled or treated by extraction. The direct problems of poverty are unemployment, low income, limited education, and inadequate diet. This leads to overcrowding, poor housing, inadequate water and sanitation, which in turn are related to infectious diseases, pollution, accidents, stress, alienation, instability and insecurity. Good health of individuals, families, and communities requires a decent environment built on a solid foundation of fairness, respect, and equality.

"Equity in health implies that ideally everyone should have a fair opportunity to attain their full potential and more pragmatically, that no one should be disadvantaged from achieving this potential, if it can be avoided"(WHO, 1986) . Inequity means injustice. Despite efforts in the past decade to make health systems more equitable, in the poorer countries and communities things are getting worse in terms of people's health and access to health care.

Health is a basic human right and oral health is a significant component of general health. they are important public health problems. However, it has not been given the attention it deserves.

An important feature of oral diseases is that effective preventive methods which are simple and cheap are available, but in many cases, these methods are not appropriately applied. If the community oral health programmes can be developed, it will provide a better chance of ultimately improving both services and community oral health. these community-based programmes are more likely to lead towards self-reliance and self-management of oral health programmes. Just because of this, the Berlin Declaration 1992 provided a guidance to programme planners for planning, implementing and evaluating of oral health care programmes aimed at improving oral health and oral health services in deprived communities.

1. 发展贫困社区口腔卫生保健项目所推荐的策略 Recommended strategies for developing oral health care programmes in deprived communities

初级卫生保健途径中的两个原则必须在所有的项目中加以考虑。这些原则是社区参与，多部门合作和一体化。达到口腔健康与口腔卫生服务平等的一个重要因素是多方合作的成功，才保证了社区的发展。

Two principles of the primary health care approach have to be considered in almost all programmes, if lasting solutions to problems are to be found. These are community participation and multisectoral cooperation and integration. An important element in achieving equity in oral health and oral health services is the success of the multisectoral approach in securing community development.

（1）口腔疾病预防的策略 strategies for oral disease prevention

预防应根据健康促进的原则：重新定向口腔卫生服务，创造支持环境，制订公众的健康政策，支持社区行动，发展应对技能。除了柏林宣言规定的一般原则外，在所有项目中还应考虑：

①依据国家的社会经济状况采取预防措施。预防项目应采取灵活的途径，允许选择适合于现时情况的措施。健康教育与预防都必须采用科学上经过试验的方法；

②在大多数贫困社区，国家与人群中，其他健康问题远比口腔健康问题更重要；

③应采用适宜技术，如自制牙刷，应使人们掌握制作牙刷的能力，鼓励自我保健，使家庭能开展自家预防活动；

④几种不同的用氟方案联合应用，并不总会导致临床上明显的累积作用。

Prevention should be based on the principles of health promotion: reorienting oral health services, creating supportive environment, building healthy public policy, supporting community action, developing coping skills. In addition to the general principles outlined in the Berlin Oral Health Declaration the following points should be considered in all programmes:

The application of preventive measures depends very much on the socio-economic situation of the country, therefore, a flexible approach to preventive programmes should be taken, which will permit adaptation to suit existing circumstance. Such adaptation must be undertaken by utilizing scientifically tested methods of health education and prevention.

In most deprived communities, countries, and population groups other health problems are much more important than oral health problems

Appropriate technology should be used (e.g. Chewing sticks) and people should be enabled to make their own toothbrushes/toothpaste. Self-care should be encouraged. Families should be enabled to carry out their own set of preventive activities.

Some combinations of different fluoride regimens do not always lead to a clinically significantly better cumulative effect.

2. 具体的策略包括 Specific strategies include

（1）氟化物的广泛应用 Fluoridation

许多国家促进使用含氟牙膏是减少龋发病的最有效方法。最主要的是生产廉价的含氟牙膏并广泛使用，应进一步推进这一策略：①应说服国际公司生产销售廉价含氟牙膏；②关于洁牙可以减少龋的健康教育信息应尽量少强调直到人们能定期得到含氟牙膏时；③国际合作机构应鼓励分配含氟牙膏。

The promotion of fluoridated toothpaste is the most appropriate way for many countries to reduce the levels of caries. The highest priority should be to make cheap fluoridated toothpaste widely available. In furtherance of this strategy therefore:

International companies should be persuaded to sell cheap fluoride toothpaste in bulk;

Health education messages about tooth cleaning for caries reduction should be given less emphasis until people can get fluoridated toothpaste on a regular basis;

International cooperation agencies should be encouraged to distribute fluoride toothpaste.

（2）健康教育 Health education

健康教育应置于健康促进之内，健康教育的同时应提供治疗性服务，并建立一种支持性环境。例如，提供清洁饮水，健康食品。

Health education should be put in a health promotional context. Thus, it should be combined with the provision of curative services and carried out in a supportive environment where there is clean water and healthy foods.

（3）一体化健康促进活动 Integration of health promotional activities

口腔健康信息与活动应包括在全身的健康信息与行动之中。一体化与共同危险因素应成为健康促进活动的里程碑，其基本概念是：①对付多种慢性疾病的共同原因；②口腔健康是全身健康的一部分；③发展人口策略而不是高危策略。

Oral health messages and activities should be included in general health messages and actions. Integration and a common risk factor approach outlined below should be the cornerstones of health promotional activities. The fundamental concepts are:

Tackling causes common to a number of chronic diseases

Including oral hygiene as part of general hygiene

Developing population rather than the high risk strategies

（4）口腔健康服务 Oral health services

计划口腔健康服务应考虑所有可能的资源，包括私人开业医的作用。为改善健康服务，始终应考虑 6 个 A 字：可利用性，可进入性，可说明性，可负担性，可提供性以及可接受性。

在健康服务中，口腔卫生人员分布不均问题几乎存在于所有的国家。最大的成功是使用牙科辅助人员，培训更多的辅助人员是提高服务覆盖率的最重要办法。建立转诊制度，发挥初级卫生保健的作用，明确各类人员的岗位职责。

In planning oral health services, all possible resources should be considered including the role of independent practitioners. The six A's should always be considered in order to improve health services. These are availability, accessibility, accountability, affordability, accommodation and acceptability.

The problem of unequal distribution of oral health personnel within the health services exists in nearly all countries. Greater success has occurred with auxiliary personnel. Training more auxiliary personnel may be an important way of increasing coverage. The development of a referral system, supporting the role of the primary care level, and job functions need to be clearly stated.

（5）社会参与 Community involvement

口腔卫生人员与社区之间的合作依据双方的尊重与信任。有必要请社区领导参与计划，实施与评价社区服务，然后发展成为全社区性服务，卫生人员提供的服务要得到社区的理解和支持。

社区现有的卫生工作者应包括在内，并发挥其宣传与促进作用。以社区为基础的口腔卫生保健项目如果没有科学的基础或者这样的项目没有社区的参与都是没有价值的。

Genuine partnership between oral health personnel and the community depends upon mutual respect and trust. It will be necessary to approach the community through local leaders and involve them in planning, implementation and evaluation of the community-oriented service as a first step. Later this should lead to the development of a fully community-based service which is perceived by the community as their service.

It is important to include the existing health workers and to define and develop their advocacy and facilitator roles within the group.

Neither the scientific basis of community-based oral health programmes nor the capacity of the community to participate in such programmes on a scientific basis should be undervalued.

（6）口腔卫生保健人员在多部门合作与一体化项目中的作用 The role of oral health personnel in multisectoral and integrated programmes

采取一体化与多部门的合作的重要机制，初级卫生保健应包括在任何项目之内。一体化也包括人员结构的调整。在不同的卫生保健服务水平上，口腔卫生保健人员有不同的作用。在全国与中级水平上口腔医师发挥重要作用。在初级水平上，辅助人员起重要作用。但这并不是说没有辅助人员在较高的水平上工作或者口腔医师对初级卫生保健没有责任，他们有监督与培训的责任。在一体化多部门合作的项目中推荐口腔卫生保健人员的作用有：①在所有服务水平上，卫生人员都有责任宣传公众的健康政策，使人们能以健康的生活方式生活；②卫生人员有责任评价他们的工作。因此，参与服务研究是所有工作者作用的一部分；③在高级与中级水平上工作的口腔卫生保健人员在计划，协调，教育，监督，指导与科学鉴定以及为转诊病人提供治疗诸方面都应发挥重要作用。

An important mechanism for getting integration and multisectoral cooperation implemented is to include primary health care in any programme. Integration would also be facilitated by the removal let inequalities in career structures between different members of the health team.

The role of oral health personnel has to be seen as being different at different levels within the health service. Thus, dentists have important roles at national and intermediate levels and auxiliaries at the primary level. This is not to say that there should be no auxiliaries working at higher levels within the health systems, or that dentists do not have important responsibilities for the primary level of care in relation to supervision and training.

The following are recommended roles of oral health personnel in integrated multi-sectoral programmes:

At all levels of service, health personnel have a responsibility to be advocates of healthy public policy, and to enable people to live healthy lifestyles

At all levels of service, health personnel have a responsibility to be critical of what they are doing. Participation in health services research is therefore an important part of all workers roles

Oral health personnel employed in the higher and intermediate levels of the service have important roles in planning and coordination; education and supervision; provision of leadership and scientific expertise; and the provision of treatment for referred level patients.

（7）教育与培训 Education and training

所有的卫生保健人员接受初级口腔卫生保健概念与公共卫生政策方面的培训是重要的。课程改革必须看其社会内容。对口腔卫生保健人员的教育需要重新定向，在与人群需要有关的内容应更多。为了使他们能掌握与健康促进行动和一体化工作方式有关的技术，有必要：①培训与教育计划应作为全面改善口腔健康的一部分；②培训应依据整体观，不只是关心32颗牙。特别是发展社区工作技能方面的理论与实践，培训学生应与国家的全国性口腔健康计划有关联；③口腔医师应接受高级与中级水平的工作培训，为转诊病人提供服务与服务管理；④学习活动应在城市、郊区与农村社区进行，参与社区调查或社会诊断与行动计划或参与社区卫生项目，以及对初级卫生保健机构的监督工作。

It is important that all health personnel receive additional training to support the concept of primary oral health care and roles in respect of public health policy. Curriculum change has to be seen it its social context. A fundamental reorientation of the education of oral health personnel is required to make it more relevant to the needs of the population.

The following are suggested as necessary in the future education and training oral health personnel to acquire the skills for health promotion action and for working in an integrated manner:

Planning of training and education of personnel in oral health should be a part of comprehensive planning for improving oral health;

Training of oral health personnel should be based on a holistic approach and not on the care of thirty-two teeth. Particularly in the development of community working skills from theory to practice. The training of students should be related to a country's National plan for oral health;

Dentists should be trained to work in the secondary and higher levels of the service, providing oral health care for referred patients and in the management of oral health services;

Learning activities should take place in an urban, suburban, or rural community and participation in a community survey or community diagnosis and action plan or in ongoing community health programmes and supervised work at the primary care facilities.

（8）适宜技术 Appropriate technology

为适宜技术工作的各类人员的知识与专长需要分担。适宜技术也包括那些在教育与管理领域的人员。因为他们与人员，方法以及学习设备用品有关。为此推荐的适宜技术应是：①更能负担得起；②建立网络，从事适宜技术工作人员的知识与专家需要分担；③应确定并公布确实应用有效的治疗方法与制剂；④在以学员为中心的方法中，适宜技术需要通过网络人员的工作使其能更广泛的传播和利用；⑤为发展能用于贫困社区的设备，材料与途径应建立研究中心；⑥有关机构应列出在各种情况下所需要的器材清单，促进器材的信息交流。

The knowledge and expertise of various people working on appropriate technologies needs to be shared. Appropriate technologies include also those in the education and administration fields. As such they involve personnel, methods, learning aids. Therefore, we recommend that:

Appropriate technologies need to be made more affordable;

The knowledge and expertise of various people working on appropriate technologies need to be shared by the creation of a net work

Popular therapies and therapeutic agents that are being used and are beneficial should be identified and publicized

Appropriate technologies in education need to be made more widely known and available through a network of people involved in such appropriate learner centred methods

Research centres should be established for the development of equipment, materials, and approaches for applying them in deprived communities.

The relevant organizations should be called upon to prepare lists of materials needed in various situations to facilitate the exchange of information on equipment and materials.

（9）研究 Research

选择与推荐的重点研究领域如下：

①研究应与人们需要改进的“技术”有关，如材料，设备，初级卫生保健，教育与管理；

②研究教育与社会因素对人们理解幸福与接受有益实践的能力的影响；

③研究人员与社区之间应共同努力研究促进人们的幸福，因为它能直接导致行动；

④研究人员首先应有奉献于社会的精神，其次才是他们的科学社会事业，研究人员必须尊重社区的意见；

⑤口腔卫生工作者应帮助社区人员进行研究，使他们了解应用研究的原则与步骤；

⑥需要深入研究窝沟封闭，ART，使更多的人了解认识，并降低含氟牙膏与牙刷的成本。

The priorities in research areas for selection and recommendation as follows:

Research should be relevant to the needs of people in terms of improving the "technologies" of materials, equipment, primary care, education and administration

It is important to do research on educational and social factors that influence people's understanding of well-being and their abilities to accept beneficial practices.

Research should always be a joint endeavour between researchers and the community, such that it promotes the well-being of people because it leads directly to actions

A researcher's allegiance is first to his/her community and second to the scientific community at large. As such, researchers must respect a community's point of view.

Dental workers should help community people undertake research by helping them understand and apply both principles and steps involved in applied research

Further research is needed to make fissure sealants, ART, more user-friendly and to reduce the cost of fluoridated toothpaste and toothbrushes

八、综合基本口腔保健 WHO integrated package of basic oral care（IPBOC）

发展中国家农村人口的口腔卫生状况无明显改变，城市人口的口腔卫生状况在恶化，甚至大多数社区的基本急诊保健都没有保障，现有的机构无任何预防，资源匮乏，缺少人力是主要障碍，增加口腔保健人员并不可行。

乳牙患龋水平太高，不能接受。现代口腔医学所采用的高科技，质量有明显改进，而成本明显增加。许多发展中国家，大多数青少年龋病得不到及时治疗，因而常有引起疼痛与扩大感染的危险。这些情况导致年轻人失牙。解决因口腔感染引起的疼痛，有些可能危及生命，贫困人群急需要治疗。而这些社区的人不看牙，不采取预防性干预或修复性治疗，以防止牙缺失。口腔卫生水平低，一般与口腔健康有关的知识，态度与习惯普遍地差。

发展中国家的大多数人还没有接触到口腔健康教育。大多数农村地区难以得到口腔卫生保健，即使有，拔牙是主要的治疗。在城市由口腔医生提供的保健服务花费大，大多数人无法得到，这种传统式口腔医学服务模式忽视了社区预防的重要性。

发达国家的口腔医学实践经验显示，只增加传统的口腔医学服务能力并不能控制口腔疾病，直到接受了口腔健康教育和引进了群体预防措施，特别是拥有含氟牙膏，龋齿与牙龈炎的患病率才开始下降。然而，牙膏，特别是含氟牙膏现在到处都有，但价格太贵，动员人们广泛定期使用的难度很大。

在口腔疾病控制中，预防途径是最值得推荐的选择。然而，在美国仅预防口腔疾病的成本就已达到近30%（590亿美元），如此高的成本在公共卫生中已变成为最难解决的问题，尤其是在发展中国家由于许多人还不能享有基本的急诊保健，如安全的无痛拔牙。

虽然大多数发展中国家和经济正在转变的国家拥有有限的卫生保健资源，包括口腔卫生服务，但其中许多仍有一定的公共卫生经费，用于培训口腔保健人员和推动口腔卫生保健。上述情况在大多数发展中国家称为从传统的口腔医学向着按初级卫生保健原则的预防口腔医学转变。这意味着更强调以社区为基础的促进口腔健康和为满足大多数人中的大量未治病例而进行干预。

由见于此，显然需要针对有限的经费，现有的机构以及察觉到的人口需要，发展基本口腔卫生系统。为帮助各省，尤其是西部和贫困的边缘地区，有效地利用即使是很少的经费，全国牙病防治指导组已经与其他组织，如WHO与工业界合作，开始建立一些试点项目，决定以最合理的方式按照一个社区的具体情况引入口腔卫生保健提供系统，这些项目体现了一种综合为一体的基本口腔保健（IPBOC）包括急诊口腔保健，口腔疾病预防与控制，可以由口腔专业人员和部分非专业人员指导。通过这些项目，打算在社区水平上进行示范，以便大量减少口腔疾病的负担。然而，我们应该清楚，没有一种单一的模式普遍适用，因此，应该鼓励各省市，各地区发展自己的IPBOC，依据具体察觉到的人群需要，利用现有的卫生保健机构。这点很重要，因为，在过去许多口腔卫生项目之所以失败，是由于重要的逻辑问题与经费问题，以及它们是离开了现有的初级卫生保健系统去组织的。

An Integrated Package of Urgent Oral Care, Oral Disease Prevention and control has been proposed which combines these essential components of an oral health service. It is felt that it is applicable for developing and developed countries as well as economies in transition. The provision of an oral health service is costly since high technology is involved. Different countries have different financing systems. It is common in the majority of countries that public funds (partly or in total) are used to cover the cost of the oral health service. Due to various situations (lack of resources, irregular visits to dentists, high cost of care) dental pain is the predominant reason for seeking help. The most common need in these patients is for urgent care of infections, which in many cases could be life-threatening. Therefore, a pain relief service should be available in all communities and public funds used to maintain this service. Guidelines for urgent oral care using an essential set of a minimal number of instruments, medicaments and material needed for different levels of oral care settings are currently being developed at WHO. Preventive activities with the use of fluoride represent the second component of the Integrated Package. Such activities are normally based on data obtained from standard analysis of the oral health situation in a particular country or community. One method of systemic fluoride administration (with water, salt or milk) is recommended in combination with fluoridated toothpaste and intensive oral health education programmes. Affordable cost fluoridated toothpaste can become available for communities with a low-income population. The third component of the package of oral care for community service is Atraumatic Restorative Treatment (ART) which is suitable for all populations at all levels of economic development. It fits very well with modern concepts of preventive and restorative oral care, which stress maximum efforts in prevention, minimal invasiveness in treatment, and the principles of primary health care.

The Integrated Package approach is believed by WHO to be of great value in delivering affordable preventive and early treatment components. The approach is in its early stages of development and use, and subject to improvements in materials, instrumentation and techniques. The impressive beginning of ACT and ART projects is encouraging for WHO's mission in oral health. thus, WHO will follow its development in implementation, modification and testing, with special interest in that which can be recommended for implementation by its Member States. Funding to implement demonstration projects in two WHO Regions are partly available and additional resources will be identified through continuous fundraising activities.

1. 示范项目的主要目标 The main objectives of demonstration programme

（1）评价人们对预防口腔疾病与基本口腔保健的需要；

（2）尝试在减少人们急诊保健需要，改善口腔健康状况方面取得成功；

（3）发展基本口腔保健模式（急诊保健，可负担得起的含氟牙膏与无创伤修复治疗），可扩展到当地其他地区，以便减少拔牙要求和治疗感染的需要。鼓励儿童采纳将有助于增进儿童时期的口腔健康并延续到成年时期的适当的口腔卫生实践。在社区水平上减少儿童主要口腔疾病的患病率。

（4）依据口腔健康的流行病学资料及其他有关资料作情况分析，确定最紧迫的口腔保健需要。

- 推荐对一个关键年龄组的儿童作口腔检查
- 问卷调查目标地区 1,000 名 12 岁，1,000 名 35 ～ 44 岁
- 应用标准统计学分析与口腔健康调查结果比较
- 记录看牙次数，理由及对现有口腔保健系统的满意程度
- 估计牙膏、牙刷的消费水平

2. IPBOC 的三个组成部分 Three essential components of IPBOC

（1）口腔急诊治疗 Oral urgent treatment, OUT

- 由于多种原因，牙疼是寻找帮助的主要理由；
- 急诊保健最普遍的需要是那些感染的病人，其中有许多病例可能会危及生命；
- 所有社区都应有缓解疼痛的服务，公共费用用于维持这种服务；
- 示范模式的推荐，其服务内容依据当地人的需求增减。而且要评估卫生中心最低数量的基本器械，药品，材料的需要；
- 应仔细分析当前的急诊保健需要与相应的服务，强化人员培训；
- 鼓励生产低成本的简易器械。

(1) Oral Urgent treatment, OUT

dental pain is the predominant reason for seeking help, due to various situations

the most common needs in these patients is for urgent care of infections, which in many cases could be life-threatening

a pain relief service should be available in all communities and public funds used to maintain this service

the recommendation of demonstration model in which the service issues will depend on the needs and demand of local people and an essential set of a minimal number of instruments, medicaments and material needed for different levels of oral care settings should be evaluated

the current needs of emergency care and its relevant services should be carefully analysed, in order to strengthen manpower training

（2）可负担的含氟牙膏 Affordable cost of fluoridated toothpaste, ACT

♦ 暴露于适量的氟化物是最有效的防龋措施；

♦ 广泛使用氟化物，每天用含氟牙膏刷牙 2 次；

♦ 由于某些原因，限制糖消耗，改变饮食习惯并不现实；

♦ 工业化国家龋病下降，而并没有减少蔗糖的消耗；

♦ 龋病下降最重要的原因是逐渐增加应用含氟牙膏，5亿人用含氟牙膏刷牙这一降低龋齿的口腔卫生措施有最大的影响；

♦ 广泛，定期使用含氟牙膏对降低龋齿有明显益处，这一预防措施还有利于牙周组织健康；

♦ 牙膏价格太贵而无力购买。1990年WHO提出为不发达地区生产可以负担的含氟牙膏；

♦ 促进使用这种牙膏，应纳入口腔健康教育的内容；

♦ 儿童时期改变习惯为成人口腔健康打好基础，尤其是学龄前儿童。

口腔健康教育需要系统培训。（幼师，护校）

①喂养习惯与方式与早期儿童龋有关；

②保护儿童乳牙，尽早用含氟牙膏刷牙；

③动员母亲关心自身与儿童口腔健康。

The first phase of an Affordable Cost of Toothpaste (ACT) Project has been successfully completed. A formula for a newly-developed fluoridated toothpaste was developed, the main ingredient being Calcium carbohydrate. A three-year clinical study of this toothpaste has shown an adequate preventive effect and these findings are reported in a WHO publication. The cost of this toothpaste is considerably lower than other brands and is currently being manufactured in Brazil and China; and from 1999 it will be available in the Russian Federation. The second phase of the project is in progress to evaluate how affordable this toothpaste could be in reality. It is also essential to identify the possibility of cooperation between consumers, health authorities and toothpaste manufacturers which will stimulate regular use of fluoridated toothpaste to improve oral health in populations worldwide. A number of countries have now agreed to introduce an Affordable Toothpaste Project (ACT) and to use public funds where needed to provide each child with the necessary fluoridated toothpaste and toothbrushes on a regular basis. Adoption of fluoridated toothpaste and regular oral hygiene are part of life-style changes propagated by industry through advertising on television and radio, cinemas and in magazines. In this way industry has been a very powerful force in strengthening the preventive message of oral health personnel.

（3）无创伤修复治疗 Atraumatic restorative treatment, ART

♦ 预防措施成本虽低，但达到人人，其速缓慢；

♦ 长期处理龋齿，需防治结合；

♦ 现代修复龋齿采用最低的干预途径，通过氟化物，封闭剂，预防性充填，具体抗菌治疗，阻止龋发展；

◆ ART技术是首选，生产玻璃离子材料，手器械，无需复杂设备，电、水，在任何场合可进行治疗；

◆ 美国公共卫生服务标准认为 ART 修复简易，快捷，恰当。

Atraumatic Restorative Treatment (ART), the least invasive of the minimal intervention approaches, which comprises preventive and restorative procedures has been developed and is currently being implemented in a number of countries. Support to launch a global project on further ART promotion ahs recently been obtained from the Government of the Netherlands and various dental material manufacturers. A consultative group of experts was set up to design the Global Project and to prepare a plan of global activities to further promote ART and other techniques and materials for a non-invasive restorative approach in oral care.

IPBOC 项目的重要目标之一是评价 ART 的效果：

◆ ART 符合预防与修复性口腔保健的现代概念；

◆ 强调最大的预防努力与最少的入侵组织；

◆ 减少疼痛与不适及使用麻药；

◆ 减少儿童惧怕压力；

◆ 可适用于基层卫生机构，学校；

◆ ART 作为可负担的治疗，补充初级预防活动；

◆ 符合 PHC 原则：预防，适宜技术，可负担的治疗以及平等分配服务；

◆ IPBOC 所有的内容可依据资源状况分别实施；

◆ 综合成一体的项目是为了口腔健康促进和减少新龋发生。

IPBOC 项目的重要内容：

◆ 评价当地卫生机构，经济能力与人们的知识，态度，习惯与有关口腔健康的需要；

◆ 评估 OUT 内容，需要最低限的器械与材料；

◆ 安排提供有效低价位含氟牙膏；

◆ 评估口腔健康教育内容，如何通过卫生人员把口腔健康教育引入妇幼保健；

◆ 评价通过口腔辅助人员为母亲及其儿童及小学儿童提供 ART 的可行性。

IPBOC 作为一种新的途径，有效利用公共经费满足社区口腔保健需要。

小结 Summary

通过本章学习帮助学生了解社会，文化，政治与经济因素都会对健康与口腔健康产生影响，熟悉初级卫生保健途径以及初级口腔卫生保健的基本概念与基本内容，社区口腔卫生保健的模式构架与实践，掌握社区口腔健康状态干预指数贫困社区的口腔卫生保健以及综合基本口腔保健的基本内容。

思考题 Review questions

1. 初级卫生保健的基本原则有哪些？
2. 社区口腔保健模式的基本构架是什么？
3. “零点”概念的实际意义是什么？

4. 社区口腔健康状况干预指数可用于哪些方面?
5. 贫困社区口腔保健的基本原则是什么?

参考文献 References

1. Cynthia M Pine. Community Oral Health. wright, 1998
2. 威廉·科克汉姆等. 医学社会学: 第七版, 华夏出版社, 2000
3. 亚历克斯·英克尔斯. 社会学是什么. 中国社会科学出版社, 1987
4. 梁浩材. 社会医学. 湖南科学技术出版社, 1987
5. 汝信. 社会科学新辞典. 重庆出版社, 1988
6. WHO/UNICEF Primary health care. Alm a Ata 1978. "Health for all" series no. 1. Geneva. World Health Organization, 1978
7. International Dental Federation and the World Health Organization: Global goals for oral health in the year 2000. Int. Dent J, 1982, 32: 74-77
8. World Health Organization: prevention methods and programme for oral diseases. Technical report series no. 713. WHO. Geneva, 1984
9. World Health Organization: Alternative system for oral care delivery. Technical Report series No. 750. WHO. Geneva, 1987
10. WHO Formulating strategies for health for all by the year 2000. WHO, Geneva, 1979
11. WHO Global strategy for health for all by the year 2000, WHO, Geneva, 1981
12. Halfdan Mahler. The meaning of "health for all by the year 2000. World Health Forum, 1981, vol2, No. 1: 5-22
13. Elizabeth T. Anderson, et al. community as partner. 3rd edition Lippincott, 2000
14. 张自宽. 卫生改革与发展探究. 黑龙江省人民出版社, 1999
15. 中华人民共和国卫生部医政司. 中国农村初级卫生保健指导手册. 沈阳出版社, 1992
16. Cynthia Pine M. Community oral health. Wright, 1998
17. Walter Mantsch. Aubrey Sheiham. Promoting oral health in deprived communities. DSE, 1995

（卞金有）

第十三章　口腔保健项目管理

Chapter XIII Programme Management for Oral Health Care

概述 Overview

本章首先介绍科学管理的基本概念与原则，阐述项目管理的三大基本职能（计划、实施与评价），重点叙述项目的计划。

This chapter is based on essential concepts and principles of scientific management, to describe three main functions of the programme management.

要点 Key points

- *Management — concepts, principles, main functions*
- *Concepts: 6M's*
- *Principles*
- *Procedure*
- *Planning*

第一节　科学管理的基本概念与原则

Section 1 Essential Concepts and Principles in the Scientific Management

许多卫生保健机构或卫生保健项目都是由医务人员负责管理的。他们负责管理许多人的活动和经费开支，并要达到一定的目标。医学专业与管理专业是两个不同的领域。因此，担任各级管理工作的医务人员都需要学习并掌握管理的基本理论知识与技能，才有可能把一个机构或一个项目运筹好，以取得预期的结果或达到既定的目标。

在知识与应用之间，总是存在着一些距离。例如，我们早已知道如何预防龋病，但是，由于我们没有及时开展口腔预防保健工作，许多儿童至今仍在患有龋病，而且出现了上升趋势。随着医学科学的发展，医学模式的转变，现在我们已经认识到，影响大众的健康因素是多方面的。除已知的生物因素外，还有环境因素、行为与生活方式以及卫生保健服务。这四大因素的相互影响与作用，问题的解决变得复杂。所以，有些知识，特别是口腔保健知识的应用，要使得大多数人都能从中获益，并不是一件简单的事情。不过，如果我们能通过发展口腔保健项目，恰当起运用现代科学管理的原则和方法，就可以帮助我们分析问题、确定适当目标、选择重点、付诸实践、使有限的资源能得到最充分的利用，人们的口腔健康状况才有可能得到改善。

一、管理学简介 Introduction of management science

自从人类有了社会，就有管理存在。人类活动的领域中，管理很重要。管理人员的基本任务是设计和维护一种环境，使处于其间的人们能在集体内一道工作，以完成预定的使命和目标。换句话说，主管人员有责任采取各种行动，使个人有可能对集体目标尽其所能地作出贡献。

The basic task of all managers is to design and maintain an environment in which individuals, working together in groups, can accomplish preselected missions and objectives. In another words, managers are charged with the responsibility of taking actions that will make it possible for individuals to make their best contributions to group objectives.

（一）为什么要管理？ Why management?

管理工作是一切有组织的协作所不可缺少的，也是一个企业的各级组织所不可缺少的。实际上，凡想用最少量的时间、金钱、物资或劳务成本，以达到的目标所作出的每一种有效的努力都有一个特点，就是它会采用管理的基本过程、原理以及技术方法。

Managing is essential in all organized cooperation, as well as at all levels of organization in an enterprise. Indeed, a characteristic of every effective group effort designed to attain group goals at the least cost of time, money, material, or discomfort is that it adopts the basic process, principles, and techniques of management.

（二）管理是一门科学还是一门艺术？ Is managing a science or an art?

虽然自古就有人类组织起来以达到共同的目标，但是管理作为一门科学只是在现代才发展起来，尤其是第二次世界大战以来，人们才逐渐开始认识到管理工作的质量对现代生活是重要的，正因为如此，才引起人们对管理过程，及其环境和技术方法进行广泛分析与研究的兴趣。管理的科学性质反映出这样的事实，它是依据一些由理论和原理组成的知识主体作为研究和进一步实验的对象，然而，作为一门科学它缺乏一门精确科学，如化学或数学那种确切的特征。实际上，管理工作如同所有其他艺术一样（不论是医学、作曲、工程学、棒球运动还是会计工作），利用了系统化的基本知识和科学，并根据现实情况加以运用，以获得期望的实际结果。这样做时，实践必定要求设计出一种能够通过工作，取得一定的实际结果的解决办法。这时，艺术就是达到一种预期结果的“诀窍”（know-how）。因此，在任何一个社会中只要人们认识到既有效果又有效率的集体协作的重要性，管理工作是所有艺术中最重要的就不会有大的争议。所以，与人的因素有关的许多变量使管理与科学相比，更像一门艺术。有效的管理总是一种随机制宜的，或因情况而异的管理。

The scientific nature of management is reflected in the fact that it is based on a more or less codified body of knowledge consisting of theories and principles that are subject to study and further experimentation. Yet, management as a science lacks the distinct characteristics of an exact discipline, such as chemistry or mathematics. The many variables associated with the human element make management as much an art as a science. Effective managing is always contingency or situational management.

（三）科学管理思想的出现 The emergence of scientific management thought

费雷德里克 · 泰勒被称为是科学管理的创始人。他认为科学管理实质上是在一定机构或行业内从事劳动的人们的一种彻底的心理革命，其基本原理可以概括为：(1)以科学（有系统的知识）代替经验法则；(2)协调集体行动，而不是相互不和；(3)达到人们的协作，而不是无秩序的个人主义；(4)为最大的产量，不是为受限制的产量而努力；(5)尽可能地发挥出工人所有的力量，从而使他们自己和他们的公司获得最大成功。

Frederick Taylor is usually called the father of scientific management. In its essence, scientific management involves a complete mental revolution on the part of the working man engaged in any particular establishment or industry. The fundamental principles that Taylor saw underlying the scientific approach to management may be summarized as follows:

(1) Replacing rules of thumb with science (organized knowledge);

(2) Obtaining harmony in group action, rather than discord;

(3) Achieving cooperation of human beings, rather than chaotic individualism;

(4) Working for maximum output, rather than restricted output;

(5) Developing all workers to the fullest extent possible for their own and their companies highest prosperity.

也许现代管理理论的真正创始人是法国工业家亨利 · 费约尔。费约尔指出管理学的原理是灵活的而不是绝对的，而且不论情况如何变化和特殊，都必须是能应用的。根据他的经验，列出十四条，概述如下：

1. 分工 Division of work

这就是经济学家所考虑的，为了有效地利用劳动力必须分工。费约尔把这个原则用于各种管理与技术工作之中。

This is the specialization which economists consider necessary to efficiency in the use of labor. Fayol applies the principle to all kinds of work; managed as well as technical.

2. 权力与职责 Authority and responsibility

费约尔在这里认为权力与职责是有关联的，职责是权力的必然结果，又是起因于权力。他把权力看作为是经理的正式职务与个人的智慧，经验，道德价值，以往服务等方面诸要素的结合。

Here Fayol finds authority and responsibility to be related, with the latter the corollary of the former and arising from it. He sees authority as a combination of official-deriving from the manager's position-and personal- "compounded of intelligence, experience, moral worth, past service, etc." -factors

3. 纪律 Discipline

是“对合同的尊重，以便达到服从，实际运用，有活力，以及人表面上的尊重”。费约尔断言纪律需要有各级水平的好领导。

Seeing discipline as "respect for arguments which one directed at achieving obedience, application, energy, and the outward marks of respect," Fayol declares that discipline requires good supervisors t all levels.

4. 统一指挥 Unity of command

这意味着雇员应该只接受一个上级的指令。

This means that employees should receive orders from one superior only.

5. 统一指导 Unity of direction

按这个原则，以同一目标活动的各个组织必须有一个领导和一个计划。与第四个原则不同，它与“法人团体”组织，而不是人员有关。(从任何意义上讲这并不意味着所有的决定都应由最高一级作出)。

According to this principle, each group of activities with the same objective must have one head and one plan. As distinguished from the fourth principle, it relates to the organization of the “body corporate”, rather than to personnel. Fayol did not in any sense mean that all decision should be made at the top.

6. 个人利益服从于总体利益 Subordination of individual to general interest

这个意义不解自明，当发现两者不一致时，管理者必须使其一致起来。

This is self-explanatory; when the two are found to differ, management must reconcile them.

7. 报酬 Remuneration

报酬与支付的方式要公平，使雇员与雇主双方都最大可能的满足。

Remuneration and methods of payment should be fair and afford the maximum possible satisfaction to employees and employers.

8. 集中 Centralization

费约尔不用“权力集中”一词，他指的是权力集中或分散的程度。依据“产生最大收益”的个别情况决定集中的程度。

Without using the term “Centralization of authority”, Fayol refers to the extent to which authority is concentrated or dispersed. Individual circumstances will determine the degree that will give the best over-all yield”.

9. 分级系统 Scalar chain

费约尔认为作为从最高层到最基层的“各级管理者”对此虽然没有必要时不违背组织程序，但当完全服从它变得不利时，就应该走捷径。

Fayol thinks of this as a “chain of superiors” from the highest to the lowest ranks, which, which not to be departed from needlessly, should be short-circuited when to follow it scrupulously would be detrimental.

10. 次序 Order

费约尔遵循一条简单的格言“各有其位（事或人)，各在其位（事或人)”把次序分成为“物质的”与“社会的”，这是安排人和事的一个基本组织原则。

Breaking this into “material” and “social” order, Fayol follows the simple adage of “a place for everything (everyone), and everything (everyone) in its (he order) place”. This is essentially a principle of organization in the arrangement of things and people.

11. 公平 Equity

对待下级管理者的厚道与公正的本分会引发下级的忠诚与热心。

Loyalty and devotion should be elicited from personnel by a combination of kindness and justice on the part of managers when dealing with subordinates.

12. 任用期稳定 Stability of tenure

他发现人员的不必要流动是管理不善的原因与后果，费约尔指出它的危害性与成本增加。

Finding unnecessary turnover to be both the cause and the effect of bad management, Fayol points out its dangers and costs.

13. 创意 Initiative

创意可陈述为想办法实施计划。因为创意是一个有智慧的人所能经历的最大满足之一。所以费约尔奉劝管理者要“牺牲个人的虚荣心”，好让下级发挥其作用。

Initiative is conceived of as the thinking out and execution of a plan. Since it is one of the "keenest satisfactions for an intelligent man to experience," Fayol exhorts managers to "sacrifice personal vanity" in order to permit subordinates to exercise it.

14. 团结精神 Esprit de corps

这是“团结就是力量”的原则，又是统一指挥原则的扩展，它强调需要团队工作和通过交流协调一致的重要性。

This is the principle that "in union there is strength", as well as an extension of the principle of unity of command, emphasized the need for teamwork and the importance of communication in obtaining it.

上述这些原则，在各项事业中用得最多，不可缺少。

二、现代管理的基本概念 Essential concepts of modern management

管理既是一门艺术又是一门科学。它是以科学为基础的一门艺术。管理科学能够通过正规教育来学习。组织理论是管理科学的一个典范，可以作为基本原理来学习。然而艺术通过这种方式只能部分获得，另一部分必须通过经历，试验与错误，通过个人的偏爱来获得。管理艺术的一个范例是时机选择，是管理决策方面的一个重要内容。

管理的概念与许多其他的复杂概念一样，意味着对不同的人是不同的事情。作为一种结果，可以发现管理一词有许多定义，当把管理作为一门学科来学习或者当讨论它与实际工作的状况的关系时，其中大多数的一个共同思路是有必要想到管理是一个过程，管理作为一个过程，可以用这一过程所包含的职能或活动范围加以分析和叙述。不同的作者给予了不同的定义，其中最简单的一个定义就是：管理就是有目的地去完成一件事情。从我们的目的考虑，管理是一个过程，包括人际与技术两个方面，一个组织或者它的部分管理目标就是通过利用人力与物力资源以及技术来完成。因此，凡是有共同劳动，合作与生活的地方都有管理活动。

管理还有另一个定义，就是有效地利用资源。按照管理学的基本原理，管理有六大要素，在国外称之为6个“M's”，即意图（包括目标策略等）、措施、方法、人力、物力、以及财力。

为了达到既定目标，人、财、物的使用必须达到平衡。平衡的实质是效率。例如，在一个口腔保健项目的开展与管理之中，人、财、物的资源总是有限的。管理的目的就是要通过制定口腔健康目标，选择适当的策略、措施和方法，通过人们协调一致的工作，使有限的资源得到充分合理的利用，从而在一个项目的目标地区内，在一定的项目周期内，产生最大的效率，即尽可能获取最佳的口腔健康效果。所以，管理还有一个更进一步的定义：就是管理是使得资源更有效地得到利用并使人们在一起协调一致地工作以便达到目标

管理是以一定的思想作指导，通过职能机构的集体努力，把思想付诸行动的连续而能动的应用过程。可以把这个过程看作为一种简单的输入——输出关系，其中输入（人力、物力资源

与技术）转化成期望的输出（完成组织的或部分组织的目标）。

Management is getting things done by its objective. Management is a process, with both interpersonal and technical aspects, through which the objectives of an organization, or that part of it being managed, are accomplished by utilizing human and physical resources and technology. Management is the efficient use of resources. There are 6 Ms in management - meaning, measurement, methods, men, materials, money. The different types of resources used for achieving objectives must be carefully balanced. The key concept in the above definition is efficiency, which is concerned with the balanced use of resources. Management is to make effective use of resources and to get people to work harmoniously together in order to achieve objectives. Management has been defined as a process of continuing, dynamic application of thought and action directed at the philosophy, function and structure of organized efforts. This process can be viewed as a simple input-output relationship in which inputs human and physical resources and technology are transformed into desired outputs accomplishment of the objectives of the organization or some part of it.

三、管理的基本原则 Principles in management

管理的原则可以用于各级组织机构，也可用于开展各种项目与活动。一个口腔保健项目，如果管理得当，能够提供必需的口腔保健服务，可以促进项目地区的目标人群口腔健康水平的提高。一般来说，管理有 9 个基本原则。

（一）目标管理 Management by objectives, MBO

目标管理或结果管理是一个计划，动员与控制的过程，在这一过程中组织的资源将集中用于达到一个总目标中的主要目标。它提供了一个框架，在这个框架内，为了达到具体的目标，要不断地评估该组织的人员与资源。它强调总体目标，认可下属机构的工作对整个组织的影响，对资源分配的决定要以最佳完成所有任务的方式进行。目标管理是一体化管理的概念，包含着计划过程、参与管理、动员与控制诸要素。它反映出对管理的系统途径，强调计划，完成，以评估输入——输出周期变化提供反馈信息的循环过程。

Management by objectives (MBO) or results management is a process of planning, motivating, and controlling in which the resources of the organization are focused on achieving the key objectives stated in the organization's overall goals. MBO provides a framework within which the personnel and the resources of the organization are assessed continually in the light of specific goal attainment. The overall goals are emphasized, the impact of the work of a unit or division on total organizational effort is recognized, and the decisions to allocate organizational resources are made in a manner that optimizes overall performance. MBO is an integrative management concept, containing elements of the planning process, participative management, motivation, and control. It reflects the systems approach to management with its emphasis on a cycle of planning, effecting, and feedback with assessment of change in the input-output cycle.

应用目标管理的主要理由是合理的组织计划更容易实现，以一种系统的方式促进上下信息交流，监督任务的完成，加强动员，明确责权相应的关系，以及确定培训的需要。因此，目标管理是管理的第一个原则。

目标管理就是首先要把完成的事情确定为一个目标。目标可以有多种。有些目标可以是今后某个时期内一个人群的口腔健康状态预期的变化，也可以是人群可以利用的服务方面或者服务覆盖某个适宜年龄组的范围；还有一些可以列出在某一周期内所要完成的任务。而所有这一切可以归纳为：

- 要完成什么；
- 完成多少；
- 在什么地方完成；
- 何时完成。

MBO is saying what one wants to accomplish is setting an objective (a goal, a purpose, a target) . There are many kinds of objectives. Some of these objectives describe an aspect of the oral health status of a population at some later time; others state the services that will be made available to that population or the coverage of some eligible group; others list the tasks that will be performed in a particular week; but all should state:

- *What is to be accomplished;*
- *How much of it;*
- *Where it is to be done;*
- *When it is to be completed.*

为什么要制订这样的目标呢？首先需要明确有目标才有可能对达标的效果进行评价。然而明确了目标，并不一定就能达到。只有经过一段时期，通过相互合作，合理分配与有效利用资源，完成总体计划中的部分目标，然后比较预期的目标与实际达标的程度，以判断其效果。效果是指既定目标达到的程度。另外，明确了目标可以使一个人决定如何达到目标，也就是说结果可以有助于选择某种手段来达到目标。目标管理的目的是有效地利用资源，产生最大效果。

（二）学习经验 Learning from experience

当目标与结果之间产生差距时，管理就是分析结果是如何达到的，找出造成差距的原因。有时有些困难不可能在短期内克服，另一些则可以设法克服。这一过程就是学习，也称为反馈。从实践中学习，获得经验，并分析成功的原因与失败的教训，从实践中获取反馈信息，决定采取某种行动。

When a gap occurs between the objectives and results (or achievement) , management makes an analysis of how the observed results were achieved, and discovers what caused the gap, sometimes the causes cannot be removed in the short run: These are usually called constraints; others can be removed or remedied, and action is taken accordingly. In this process, learning takes place. This process is sometimes called feedback (of information from experience to decision for action) . There are other kinds of feedback from which management learns from experience.

（三）劳力分工 Division of labour

管理的总原则正常地称作劳力分工，即分工明确，各负其责。也就是说工作必须由各类不同的技术人员来分担，每个人都具有其达标的技能，所以，需要明确规定各自的职能，平衡和协调各类人员的作用。

当这个原则正确地用于一组成员中的分工或工作分配时，这个组就成为一个团队。在一个团队中，当有专门化与劳力分工时，每一类人员发挥各自的技能以便达到目标，管理就存在于把权限分配到每一类人员所负责的工作之中。团队途径是管理试图使有关的各种不同的人员之间达到平衡的一种方式。但是在其他资源之间也必须保持平衡。例如，器械不够或供应不足或经营经费短缺等。

Work must be shared by or divided among, a number of different categories of technically skilled people. When this principle is correctly applied and work is divided, or distributed, among members of a group, the group becomes a team. In a team, and generally when there is specialization and division of labour - each kind of manpower exercising its own skills towards achieving the objectives, management will consist in assigning the right (balanced) proportion of each kind of staff to the job in hand.

（四）资源替换 Substitution of resources

主要指劳力与物资的替换，特别是在人力、物力短缺的地区，使用辅助人员取代口腔专业人员完成某些口腔保健工作。

Often, when the resources that are normally used to provide services become scarce or too expensive, different resources or a different balance of the resources may be used to produce the intended results. One particular type of substitution of resources is labour substitution.

（五）工作趋同 Convergence of work

工作趋同的原则意味着为了共同的目标一起工作，各项工作与各种活动应相互支持，以便达到目标。这里包含着工作关系应有助于每项活动的成功，体现出总体效果。一般来说，卫生保健活动在三个方面带有学习性，叙述性和提供性：服务、发展以及支持。服务活动（如窝沟封闭）通常需要一些前期的开发活动（如培训操作人员）以及一些连续的支持活动（如供应）。这些都需要管理使保证适当的趋同一致，资源平衡，工作关系协调，最终产生预想的结果。这些具体的活动彼此之间必需有一定的逻辑关系，时间关系或程序关系，以及活动之间的空间场所关系。所以组织协调很重要。

This means that work activities should be so designed and directed to support each other towards the achievement of objectives. It also implies that working relations should contribute to the success of each activity, and so to general effectiveness.

（六）职能决定结构 Functions determine structure

人与人之间的工作关系常用职能与结构来叙述。职能关系直接从工作的技术性质衍生而来，例如，一个牙防小分队的工作关系。结构关系适合于管理规章与标准，特别是与分配给个人的职权有关，例如，谁有权雇用与解雇工作人员，一个口腔保健医师的职权范围，一个保健护士必须向谁汇报工作等。当人们的岗位职权范围确定之后，相互之间的工作关系也就确定了。工作关系的要点是在必要的地方必要的时间由最合适的人作出决定。在紧急情况下，一个卫生工作者如果还固守规定，什么也不做，将会受到责备。这需要从劳力分工、职能决定结构以及授权的原则来理解。工作关系的一个主要着眼点是在必要的时候和适当的地方由最适合的人来作出决定。

The working relations between people are usually described as functional and structural. Functional relations are derived direct from the technical nature of the work; and where, when, and in which sequence it takes place; e.g., the working relations of a team. Structural relations pertain to administrative rules and standards, and in particular to the authority and responsibility assigned to individuals.

In this area of relations between people and their activities and the resources they use, management is based on one major principle of organization: when work is clearly defined, working relations are easily determined. This may be briefly stated as functions determine structure. A major concern in working relations is to enable decisions to be made where and when necessary, by the most suitable person.

（七）授权 Delegation

把某个人的权利委托给另一个人时就产生了授权。授权就是把权利委托给人或机构代为执行。这可以是有条件的，或者是无条件的，只要机会存在，就可使人负起责任。当管理工作繁忙时，用授权方式解决尤为重要。

It states that responsibility or authority is delegated to the lowest level at which it can be competently discharged. Delegation takes place when somebody's authority is lent to another person, conditionally or not, so as to enable that person to take responsibility when the occasion arises. Never do yourself what another can do for you as well as you would.

（八）例外管理 Management by exception

掌握异常情况，抓住关键信息，作出决定或采取某种行动。其含义是掌握的信息一定要经过选择，不必过多。同时，首先要作出重要决定，决定过多意味着对重要决定的决定。因此，例外管理的原则是对信息的选择与重点决策。

It is important to note that management need not know everything that takes place. In particular, a programme that runs well does not call usually for control decisions. It is more important to be informed about exception, i.e., things that do not go so well, which may require urgent decisions. The first of the two management principles that deal with information is management by exception.

In effect this means two things: First: do not be overloaded with routine, unnecessary information. Be selective. Keep your mind available for critical information, on which you will be required to act. Second: make big decisions first. Being overloaded with petty decisions may mean neglect of more important ones, or what has been called "postponing decisions until they become unnecessary". In short, management by exception means selectivity in information and priority in decision.

（九）决策捷径 Shortest decision-path

由处于最佳决策地位的人作决定。这一原则意味着决策必须及时，尽可能接近并及时影响决策对象。这样做，可节省时间，简化程序，符合实际情况，产生有效作用。

The last management principle deal with the issue: WHO should make which decision? It means that decision must be made as closely as possible in time and place to the object of the decision and to those affected by it. This saves time and work (e.g. to transmit information) and also ensures that decisions can take full account of the actual circumstances which demand the decisions and in which they are put into effect.

Therefore, to be effective and efficient, health care activities should support each other; this is the convergence principle. The working relations of health workers should be guided by the principle that function determine structure. From this follows another principle-the delegation of authority.

Dealing with the information needed for management, we highlight two principles: management by exception, for selectivity and priority; and the shortest decision-path, which indicated who is in the best position to make decisions, in relation to the object and the circumstances of the decisions.

四、口腔保健项目管理的基本程序 Basic procedure of programme management for oral health care

项目管理是通过有组织的运用系统理论和方法对项目及其资源进行计划、组织、协调与控制的过程，旨在实现项目的特定目标。卫生项目管理是一项临时性有组织的活动，建立并开展一项新的或经过改进的服务活动，以达到减少与健康有关的问题的目的。这种有组织的活动围绕着一个明确的目标，并且有一定的达标日期限制。

Programme or project management is a process through an organized efforts, by using the systemic theory and methods in planning, organizing coordinating, and controlling the programme and its resources in order to achieve the specific objectives of the programme. Health programme management is a temporary organized effort to set up and put into operation a new or revised service that will result in the reduction of specific health and health-related problems. Programme management for oral health care always follow these basic concepts, principles and steps, if we want to make it successfully and effectively.

为了有效地开展口腔保健项目，应该遵循四步必要的程序：（需要）评估、计划、实施与（结果）评价。不论是在社区，还是在其他非社区的人群，甚至是口腔保健机构，通过项目管理的模式提供适当的口腔保健服务都需要熟悉和利用这四步程序或者称为项目管理的基本内容。这是任何项目管理获得成功的基本保障。

（一）需要评估 Needs assessment

需要评估是通过一种有组织的系统途径确定目标人群和现时人群口腔保健需要的程度和严重性。

Needs assessment is an organized and systemic approach to identify a target group and to define the extent and severity of oral health needs present.

（二）计划 Planning

计划是对减少或消除一个或多个问题作出的有组织的反映。

Planning is an organized response to reduce or eliminate one or more problems.

（三）实施 Implementation

实施包括按计划采取行动的过程以及监督计划活动，人员，设备资源以及供应。这个步骤应包括来自专业人员与参与者还有进行评估机制的反馈信息。

Implementation includes the process of putting the plan into action and monitoring the plan's activities, personnel, equipment, resources, and supplies. This step should include feedback from personnel and participants as well as ongoing evaluation mechanisms.

（四）评价 Evaluation

评价是针对早期计划阶段制订的目标测量项目结果的方法。这个过程在进行之中应明确存在的问题与解决问题的办法，在需要时可以帮助修改项目。它还可分为中期评价或称为过程评价，以及终期结果或称结果评价。

1. 中期评价或称为项目的内部评价，因为评价是在项目进行之中进行的，是对项目过程或活动的一种检查。

2. 总结评价或称评价，涉及在项目实施完成之后判断项目的成就或价值。这个步骤是试图决定整个项目的实施是否适合于制定的目标。

Evaluation is the method of measuring results of the programme against objectives developed during the early planning stages. This process is ongoing and should identify the problems and solutions to assit in revising the programme as needed.

a. Formative evaluation, or the internal evaluation of a programme, is an examination of the processes or activities of a programme as they are take place.

b. Summative evaluation involves judging the merit or worth of a programme after it has been in operation. This step is an attempt to determine whether a fully operational programme is meeting the goals for which it was developed.

（1）需要评估 Needs assessment

评估需要的相对重要性可能是一个复杂的过程。这取决于人的价值观，其中有些需要是普遍公认的，而另一些则是有较多矛盾的。虽然许多人会认为影响大多数人的需要一定要作为重点，而另一些人则考虑到其他因素，如年龄、对社会未来的影响等。

For example, a need that involves life or death generally receives higher priority; however, a choice between a health need that might affect the lives of a few people and one that affects the lives of large numbers of people is less clear-cut. For example, a community may need to decide about initiating a free influenza vaccine programme for its old population, enhancing the immunization programme for children, or adding a clinic offering reduced dental care for indigent families.

确定健康重点问题的指导原则是：

Guiding principles —— Establishing Health priorities

- *What is the magnitude of the problem? (Does it cause death or disability?)*
- *How many people are affected (one person, small community, whole country?)*
- *What type of resources are available (personnel, money, facilities, technology?)*
- *What has already been done in the community?*
- *What are the prevailing attitudes towards the problem?*
- *Which groups are expressing the most interest in the problem?*
- *What are the legal constraints?*

确定健康需要的重点问题，事实上每个人按照其自身的价值与想法都是不一样的。问题常由想法引起，很明显解决这个难题涉及在疏忽与过分关注之间找到适当的平衡。

If a community's basic need for food and security are not being met, dental needs assume a low priority. if a community's perception of needs is adhered to exclusively, actual clinical health problems may go untreated because the people are not knowledgeable about many areas of health care. Although it is unethical to impose one's own perceptions on a community, it is the professional's responsibility to inform people of existing problems and their consequences.

对需要的评估能够帮助发现问题。指导进行社区需要评估可能要花费很多劳力与经费。口腔调查是由牙学院、地方和国家卫生部门以及社区健康中心进行的。因此，可以利用各种方法获取资料和分析资料，在完成需要评估之后，制定适当的目标就是下一步的工作。

The assessment provides information not only about the problem but also about the community profile that will assist in finding the appropriate solution. If funds are not available, coordination with other agencies interested in obtaining similar health information on the given population may be the solution. Another possibility is to investigate dental surveys that have been done by other organizations. Coordination with other agencies and organizations to know what has been done and what need to be accomplished can prevent duplication of services.

（2）计划 Planning

制定总目标、具体目标与项目活动是计划过程的一部分在这个阶段，要有社区参与。制定项目的目标是一个积极的过程，为了改变社区的状况而提出具体的建议。这些改变针对需要评估中确定的重点问题。

Developing goals, objectives, and programme activities are part of the planning process. The formulation of programme goals and objectives is an active process, offering specific proposals for changes to be made in the community. These changes address the specific problems identified in the needs assessment.

总目标（Goals）对将作出什么样的改变作大体概述，以此为据，制定具体目标。

具体目标（Objectives）比总目标更具体；以可测量的，项目活动的预期结果。

Goals provide a broadly based statement of what changes will take place, from which specific objectives are developed. For example: the school-based fluoride mouthrinse programme will improve the oral health of school aged children.

Objectives are more specific than goals; they describe, in a measurable way, the desired end result of programme activities.

完成是一个可测量目标的关键。这是一个动作词，例如“书写”“示范”，或“叙述”。目标的另一个要素是情况。说明活动在什么情况下展开，以及标准，说明活动必须达到什么程度，在书写具体目标时，完成动词是主要的，目标包括情况与标准，使目标更具体而有用。

In Summary:

1. A performance verb tells the activity and outcome.

2. A condition tells under what circumstance the outcome will occur.

3. A criterion tells how well the action and outcome must e accomplished to be effective.

An example of an objective for the aforementioned goal would be as follows: upon completion of today's six-step demonstration of how to rinse, the children will demonstrate the six steps without error.

Performance verb: demonstrate

Condition: upon completion of today's six-step demonstration

Criterion: without error

一旦问题得到确认，用一种解决问题的方式叙述项目总目标与具体目标，下一步是陈述如何达到预期的结果，提出项目的活动，叙述怎样完成项目的具体目标。在计划这些项目活动中，必须仔细考虑项目可以利用的资源种类，还有制约因素。计划对于一个项目的成功是至关重要的因素。一个计划得很好的社区口腔保健项目，有具体的活动，又考虑到资源与制约因素，在实施中通常是会成功的。

Once the problem has been identified and programme goals and objectives have been established with a description of a solution, the next step is to state how to bring about the desired results.

In planning these programme activities, one must carefully consider the type of resources available as well as programme constraints. For example, in planning a school fluoride mouth rinse programme in which the chosen activity would be weekly rinsing, resources might include selecting (1) the site at which the rinsing is conducted, (2) personnel, (3) supplies, and (4) the financial means to pay for the supplies. Constraints might include (1) availability of dental personnel to conduct screenings, (2) negative attitudes from some patients, (3) the amount of time it takes to rinse, or (4) lack of funding.

Planning is a crucial element to a successful programme. A community oral health programme that is well planned, with specific activities and consideration to resources and constraints, is usually successful in terms of implementation.

(3) 实施 Implementation

实施是把计划付诸行动的过程。在实施进展阶段，应该进行监督与评价，以确保项目的效果。实施同计划一样，涉及个人、机构与社区一起工作。

The process of putting the plan into action, the implementation phase, is ongoing and should be supervised and evaluated to ensure programme effectiveness. Implementation, like planning, involves individuals, agencies, and the community working together.

The strategy should answer the following questions:

1. Why: the effect of the objective to be achieved

2. What: the activities required to achieve the objective

3. Who: the individuals responsible for each activity

4. When: the chronological sequence of activities

5. How: the materials, media, methods, and techniques to be used

6. How much: a cost estimate of materials and time

为了有助于这些问题的解决，许多社区口腔保健项目先从小范围开始。在较小的人群中开展的试验研究称为预试验。这种实施策略允许有机会测试项目的效果，并且容易提供项目活动的控制与监督。预试验项目可以提供有用的信息，用于对未来的项目作出决定。预试验是评价项目实施的一种形式。

pilot testing. In a pilot test for a fluoride mouth rinse programme, for instance, only one school would be involved the first year and the programme would be expanded to included two or more schools the following year.

(4) 评价 Evaluation

评价是对有关项目价值的一种判断。第一步是评阅项目的总目标，然后检查具体的可测量的目标。每一个目标都应该评阅，以便确定达到总目标的程度。评价是为了确定项目是否是按设计完成的。总结完成的好与否，或者依据直觉判断作出结论。

Evaluation is a judgment of merit or worth about the programme. The first step is to review the programme goals and then to examine the specific measurable objectives. Each objective should be reviewed to determine how well it is meeting the programme goals. Evaluation determines whether the programme accomplishes what it was designed to accomplish (e,g., were the objectives of this study or programme successfully met? If not, why not?

这个途径的一个内在特点是形成相反结果的可能性。如果作出没有达标的结论，并不意味着项目已经失败。如果评价恰当，负面结果可以变成学习经验，对未来的项目指标，研究都有好处，因此有一定的成功之处。在实施过程中的中期评价可以帮助指出问题，尽早提供改正的机会。终期评价实际上是测量项目开始时提出的问题是否取得成功。

项目评价是应用性研究的一个案例。基础（临床）研究涉及获得关于事实，行为，关系与原则的真实性。应用性研究具有相同的概念，但是强调应用知识和发展对问题的解决办法。项目评价的根本目的是帮助决定项目的总体效果。

For example, a basic researcher would be concerned with the effectiveness of the fluoride mouth rinse on the teeth and which concentration to use. A programme evaluator would be concerned with the effect of the programme operation and its ability to met the programme objectives.

项目管理人员在项目的需要评估、计划、实施与评价中将起到重要作用。通过了解如何有效地组织一个社区的口腔保健项目，并直接参与实施，对于达到为了所有人的口腔健康目标有重要影响。

第二节　口腔保健项目的计划

Section 2 Planning for oral health programmes

微生物学家Rene Dubos指出人类历史的大部分是意外与盲目选择的结果。当危机发生时，我们的解决办法总是即刻作出一点点努力而不是经过精心的计划。因此，最大的重点是需要发展我们预测、计划，从而防止相同危机再次发生的能力。

Microbiologist Rene Dubos has suggested that most of human history has been a result of accidents and blind choices. When a crisis occurs, our solutions are immediate and involve piecemeal efforts rather than considered and thoughtful planning. The need to develop our ability to predict, plan, and thus prevent the same crisis from recurring should have the highest priority.

按照字典的定义："计划是用一种详细的方法建立行动的基础"换句话说，计划是通过一种系统的方式，确定问题、建立重点、形成目标、决定策略选择、并决定如何使计划付诸行动。

Planning is the use of a detailed method to create a basis for action) 。E.C. Banfield presents a much more explicit definition of the term "planning is a decision about a course of action". A plan is an approach to defining the problem, setting priorities, developing specific goals and objectives, determining alternative strategies, and then deciding how to put the plan into action.

健康计划有多种类型。因影响健康系统的因素不同而不同，例如，一个地区的地理状况、人口的社会文化背景、经济状况以及政治状况。Spiegel 提出了几种类型，简述如下：

1. 解决问题的计划涉及确定和解决一个问题

Problem-solving planning involves the identification and resolution of a problem. An example of problem solving was the appearance of dental fluorosis among residents of a community. This enamel disorder was identified through a scientific study of possible causative factors.

2. 项目计划需要对一个限定的健康问题设计如何采取行动的过程

Programme planning entails designing a course of action of a circumscribed health problem. School-based fluoride rinse programmes are an example of designing a course of action for the problem of dental caries within a community setting.

3. 协同努力开展活动目的在于提高活动与项目的可利用率、效率、生产力、效果及其他方面。这个阶段常常涉及一个调整的过程，例如，一种服务与设施的合并或者重新组合。

Coordination of efforts and activities aims to increase the availability, efficiency, productivity, effectiveness, and other aspects of activities and programmes. This stage often involves an adjustment process, such as a merger or a closing of services and facilities. An example is the closing of preventive and pediatric clinics in a dental hospital located in areas with a declining dental caries in children.

4. 当资源有限时，资源分配计划涉及选择最佳方案达到预期目标。计划人员要求在一个系统内分配预算、劳力与设施，这样可以满足现时的需求。

Planning for the allocation of resources involves selecting the best alternative to achieve a desired goal when the amount of resources is limited. Planners are called on to allocate the budget, the labor, and the facilities in a system so that it may meet existing needs and demands. An example is the decision by a provincial government with limited financial resources for the provision of dental services to cut services to medically indigent adults based on the cost-effectiveness of providing preventive dental care to a younger population.

5. 制定一个涉及发展的计划或行动方案包括推荐与支持性资料。这一项工作或具体任务对于计划的制定是具有普遍性的。一个社区的口腔健康计划叙述那个社区人群的口腔健康状况与口腔保健服务的分布是这种计划的一个范例。

Creation of a plan involves the development of a blueprint or proposal for action containing recommendations and supporting data. It is common for a commission of specific task force to be created to prepare the plan. A community oral health plan that describes the oral health status and the distribution of oral health services for the population in that community is a good example of such planning.

6. 设计标准操作程序，要求计划人员提出一套实践标准或者操作与评价标准。这可能是一项法规，或者可能是有关部门自愿制定的。

Design of standard operating procedures requires planners to come forth with a set of standards of practice or criteria for operation and evaluation. This can be a result of legislation, or it can be created voluntarily by the parties concerned. Guidelines for evaluating the quality of dental care as part of a continuous quality improvement programme for a health authority is one example.

采用系统的方式计划口腔保健项目，应当用这一计划过程，通过选择适当的口腔疾病预防策略和方法作为指南解决特殊的问题。对不同的社会，面临着不同的疾病发病状况，不同的社会文化、经济与环境条件以及可利用的资源，应当选择适当的预防步骤，并给予适当的技术指导。计划的目的是在既定的项目目标下，一定量的资源范围内获取最大的效果。必须把计划看作为一个过程，包括一个计划人员应采取一系列合乎逻辑的步骤建立一个唯独适合于这一具体情况或系统的计划。

The aim of planning is to obtain the maximum effectiveness of a given amount of resources in terms of the stated goals of a programme. Planning has to be seen as a process involving a sequence of logical steps which should be used by a planner to create a plan that is unique for the specific situation or system.

计划过程有能动的连续性。现在口腔健康状况已发生了鲜明的变化，工业化国家变得越来越好，而大多数发展中国家正在变坏。所以实施项目建立在一次就解决所有问题的基础上是不行的，一个项目的成功将会改变疾病的水平，那么，采用另一种不同的策略可能会更适当而有效。世界卫生组织推荐的快速而经济的监测性预调查能够保证尽早地认识到这种趋势，采取适当的行动来改变这种状况，然而，为了后代人的利益，这些有效活动应该是连续的。

The process of planning is a dynamic continuer. Thus, it is not sufficient to implement programmes on a “once-and-for all” basis, because the success of a programme will change disease levels and a different strategy may then be more appropriate and efficient. Rapid and economical monitoring surveys of the WHO pathfinder type can ensure that such trends are recognized early and appropriate action undertaken to respond to the changed situation. However, effective activities should be continued for the benefit of future generations.

因此，在一个起伏不定的，不断变化的系统内，这一过程本身必须保持机动灵活，反映提出的新问题。

计划项目的过程必须按照以下的逻辑过程与步骤进行：

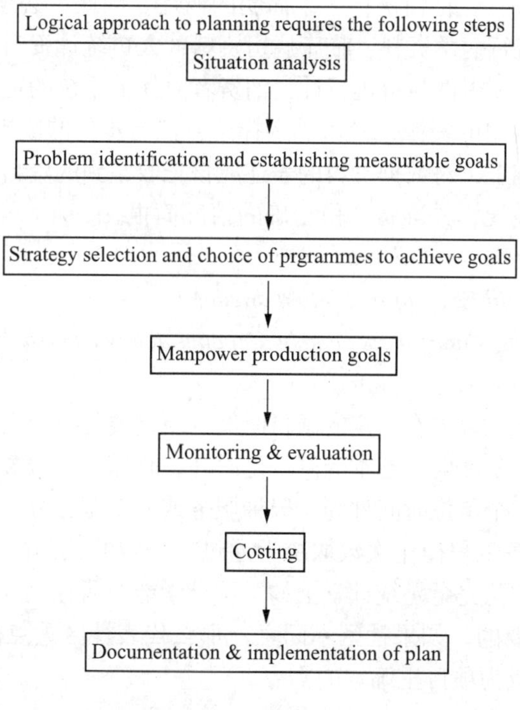

一、情况分析 Situation analysis

应该对情况进行仔细分析，以便确定口腔保健需求以及限制项目选择的制约因素。这样做有几方面的原因：

(1) 主要原因是明确问题以及确定问题的范围与严重程度；

(2) 了解社会概貌，弄清为什么问题存在，即产生这些问题的原因，这种信息将为问题的解决提出适当的目标；

(3) 评价项目的效果，通过获得基础资料，检查在具体问题的解决方面取得的进展数量来进行评价。

A carefully conducted situation analysis should be undertaken to identify oral health needs and demands and the constraints that limit choice of programme. There are several reasons for doing so:

(1) The primary reason is to define the problem and to identify the extent and severity of the problem;

(2) To obtain a profile of the community to ascertain why the problem exists, that is, the causes of the problem. This information will help in developing the appropriate goals and objectives in the problem solution;

(3) To evaluate the effectiveness of the programme. This is accompanied by obtaining baseline data and over time, measuring the amount of process achieved in solving the specific problem.

An analysis of the situation is essential.

分析目标地区的具体情况是项目计划的基础。通过具体的情况分析，要确定现时目标人群的口腔健康状况，估计现时的口腔卫生服务提供系统的完成状况，然后用文字尽可能全面清楚地描述现时的状况，并且，把情况作一个简明的概述。因此，必须要获得所需要的数据资料。这些数据资料包括：流行病学资料、临床病历资料、人口统计资料、选择的社会经济指标、提供的口腔保健设施的可利用性与可进行性、消费者对保健系统的行为与态度、与口腔健康问题有关的病因学或可以利用的资源以及可供选择的方法与步骤的成本与效果。

在情况分析的基础上，对数据资料的表述应该把收集到的资料编成一个文件。尽可能清楚而完整地叙述现时的情况，并准备一份正确的情况简报。

Presentation of data on situation analysis

Data collected should be compiled into a document

Describe the existing situation as clearly and completely as possible

Prepare a concise summary of situation

采用数学方法可以计算出在一定的项目时间内所需要的口腔资源，然后把这些数据资料转化成时间，人力以及设备需要。基本的测量是时间，临床口腔服务需要以及医务人员的能力都可以用时间来表示，这个单位时间称为一分钟服务或一个服务分。口腔医生及辅助人员数还有为人口治疗所需的设备数和操作次数取决于通过在一定的人群内所需要的总服务分钟数来确定。在性质上，这种方法完全是统计学上的，统计学能对所存在的问题建立参数，但是人的价值观与态度同样是重要的，如果社区不同意，那么代表社区重点需要的统计学上的一系列数据，几乎不可能转变成为项目里确定的需要。

二、确定重点 Determining priorities

确定重点就是利用人的价值方法以及原始资料，加之有限的资源，判断什么重要，必须建立重点，这样可以使资源得到最充分的利用。如果不确定重点，项目就无法保证那些最需要得到保健的人享有这种服务。

在确定重点时，有些因素应该考虑到：

1. 影响大多数人的问题与影响少数人的问题相比，前者应成为重点；

2. 影响大多数人的问题与影响少数人的问题发生对抗，那么，比较严重的问题应成为重点；

3. 帮助确定重点时，社区应该参与；

4. 应该建立健康顾问委员会或代表消费者的服务机构，社区领导与保健提供者一起帮助制定政策和确定重点；

5. 与社区代表一起制定的计划将有助于项目的执行与接受；

6. 当牙病问题影响到一个以上目标人群时，一般来说下列人群是最需要的，学龄和学龄前儿童、残疾人群、 慢性病患者、老年人、妇女以及低收入人群；

7. 如果龋病是首要问题，那么比较容易患龋的人群是学龄前与学龄儿童以及收入低的人群。

当依据牙病问题确定了目标人群之后，就可以确立项目的类型。

Certain factors should be considered in determining priorities

A problem that affects a large number of people generally takes priority over a problem that affects a small number of people;

If the problem affecting a large number of people competing with the problem affecting a few people, then the more serious problem should take priority;

The community should be involved to assist in the establishment of these priorities;

A health advisory committee or task force representing consumers, community leaders, and providers should be established to assist in the development of policies and priorities;

Planning with community representative will aid in the implementation and acceptance of programme;

When the health problem is dental disease there is generally more than one target group that is affected. The following are target groups commonly associated with high-risk dental needs:

Preschool and school-age children

Mentally and/or physically handicapped persons

Chronically ill and /or medically compromised persons

Elderly persons

Expectant mothers

Low-income minority groups (urban and rural)

If dental caries is first problem, the special groups that are more susceptible to dental caries are preschool and school-aged children and low-income minority groups.

Once the target group has been identified based on dental problem, the type of programme should be established.

三、形成项目目标 Development of programme goals and objectives

项目总目标是针对确定的问题概括整个项目的目的，例如，在学龄儿童中间存在着龋病问题，一个社区项目的目标可以是“改善这个社区学龄儿童的口腔健康状况。

Programme goals are broad statements on the overall purpose of a programme to meet a defined problem. An example of a programme goal for a community that has an identifiable problem of dental caries among school-aged children would be “To improve the oral health of the school-aged children in community.

项目的具体目标是用一种可以检查的方式、更为具体地叙述项目活动所期望达到的最终结果。其具体目标应作如下说明：

Programme objectives are more specific and describe in a measurable way the desired end result of programme activities. The objectives should specify the following:

1) What: the nature of the situation or condition to be attained;

2) Extent: the scope and magnitude of the situation or condition to be attained;

3) Who: the particular group or portion of the environment in which attainment is desired;

4) Where: the geographic areas of the programme;

5) When: the time “at” or “by” which the desired situation or condition is intended to exist.

An objective might state “By 2010 more than 95% of the population aged 5 ～ 18 years in the community × will retain all their teeth, and at least 60% will be caries-free”.

这个目标是一种结果目标，它提供了一种手段，用以测量具体目标的数量结果，这种途径帮助评价者和社区知道项目的起点以及项目预期要解决的一定问题的终点。它也帮助确定了一个减少或预防主要健康问题的时间表。

This is known as an outcome objective and provides a means of measuring quantitatively the outcome of the specific objective. This approach helps the evaluator and the community know both where the programme is and where it hopes to be with respect to a given health problem. It also aids in establishing a realistic timetable for reducing or preventing principal health problems.

第二种目标是实现总目标的具体途径。这种过程目标叙述一个具体过程，通过这一途径能够减少或预防一个公共卫生问题。例如，到 2005 年某社区实施一种群体用氟项目，确保通过以下途径达到适当的氟暴露。

Second, objectives are the specific avenues by which goals are met. Process objectives state a specific process by which a public health problem can be reduced and prevented. For example, by 2005 community × will have a public fluoride programme to guarantee access to fluoride exposure with the following:

Fluoridation of the public water supply to the optimum level

Fluoridation of school milk supplies in areas where community fluoridation is impossible or impractical

Initiation of the most cost-effective topical or systemic fluoride supplement programmes available to all schools if both objectives 1 and 2 are impossible.

Provision of topical fluoride application for persons with high caries and use of pit and fissure sealants where indicated.

一旦问题确定，项目的总目标与具体目标确立，叙述了解决或减少问题的办法。下一步就是陈述如何达到预期的结果，项目计划的这一步是提出项目开展的活动，叙述如何完成项目的目标。

Activities include three components:

(1) What is going to be done

(2) Who will be doing it

(3) When it will be done

Activity 1: Beginning January 1, 2005, two dental nurses will be hired to administer a self-applied fluoride rinse programme within the public school systems.

Activity 2: on March 1, 15 and 30, 2005, a series of 1-day training workshops for school teachers will be conducted by one dentist at selected public schools in community ×.

在计划开展这些项目活动时，重要的是考虑到项目可利用的资源和制约因素。

四、确立资源与制约因素 Identifying resources and constraints

确定了总目标与具体目标之后就是项目活动，包括三个方面：(1) 将要做些什么；(2) 由谁去做；(3) 什么时候完成。当计划开展这些活动时，应仔细考虑可利用的资源以及项目的制约因素。

Once the problem has been identified and programme goals and objectives have been established describing a solution to, or a reduction of, the problem. The next step is programme activities, including three components: 1) what is going to be done; 2) who will be doing it; 3) when it will be done. When planning these activities, careful consideration should be made to the type of resources available as well as to the programme constraints.

（一）确立资源 Identifying resources

要根据完成目标什么是最有效果的、最有效益的、最适当而又最合适的来决定人员、器械与供应、设施与经费。

Personnel, equipment and supplies, facilities, and financial resources, must be determined by consideration of what would be most effective, adequate, efficient, and appropriate for the tasks to be accomplished.

（二）确立制约因素 Identifying constraints

任何项目都有限制因素，与需要有关的资源通常是缺乏的，因此必须要作出选择，在计划阶段尽早确立这些制约因素，就能修改项目设计，从而可以制定一个更加实际可行的项目计划。

A planner seldom operates without limitations, his resources are usually scarce in relation to needs. Hence the necessity of making choices. By identifying these constraints early in the planning, one can modify the design of the programme, thereby creating a more practical and realistic plan.

通常有以下 4 种主要制约因素：

1. 行为方面：一个系统给予人的服务内容不会超过人们所希望得到的，即便服务是免费的。因此，必须了解各种类型的“顾客”的意见、态度、价值观与行为，以便估计如果开展预防性服务，有多少可能的要求可以变为有效的要求。

2. 经济方面：可以在口腔预防性服务方面花费多少总是有一个上限。

3. 社会，政治与行政管理方面：口腔保健系统是整个卫生保健系统的一个组成部分，其本身又与公共部门，管理系统联系在一起的，政治决策和社会政策可以影响卫生服务。

4. 专业人员方面：专业人员的价值观转变成为道德观以及他们对提供卫生保健的意见和态度，对任何一个计划的成功都有重要作用。

The system cannot do more for people in terms of services that what they are willing to receive, even if services are free. The opinions, attitudes, values and behaviour of the various types of "client" have to be known in order to estimate how much of potential demand could be transformed into effective demand if the preventive services were made available.

There is always an upper limit to how much can be spent on oral preventive services.

The dental care system is an integral part of the overall health system, which in turn is bound, in the public sectors, to the administrative system. Political decisions and social policies may affect the health services.

The values cherished by the profession and translated into ethical codes, as well as currently held opinions and attitude about the delivery of health care, have an important bearing on the success of any plan.

One of the best way to identify constraints is to bring together a group of concerned citizens who might be involved in or affected by the project. As a group that is familiar with the local politics and community structures, these individuals not only can identify the constraints but also can offer alternative solutions to and strategies for meeting the goals.

五、确定策略选择 Establishing alternative strategies

口腔保健项目可以利用的人员、资金、材料和器械等各不相同，这些可利用的资源大致可以分为少量的、稍有增加的、中等的、中等而有增加的以及大量的。而有关龋病与牙周病的一般情况至少可分为三种：1）龋病患病率从很低到低水平，但有增加趋势，牙周病患病率从中等到高水平；2）龋病患病率从低到中等水平，但有增加，牙周病患病率从中等到高水平；3）龋病患病率从高以很高水平，并且稳定或有减少趋势，牙周病患龋率从低到中等水平。

The personnel, funds, material, and equipment available for oral health programmes will vary greatly from one situation to another. The available resources are broadly classified as minimal, minimal increasing, moderate, moderate increasing and plentiful. There are at least three general situations with regards to dental caries and periodontal diseases: it may be (1) the prevalence of caries is very low to low, but increasing. The prevalence of periodontal diseases is moderate to high; (2) the prevalence of caries is low to moderate and increasing, the prevalence of periodontal diseases is moderate to high; (3) The prevalence of caries is high to very high and either stable or decreasing, the prevalence of periodontal diseases is low to moderate.

下面提出的一些策略与步骤可以作为在不同的疾病水平、可利用的资源以及规定的目标情况下的行动指南。

1. 具有少量资源，龋病患病水平低或很低，并且没有增加的指征，牙周病患病率高或很高的社区

策略——监测疾病水平，抓住每一个机会提高群众的认识，特别是初级卫生保健这一类活动。

Community with minimal resources, low and very low caries prevalence, with no indication of increases, and high or very high periodontal disease prevalence.

Strategy-monitor disease levels and take every opportunity to increase public awareness of the value of a clean and healthy month, particularly by including this activity in primary health care activities.

2. 具有少量的，但是有增加的资源，龋病患病率低，但有增加，牙周病患病率中等到很高水平的社区

策略——除了上述推荐的方式之外，应培训初级卫生保健人员，去除龈下牙石及牙菌斑，并给予口腔卫生指导。如饮水或食盐氟化可行，则应采取，并应鼓励使用含氟牙膏，但除了在城市学校里可以采用氟水含漱项目之外，无需再开展其他控制龋病的项目。

Communities with minimal by increasing resources, low but increasing caries prevalence, and moderate to very high periodontal disease prevalence. Strategy-in addition to the approach recommended in section 1. primary health care personnel should be trained to remove sub gingival calculus and plaque and give oral hygiene instruction. If water or salt fluoridation is feasible, it should be used use of fluoride toothpaste should be encouraged, but no other programmes of caries control except, possibly, mouth rinsing in urban schools, would be advised.

3. 具有低／中等资源，龋病水平可以是低的或甚至由中等到高水平，而且有增加趋势，牙周病患病水平从中等到很高的社区。

策略——在可能的地方应采用社区饮水或食盐氟化，应当适当地鼓励使用含氟牙膏，应在监督之下，引入氟水含漱，尤其在城区或其他高危人群。尽一切努力来控制每年的糖消耗量低于每人 20 公斤，并且对能起到关键作用的人群（卫生人员，教师）进行有关经常消耗含糖食物与饮料有害于口腔健康的教育。可能的话，制定规章劝阻儿童进食含糖点心。

Communities with low /moderate resources, with caries already at low or even moderate-to-high level and increasing, and moderate-to-very high periodontal disease.

Strategy-Community wide water or salt fluoridation should be used where possible. The use of fluoride dentifrices should be encouraged where appropriate and fluoride mouth rinsing should be introduced, under supervision, especially in urban areas or for other high-risk groups. Every effort should be made to keep annual sugar consumption below 20Kg per person and key groups (health workers, teachers) should be educated about the dangers of frequent consumption of food and drink containing sugars. Where possible, regulations should be introduced to control advertising that encourages children to eat sugar snacks.

4. 具有中等以及增加的资源，龋病患病率低／中等或高，并有增加，牙周病患病率从中等到很高的社区

策略——除上述之外，在饮水或食盐氟化不能进行的地方，应引入氟水含漱项目。如果含氟牙膏使用广泛，提供氟水含漱项目可以额外减少患龋率，但可能是不经济实用的。如果发现窝沟龋增加占优势，应考虑培训口腔辅助人员或非口腔人员应用窝沟封闭，或者也可培训非口腔专业人员提供口腔卫生指导，去除龈下牙石。在每人每年糖消耗量超过 20 公斤的地方，应鼓励市场上销售低糖食品或无糖甜食，由非口腔专业人员进行口腔卫生指导。

Communities with moderate and increasing resources, low/moderate or high and increasing caries prevalence, and moderate to very high periodontal disease.

Strategy-in addition to the approaches described in section 3, fluoride rinsing should be introduced where water or salt fluoridation is not possible. If fluoride toothpaste is in widespread use, fluoride mouth-rinsing programmes may provide some additional caries reduction, but may also be uneconomic. If increasing caries is found predominately in pits and fissures, the training of auxiliaries or non-dental personnel to apply fissure sealant should be considered. Auxiliaries or other non-dental personnel could also be trained to provide oral hygiene instruction, and to remove subgingival calculus, if resources allow. Where annual sugar consumption is above 20 Kg per person, the marketing of low-sugar foods and snacks containing non-sugar sweeteners should be encouraged. Oral hygiene instruction programme should be introduced, using supervised non-dental personnel.

5. 具有丰富资源，龋病患病率增加或高水平，牙周病患病率从中等到高水平的社区。

策略——除上述外，在食盐或饮水氟化不能推行的地方，可以引起学校饮水氟化，氟水含漱或其他项目，如用含氟牙膏进行有指导的刷牙，在经济上是可行的，并且可以提供额外的好处。应培训人员对龋易感儿童进行窝沟封闭，同时开展清洁牙齿及口腔卫生指导项目。

Communities with plentiful resources, increasing or high caries prevalence, and moderate-to-high periodontal disease prevalence.

Strategy-in addition to the approaches described in section 4. school water fluoridation may be introduced where salt or water fluoridation is not possible. Fluoride mouth rinsing, or other programmes, such as supervised brushing with fluoridated toothpaste, should be economically feasible and provide added benefit. Personnel should be trained to apply fissure sealants to the posterior teeth of caries susceptible children, and they can also be used in programmes of tooth cleaning and oral hygiene instruction.

6. 患龋率低或中等并且正在减少，牙周病患病率低／中等或高水平的社区。

策略——上述项目应继续，当12岁的患龋率，龋均（DMFT）水平下降到2.6以下时，氟水含漱项目应停止，因为从这一项目获得的额外利益与其经营成本相比不再有价值。随着患龋率的下降，大部分的病损是窝沟龋，想从氟化物获益证据已不充分。实际上，在这样的龋病发病水平，采用窝沟封闭项目有好处，并且可能是经济的，还可以利用口腔辅助人员开展专业性洁牙项目，以及口腔卫生监督与指导项目。在这种情况下，为了保证有效的防龋项目不被抛弃，适当地注意监测以及健康促进与教育仍然是基本的，虽然看来似乎不再需要。但仍应继续

加强。

Communities with low or moderate and decreasing caries prevalence, and low/moderate or high periodontal disease prevalence.

Strategy-the programmes described in section 5. should be continued, except that fluoride-rinsing programmes should be stopped when caries prevalence levels of 12-year-old drop below DMFT=2.6, since the added benefit from the rinsing programme may not be worth, the cost of operating it; as caries prevalence drops, the residual lesions are almost entirely pit and fissure lesions, and less amenable to the beneficial action of fluoride. At these caries levels, in fact, programmes of fissure sealant application should be beneficial and may be economic. Auxiliary personnel can also be employed in programmes of professional tooth-cleaning and in oral hygiene monitoring and instruction. Adequate attention to monitoring and to health promotion and education is still essential in this situation in order to ensure that effective caries prevention programmes are not abandoned because they appear to be no longer needed; continued reinforcement is essential.

六、选择推荐的口腔疾病预防方法 Selecting methods recommended for oral disease prevention

预防和控制口腔疾病，特别是龋病与牙周病，所推荐的方法在以社区为基础的项目中，清楚地证实了它们的效果与效益。在任何一个特定的社区里，选择与应用一种或多种方法必须依据需要与资源，就这点而论，在计划中，方法与步骤选择的成本——效果非常重要。选择的限制条件主要在于缺乏可以利用的措施的成本——效果方面的信息。例如，比较由不同人员组成的口腔卫生保健小分队在口腔健康教育方法，氟水含漱项目，局部用氟，以及口腔洁治等方面的效率，由于成本不是容易直接测量，不得不寻找可能表明其成本——效果的可供选择的方法。

The methods recommended for the prevention and control of oral diseases, particularly dental caries and periodontal diseases are clear evidence of their efficiency and effectiveness in community-based programmes selection and application of one or more of the methods must be based upon needs and resources in any given community. In this connection cost-effectiveness of alternative methods and procedures is of crucial importance in planning. The limitation, here, lies mainly in the shortage of information on the cost-effectiveness of available measures, such as comparative oral health team efficiency in using different combination of personnel, oral health education techniques, mouthrinse, topical applications of fluorides and oral prophylaxis, etc. since cost is often not directly measurable, alternative ways may have to be found to express cost-effectiveness.

1. 防龋方法 Methods for preventing dental caries

应用氟化物防龋是社区项目的最有效手段。包括：

The use of fluoride is recognized as the most effective means available for the prevention of dental caries in community-based programmes.

（1）公共饮水氟化 Fluoridation of public water supplies

（2）食盐氟化 Salt fluoridation

（3）学校饮水氟化 Water fluoridation in school

（4）牛奶氟化 Milk fluoridation

（5）氟片与氟滴剂 Fluoride tablets and drops

（6）氟水含漱 Mouth-rinsing with dilute solutions of fluoride

（7）含氟牙膏 Fluoridated toothpastes

（8）由专业人员应用的氟化物 Operator-applied fluoride compounds

（9）其他控制龋的方法 Other methods of caries control

①窝沟封闭剂 Pit and fissure sealants

②非创伤性修复治疗 Atraumatic Restorative Treatment（ART）

③控制致龋食物 Control of cariogenic foods

④ 口腔卫生指导 Oral hygiene instruction

2. 预防与控制牙龈炎及牙周病的方法 Methods for the prevention and control of gingivitis and periodontal disease

整个一生之中，牙周病的初级预防需要坚持彻底清除牙菌斑。

Primary prevention of periodontal disease requires consistent thorough removal of plaque on a lifetime basis.

（1）个人用机械方法清除牙菌斑 Mechanical plaque removal by the individual

个人自我保健是牙周健康的关键。个人的努力意味着用牙刷刷牙清除牙菌斑，还有其他用品如牙线，邻间刷，以及本质牙签。应该强调的是洁牙的效果而不是次数或方法。

Self-care by the individual is the key to periodontal health. individual effort means mechanical plaque removal with the toothbrush and aids like dental floss, the interproximal brush, and wood points. The emphasis should be placed on effectiveness of cleaning rather than frequency or methods.

（2）专业人员用机械方法清除牙菌斑 Mechanical plaque removal by professionals

由口腔专业人员定期彻底地清除病人的牙菌斑能够成功地控制牙周病，但所需要的次数与彻底性是值得考虑的。

Periodontal disease can be successfully controlled when dental professional carry out regular and thorough plaque removal for their patients, but the frequency and thoroughness required are considerable.

（3）化学治疗方法清除牙菌斑 Plaque removal by chomotherapeutic methods

用力学方法控制菌斑的操作作为控制牙病的主要措施已得到肯定。然而，因人而异，由于多种因素的影响使结果不能完全成功。多年的研究已提示出用化学方法清除菌斑，即使有部分特别成功的产品，也只能在特殊情况下应用。其中有二种产品已为美国牙科学会接受-洗必太与施德林。

Mechanical plaque control procedure are the established mainstay for controlling dental disease. However, these effort vary individually and depend on a number of influences that often result in the outcome being less than completely successful. Research over many years, has uncovered a chemical method of plaque removal even some particularly successful products that can be of use in special circumstances. Of this group, two products are accepted by the American Dental Association-chlorhexidine and Listerine.

在社区内，群众性的健康教育项目应继续强调需要个人口腔卫生措施和定期看牙。同时也需要口腔专业人员砍定期为成年病人做彻底的预防性治疗的必要性。广泛接受这种指导思想对口腔教育，口腔保健提供，有深刻影响，同时会改善社区的牙周健康。

In the community, public health education programmes should be continuous and stress the need for personal oral hygiene measures and regular dental visits. By the same taken, dental professionals themselves need to be convinced of the necessity for thorough prophylaxis for their adult patients at regular internals. Widespread acceptance of this philosophy could have profound implications for dental education and the provision of care, as well as leading to improved periodontal health in the community.

3. 其他口腔病况的预防和控制 Prevention and control of other oral conditions

（1）口腔癌与癌前病变 Oral cancer and potentially precancerous lesions

口腔癌作为一个公共卫生的重点非常重要。口腔癌最常见的病因是应用烟草。在一些发展中国家，嚼烟草是引起口腔癌 最重要的原因。口腔白斑是最常见的黏膜病变，口腔最常见的癌前病变。口腔癌可以预防，各种因素可以排除。因此，推荐减少病原因素作为预防性措施。

As a public health priority, oral cancer is very important, and the commonest cause of oral cancer is tobacco is by the most important cause of oral cancer. Leukoplakia was the most common mucosal lesions, and the most frequent precancerous lesion of the mouth. The varied factors can be eliminated and oral cancer could be prevented. Therefore, preventive measures for reduction of etiological factors would be recommended.

（2）艾滋病 AIDS

口腔念珠菌感染与口腔“毛状”白斑已经确认为是艾滋病综合征的早期症状，卡波济肉瘤经常发生在艾滋病人的口腔内，并且已经认为是这种病的早期症状。

上述研究表明，口腔癌、白斑与艾滋病的口腔表征都应包括在所有的口腔保健项目内。

Oral candidiasis and oral “hairy” leukoplakia have been suggested as early signs of the AIDS syndrome, Kaposi’s sarcoma frequently occurs in the oral carity in patients with AIDS, and has been recognized as an early sign of the disease.

The above studies indicated that oral cancer, leukoplakia and oral manifestations of AIDS should be involved in all oral health care programmes.

4. 健康教育与促进的作用 Role of health education and health promotion

健康教育与促进是达到个人与整个社区口腔健康必不可少的，两者不能分开，无论何时应成为所有项目计划，实施与评价的一部分，必须与其他影响健康的因素－经济、社会、立法、环境结合在一起，这一切都影响到群众的介入与接受预防项目。

促进口腔健康有许多可以利用的措施，如饮食或食盐氟化、其他用氟方法控、制糖消耗频数、指导有监督的口腔卫生活动、提供常规口腔保健服务，以及带有强制性的涉及预防措施的规章制度。

不论健康教育还是健康促进，对开展并保持口腔卫生预防项目的成功都是基本的。

Health education and promotion are indispensable in achieving both individual and community oral health. They are inseparable from one another and should at all times form part of all programme

planning, implementation and evaluation. It must be integrated with other influences on health-economic, social, legal and environmental-all of which affect public access to, and acceptance of, preventive programmes.

There are numerous measures available for promoting oral health, such as water or salt fluoridation or other fluoride regimens, controlling the frequency of consumption of sugar, conducting supervised oral hygiene activities, provision of routine dental services, and legislation or regulation making a preventive measure mandatory.

Both health promotion and health education are essential for initiating and maintaining successful, effective, preventive oral health programmes.

七、实施、监督、评价与调整 Implementation, supervision, Evaluation and Revision

项目实施过程与计划过程一样，涉及人员，组织机构与社区，整合所有的外部变量，以便实现综合的计划和实施需要通过一种“生态学”途径，只有通过人员与环境之间的团队工作才能成功地实施项目。

制定实施策略必须回答以下的问题：

1. 为什么要达到这样的目标？
2. 为达到目标所需要的活动是什么？
3. 由谁负责每一项活动？
4. 按时间程序如何排列活动？
5. 如何应用材料、媒体、方法与技术？
6. 估计材料与时间的成本是多少？

The implementation process, like the planning process, involves individual organizations, and the community. Integrating all the external variables to achieve comprehensive planning and implementation requires an “ecologic” approach; only through teamwork between the individual and the environment can the implementation be successful.

Developing an implementation strategy for each activity is complete when the following questions have been answered:

1. Why: the effect of the objective to be achieved.
2. What: the activities required to achieve the objective
3. Who: individuals responsible for each activity
4. When: chronologic sequence of activities
5. How: materials, media, methods and techniques to be used
6. How much: a cost estimate of materials and time

（一）项目实施的规则

1. 清楚地说明活动（由谁为谁做什么）；
2. 确保某人负责整个活动并协调执行不同任务的人员；
3. 在活动开始前确定所有的准备步骤（即准备培训手册、材料、写文章、设备、培训志愿者、决定治疗方案）；

4. 一定要按顺序列出必须进行的步骤；
5. 检查是否有遗漏的步骤；
6. 决定每一步骤开始与结束的时间；
7. 检查日期确保时间准确；
8. 咨询影响活动的有关组织，确定可能的问题，机会等；
9. 说明所需要的资源及其来源；
10. 确保所有参与的人都知道对他们的期望是什么，以及到什么时候完成。

Rules for programme implementation is:

- *Specify clearly the activity (who does what for whom).*
- *Be sure someone is responsible for the whole activity and coordinates individuals who may carry out the different tasks.*
- *Identify all the preparatory steps before doing that activity (e.g.) prepare training manual, prepare materials, write papers, acquire equipment, training volunteers, determine treatment protocol.*
- *List steps in the order in which they must occur.*
- *Check for missing steps that must be added.*
- *Determine when (date) each step should begin and end.*
- *Check the dates to make sure the correct amount of time has been allowed.*
- *Consult with organizations affected by the activity, identify potential problems, opportunities, and so on.*
- *Specify what resources will be needed and their source.*
- *Specify what constraints must be addressed.*
- *Make sure all people involved know what is expected of them and by when.*

（二）监督、评价和调整项目 Monitoring, evaluating and revising the programme

一旦项目开始，所有的项目活动都需要不断的监督。项目的成功取决于监督个人如何完成其任务，设备的功能，设施的适当程度。在任何方面出现问题之前，必须作出判断并适当调整项目。

Once it has been implemented, the programme requires continuous surveillance of all activities. The programme's success is determined by monitoring how well the programme is meeting its stated objectives, how well individuals are doing their jobs, how well equipment functions, and how appropriate and adequate facilities are. Before problems arise in any of these areas, adjustments must be made to time-tune the programme.

评价包括非正式的与正式的评价，是项目的一个必要的和重要的方面。评价使我们可以（1）测量每项活动的进展；（2）测量每项活动的效果；（3）确定活动进行中的问题；（4）计划调整与修改；（5）判断管理项目的成本，如有必要，寻找额外的经费。应定期检查每一个目标以便确定是否符合项目的总目标。目标应用可以测量的词汇，这样可以比较打算完成的目标和实际完成的目标。评价应提出完成的质量。例如，如果活动之一是为学龄儿童的特定牙作窝沟封闭，评价者要评估封闭剂封闭的是否完好，牙齿选择是否适当，以及封闭牙的时间。

Evaluation, both informal and formal, is a necessary and important aspect of the programme.

Evaluation allow us to (1) measure the progress of each activity; (2) measure the effectiveness of each activity; (3) identify problems in carrying out the activities; (4) plan revision, and modification, and (5) justify the dollar costs of administering the programme and if necessary, justify seeking additional funds. Each objective should be examined periodically to determine how well it is meeting the programme goals. The objective should be stated in measurable terms so that a comparison can be made of what the objective intended to accomplish and what it actually accomplished. Evaluation should address the quality of what is being done.

应该检查项目接受者的态度，以便决定项目是否为他们所接受的，许多项目，项目的负责者认为是成功的，而接受者可能对有些事的看法完全不同。

The attitude of the recipients of the programme should be examined to determine whether the programme was acceptable to them. Many programmes are considered successful by those who run the programme, however, the people who have been the recipients of the service may have wanted something very different.

21世纪要求口腔保健专业人员，除了提供临床服务之外，必须有社区口腔保健的意识。根据社区需要指导开始社区项目以及强调预防的重要。当然，计划是为了改变现状而开展的活动之一。卫生专业人员应具备这方面的能力，在地方，省与全国水平上发挥其作用，这种作用要求毕业生具备评估、计划、实施项目及开展活动的能力以便使全体人员从中获益。

The twenty-first century requires that oral health professional, in addition to the delivery of clinical services, must demonstrate awneness of community health issues and provide leadership in the development of programmes that address community needs and stress the importance of prevention. Planning is, of course, one of the activities that proceed the implementation of change. The oral health professional must express their competencies and play their role at the local, provincial and national levels. This role requires the graduate dentists to assess, plan and implement programmes and activities to benefit the general population.

小结 Summary

通过本章学习，学员应该知道管理的基本概念和原则、项目管理的三大基本职能尤其是项目计划的基本步骤。

思考题 Review questions

1. What steps should be considered when planning an oral health programme for a community?

参考文献 References

1. George M. Gluck, et al. Jong's Community Dental health (5th edition). Mosby, Inc, 2003
2. Cynthia Pine M, et al. Community Oral Health. wright, 1998
3. WHO Regional office for Europe. Planning and evaluating Dental health services, 1971
4. John K. Bainbridge, et al. Health project management: A manual of procedures for formulating and implementing health projects. WHO/HQ Geneva, 1974

5. WHO/HQ Geneva Prevention methods and programmes for oral diseases: technical report series 713, 1984
6. Arnold D. Kaluzny et al. Management of health services. Prentice-hall, Inc. Englewood cliffs, New Jerseey 07632, 1982
7. 卞金有主编. 预防口腔医学. 第 4 版, 人民卫生出版社, 2003
8. WHO. Regional Office for Europe (1972) planning and evaluating dental health services: Report on a working group, OSLO, 1971
9. George M. Gluck, Warren M. Morganstein. Jong's Community Dental Health. 5th edition Mosby, 2003 (10)

（卞金有）

第十四章　感染性疾病对口腔临床实践的影响

Chapter XⅣ The Impact of Infection Disease on the Practice of Dentistry

概述 Overview

本章以传统的“医院感染及其控制”概念为契机，按照未来的临床实践，扩大社会卫生服务以及公共卫生实践理念，介绍几种与口腔医学实践密切相关主要感染性疾病，并阐述这些医源性感染的传播途径，并从个人保护，无菌术，消毒与灭菌以及废物处理等方面，简要介绍感染控制的目标，策略与方法，以帮助各级口腔医务人员增强应对公共卫生突发事件，以及在提供口腔公共卫生服务过程中，控制感染的安全意识，责任，与能力，达到最大限度保护公众健康的目的。

This chapter is based on the traditional concept of "hospital infection and its control" as a turning point, and following the new concepts of clinical practice, outreach health services, and new public health movement, to briefly describe several main infectious diseases which are closely related to dental practices and their transmissible approaches through the process of dental services. Finally, a brief introduction in the objectives, strategies, and methods of infection control, such as personal protection, instruments sterilization and disinfection processing, surface and equipment asepsis and waste management, in order to strengthen the awareness of safety, responsibilities and empowerment in deal with sudden happenings in public health and offering dental public health services to reach the objective for protecting the public's health.

要点 Key points

- 感染性疾病 infectious diseases
- 医院感染 hospital infection
- 外源性感染 exogenous infection
- 感染控制 infection control
- 防护屏障 protective barrier
- 无菌术 asepsis
- 无菌 sterilization
- 消毒 disinfection

医学实践中的感染问题是当前医学发展中存在的重大问题，也是医学界及社会各界十分关注的问题。在 口腔医学中，感染性疾病是重要的。疾病的感染通常可分为社会感染和医院感染两个方面。发生在医院的一切感染称为医院感染（Hospital Infection，HI；Nosocomial

Infection，NI)，或医院内获得性感染（Hospital Acquired Infection，HAI)。就其病原体而言，可分两类。一类是外源性感染，又称交叉感染。病原体是来自病人以外的地方，如其他病人或外环境等。另一类是内源性感染，亦称自身感染。病原体来自病人本身，如病人的正常菌群。医院感染可以影响到所有在医院里的人，包括病人及其家属，所有的医务人员与非医务人员。因此，医院感染是医院医疗质量的核心问题之一，是随着医院的建立而发生并与医院相依并存的。从非典（SARS）的经验教训中可以得到启示，医院感染不仅影响患者的康复、增加患者的痛苦、使死亡率上升、住院时间延长，经济负担加重，同时也影响到医务人员的健康和医院的正常工作，增加国家和社会的负担，造成社会的不安定。因此，控制感染是现代医院质量管理的重要目标之一，是现代医学的重点研究课题。控制感染已形成为涉及基础医学、临床医学、预防医学和、医院管理以至整个社会关注的焦点问题。

一、医院感染的定义 Definition of Hospital Infection

所谓医院感染即指病人在入院时不存在、亦不处于潜伏期，而在医院内发生的感染，包括在医院获得，在出院后发病的感染。这是一种传统的概念。现代的概念包括一切发生在医院里的感染都称之为医院感染。

Nosocomial infection：An infection acquired in hospital by a patient who was admitted for a reason other than that infection. An infection occurring in a patient in a health care facility in that whom the infection was not present or incubating at the time of admission. This includes infections acquired in the hospital but appearing after discharge, and also occupational infection among staff of the facility.

美国疾病控制中心（CDC）定义（1980）为：医院感染是指住院病人发生的感染，而在其入院时尚未发生此感染也未处于感染的潜伏期。对潜伏期不明的感染，凡发生于入院后皆可列为医院感染。若病人入院时已发生的感染直接与上次住院有关，亦列为医院感染。

中华人民共和国卫生部下发的《医院感染管理规范（试行)》中对医院感染的定义是：“医院感染是指住院病人在医院内获得的感染，包括在住院期间发生的感染和在医院获得出院后发生的感染；但不包括入院前已开始或入院时已处于潜伏期的感染。医院工作人员在医院获得的感染也属于医院感染”。

医院感染定义中包括了感染的地点、时间、对象等，既①明确规定了感染发生的地点必须是在医院，它排除了在医院外受到感染而在医院期间发病的病人，包括了在医院感染而在出院后转至其他医院后发病的病人。②感染和发病是发生在不同阶段，顺序是感染→潜伏期→发病。因此，疾病的潜伏期是判定感染的发生时间和地点的主要依据。但由于潜伏期的变动幅度较大，因此，判定时必须参考其他因素，如病原学及流行病学等资料等。③医院感染包括一切在医院活动的人群，如住院患者、门诊患者、医院工作人员、陪住者以及探视者。

二、医院感染分类 Types of Hospital Infection

医院感染按其病原体的来源可分为外源性医院感染和内源性医院感染两大类：

1. 外源性医院感染 Exogenous nosocomial infections

外源性医院感染（exogenous nosocomial infections)，亦称为交叉感染（cross infection)，是指从病人到病人、从病人到医务工作者、从医务工作者到病人的直接感染，或通过物品对人体的间接感染。病原体通常来自被感染者体外，如其他病人、病原携带者（包括医务工作者及探视者）、未彻底消毒灭菌或被污染的医疗器械、血液、血液制品、生物制品、医院环境等。也有些学者将外源性医院感染进一步分类，将引起医院感染的病原体来自其他病人的称为交叉感染；病原体来自医院环境的称成为环境感染；病原体来自未彻底消毒灭菌或被污染的医疗器具、污染的血液或血液制品和药品的称为医源性感染（iatrogenic infections）。

通过加强消毒、灭菌、隔离和屏障护理等控制措施，可以达到有效地预防和控制外源性感染，因此又称为可预防性感染。

Cross infection may be defined as the passing of harmful microorganisms from one place or person to another place or person

2. 内源性医院感染 Endogenous nosocomial infections

内源性医院感染（endogenous nosocomial infections）也称自身感染（autogenous infections）。是指病人自身抵抗力降低，对本身固有的细菌感受性增加而发生的感染。引起这类感染的微生物来自病人体内或体表的正常菌群或条件致病菌，包括虽从其他病人或环境中来，但已在该病人身上定植（colonization）的微生物，例如肠道、口腔、呼吸道、阴道、尿道及皮肤等部位常构成内源性感染微生物的“储藏库”。通常定植在这些部位的正常菌群对宿主不致病，形成相互依存、相互制约的微生态体系；当宿主抵抗力下降或免疫功能受损时，原有微生态平衡失调，宿主对自身固有的菌群感受性产生变化而发生感染。研究发现，导致内源性医院感染的微生物大部分来自医院，多数是在入院早期从医院环境或其他病人、医务工作者处迁移到病人身上，并定植于适宜部位，即外来菌群取代了宿主原有的正常菌群。尤其是抗菌药物的应用，干扰了宿主机体的正常菌群，使宿主对医院环境中出现的耐药菌株更加易感。内源性医院感染多呈散发性，发病机制复杂，但也与病人的机体免疫功能、基础病、诊疗措施等多种因素相关，预防内源性医院感染较困难，因此又称为难以预防性感染。

三、与传染病学的区别 Distinction of communicable diseases

传染病（communicable disease or contagious disease）是指能够在正常人群中引起流行的感染性疾病（infection disease），由病原微生物引起，大多也能传播给他人。对人类有致病性的病原微生物约在500种以上，包括病原微生物如病毒、依原体、立克次体、支原体、细菌、螺旋体、真菌及寄生虫如原虫、蠕虫等，二者统称为病原体（pathogen）。某种病原体克服机体的防御机能，侵犯或侵入机体的特定部位，并能在入侵处或其他部位生长繁殖者，称为感染（infection）。感染在宿主机体发生、发展及转归的过程称感染过程。医院感染学与传染病学的区别见表 14-1。

表 14-1 医院感染学与传染病学的区别

传染病学	传染病学	医院感染学
病原体		
病原体	典型致病菌	条件致病菌为主
病原学诊断	易于判定	不易判定

续表

传染病学	传染病学	医院感染学
流行病学		
感染源	外源性	外源性 + 内源性
传播方式	常见途径（如空气、水、食物）	常为特殊方式（如插入性操作等）
感染对象	健康人群	病人，特别是免疫功能低下人群
爆发频率	多而明显	少而不明显
传染性	高	低
隔离意义	病原性隔离（保护外界易感人群）	保护性隔离（保护病人）
临床疾病学		
临床表现	单纯和典型	复杂和不典型
诊断	临床和流行病学分析可确诊	需要微生物学定性、定量、定位分析
治疗	较易	较难

第一节　感染性疾病对口腔实践的影响

Section 1 The Impact of Transmissible Disease on the Practice of Dentistry

我们的生存环境有由许多生命和物种组成如，哺乳类、鱼类、鸟类、爬行类、昆虫以及数以千计的其他物种。它们中大多数都可被是肉眼看得所见的，但也存在一些肉眼不可见、被称作“微生物”的生命。微生物无随处不在可见，以多种方式生存在环境中，如食物、水、地层深处、高空、甚至在超过 90℃的温泉和汽油桶中。

人体是在许多微生物的协调之中生存的，在这些微生物中只有外来菌和条件致病菌才可使人体患病，所以又将这些微生物分为致病菌和非致病菌。有些微生物消毒（disinfection）不是很敏感，但所有微生物都可通过灭菌（sterilization）的手段消灭。由于微生物不为肉眼所见，因此在临床工作中必须建立一套保护医患的工作程序，也就是说在每位就医患者之间必须采用一定的方法消灭那些有致病危险或可引起交叉感染的微生物。

口腔环境是口腔医疗保健中潜在的病原体来源，包括血源性疾病、口腔疾病、系统性疾病的口腔病损及呼吸道疾病。表14-2是口腔临床工作中可能遇到的多种感染性疾病，包括呼吸感染，儿童时期的疾病，以及性传播疾病等。

表 14-2　Various infectious diseases possibly transmitted in dental environment

Diease	Agent	Route	Potential Complications
AIDS	Retrovirus	bxs	Death
Candida	Fungus	s	Oesophagitis/systemic
Chicken pox	Virus	bsd	Shingles
Common cold	Virus	bsd	Temporary disability
Gonorrhoea	Bacteria	x	Sterility, arthritis
Hepatitis A	Virus	of	Disability

续表

Diease	Agent	Route	Potential Complications
Hepatitis B	Virus	bsd	Disability, death
Hepatitis C	Virus	bsd	Disability, death
Hepatitis D	Virus	bsd	Disability, death
Herpetic conjunctivitis	Virus	bsd	Potential blindness
Herpes simplex II	Virus	bsx	Painful lesions
Herpetic whitlow	Virus	bsd	Painful, disability
Infectious mononucleosis	Virus	bsd	(Temporary) disability
Influenza	Virus	sd	Death
Legionellosis	Bacteria	r	Death
Measles (rubella)	Virus	snd	Disability, encephalitis
Measles (German)	Virus	snd	Congenital defects
Mumps	Virus	r	Disability, sterility
Pneumonia	Mycobacteria and virus	rb	Death
Staphylococcus infections	Bacteria	sd	Skin lesions, death
Streptococcus infections	Bacteria	bsd	Rheumatic heart conditions, death
Syphilis	Treponema	xb	CNS damage, death
Tetanus	bacteria	o	Disability, death
Tuberculosis	bacteria	sd	Disability, death

b = blood; s = saliva; d = airborne respiratory droplets; x = sexual contact; n = nasal; o= open wound;
o = open wound; r = respiratory.

一、人类免疫缺损病毒疾病 Human immunodeficiency virus HIV

人类免疫缺损病毒（human immunodeficiency virus, HIV）引起的疾病称为 HIV 疾病，包括 HIV 感染及后期的获得性免疫缺损综合征（acquired immunodeficiency syndrome, AIDS）。自 1981 年报道第一例 AIDS 病例至今，全世界大约有 3100 万人被感染此疾病。中国 1985 年 6 月发现首例艾滋病患者以来，艾滋病于近年来蔓延迅速，根据卫生权威部门统计，我国现有艾滋病病毒感染者约 84 万人，其中艾滋病病人约 8 万例。

HIV 疾病破坏机体的免疫系统，从最初的 HIV 感染到疾病终期（AIDS），大约是 2 到 12 年，平均接近 10 年。HIV 是一种 RNA 病毒，其中 HIV-1 型病毒是最常见的引起 HIV 疾病的病毒。HIV-1型病毒首先感染淋巴调节系统的T_4淋巴细胞，病毒RNA迅速转变成为病毒DNA，此病毒 DNA 结合进入淋巴细胞染色体，这样淋巴细胞就被永久性地感染上了 HIV-1 型基因。在淋巴细胞内这些基因可诱导生成新的病毒颗粒，病毒产物破坏淋巴细胞，同时可侵入感染更多的淋巴细胞，最终破坏肌体所有的 T_4 淋巴细胞，因此只有当 T_4 淋巴细胞水平相当低的时候才出现临床症状。HIV-1型可以有基因突变，形成不同的基因型，在淋巴细胞内复制形成不同的基因型，这也为疫苗预防 HIV 感染造成困难。

1. HIV 感染症状 Symptoms of HIV infection

HIV 感染症状

人类在感染 HIV-1 型 4 周后，可以出现咽喉疼痛、发热、腺体肿大、腹泻以及关节疼痛。这些症状可称之为反转录病毒综合征，或急性HIV综合征。与其他病毒感染不同，这些症状可以很轻微，通常不被注意。在 HIV-1 感染人类 6 ~ 12 周后出现抗体，但这种抗体不能抵抗这种疾病，只能为疾病的诊断提供依据。带有HIV抗体的人，可以证明此人被HIV感染。HIV急性感染后，在数月以至数年内大多数患者没有进一步的临床症状，但此期间具有传染性。

AIDS

Replication of HIV type 1 in T4 lymphocytes kills the lymphocytes, and as more and more cells are killed, the immune system becomes progressively weaker. This immunodeficiency results in increased susceptibility to opportunistic disease agents that normally do not cause infections or cause less severe infections in those with healthy immune systems. When an HIV-positive patient experiences one or more of these indicator opportunistic infections or a cancer, the patient is diagnosed as having AIDS. The symptoms experienced depend on the type of infection or cancer that occurs, examples of which are list in table (表 14-3). The symptoms experienced depend on the typed of infection or cancer that occurs. Eventually, one of these diseases causes death. The infectious diseases may be caused by bacterial, viral, fungal, or protozoan agents; the leading cause of death in an AIDS patient is Pneumocystis carinii pneumonia.

表 14-3 Examples of diseases associated with HIV disease

Bacterial		Bacterial	
	Mycobacterium avium-intracellulare	Fungal	
	Mycobacterium tuberculosis		Candidiasis
	Salmonella spp.		Histoplasmosis
	Shigella flexneri		Cryptoxoxxosis
	Clostridium difficile		Coccidiodomycosis
	Streptococcus pneumoniae	Cancers	
	Norcardia asteroids		Kaposi's sarcoma
	Legionella pneumophila		Non-Hodgkin's lymphoma
Protozoan		Others	
	Pneumocystis carinii pneumonia		HIV encephalopathy
	Toxoplasmosis		Aseptic meningitis
	Giardiasis		Persistant generalized lymphadenopathy
	Cryptosporidiosis		HIV wasting syndrome
Viral			
	Herpes simplex infections		
	Cytomegalovirus infections		
	Hairy leukoplakia		

2. AIDS 的口腔表现 Oral manifestations

AIDS的早期表现多发生在口腔：真菌性疾病有念珠菌病、组织胞浆菌病、地丝菌病和隐球菌病；病毒性疾病有疣状和、毛状白斑班和I型疱疹病毒感染；细菌性感染有快速进展性牙周炎和牙龈炎，肿瘤性疾病包括卡波希肉瘤和非何杰金淋巴瘤。

3. HIV 的传播 Transmittion of HIV

HIV-1 型通过以下方式传播：

- 密切的性接触（阴道、直肠、口腔），体液的接触包括精液和阴道分泌物。
- 接触血制品及血液污染的体液。
- 围产期接触（感染从母亲到孩子）

其他的传播方式都是在这三种基本方式之中，日常接触不会引起 HIV 感染。

虽然在体内不易消灭HIV，但在体外通过高温蒸汽灭菌、普通液体灭菌和表面消毒都可消灭各种 HIV。

4. 口腔科 HIV 医患被感染的危险性程度：Risks of HIV infected health personnel and patients in dental pracrice

口腔工作人员存在着被患者感染的可能，感染大多数是由于皮肤或黏膜损伤暴露于HIV阳性血液造成。口腔科患者在口腔诊室感染HIV的程度同样相当小。通过极少数医患间发生感染病例的研究结果显示，医患间HIV直接传播的危险性大于经被污染的口腔器械、设备等的间接传播的危险性。

二、病毒性肝炎 Viral hepatitis

There are at least six hepatitis viruses that cause clinically similar diseases: hepatitis A, B, C, D, E and G. Hepatitis A and E are mainly transmitted through contaminated food and water (fecal-oral route of spread); hepatitis B, C, D, and G are bloodboren diseases usually transmitted by direct contact with infected body fluids.

1. 乙型病毒性肝炎（Hepatitis B）

简称乙肝，是导致急慢性肝炎、肝硬化和肝癌的主要原因，是世界范围的地方性疾病，其流行程度目前还在增加，估计世界上约有2亿HBV携带者。我国是乙型病毒性肝炎的高发区，每年报告乙型肝炎新发病例约数约 50 万，目前全国有现患慢性病毒性肝炎患者约 2000 万人，每年死于与乙型肝炎相关的肝病约 28 万人，其中 50% 为原发性肝细胞癌。

HBV是一种带有囊膜的DNA病毒，感染肝细胞并在肝细胞中繁殖。在感染过程中，病毒颗粒和含有病毒颗粒的细胞作为病源性感染物质进入循环系统。感染患者的1ml血液中，含有一亿病毒颗粒，这也意味着很小量的体液就足以将疾病传播给他人。病毒有三个重要抗原成分，分别是乙型肝炎表面抗原-HBsAg；乙型肝炎核心抗原-HBcAg和乙型肝炎e抗原-HBeAg。使用普通的消毒和灭菌方法可以杀死或灭活乙肝病毒，包括高压蒸汽、1∶16戊二醛、70%异丙醇等。在体外只要化学药物能够直接接触到乙肝病毒就能比较容易消灭它。

HBV 感染者中 90% 可以恢复正常，5% ～ 10% 的感染者成为病毒携带者，这些人中病毒携带者的50%可以在两年半时间内清除体内病毒，其余1/2的感染者成为慢性肝炎患者。HBsAg阳性患者具有传染性，HbeAg阳性患者血液中含有高浓度病毒，有高度传染性。其传播主要通过血清及日常密切接触而传播。血液传播途径除输血及血制品外，如注射、刺伤、共用牙刷、剃刀、外科器械等方式，经微量血液也可传播。由于在患者的唾液、精液、初乳、汗液、血性分泌物中均有病毒颗粒存在，故密切生活接触可能是重要传播途径。另一种传播方式是母婴传播。高危人群是：共用污染的静脉注射器者；有多个性伙伴的同性、异性及双性恋者；被血液或体液污染的器械刺伤者；伤口暴露于感染的血液或体液者。乙肝病毒可通过血液或其制品传播，但目前对献血者乙肝病毒筛查制度的建立，此种传播少见；大约有40%的乙肝患者的传播途径不十分清楚。

对口腔工作者最大的危险是：被污染的锐器刺伤（针头、穿刺器械、刀片、钻头）；血液或唾液污染了皮肤损伤处；裸露皮肤或手套破损部位；血液或唾液飞沫接触到皮肤病损或飞溅到黏膜上。一些调查结果表明：13%口腔助手、17%口腔卫生士、14%实验室技术人员、9%～25%牙科医生被感染乙型肝炎，被感染程度是正常人群的2～5倍。目前虽然使用手套、口罩、帽子和眼镜来防护血液或体液的污染，但被污染器械刺伤在所难免。由于没有有效的治疗乙肝的措施，因此建议口腔医务工作者最好使用乙肝疫苗。口腔患者从口腔医务工作者感染乙肝的可能性非常低。上个世纪 80 年代曾有报道患有乙肝口腔医务工作者将感染传播给患者（自身带有高浓度的HbeAg，并在诊疗过程中没有防护措施）的报道，但目前这种情况已十分罕见。

2. Hepatitis C

Hepatitis C was previously called parenterally transmitted non-A, non-B hepatitis. The hepatitis C is a bloodborne disease. Approximately 50% of hepatitis C cases are associated with intravenous drug abuse, 13% are associated with sexual activity, 3% with blood transfusions, and 1% with occupational in health-care workers. The remaining cases have unidentified routes of transmission. Hepatitis C has been transmitted to health-care workers through needlestick injures.

An alarming fact about hepatitis C is that at least 50% of those infected apparently become chronic carriers. Until recently, hepatitis C was diagnosed by indirect means showing that the patient did not have type A or type B hepatitis. The causative virus was first isolated in 1989, and a blood test for antibodies to hepatitis C virus (HCV) was designed in 1991. This test aids in diagnosing the disease , identifying those who are or have been infected, and in screening potential blood donors. As yet there is no vaccine for hepatitis C but development of the badly needed test for HCV is leading to more firm information on modes of spread of the virus. Neither the hepatitis A nor the hepatitis B vaccines provide any protection against hepatitis C.

3. Hepatitis D

Infection with hepatitis D virus (HDV) , also known as the Delta agent, can apparently be regarded as a complication of hepatitis B. This virus may cause infection only in the presence of an active HBV infection. HDV is a defective virus that needs a part of the HBV to complete its life cycle. Infection with HDV may occur as a coinfection with HBV (both HDV and HBV infect simultaneously) or as a superinfection of HDV in an HBV carrier. Both instances usually result in clinical acute hepatitis and coinfection usually resolves, whereas superinfection frequently causes chronic HDV infection and chronic active hepatitis. Hepatitis D virus is transmitted by routes similar to those of HBV, and outbreaks of hepatitis D have been reported in the United States. Thus those who are susceptible to HBV infection, occupationally or otherwise, are also susceptible to HDV infection. Successful vaccination against hepatitis B also should prevent hepatitis D.

4. Hepatitis G

Hepatitis G is the most recently described viral hepatitis, being first recognized in 1995. Very little information is available about the virus or the disease but transmission is thought to at least involve bloodborne spread.

5. Hepatitis A and E

Hepatitis A and E does not pose a particular risk to dental workers or patients because this form of hepatitis is primarily spread by the fecal-oral route involving consumption of contaminated food or water. There is a vaccine available for hepatitis A.

三、结核 Tuberculosis, TB

结核病是由结核杆菌（mycobacterium tuberculosis）感染所致的感染性疾病，对人类危害已有数千年，可累及全身各脏器器官，是世界范围的主要卫生问题。近几年不管是工业发达国家还是发展中国家都出现结核病流行的大回升，结核病已排列于是传染病的首位杀手。WHO于1993年4月23日宣布“全球结核病紧急状态宣言”。这也是世界卫生组织首次作出紧急宣言，号召全球紧急动员，加强结核病控制工作。

我国结核病人数居全球第二位，75%的肺结核病人年龄在15～54岁之间；80%的肺结核病人在农村，成为农村因病致贫、因病返贫的重要原因。西部地区人口数占全国的四分之一，而传染性肺结核病人数却占全国的三分之一。

结核病主要是以空气为传播因子的呼吸道传染，还有消化道传染、皮肤传染等其他途径，后者如胎盘传染、生殖器官传染等；皮肤传染和其他途径极为罕见，无流行病学意义。通过消化道虽也可传染，但消化道对结核菌有较强抵抗力，只有摄入被严重污染的食品如牛乳等，使大量结核菌进人体内，才能造成感染，不是常见的传染途径。呼吸道传染的方式是：带菌体排出大小不一的带菌飞沫，大飞沫（＞10μm）咳出后很快坠落于地面；小飞沫可在空气中停留数分钟，待蒸发后成为飞沫核（1～10μm）浮游于空气中，如通风不好，可悬浮5小时之久。带菌大飞沫如接触到健康人的皮肤或黏膜，结核菌不会侵入组织内，即使进入呼吸道，则降落在支气管黏膜纤毛上面而被排出。只有带菌的飞沫核，由于其微小，才能进到肺泡内，导致感染。

实验证明：病人将痰吐在地上，痰干后结核菌随尘埃飞扬在空气中，成为带菌的尘埃粒子，如不被人们吸入并不易构成感染。病人衣服和被褥被带菌的痰液所污染，也由于其粒子较大，不能吸入肺泡内，因而在传染上无重要意义。

由此看出，结核病的传染性同带菌粒子的大小有直接关系。此外，还同带菌粒子的密度有关。带菌粒子飘在空气中可以游散，所以距离病人越近，传染性越大，距离越远则传染性越小；室内通风良好或阳光充足，带菌粒子易被稀释或被紫外线消毒，传染性也就随之减小。实验表明，每小时换气6次，可将空气中带菌浓度在45分钟内减到原来的1%。除这些环境条件的影响外，带菌粒子密集更取决于病人呼出气的速度。平息平静呼吸时呼出的粒子不多，而一次咳嗽呼出的粒子等于5分钟说话的呼出量，打一次喷嚏排出的粒子量高于咳嗽许多倍。

除青少年结核发病高外，60～70岁的老年人亦呈发病高峰。未注射过疫苗的医务工作者，接触开放性结核病人时有被感染的危险。

The risk for the dental team of acquiring TB is low because prolonged exposure to an infectious environment is usually required for infection to occur and brief contact appears to be of little risk. Spread from one person to another relates to closeness of contact and the duration of exposure to infectious droplets. Thus the key factor in spread is the concentration of infectious particles in the inhaled air. Respiratory aerosols remain airborne for several hours but the concentration of the infectious particles decreases with time from dilution with "clean" air and eventual settling. Nevertheless, TB is acquired by breathing in respiratory droplets from an infectious person with active pulmonary TB, and this must be given concern by the dental team.

The dental office should have a protocol for identifying patients who possibly have active pulmonary TB. These patients should be immediately referred for medical evaluation and have their dental care deferred until the TB is inactive or has been treated and is no longer infectious. Dental personnel should not treat patients with active TB unless they institute special isolation precautions that are usually only available in hospital clinics.

Risk factors for TB and symptoms of active TB are shown in table (表 14-4). This table also describes questions on a medical history that may help identify dental patients that possibly have active TB.

表 14-4 Risk factors, symptoms, and medical history questions related to tuberculosis

	Close/prolonged contact with known active TB case
	Residency in prisons, mental institutions, nursing homes, certain health-care facilities
	HIV disease
	Alcoholism
	Intravenous drug abuse
	Homelessness
	Old age
Symptoms	
	Malaise
	Productive cough for more than 3 weeks
	Blood in sputum
	Headache
	Fever, night sweats
	Weight loss
Medical History Questions	
	Previous diagnosis of TB?
	Previous treatment for TB?

续表

Positive TB skin-test?
Productive cough for more than 3 weeks?
Blood in your sputum?
Headache, fever, chills, night sweats?
Recent weight loss, anorexia, fatigue?
HIV-disease?
Other systemic diseases?
Immunosuppressive therapy?
Alcoholism?
Intravenous drug use?
Relatives or close friends with active TB?
Visited anyone in hospital with active TB?

四、人疱疹病毒 Human herpes virus

人疱疹病毒分为一型（HSV-1）和二型（HSV-2）两类。一型疱疹病毒，又称单纯疱疹病毒，可以引起口腔，皮肤，眼，生殖器的感染，免疫系统低下的人可以有广泛的感染。二型疱疹病毒，又称二型单纯疱疹，约 90% 引起生殖器疱疹感染，但偶见于口腔感染。

Human herpes viruses (HHV) cause several diseases. Human herpes virus type 1 (herpes simplex virus 1 [HSV-1]) may cause infections of the mouth, skin, eyes, and genitals, and those who have depressed immune systems (immunocompromised) may have a widespread infection.

About 90% of adult have been infected with HHV-1. Only of 10% of infected persons (usually children) experience the typical symptoms of oral herpes (primary herpetic gingivostomatitis) . In this disease, vesicle-type lesions occur in the mouth. Most (if not all) herpes viruses cause recurrent diseases (periodic re-occurrence of the disease) . An example is herpes labialis, sometimes called fever blisters, with lesions periodically appearing on the lips. Vesicles during active HHV-1 infections at any site of the body contain the virus that may be spread to others by direct contact with these lesions. Also, the HHV-1 may be present in saliva in those with oral or lip lesions and in a small percent of those who are infected but have no active lesions. In such instances, direct contact with lesions may cause infection of the skin or sprays or aerosols of the saliva may result in spread of the virus to unprotected eyes of the dental team. Entrance of the virus through breaks in the skin on unprotected hands and fingers can lead to vesicle development at these sites called herpetic whitlow. A vivid example of how the HHV-1may be spread from a lip lesion of one patient to the mouths of other dental patients via the ungloved hands of a dental hygienist.

Human herpes virus type 2 (herpes simplex virus 2 [HSV-2]) cause about 90% of genital herpes infections but occasionally causes oral infections. Although most infections are asymptomatic, HHV-2 can cause vesicle type lesions in the mouth or on the skin in the male and female genital and anal areas or internally in the female. As with other herpes virus infection, these vesicles may periodically recur. The vesicle contain the virus and are contagious on contact but the virus can also be spread in the absence of symptoms. Genital herpes is one of the most common sexually transmitted disease (STD).

第二节 感染与控制
Section 2 Infection and Control

口腔医疗实践中控制感染的基本原理就是在口腔医疗行为场所内干扰、阻断感染性疾病传播的过程，也就是杜绝或减少病原体的传播。对口腔操作中感染的诸多因素有足够的认识才能达到有效控制感染的目的。

一、感染传播的路径 The ways of infection

在研究感染性疾病的传播与控制上主要从以下几个方面考虑：

①病原体从患者传播到口腔医务工作者

②病原体从口腔医务工作者传播到患者

③病原体从患者传播到患者

④病原体从医疗行为场所传播到社会

⑤病原体从社会传播到患者

1. 病原体从患者传播到口腔医务工作者 Pathogens transmitting from patients to oral health workers

在医疗过程中患者的病原体可以轻易感染口腔医务工作者，这是一条难以控制的感染路径。直接接触（direct contact）感染是指被感污染的患者的血液、唾液经直接接触（direct contact）破损的皮肤伤口感染医务工作者，这也包括一些肉眼不可见的一些伤口，特别是指甲周围。患者口腔中的病原体可以飞沫感染（droplet infection）医务工作者受伤的皮肤、眼、鼻、口腔黏膜或被吸入体内。间接接触（indirect contact）感染是指患者的病原体可以污染物体表面如：手术器械、针头、钻针或文件表面，这些物品接触医务工作者破损的伤口进入体内。另一种比较少见的感染传播方式是患者病变或破损的皮肤或直接接触医务工作者手部破损的部位，从而引起感染。

2. 病原体从口腔医务工作者传播到患者 Pathogens transmitting from oral health workers to patients

病原体从口腔医务工作者传播到患者多发生在医务工作者忽略了医疗行为过程中某些防护环节。例如医务工作者手部皮肤带有病变或破损，在没有防护的情况下进入患者口腔内操作，病原体直接接触口腔黏膜或其他开放的组织，引起感染。另外医务工作者的血源性病原体也可通过污染器械等，间接接触患者口腔黏膜，引起感染传播。飞沫感染也同样可以从医务工作者到患者。

3. 病原体从患者传播到患者 Pethogens transmitting from patients to patients

一名患者的病原体可以通过未经严格消毒、灭菌的器械、手机或医务工作人员的手等途径间接接触感染另一名患者。有研究证实 HSV 可以通过口腔卫生人员的手传播给数名患者。

4. 病原体从医疗行为场所传播到社会 Pathogens transmitting from medical behavioural settings to the socisty

如果被患者病原体污染的物品或器械流入社会或转移出医院诊所范围以外，就有可能引起间接接触感染。例如被病原体污染的印模、义齿等进入实验室或义齿加工中心，可以导致实验室人员或技术人员的职业性疾病，乙肝等。另外医务工作者的工作服也是病原体的载体。医务工作者也可把被感染病原体带向社会、家庭。没有妥善处理或保存的医用废弃物是很危险严重的感染源。

5. 病原体从社会传播到患者 Pathogens transmitting from the society to patients

主要是指寄生在口腔综合治疗台给水系统中的水源性病原体导致患者感染某些疾病。这些水源性微生物定殖在供水系统管线内部形成生物膜（biofilm）。在使用三用枪、涡轮手机或超声洁治器时，水流将病原体带入患者口腔中。虽然到目前为止还没有证据表明污染的治疗用水给患者带来严重危害，但在口腔医疗过程中使用严重污染的供水不利于感染的控制。

感染控制的目标 Goal of Infection Control

After microorganisms enter the body, there are three basic factors that determine if an infectious disease will develop: virulence (pathogenic properties of the invading microorganism) , dose (the number of microorganisms that invade the body) , and resistance (body defense mechanism of the host) . These factors are called determinants of an infectious disease and their interaction determines the outcome of an infection, as follows:

$$\text{Health or disease} = \frac{\text{Virulence} \times \text{Dose}}{\text{Body resistance}}$$

Health is favored by low virulence, low dose, and high resistance; disease is favored by high virulence, high dose, and low resistance. Prevention of infectious diseases involves influencing the determinants to favor health.

Unfortunately, virulence of microorganisms in their natural environments cannot be easily changed. Thus our body defenses must deal with whatever microorganism presents itself, be it one with high virulence or low virulence. We can enhance our resistance to infectious diseases through specific immunization (e.g., hepatitis B, tetanus) but immunizations are not available against all of the diseases we would like to prevent. Thus the only disease determinant we can effectively manage is the dose, and management of the dose is called infection control. Therefore the goal of infection control is to eliminate or reduce the dose of microorganisms that may be shared between individuals or between individuals and contaminated surfaces. The more the dose is reduced, the better the chance for preventing disease spread. Procedures that minimize spraying or spattering of oral fluids (e.g., rubber dam, high-volume evacuation, preprocedure mouth rinse) reduce the dose of microorganisms that escape from the source. Hand washing and surface precleaning and disinfection reduce the number of microorganisms that may be transferred to surfaces by touching. Barriers such as masks, gloves, and protective eyewear and clothing reduce the number of microorganisms that contaminate the body or other surfaces.

Instrument precleaning and sterilization eliminate or reduce the number of microorganisms that may be spread from one patient to another. Proper management of infectious waste by using appropriate containers for disposal eliminates or reduces the number of microorganism that may contaminate people or inanimate objects. Disease prevention is based on reducing the dose and increasing the body's resistance.

二、防护屏障 Protective barriers

在医疗工作中避免接触病原体是最好的预防医院感染的方法，可以分为两种途径。一种是将病原体限制在它的发源地，例如对于口腔病患者而言，其病原体发源地就是口腔。由于口腔治疗需要医务工作人员的手指、医疗器械等进入口腔内进行操作；三用枪、高低速手机、超声洁治器的使用都不可避免的要将患者口腔内病原体通过直接接触、间接接触、飞沫等形式带出病源地，因此在口腔医疗过程中将病原体限制在发源地是不可能的。另一种途径是使用防护屏障，防止医务人员暴露于病原体，在口腔医疗工作中一般包括工作服、口罩、防护镜、手套等，称这些设备为“个人防护设备”（personal protective equipment）。

1. 手套（Gloves）

手套可以防止医务工作者直接接触患者口腔中或污染物表面的微生物；同时也可以防止患者不受医务人员手部微生物的侵害。

（1）对医务人员的防护

虽然没有损伤的皮肤是良好的天然屏障，但对于微生物而言即使是肉眼不可见的损伤也是入侵的通道，引起这些皮肤伤口感染或导致更广泛的病变。对医务人员而言没有防护的手部皮肤的伤口是引起乙型肝炎的重要原因。口腔医务人员由 HSV 引起的甲沟炎患病率高于普通人群。手套还可以防止一些化学试剂、药品及一些口腔材料侵蚀。

A study in 1982 shows that fourth-year dental students had an average of fours areas of trauma on their hands; 12%of the traumas became painful on contact with alcohol, suggesting open skin (cut or abrasion) . Also, some visually intact areas give a painful response with alcohol, particularly around the fingernails. Thus even a close visual inspection of the hands may not detect all possible portals of entry for microorganisms.

（2）对患者的防护

微生物有时会存在于医疗场所中没有清洁或消毒的物品表面，没有戴手套的手由于接触这些的表面而被污染，如果进行口腔医疗操作没有手套覆盖带有微生物的手，感染物同样会传播给患者。研究表明，即使在洗手的情况下，指甲沟中残留的血液也会保留数日，成为下一位患者的感染源。因此戴手套即可防止自身被污染，也可防止成为感染源。

体内存在的微生物可以通过皮肤的破口渗出体外，特别是当不带手套在患者潮湿的口腔中操作时，将更能增加患者感染的机会，也可以部分解释不带手套进行治疗的口腔医务人员可以将自身肝炎病毒传播给患者。

在治疗过程当中自始至终都应戴手套，防止病原体对医患双方造成危害。使用过的手套不可再用于下一位患者。在口腔治疗前可用清水冲净手套上的粉剂，但不可应用清洁剂、化学药品清洗手套，这些化学药品能减弱手套的稳定性，增加手套的易破损性。

暂离治疗区域时，要摘下污染手套；返回后必须再更换一副新手套。这样既就可以预防手套上的病原体污染其他区域，同样也可以避免其他地方的微生物感染患者。治疗期间如果发现手套破裂，立即脱下手套、洗手、更换新的手套。

One of the most clearly documented cases of disease spread in a dental office occurred as a result of not routinely gloving for patient care. An ungloved hygienist with dermatitis on her hands and fingers cared for a patient with active herpes labialis (herpes simplex infection of the lips) . About a week later, vesicles of herpetic whitlow developed on the hygienist's hands. Before any sign of her infection appeared, however, she unknowingly spread the virus to at least 20 other patients, who developed intraoral herpes lesions. When the vesicles appeared on the hygienist's hands, she began to routinely wear gloves, which prevented further spread of the virus to any more patients.

This case demonstrates three modes of disease spread in the office: first, from patient to dental team member; second, from dental team member to patient; and third, from patient to patient. In this instance, all three modes of disease spread could have been prevented by routine gloving with every patient. Another important point demonstrated by this case is that dermatitis greatly reduces the effectiveness of hand washing in removing contaminating disease agents. Less vigorous handwashing is performed because of the painful dermatitis, and the dermatitis itself provides additional places on the hands where microorganisms can "hide" from the mechanical action of handwashing.

手套的类型见表 14-5：

表 14-5 Types of gloves in dentistry

Patient Care Gloves	Sterile latex surgical gloves
	Sterile neoprene surgical gloves
	Sterile styrene surgical gloves
	Sterile synthetic copolymer gloves
	Sterile reduced protein latex surgeon's gloves
	Latex examination gloves
	Vinyl examination gloves
	Synthetic copolymer examination gloves
	Nitrile examination gloves
	Stryene-butadiene examination gloves
	Powderless gloves
	Flavored gloves
Utility Gloves	
	Heavy latex gloves
	Heavy nitrile gloves
	Thin copolymer gloves
	Thin plastic（"food handlers"）gloves
Other gloves	
	Heat-resistant gloves
	Dermal（cotton ）gloves

2. 洗手（Handwashing）

在疾病传播过程中手是微生物重要的来源。对个人而言洗手是良好重要的卫生习惯，对医务人员而言是疾病初级预防的必要步骤。洗手可以明显减少病原体的数量传播，减少经手传播病原体的几率及其引起的疾病，对医患双方都有保护作用。

洗手的步骤和清洗剂

洗手时的机械作用很重要，通过手的相互摩擦可以使污物和微生物脱离皮肤，轻易地被水带走。普通清洗剂不含有抗生物活性，可以祛除污物和一些暂住菌，但对常住菌几乎没有作用。卫生人员使用的清洗剂含有低到中等浓度的抗菌物，10 ~ 30 秒的清洗可以最大限度的减少暂住菌，部分减少常住菌。

At Beginning of day

1. Remove jewelry and gently clean fingernails.

2. Scrub hands, nails, and forearms with a liquid, antimicrobial, handwashing agent and soft sterile brush or sponge for one minute and rinse with cool to lukewarm water for 10 seconds.

3. Vigorously lather hands and forearms with the germicidal agent for 20 seconds and rinse with cool to lukewarm water for 10 seconds.

4. Dry hands, then forearms, with clean paper towels and use the towels to turn off hand-controlled sink faucets

Routine handwashing during the day

1. Vigorously lather hands and forearms with a liquid, antimicrobial, handwashing agent for 20seconds and rinse with cool to lukewarm water for 10 seconds

2. Repeat lathering and rinsing

3. Dry hands, then forearms, with clean paper towels and use towels to turn off hand-controlled sink faucets

There are two types of microbial flora on the hands: resident and transient skin flora. The resident skin flora consists of microorganisms that colonize the skin and become permanent residents. They are always there and can never be totally removed even with a surgical scrub (Likely because the resident flora can exist even several layers under the surface in the stratum corneum) but their numbers can be reduced. Although members of the resident skin flora can cause infection when directly or indirectly spread to others, they are likely less important in disease spread than the second type of skin flora, the transient skin flora. The microorganisms of this flora contaminate the hands during the touching of or other exposure to contaminated surfaces. They do not usually colonize and survive on the hands for long periods; thus they are called members of the transient flora (they "come and go") . The transient flora serves as a source of disease spread because it can contain just about any pathogenic microorganism, depending on how the hands become contaminated. Fortunately, the transient flora can be removed or greatly reduced by routine handwashing, usually because the contaminating microorganisms remain primarily on the outer layers of the skin.

Common antimicrobial agents in handwashing products include chlorhexidine digluconate (CHG), povidone iodine (PI), para-chlorometaxylenos (PCMX), and triclosan (TLS). Chlorhexidine digluconate is well known for its widespread antimicrobial activity and its residual activity (prolonged antimicrobial effect). CHG binds to the skin to give prolonged release of antimicrobial activity. TLS also may have a prolonged effect, whereas persistence of PCMX on skin may be less. PI does not exhibit prolonged activity. It is very important to wash hands every time before gloving and after removing gloves. When the skin is occluded (tightly covered up) with gloves, members of the resident flora, and to a lesser extent the transient flora, dramatically increase. This increase may be as great as 4,000-fold per hour. This increased growth of microorganisms in the warm, moist environment under gloves can cause skin irritation. Washing after removing gloves reduces the number of those that have increased, as well as the transient microorganisms that may have contacted the skin through defects in the gloves. Handwashing after gloves are removed also helps remove any powder containing latex protein.

3. 口罩（Masks）

口罩最初是为了减少手术病人感染呼吸道微生物而设计的。虽然不能肯定口罩能否真正起到预防呼吸道微生物感染的目的，但在目前阶段为了防止呼吸道传播性疾病，口罩仍是标准的预防步骤之一。对口腔医务人员而言，口罩可以保护口腔、鼻黏膜，避免直接接触口腔治疗过程中的液体飞沫或化学药物，这些飞沫中可能混有一些致病性微生物；同时口罩也可以在一定程度上保护患者免受医务工作者的病原体感染。

Face masks are composed of synthetic material that serves to filter out at least 95% of small particles that directly contact the mask. Face masks do not provide a perfect seal around their edges, and exhaled and inhaled air that is not filtered can pass through these sites. Thus it is important to select a mask that fits the face well to minimize passage of unfiltered air. Also, when a mask is wetted form moist exhaled air, the resistance to airflow through the mask increases, causing more unfiltered air to pass by the edges of the mask. Thus wet mask should be replaced, maybe every 20 minutes. To maintain high filterability. The mask should be changed with every patient because its outer surface becomes contaminated with droplets from sprays of oral fluids from the previous patient or from touching the mask with saliva-coated fingers.

4. 防护镜（Protective eyeglasses）

许多微生物都可以通过眼部或其他黏膜部位侵入体内引起系统性疾病，例如HSB和HBV都可通过黏膜感染。防护镜对眼睛的防护不仅是对微生物的防护，也可以是对物理或化学性物质的防护，如牙齿的碎屑、充填物质、打磨物、抛光物，以及清洁剂、消毒剂等。

在使用旋转器械操作时或接触病人体液、化学药品时都应使用防护镜。在每位患者治疗完成后应清洗防护镜。患者也应在治疗时戴防护镜，资料表明患者眼睛也同样可以被物理、化学物质损伤。介绍防护镜的特点：

表 14-6 Comparison of eye protection devices

Type	Front Splash Protection	Side Splash Protection	Front Impact Protection	Side impact Protection	Neck and Face Protection
Goggles	Excellent	Excellent	Excellent	Excellent	Poor
Glasses (no shields)	Good	Poor	Excellent	Poor	Poor
Glasses (with shields)	Good	Good	Excellent	Fair	Poor
Face shield	Excellent	Good to Excellent	Variable (depends on thickness)	Variable (depends on thickness)	Variable (depends on thickness)

5. 防护服（Protective clothing）

含病原微生物的飞沫不仅可以感染没有防护的眼、鼻和口腔黏膜，也可以污染医务工作者的前胸和前臂的区域，大的液体飞沫还可降落在腿部。在没有防护服的情况下，带有病原体的液体飞沫可以感染医务工作者，或者被医务工作者从工作环境带入家庭、社会。

防护服是最外层的服装，覆盖皮肤、外衣、内衣等，应能抵御其下方的部分不被感染物所污染。医务工作者一旦进入工作环境，也就是皮肤或衣物有可能被带有病原体的飞沫污染时，就应该穿戴防护服，离开医疗环境时应脱去防护服。

穿脱防护服的步骤：

- 穿戴：防护服→防护镜→口罩→手套
- 摘脱：防护服→手套→防护镜→口罩

三、器械处理 Instrument processing

口腔医用器械使用后，被患者、医务工作者、周围环境等病原体污染，必须进行处理后才可继续使用，但同时必须使器械损伤降低到最小程度。

表 14-7 Instrument processing

1. Holding（Presoaking）
2. Precleaning
3. Corrosion control, drying, lubrication
4. Packaging
5. Sterilization
6. Sterilization monitoring
7. Handling processed instruments

As with other medical and surgical instruments, dental instruments are classified into three categories - critical, semi critical, or no critical - depending on their risk of transmitting infection and the need to sterilize them between uses. Each dental practice should classify all instruments as follows:

Critical: Surgical and other instruments used to penetrate soft tissues or hardbone tissues are classified as critical and should be sterilized after each use. These devices include forceps, scalpels, bone chisels, scalers, and burs.

Semicritical: Instruments such as mirrors and amalgam condensers that do not penetrate soft tissues or bone but contact oral tissues are classified as semi critical. These devices should be sterilized after each use. If, however, sterilization is not feasible because the instrument will be damaged by heat, the instrument should receive, at a minimum, high-level disinfection.

Noncritical: Instruments or medical devices such as external components of X-ray heads that come into contact only with intact skin are classified as non critical. Because these non critical surfaces have a relatively low risk of transmitting infection, they may be reprocessed between patients with intermediate-level or low-level disinfection or detergent and water washing, depending on the nature of the surface and the degree and nature of the contamination.

1. 灭菌和消毒 Sterilization and disinfection

灭菌（sterilization）是指消灭存在于任何非生命体或器械上的所有生活的微生物。所说的无生命，不是指活着的人体组织，如我们不能在皮肤上灭菌。日常工作中很难判断是否消灭了所有微生物，因此通常选择一种抵抗力强的微生物作为标准，如果消灭了这个微生物，就意味着完成灭菌过程。细菌芽孢对热和化学药剂有较强的抵抗作用，通常被选作为标准物。也存在一些其他较难消灭的微生物有，如结核杆菌、肝炎病毒、真菌孢子、疱疹病毒和、葡萄球菌等。

消毒（disinfection）是指杀灭病原微生物，但不一定杀灭细菌芽孢的方法。理论上应杀灭一切具有生长能力的微生物，但实际工作中，是以减少致病因子，使其不能达到可引起感染的数量水平为目的。消毒剂的作用机理：①使细菌细胞膜通透性受损；②使菌体蛋白变性和凝固，失去其生物活性，导致细菌死亡；③破坏或改变蛋白质与核酸功能基团，使菌体酶蛋白失去酶的活性。影响消毒剂作用的因素：①消毒剂浓度和作用时间；②温度；③细菌种类和数量；④被消毒物的性质。

一种理想的消毒剂应具有抗谱广、作用快、不受物理因素影响、无毒、表面相容、应用简便、受处理表面无残留作用、容易应用、无异味、价格低等特点。但是没有一种消毒剂能满足根据上述要求，没有一种是完美的。根据各种消毒剂的不同特点与污染程度，可把消毒用化学物品分为三类：①高效水平消毒剂：与杀芽胞药相类似，能使细菌芽胞失活，还可杀灭其他微生物；②中等水平消毒剂：不能使细菌芽胞失活，但能杀灭其他微生物，特别是结核杆菌；③低效水平消毒剂：抗微生物范围最窄，常用于清洁环境表面，虽能使亲脂类病毒与细菌繁殖体失活，对真菌也有一定作用，但不能杀灭结核杆菌、细菌芽胞和非脂质病毒。

（1）戊二醛（glutaraldehyde）：为无色或浅黄色油状液体，可按任何比例溶于水和醇，水溶液呈酸性（pH4-5），较稳定。对橡胶、塑料、透镜及结合剂、金属器械等多数物品无腐蚀性。推荐使用2%水溶液作浸泡消毒，穿透力强，具有广谱、高效、快速杀菌特点，依浸泡时间达到高水平消毒作用，3 小时可杀灭细菌芽胞。WHO 肝炎小组将 2% 水溶液推荐为 HBV 污染物的消毒剂，一般 5 ~ 10 分钟可使 HBV 灭活。国产中性与碱性戊二醛具有相同的杀菌能力，使用期可延至 4 周，且无酸性戊二醛的腐蚀性。

戊二醛—酚是碱性戊二醛与石碳酸钠缓冲到pH7.4形成的戊二醛与酚的复合物，是高效消毒剂。临床使用1∶16配比稀释溶液。副作用及注意事项：未稀释溶液对眼睛、皮肤和呼吸道黏膜有刺激。混合使用时应戴眼镜、厚手套和穿工作服，应在通风好的地方使用，容器应覆盖。不推荐用于表面消毒。

（2）含氯的配方（chlorine preparations）：①次氯酸钠溶液（sodium hypochlorite solutions）为白色或无色液体，属强氧化剂，杀菌作用快但不稳定；商品含有效氯8%～12%。抗感染溶液0.5%，应每日制备新液。暴露于空气中不稳定，与有机物质发生反应可使效力减弱，可用于表面消毒。副作用为对眼睛和皮肤黏膜有刺激，且对金属有腐蚀作用（特别是铝），使衣物脱色；②亚氯酸和二氧化氯（chlorous acid and chlorine dioxide）将氯化钠和有机酸结合产生，作为 3 分钟的强消毒剂，可喷擦表面，长期反复使用可导致一些金属表面氧化。

（3）酚类：1∶32稀释液可作为消毒剂。对细菌、病毒、结核菌等都有杀灭作用，但对芽胞无此作用。作为表面和浸泡消毒，需 10 分钟接触时间，应每日新鲜配制，无臭，但可能损坏塑料和橡皮，对皮肤、眼睛有刺激。

（4）碘伏：是一种有机复合物。原液稳定，毒性及腐蚀性低。多用 1∶213 的稀释溶液，应每日新配制，较之醇溶液更有活性。用作表面消毒或浸泡，对大多数微生物有效，包括结核、HBV。用作表面消毒时可将表面喷射湿润，保持 10 分钟。碘伏常用于外科手术前的皮肤、黏膜以及医疗器械、玻璃制品的消毒，医疗器械浸泡 1～2 小时。一般安全，无刺激，但对一些人的皮肤有染色或刺激，混合溶液时应使用手套、眼镜和工作服。

（5）酒精：不推荐作为表面和浸泡消毒。对细菌芽胞无效，抗病毒活力参差不齐，挥发快，残留作用小，有机物容易使其失去活力。但是，结合低浓度的合成酚可用于表面消毒或预清洁。

2. 器械处理的步骤 Steps of instrument processing

（1）浸泡（holding, presoaking）

为防止附着在器械上的唾液或血液干燥不易清洗，在清洗前，将器械浸泡于溶液之中，易于清洗，同时防止感染物质扩散。为防止器械腐蚀，浸泡器械时间不宜超过数小时。1∶32稀释的合成酚溶液是理想的浸泡溶液，应每日更换。

（2）预清洗（precleaning）

在器械灭菌与消毒之前，预清洗是必须的步骤。可减少微生物数量；祛除血液、唾液以及其他可以阻碍灭菌或消毒效果的物质。带有污染物的器械不能灭菌，而且患者永远不会认可带有污染物的器械是安全的治疗工具。

Ultrasonic cleaning, compared with scrubbing instruments by hand, reduces direct handling of the contaminated instruments and the chances for cuts and punctures. It is also an excellent cleaning mechanism, and staff can do other tasks while the instruments are being cleaned. The ultrasonic energy produces billions of tiny bubbles in the cleaning solution that collapse and create high turbulence at the surface of the instruments. This dislodges the debris and suspends it in the solution or it dissolves. Very few instruments cannot be ultrasonically cleaned. One exception is some high-speed handpieces, although others can withstand ultrasonics.

Manual scrubbing of contaminated instruments by hand is dangerous even though it is a very effective method of removing debris, if performed properly. All surfaces of all instruments should be thoroughly brushed while the instruments are submerged in a cleaning solution to avoid spattering. It is also best to use a long-handled brush to keep the scrubbing hand as far away from the sharp instrument tips as possible. This is followed by thorough rinsing with a minimum of splashing.

Routine manual scrubbing of instruments is not recommended, however, because it requires maximum direct contact with the contaminated instruments, increasing the chances for cuts or punctures through the gloves. Also, there is no real need to hand scrub and ultrasonically clean all instruments if the ultrasonic cleaner is working properly; occasionally, however, an ultrasonically cleaned item may need additional hand cleaning to remove some cements.

Instrument washers designed to clean medical and dental instruments are used in some large facilities (hospitals, dental schools) and in some smaller dental offices. These units automatically provide cleaning and rinsing and some (called washer-disinfectors) use very hot water and achieve disinfection of the instruments with cleaning. Household dishwashers are not recommended for use on contaminated instruments because their manufacturers did not design them for this purpose.

(3) 防腐、干燥、润滑（Corrosion control, drying, and lubrication）

高压蒸汽灭菌会造成某些器械或零件的腐蚀，如碳钢钻针、非不锈钢的釉凿、釉斧、镊子、正畸克断钳等。虽然防腐剂可以减少这些器械的腐蚀，但最好的方法是不使用高压蒸汽灭菌法，代之以彻底的干燥，使用干热灭菌法或不饱和化学蒸汽灭菌法为好。

器械在高压蒸汽灭菌前应尽量干燥，以避免残留水分浸湿纸性包装物，造成外包装破损，影响灭菌效果。旋转器械在灭菌前应适当润滑。

(4) 包裹（Packaging）

器械包裹是保持灭菌后的器械在使用之前始终处于无菌状态。为了防止灭菌后的器械污染，器械包裹应在灭菌步骤前进行。未包裹的器械在脱离灭菌环境后立即处于被空气中灰尘、飞沫、触摸等污染的状态中。包裹应按器械功能分类，将器械装入袋状、盒状物中，每件包裹好的物品都应用变色指示条封闭，当达到设定的时间与温度时即变色。

General packaging procedures Onlyonly use packaging material or open containers that have been designed for use in sterilizers, and use the appropriate sterilization packaging materials for the sterilization method being used (table 56-8). Other wrap, plastic bags, containers, or paper may melt, prevent the sterilizing agent from penetrating to the instruments inside, or may release unwanted chemicals into the sterilizer chamber. Sterilization pouches, wraps, or bags should never be sealed with metal closures, including staples or anything that can puncture the material and breech sterility.

Closed containers such as trays or pans with solid tops and bottoms, capped glass vials, or wrap such as aluminum foil should never be used to package items for sterilization in steam or unsaturated chemical vapor sterilizers. The steam or hot chemical vapor will not penetrate these containers or materials to reach the items inside. These may be appropriate for sterilization in dry heat, however, if sufficient exposure time is used. Sharps containers and biohazard bags containing regulated waste that will be sterilized before disposal must be left open during the sterilization process and then closed after removal from the sterilizer.

(5) 灭菌（Sterilization）

口腔医疗常用的有三种灭菌方法：

①热灭菌法（Heat sterilization），

②气体灭菌法（Gas sterilization），

③液体化学灭菌法（Liquid chemical sterilization）。

热灭菌法（heat sterilization）最常用，它包括高压蒸汽灭菌法（autoclave）、干热灭菌法（dry heat）和不饱和化学蒸汽压力灭菌法（unsaturated chemical vapor）等三种灭菌方法。

高压蒸汽灭菌法用于口腔器械灭菌安全系数最大，是在高温、高压下通过饱和蒸汽完成灭菌过程。这类灭菌法能有效破坏细菌及其芽孢。高温蒸汽灭菌法适用于下列物品灭菌：优质不锈钢器械、耐高温消毒手机、布类、玻璃杯，大吸唾管、包扎的器械以及耐热塑料器械。高温蒸汽灭菌法的缺点是对碳金属器械有腐蚀作用，在灭菌前可使用无毒润滑油以减少器械的腐蚀。针头、油类、酚类、蜡类不能应用高压蒸汽灭菌法高温灭菌。

干热灭菌法是一种有效的灭菌方法。由于在干热的条件下灭菌较湿热条件下困难，所以此方法不适用于频繁口腔临床周转器械。但由于没有水蒸气的影响，故适用于金属器械、玻璃制品和、不能被水蒸气干扰的物品的灭菌。

不饱和化学蒸汽压力灭菌法是利用低湿蒸汽或同时导入化学物气体进行消毒的一种装置。通过加热甲醛、乙基甲基酮等溶液将器械放在一密封内胆中灭菌。它有三个优点：①相对循环周期短，7～30分钟可完成未包扎物品灭菌；②器械不会变钝、生锈、腐蚀，可延长使用寿命延长；③器械在灭菌后即干燥。不饱和化学蒸汽压力灭菌法适用的器械包括全部牙科手用器械、高速手机、碳钻或金刚石车针、根管器械、正畸钢丝和锁槽。缺点是需要花费额外的费用购买溶液，要求通风条件良好，以排出化学气体。

表 14-8　Type and use of sterilization packaging materials

Sterilization Method	Packaging Material	Precautions
Steam autoclave	Paper wrap	No closed containers
	Nylon “plastic” tubing	Thick cloth may absorb too much Steam
	Paper/plastic peel pouches	Some plastic containers melt
	Thin cloth	Use only material approved for
	Wrapped perforated cassettes	steam
Dry heat sterilizers	Paper wrap	Some paper may char
	Appropriate nylon “plastic” Tubing	Some plastic containers melt
	Closed containers	Only use material approved for dry heat
	Wrapped perforated cassettes	
	Aluminum foil	
Unsaturated chemical sterilizer	Paper wrap	No closed containers
	Paper/plastic peel pouches	Cloth absorbs too much chemical vapor
	Wrapped perforated cassettes	Some plastic containers melt
		Use only material approved for chemical
		vapor

Ethylene oxide gas sterilizers that operate at 72°F to 140°F (much lower than heat sterilizers) also can be monitored with bacterial endospores but this type of sterilization is not commonly used in dental offices because of the long exposure time required for sterilization, the high cost of gas sterilizers, and the required special handling of the ethylene oxide gas sterilant.

Liquid chemical sterilizations used on items that are damaged by heat sterilization. The liquid chemical sterilant used is 2.0% to 3.4% glutaraldehyde, and although it can be shown to be sporicidal in controlled laboratory testing, the microbial killing that occurs during actual use in the office cannot be routinely determined. Spore tests for biologic monitoring have not yet been developed for office-testing of liquid sterilants. The best that can be done is to chemically estimate the concentration of active glutaradehyde remaining in the used solution. It slowly becomes inactive.

(6) 灭菌的监测（Sterilization monitoring）

成功的灭菌意味着消灭所有微生物，检测的唯一标准是验证所有微生物是否被消灭，但到目前为止没有任何方法或步骤能绝对证明所有微生物被消灭，灭菌后仍有存活微生物的风险。目前口腔医疗常用的灭菌方法都能很好消灭DAN和RNA病毒，有效清除污染病毒的特异性蛋白和核酸，表明所用灭菌、消毒手段在预防病毒的感染方面已经较为有效。常用的三种监测方法有：生物监测（biologic monitoring）、化学监测（chemical monitoring）和物理监测（physical monitoring）。

Biologic monitoring provides the main guarantee of sterilization. It involves processing highly resistant bacterial spores through the sterilizer and then culturing the spores to determine if they have been killed. Biologic indicators (BI) contain the bacterial endospores used for monitoring. The spores used are Bacillus stearothermophilus (for testing steam or chemical vapor sterilization) or Bacillus subtilis (for testing dry heat or ethylene oxide gas sterilization) . There is no BIs available to routinely test liquid chemical sterilants or disinfections during use in the office.

Chemical monitoring uses heat-sensitive chemicals (rather than live spores as in biologic monitoring) to assess the physical conditions during the sterilization process. Chemical monitoring involves the use of indicators that change color or physical form when exposed to certain temperatures. There are two types of chemical indicators. The rapid-change indicator changes color rapidly after a certain temperature has been reached (e.g., autoclave tape and special markings on pouches and bags) . Thus it demonstrates only that an item has been exposed to a certain temperature for some length of time. The second type of chemical indicator is called a slow-change or integrated indicator that changes color or form slowly, responding to a combination of time and temperature or time, temperature, and the presence of steam.

Physical monitoring of the sterilization process involves observing the gauges and displays on the sterilizer and recording the sterilizing temperature, pressure, and exposure time. Although correct readings do not guarantee sterilization, incorrect readings give the first indication that a problem has likely occurred. Many small office sterilizers now have recording devices that print out these parameters, providing a physical monitoring record for each run. It must be remembered that sterilizer gauges and displays indicate the conditions in the sterilizer chamber rather than conditions within the packs, pouches, or cassettes being processed. Thus physical monitoring may not detect problems resulting from overloading, improper packaging material, or use of closed containers.

(7) 器械保管（handling processed instruments）

器械保管是器械处理的重要步骤。在保管前应将灭菌后物品烘干，因为潮湿环境有利于微生物生长，包裹易损坏。应缓慢降温，以防器械表面形成负压，造成污染。保存场地应是干燥、密闭、低灰尘区域。打开器械包裹前，应检查包裹是否破损，打开时禁止触摸内部物品。

四、表面与设备无菌术 Surface and equipment asepsis

在治疗期间病原体可以污染设备表面，如被医务工作者带有血液、唾液污染的手套所接触的区域，患者口腔唾液及分泌物形成的飞沫可污染的治疗区域。因此在两位患者治疗间隙期间，必须进行适当的表面消毒处理，防止病原体的传播。易被污染区域见表 14-9。

不同微生物在表面环境中生存时间不同，如结核杆菌可生存数周，单纯疱疹病毒最多只可生存数分钟。另外温度、湿度、所在环境中是否有营养性（唾液、血液等）物质等都可影响微生物生存时间。由于上述诸多不确定因素，不可能准确预测口腔治疗环境中微生物的生存状况。因此预防感染传播的有效方法是在每位患者治疗结束后，祛除或消灭治疗区表面微生物。表面无菌术有两种方法：一种是表面覆盖（surface cover），隔绝感染；另一种是对污染区域进行预清洁（preclean）、和消毒（disinfection）。

Surface cover can prevent contamination before there is an opportunity for contamination. Surface covers should be impervious to keep microorganisms in saliva, blood, or other liquids from soaking through to contact the surface. Examples of appropriate material for surface covers include clear plastic wrap, bags, or tubes, and plastic-backed paper. Some plastics are designed specifically for use as surface covers in the office in that they have the shape of the item to be covered (e.g., air/water syringe handle covers, hose covers, pen coves). Some sheets of plastic also have a slightly sticky substance on one side so they will be held on the surface. Other plastics (e.g., some food wraps) have a natural "clinging" ability on contact with a smooth surface. Some plastic bags are available with drawstrings that will hold them around an item to be protected. To reduce costs, thin rather than thick plastic sheets or bags can be used as long as they are not punctured by the surface being covered. Patient bibs are made of plastic backed paper and also can be used to cover flat operativeory surface, although thin plastic sheets may be less expensive.

Precleaning must be done before the disinfection. This reduces the number of contaminating microorganisms and the blood or saliva present (referred to as bioburden) and facilitates action of the disinfecting chemical. The organic material in blood and saliva will insulate microorganisms from contact with a disinfecting chemical and also may inactivate a portion of the active chemical in the disinfectant. During the precleaning process, regular soap and water may be used but it is best to use a surface cleaner/disinfectant that contains detergents for both the precleaning step and the disinfecting step.

The disinfection procedure is intended to kill disease producing microorganisms that remain on the surface after precleaning. Spray the disinfectant on the precleaned surface and let it remain moist for the longest contact time indicated on the disinfectant label. If moisture remains, wipe it away with a towel.

表 14-9 Examples of surface susceptible to contamination during patient care activities

Headrest on chair	Drawer handles
Chair control buttons	Countertops
Light handles	X-ray unit handle and cone
Light switch	X-ray unit controls
Bracket table	X-ray view box switch
Handpiece control switches	Dental team chair backs
Handpiece hoses	Supply containers and bottles
Evacuator hoses	Light curing handle and tip
Evacuator control	Mirror handles
Air/water syringe handle	Faucet handles
Air/water syringe hoses	Shade guides

五、废弃物管理 Waste management

医务部门及医务工作者必须遵守各级卫生机构制定的医疗废物管理规定，掌握各种医疗废物的概念及处理方法。

Many people mistakenly consider the terms "hospital waste," "medical waste," and "infectious waste" as being synonymous. "Hospital waste," like "dental office waste" or "household waste," refers to the total discarded solid waste generated by all sources within a given location (Table 14～10). In a hospital, this includes biologic waste materials, such as clerical paper and plastic items. "Medical waste" includes materials generated during patient diagnosis, treatment, or immunization. "Infectious waste" is a small subset (estimated at 3% of the total) of "medical waste" that has shown a capability of transmitting an infectious disease. It should be noted that factors such as the number and virulence of the microorganisms present, host resistance, and the presence and availability of portals of entry have important roles in whether and infection occurs.

有些医疗废物需要特殊处理，如口腔医疗产生的血液或血液污染的物品、病理性废弃物、锐利器械等。血液或血液污染物包括液体、半液体血液，接触这些液体时可以被病原体感染。治疗过程中唾液中经常混有血液，因此唾液同样是感染性废弃物。牙齿和其他被分离的组织是病理性废弃物，存在潜在的感染性，使用高压蒸汽灭菌或不饱和化学蒸汽灭菌均可达到理想灭菌效果。针头、钻针等尖锐器械应放在硬包装的容器中，应用专门器械处理。

表 14-10 Definitions of waste

Term	Definition
Contaminated waste	Items that have had contact with blood or other body secretions
Hazardous waste	Waste posing a risk or humans or the environment
Infections	Waste capable of causing an infectious disease
Medical waste	Any solid waste that is generated in the diagnosis, treatment, or immunization of human beings or animals in research pertaining thereto or the production or testing of biologicals. The term does not include, hazardous waste or household waste. Only a small percent of medical waste is infectious ans needs to be regulated
Regulated waste	Infectious medical waste that requires special handling, neutralization, and disposal.
Toxic waste	Waste capable of having a poisonous effect

小结 Summary

口腔保健实践中的感染与控制问题不是单纯依靠医疗技术就能解决的，它涉及流行病学、社会学、心理学等诸多方面，必须只有在各个方面进行多方位、多层次的综合管理和质量控制之后，才可能避免医院感染现象的发生，有效保护医患双方的利益。通过本章的学习，了解口腔医疗保健中的感染、感染传播方式及其特点，熟悉个人保护、无菌术、消毒、灭菌等控制医院感染的相关知识，以利在口腔医疗工作中运用。

思考题 Review questions

1. 什么是医院感染？
2. 医院感染主要研究对象？
3. 外源性感染的主要特征。
4. HIV 的传播途径。
5. 个人防护的措施。
6. 什么是灭菌与消毒。
7. 简述表面无菌术的方法。
8. 口腔医疗废弃物处理方法。

参考文献 References

1. 卞金有主编. 预防口腔医学. 北京: 人民卫生出版社, 2004
2. 王力红主编. 医院感染学. 北京: 中国协和医科大学出版社, 2002
3. CDC Infectin Control Guidelines for Dentistry. MMWR, 1993, 41: 1-12

（陈霄迟）

第十五章　循证医学与口腔保健

Chapter XV　Evidence-based Medicine and Oral Health Care

概述 Overview

本章分为四个部分简要叙述循证医学与口腔保健的关系。第一部分是关于循证医学的基本概念，包括随机对照的流行临床试验（RCT）；第二部分介绍评价结果真实性应具备应具备的基本条件。包括系统评价与Meta分析；第三部分分为证据质量评价与循证推荐；最后一部分介绍循证预防口腔医学的概念与实践。

This chapter is divided into four parts which briefly describes the relationship between the evidence-based medicine and oral health care. The first part is related to the basic concepts of evidence-based medicine, including the randomized controlled trial (RCT); The second part introduces the basic qualifications possessed in the validity evaluation of the results from studies, including the systematic review and Meta-analysis; The third part is about the assessment of quality of evidence and evidence-based recommendations; The last part introduces the concept of evidence-based preventive dentistry.

要点 Key points

- *Concepts of evidence-based medicine (EMB)*
- *Randomized controlled trial (RCT)*
- *Blindness*
- *Systematic review*
- *Meta-analysis*
- *Evidence-based preventive dentistry*

传统的医学模式以经验与推理为基础。20世纪80年代以来引入了循证医学的全新概念-以证据为基础的概念与模式，它要求对疾病的防治干预建立在有充分的科学证据的基础之上。不但评价药物或非药物手段对替代终点的作用，例如，从口腔菌斑与唾液pH值的变化推论某种制剂对龋病的预防作用，而且强调评价它对预后终点的作用，如疾病主要事件，龋病发病率，龋均，生活质量，成本-效益比等。循证医学模式强调防治疾病的科学规范，既有效，又合理使用医疗保健费用。如今，循证医学已不仅仅局限于临床病人诊治的范畴，而是扩展到整个医疗卫生保健系统，因而提出了循证保健（evidence-based health care, EBHC）的全新概念。

Traditional medical model is based on the experience and inference. Since 80's of 20th century. Evidence-based medicine as a completely new concept was introduced-evidence-based concept and model. It requires that the intervention of disease prevention and treatment should be established on the basis of sufficient scientific evidences, not only evaluating the effect by drug or non-drug approach at surrogate end -point, for example, from the change of pH values in dental plaque and saliva to inference the preventive effect of dental caries by some agents but also emphasize on evaluation of its effect at the outcome end-point, such as main events of disease, the caries incidence rate, mean DMFT/dmft, quality of life, and cost-benefit ratio, etc. evidence-based model emphasizes the scientific regulations to disease prevention and treatment, both effective and reasonable use of medical care fee. At present time, evidence-based medicine is not just limited in clinical field of diagnosis and treatment for patients. And extended to the whole medical and health care system. Therefore, evidence-based health care, EBHC as a completely new concept is proposed.

第一节　循证医学的基本概念
Section 1 Basic Concepts of Evidence-based Medicine (EMB)

循证医学的哲理起源于19世纪中叶的巴黎，较早的成为临床学家，公共卫生学家，采购与计划人员，还有公众的热门话题。现在经常有关于如何实践，如何教育的研讨会，大学生，研究生的培训项目也纳入了循证医学，在英国与其他国家建立了包括牙医学在内的许多循证医学中心。1996年著名的临床流行病学家Sacket在英国医学杂志上发表了关于循证医学的文章（Evidence-based medicine, EBM: what it is and what it isn't）.

一、循证医学的概念 The concept of Evidence-based medicine, EBM

循证医学是“医生认真，明确而审慎地应用当前所能得到的最佳证据为各个病人的医疗保健作出具体处理决定。”

实践循证意味着医生个人临床工作能力与来自系统研究的最佳的可以利用的外部临床证据相结合。

Evidence-based medicine, whose philosophical origins extend back to mid-19th century Paris and earlier, remains a hot topic for clinicians, public health practitioners, purchasers, planners, and the public. There are now frequent workshops in how to practice and teach it; undergraduate and postgraduate training programmes are in cooperating it; British and other countries centres for evidence based practice have been established in many health sectors, including dentistry. In 1996, a paper titled evidence based medicine: what it is and what it isn't was published in the British Medical Journal by Professor David I. Sacket, et al.

(1) The concept of Evidence-based medicine, EBM

Evidence-based medicine is the conscientious, explicit, and judicious use of current best evidence in making decisions about the care of individual patients. The practice of evidence based medicine means integrating individual clinical expertise with the best available external clinical evidence from systematic research.

通过医生个人的临床工作能力，我们认为是各个临床医生通过临床经验与临床实践达到的精通与判断力。提高临床工作能力反映在许多方面，特别是在更加有效的诊断，更加深思的确定以及更有同情心地利用各个病人的处境、权利和优先考虑作出关于病人保健的临床决定。

通过医生最佳的利用外部临床证据，我们认为临床上的相关研究经常来自医学的基础科学，特别是来自以病人为中心的临床研究，准确而正确的诊断试验（包括临床检查），预后标识的功效，以及治疗，康复与预防项目的效果与安全方面的研究成果。外部的临床证据包括以前接受的证据不足的诊断试验与治疗以及取而代之的新的更有力、更准确、更有效和更安全的证据。

好的医生善于运用个人的临床工作能力与最佳的可以利用的外部证据缺一不可。没有临床工作能力，实践的危险在于因为有证据而变得专横，即使有最佳的外部证据，对个别病人也可以不能用或者不适用。

而没有当前最佳的证据，实践的危险很快变成不利于病人。

这种对循证医学的叙述会帮助我们澄清什么不是循证医学。

By individual clinical expertise we mean the proficiency and judgment that individual clinicians acquire through clinical experience and clinical practice. Increased expertise is reflected in many ways, but especially in more effective and efficient diagnosis and in the more thoughtful identification and compassionate use of individual patients' predicaments, rights, and preferences in making clinical decisions about their care. By best available external clinical evidence we mean clinically relevant research. Often from the basic sciences of medicine, but especially from patient centred clinical research into the accuracy and precision of diagnostic tests (including the rapeutic, rehabilitative, and preventive regimens. External clinical evidence both invalidates previously accepted diagnostic tests and treatments and replaces them with new ones that are more powerful, more accurate, more efficacious, and safer.)

Good doctors use both individual clinical expertise and the best available external evidence, and neither alone is enough. Without clinical expertise, practice risks becoming tyrannised by evidence, for even excellent external evidence may be inapplicable to or inappropriate for an individual patient.

Without current best evidence, practice risks becoming rapidly out of date, to the detriment of patient.

This description of what evidence based medicine is helps clarify what evidence based medicine is not.

二、随机对照（临床）试验 Randomised controlled trial, RCT

1. 临床试验的定义 The definition of clinical trial

一项临床试验规定为一项正式计划的，前瞻性研究在人体进行的有对照的干预的作用与价值。这项研究必须是前瞻性的，从应用干预作评价之前确定的基线测量及时向前推进。这种临床试验必须评价一种或多种干预，在性质上可以是诊断性，预防性或治疗性，包括制剂，方法，步骤或方案。在研究开始时，试验必须要有对照组，尽可能与治疗组相似，因而随后的健康状况发生的变化可以合理地归之于进行测试干预的结果。

A clinical trial is defined as a formally planned, prospective study comparing the effect and value of an intervention (s) against a control in human beings. The study must be prospective, moving forward in time from baseline measurement established just prior to the application of the intervention to be evaluated. The clinical trial must evaluate one or more interventions that may be diagnostic, properly lactic or therapeutic in nature, comprising agents, devices, procedures or regiments. The trial must incorporate a control group that at the outset of the study is sufficiently similar to the treatment group (s) so that subsequent changes in health status may be reasonably ascribed to the intervention being tested.

三期临床试验是大多数临床学家们熟悉的普遍的，大范围的随机双盲临床试验。可以称作为随机临床试验（RCTs）或对照临床试验（CCT）。

2. 道德内容 The ethical issues

当试图进行一项临床试验时，总是会适当考虑道德问题，因为人参与的安全性与尊严一定非常重要。考虑的内容有许多不同的方面，难免包括得到受试者参与的过程，完成与理解知情同意，研究设计的适当，所测试制剂可能的有害作用以及可能削弱有益的治疗。在口腔科学文献中包含着许多口腔临床试验涉及的道德问题的讨论。因为随机临床试验的真正本质是提供口腔专业，牙科工业与公共卫生机构用于病人保健的较好的治疗知识。在龋病临床试验中安慰剂对照的可能作用也可以引起一种道德问题。

Phase III clinical trials represent the common, large-scale, randomized, double-blind clinical trials well known to most clinicians. It may be referred to as randomized clinical trials (RCTs) or as controlled clinical trials (CCT) .

Ethical Issues Ethical concerns always and properly, arise when a randomized clinical trial is contemplated, because the safety and dignity of the human participants must be paramount. The issues to be considered are many and varied but inevitably include concerns about the process for gaining people's participation, completeness and understanding of informed consent, adequacy of study design, potentially harmful effects of the agent being tested and possible with holding of beneficial treatment. The oral science literature contains a number of excellent discussions of ethical issues in dental clinical trials. Since the very essence of randomized clinical trials is to provide the dental profession, the dental industry and public health agencies with better therapeutic knowledge to apply in patient care. The potential role of placebo controls in caries clinical trials may also arise as an ethical issue.

面对问题的具体实例包括：①为得到允许在规定的国际机构内进行研究而给予过多的奖励；②为了得到个人知情同意而提供不适当的经济奖励；③参照具体人权，反对知情同意书中的用词；④作为研究的临床检查的一部分，当发现口腔疾病时可能没有能力提供保健或者转诊保健。

Specific examples of problems faced include: ①excessive economic incentives to obtain permission to conduct the study in defined international settings; ② inappropriate economic incentives for gaining individual informed consent; ③ objections to working in informed consent forms with specific reference to human rights, and ④ potential inability to provide or refer for care when dental disease is discovered as part of the study's clinical examinations.

3. 临床试验中的随机化 Randomization in clinical trials, RCT

RCT的一种明显而唯一的特征是作为前瞻性研究，通过一种正式的随机化程序把进入研究的受试者分配到一个或多个实验组与一个具有共同点的对照组。随机化的目的是确保在研究开始时，实验组与对照组尽可能相似。在RCT实际进行期间，研究方案的作用是保持除了研究的干预因素之外，两组的所有其他因素都具有可比性。

研究参与者的随机化可以通过几种方法之一来达到，每一种方法都有其固有的优点和缺点。随机化方法包含相当公平和花费人力，但对RCT来说都是基本的，有几个主要理由，如下：

首先，所有适当的随机化程序避免了选择性偏差，那就是说随机化的把干预方法分配给研究参与者是不可预知的，这样一旦受试者同意参与试验，排除了分配干预方法可能出现的偏差，例如，在龋病的临床试验中可以确保一种有效的预防措施不是不均衡地分配给大多数需要的受试者，即使不是有意的，或者反之亦然。

第二个优点是随机化趋向于平衡各个实验组关于可能与龋病结果有关的预知因素或者共变因素。这一优点明显地控制着事先是否知道这些预知因素，例如，分层随机化将平衡研究组的有关年龄一种已知龋病增加预知变量。然而，很清楚，这也可以在其后面通过应用协方差分析达到。

第三个优点是随机化可以为统计学程序的应用提供某些理论基础，在实践中，这意味着，研究者可以用试验产生的数据进行适当的统计学检验。在分析结果的 ，可以对干预作用观察到的差异，分配统计学的显著性水平。

因此，适当应用随机化过程是非常重要的。

Randomization in clinical trials

A distinguishing and unique feature of the RCT is that it includes. For prospective investigation, one or more experimental group (s) and a concurrent control group to which subjects who enter the study are allocated by a formal randomization procedure. The purpose of randomization is to ensure that, at the outser of the study, the experimental and control group are as alike as possible. During the actual conduct of the RCT, it is the role of the study protocol to maintain the comparability of the two groups on all factors other than the intervention being investigated.

Randomization of study participants may be attained through one of several methods, each of which may be associated with inherent advantages and disadvantages. For details concerning these techniques and indications for their use, good reference materials may be consulted. Randomization methods may be fairly involved and labor intensive, but are also essential to the RCT for several key reasons, as follows.

First, all proper randomization procedures avoid selection bias. That is, randomized assignment of treatment to study participants is unpredicted, thus eliminating bias from the assignment of treatment once the study subject has agreed to enter the trial. In caries trials, for example, this would ensure that a potentially effective preventive is not disproportionately assigned, even subconsciously, to subjects most in need, or vice versa.

A second advantage is that randomization tends to balance the treatment groups with respect to prognostic factors or covariates that may be related to dental caries outcomes. Significantly, this advantage holds whether such prognostic factors are known or unknown in advance. For example, stratified randomization will balance study groups with respect to age, a known prognostic variable for caries increments. It is clear, however, that this could also be accomplished post hoc by the use of covariance analysis.

A third advantage to randomization is that it provides some of the necessary theoretical underpinnings for the statistical procedures to be employed. In practice, this means that the investigator may apply the appropriate statistical tests to the data generated by the trial, and on observed differences in treatment effect.

Therefore, much more important is that a proper randomization process be employed.

4. 盲法 Blindness

当随机化排除了RCT开始时的偏差之后，应用适当的盲法或者隐蔽技术作为研究方案的一部分在数据产生的过程中保持不出现偏差是基本的。两种普遍应用的方法是单盲与双盲研究设计，在双盲法可行的那些病例中双盲法比单盲法更可取。需要设置的盲法应仔细计划与监测。特别是双盲程序是复杂而脆弱的，研究都应确保整个研究过程保持程序的整体性，否则，应用这一技术就会造成很大浪费。

为了保持龋病临床试验适当的双盲程序，必须对制剂的包装与标记给予最大的关注并作出评价，目的是确保实验组与对照组的制剂对受试者与临床检查者都无法辨认，如制剂的物理性能，包括颜色、味道、粘性等应该相似，无法区分活性成分越多，问题越复杂，保持受试者与检查者双盲要作评价，引起这个问题的原因是因为难以使一个阳性对照组与多个实验组完全保持一致，遇到的同样困难是检测防龋产品具有相等的防龋效果时。Friedman建议一种复杂而有独创性的努力来处理这部分临床试验的问题。

Blindness

While randomization eliminates bias at the outset of a RCT, the employment of appropriate blinding or masking techniques as part of the ongoing study protocol are essential to maintain freedom from bias in generating the data. Two common methods are the single-blind and the double-blind study designs, with the latter being preferred to the formed in those cases where double-blinding is feasible. The need for and the method of blinding should be carefully planned and monitored. In particular, since the double-blind procedure is complex and fragile, the investigators should ensure that the integrity of the procedure is maintained throughout the study. If not, the effort and expense devoted to employing the technique in the first place will be largely wasted.

To maintain the proper double-blind procedure in caries clinical trials the greatest attention must be paid to basic matters such as the packaging and labeling of the therapies to be evaluated. The object must be to ensure that treatment and control therapies are indistinguishable from each other to the participant and the clinician examiner alike. The physical characteristics of the therapies, including the color, flavor, viscosity et cetera should be similarly indistinguishable. Maintaining subject and examiner blindness becomes more problematical the greater the number of active therapies being evaluated. This problem arises because it is difficult to produce a positive control therapy that conforms to the characteristic of multiple treatment groups simultaneously. This same general difficulty is encountered when testing caries preventive products for equivalency in caries prevention effectiveness. Friedman et al suggest a complex but ingenious effort to cope in part with this type of clinical trial problem.

This trial helps to evaluate the effectiveness by an intervention is called "golden standard" to obtain the reliable evidence.

第二节 评价研究结果真实性应具备的基本条件

Section 2 The Basic Qualifications Possessed in The Validity Evaluation of the Results From Studies

一、研究设计合格的临床试验的检索标准 Criteria for searching eligible clinical trials of the study design

①在人体进行的卫生保健的处理方法/干预措施的比较研究；

②在性质上是前瞻性研究，即在试验开始之前计划的处理方法/干预措施；以及暴露于每一项干预措施都是在研究人员的控制之下进行的；

③两组或多组处理方法/干预措施与另一组作比较（或者一个组可以是无处理方法的对照组）；

④最重要的方面是打算分配到一个特殊的处理方法/干预措施组是随机的，即不以任何方法作故意的选择。随机化的单位可以是个人，小组（社区，学校或医院）器官或身体其他部位(如牙)。

Criteria for searching eligible clinical trials of the study design

① the study compares health care treatment /intervention in human beings;

② the study is prospective in nature, i.e., the treatments/interventions are planned prior to the experiment taking place, and exposure to each intervention is under the control of the study investigators;

③ two or more treatments/interventions are compared to one another (or one may be treatment control group);

④the most important aspect is that assignment to a particular treatment/intervention is intended to be random, i.e., not deliberately selected in any way. Units of randomization may be individuals, groups (communities, schools, or hospitals) , organs or other parts of the body (such as teeth).

二、金标准临床试验的特征 The characteristics of golden standard for clinical trials

(1) 随机性 (randomization)

①受试对象随机分配到各组

②操作顺序随机安排

③影响结果的非处理因素，条件均随机化，保证组间均衡，齐同性

④抽取样本代表总体：每个受试者接受每个处理的机会完全相等，即样本由总体任意抽取，每个受试对象都有同等机会被抽取

(2) 安慰剂对照 (Placebo controlled)

用于对人进行的试验。对照组接受无任何药理作用的“对照药物”- 安慰剂

(3) 双盲法 (Double-blind)

受试者与施加处理因素的人员均不知组间的区别

(4) 同质性（Homogeneity subjects）

即相似性，均衡性。除处理因素外，组间其他条件均衡一致（如性别、年龄、健康状况、病情程度、经济条件，行为生活方式等），如果研究结果的不同并非由于机会的作用，则此研究是同质的，同质性与异质性相对立

(5) 有效样本量（Effective sample size）

保证研究结果有一定可靠性的条件下，确定最少的受试单位数。过少，所得指标不稳定，结果缺乏充分根据；过多，增加工作难度，不易控制条件，造成浪费

(6) 准确的终点，称为结果终点（Outcome end-point）

循证医学即“以证据为基础”的概念和模式要求对疾病的防治干预建立在有充分科学证据的基础之上，强调评价对结果终点的影响，如疾病的发病率，成本 - 效果比等。

传统的临床医学模式以经验与推理为基础，评价药物或非药物手段所用的指标是替代终点（surrogate end-point）。例如用生物、微生物等指标推论其对疾病的防治作用

(7) 一致的结果（效果）（Consistent results）

临床效果的决定因素依据随机对照试验的结果，同类试验的结果应是基本一致的

三、系统评价 Systematic review

衡量各种问题研究的临床证据的“金标准”是对各种原始临床试验结果进行的系统评价，以及如果适当，进而进行的数量meta-分析，但是系统评价本身可以做的有好有坏。系统评价的一个规定，特征是用一套方法允许读者评估各个作者经过严格的二次研究已经达到目标的程度。换句话说，系统评价的结果才是循证医学所称为的科学证据。系统评价的程序，如Cochrane循证医学中心所提出的：

①陈述评价的目标，并概述合格的标准

②检索符合合格标准的各种研究项目

③列表确定每项研究的特点并评估其方法学的质量

④应用合格标准，并对任何排除项目作出判断

⑤如有可能与研究人员共同重组可能最完整的数据组合

⑥如果适当而又可能，采用统计学的数据汇总方法 meta- 分析，分析合格的研究结果

⑦如果适当而又可能，完成敏感性分析与分组分析

⑧准备一份规范的评价报告，陈述目的，叙述材料与方法，并报告结果

Systematic review

The “gold standard” in clinical evidence for most types of research questions is the systematic review of original research trials, with numerical meta-analysis if appropriate. But systematic reviews can themselves be done well or badly. One defining feature of a systematic review is the presence of a methods section that allows the critical reader to assess how far the authors have achieved the goal of rigorous secondary research. Another words, the results from systemic review is just the perspective of scientific evidence in evidence-based medicine.

A systematic review is a review of a clearly formulated question that uses systematic and explicit methods to identify, select and critically appraise relevant research, and to collect and analyse data from the studies that are included in the review. Systematic review may include a statistical technique known as meta-analysis to pool the data from the individual studies included in the review. The term meta-analysis is often used as synonym for systematic review.

The procedure of systematic review is proposed by the Cochrane collaboration as follows.

State objectives of the review, and outline eligibility criteria

↓

Search for studies that seem to meet eligibility criteria

↓

Tabulate characteristics of each study identifies and assess its methodological quality

↓

Apply eligibility criteria, and justify any exclusions

↓

Assessable the most complete dataset feasible, with involvement of investigators, if possible

↓

Analyse results of eligible studies, use statistical synthesis of data (meta-analysis) , if appropriate and possible

↓

Perform sensitivity analyses, and subgroup analyses, if appropriate and possible

↓

Prepare a structured report of the review, stating aims, describing materials and methods, and reporting results

四、Meta- 分析 Meta-analysis

Meta-分析是对系统评价的数据进行定量统计合并的一种统计学方法。Meta的意思是更加全面综合，通过 Meta- 分析可以达到：

提高统计检验效能

评价结果的一致性，解决单个研究间的矛盾

改进对作用效应的估计

解决以往单个研究未明确的新问题

Meta-analysis is a statistical approach to integrating the results from two or more studies on a particular subject. Other terms used to describe this technique include: overview. Pooling, data pooling, literature synthesis, data synthesis, quantitative synthesis and quantitative review. This approach is more advantageous then traditional narrative review of a body of evidence, which may suffer from bias in selecting articles, lack of objectivity in evaluating the evidence and impressionistic synthesis of findings.

Formal methods for systematically reviewing published research and synthesizing data may help address some of these issue. By using the recently developed quantitative method of meta-analysis and

systematic review, one can accumulate results from prior research and view and combine these results in ways that identify similarities and differences among the studies. In a meta-analysis, the study, not the patient becomes the unit of analysis.

There are two conceptually distinct aspects of meta-analysis: systematic review of the literature and quantitative synthesis of the findings.

Quantitative synthesis of data may provide additional information.

① a primary benefit of quantitative summarization is that a data set having adequate statistical power can be created from a group of studies with sample sizes that are too small for detecting clinically significant differences.

② meta-analysis can help narrow the confidence limits on estimates of treatment effect.

③ meta-analysis can help identify future research needs and

④ may help determine whether the overall body of studies is sufficient to answer the question without conducting another clinical trial combining data from a number of smaller clinical trials is an attractive and economical alternative.

⑤ meta-analysis also can help clarify apparent contradictions in the literature

⑥ meta-analysis allows classification of such variables by systematically organizing studies according to specific classification factors such as treatment characteristics and research methods employed.

1. Meta- 分析的基本步骤 The basic steps in a meta-analysis

系统评价 systematic review 和数量综合 The quantitative synthesis

①规定提出的问题与正确的评价目的

②具体列出进入评价的入选研究标准

③检索文献与确定相关的研究

④评估研究的质量，满足入选标准的要求

⑤评估可以合并的研究并提取研究的数据

⑥选择最适当的方法统计分析汇总的结果或陈述的结果

⑦完成分析并得出结论

The Basic steps in a meta-analysis

systematic review and quantitative synthesis

① Define the problem to be addressed and the exact purpose of the review

② Specify criteria for selection and inclusion of studies in the review

③ Search the literature and identify relevant studies

④ Assess the quality of the studies that satisfy the inclusion criteria

⑤ Assess combinability of the studies and extract data from the studies

⑥ Select the most appropriate methods for statistical analyses of pooling or for presentation of results

⑦ Perform the analysis and reach conclusions

2. Meta- 分析的限度 The limitations in meta-analysis

难以确定相关的研究

识别研究的不同质量

关于合并一定的研究结果

发表偏差

难以确定应包括在 meta- 分析中的相关文章

meta- 分析不能增加研究质量差的报告数据的应用

确定相关文章与评价这些文章的质量不能确保从这些研究引用的数据能够加以合并

The limitations in meta-analysis

① Difficulty in identifying relevant research

② The varying quality of the studies identified

③ Concerns about combining certain study results and publication bias

④ Identification of relevant articles that should be included in a meta-analysis can be difficult

⑤ Meta-analysis cannot enhance the usefulness of data reported from poorly conducted studies

⑥Identification of relevant articles and assessment of the quality of these articles do not ensure that the data from the studies cited can be combined

第三节　证据质量评价与循证推荐

Section 3 Assessment of Quality of Evidence and Evidence-based Recommendations

一、证据质量评价 Assessment of evidence quality

Goldbloom 与 Battista 早在 1986 年加拿大医学杂志发表的定期健康检查一文中提出了证据水平与推荐分类

1. 证据水平 Levels of evidenc

1）至少来自一项适当的随机对照的临床试验提供的证据

2）至少由一项设计好的有对照的临床试验，没有随机化，可以是群组或病例对照分析性研究提供的证据，以一个中心以上，多个时间系列，或者在无对照的实验中取得的显著结果更可取

3）由受尊敬的权威们依据临床经验，描述性研究或专家委员会报告的意见提供的证据

2. 推荐 Recommendations

1）良好的证据支持一项推荐应用

2）中等水平的证据支持一项推荐应用

3）依据较差的证据推荐或者反对应用

4）中等水平的证据支持反对推荐应用

5）良好的证据支持反对推荐应用

6）无可利用的证据作推荐（Table15-1）

表 15-1　Levels of evidence and classification of recommendations

Level of Evidence	
I	Evidence from at least one properly randomized controlled trial
II	Evidence from at least one well-designed controlled trial without randomization, from cohort or case-control analytic studies, preferably from more than one centre, from multiple time series, or from dramatic results in uncontrolled experiments
III	Evidence from opinions of respected authorities on the basis of clinical experience, descriptive studies, or reports of expert committee
Recommendations	
A	Good evidence to support a recommendation for use
B	Moderate evidence to support a recommendation for use
C	Recommendation for, or against use based on poor evidence
D	Moderate evidence to support a recommendation against use
E	Good evidence to support a recommendation against use
NR	No evidence available to make a recommendation

*Adapted from Goldbloom and Battista

1998 年 Godon 依据三个证据水平分成为 6 级作为推荐的标准

3. 评价证据水平 Evaluating the levels of evidence

1999 年美国医学会杂志也提出了分析 RCT 质量特征的最低标准（Table15-2，3，4）。

1）证据强有力的定义包含有随机分配，安慰剂对照，双盲或单盲，样本量大，或者来自 RCT’s 的资料的 meta- 分析，多中心的，准确终点的，前瞻性设计以及受试者同质（表 15-3）。

2）证据弱的定义是来自观察性研究，非随机同时进行的群组研究，和非随机回顾性群组研究（表 15-4）。

3）方法学强度分级见表 15-5。效益与风险的权衡见表 15-6。证据来源分级见表 15-7。

表 15-2　Gordon’s recommendation on grades based on evidence levels（chest 1998）(modified)

Level of evidence	grade	Of recommendation
Level I	Grade A1	Methods strong Results consistent Benefit/risk clear
	Grade A2	Methods strong Results consistent Benefit/risk equivocal
Level II	Grade B1	Methods strong Results consistent Benefit/risk clear

续表

Level of evidence	grade	Of recommendation
	Grade B2	Methods strong
		Results consistent
		Benefit/risk equivocal
Level III	Grade C1	Methods strong
		Results consistent
		Benefit/risk less clear
	Grade C1	Methods strong
		Results consistent
		Benefit/risk equivocal

表 15-3 Definition of methods strong

randomized（randomly assigned to）
placebo-controlled
double/or single blind
large sample size or meta-analysis of RCTs
multicentre
exact end points
prospective design
homogeneity subjects

表 15-4 Table 4 definition of methods weak

observational studies
nonrandomized concurrent cohort studies
Nonrandomized historic cohort studies

表 15-5 Table 5 Methodological strength

Meta-analysis or a large randomized trial with consistent results
Randomized trials with inconsistent results
Observational studies
Laboratory and animal tests only（no any type of clinical human studies）

表 15-6 Table 6 Trade-off between benefits and risks

Clear enough
Less clear
Questionable

表 15-7 Table 7 Evidence from

RCTs
Published studies
Online resources
Expert panel opinions
Opinions from outside experts in the field related to prevention

评价证据水平的目的是为了提高临床试验的质量，并作为一种正确的推荐。

第四节 循证预防口腔医学的概念与实践
Section 4 The Concept and Practice of Evidence-based Preventive Dentistry

一、什么是循证医学？ What is the evidence-based medicine?

循证医学规定为“追踪发现，客观评价（其有效性与用途），以及把快速增长的证据用于临床实践的能力”。临床试验，尤其是称为金标准的“随机对照临床试验”（RCT）的增加，意味着现在拥有大量的证据有可能用于医疗实践。问题是在病人保健第一线是否应用它。但是不论研究的证据怎么好法，必须与临床经验相结合。缺一不可。

What is evidence-based medicine, EBM?

EBM has been defined as the “ability to track down, critically appraise (for its validity and usefulness), and incorporate a rapidly growing body of evidence into clinical practice (sackett and Rosenberg 1995). The rise of clinical trials, particularly the so-called “gold standard” randomized controlled trial (RCT) means that there is now an abundance of evidence with the potential to inform medical practice. Sackett and Rosenberg (1995), however, have questioned whether it is being implemented in the “front line” of patient care. But no matter how good the research evidence is, it must be combined with clinical experience. Neither is sufficient alone.

二、什么是循证牙医学？ What is the evidence-based dentistry?

循证牙医学被规定为“考虑临床问题而重新开辟途径的过程”，具有“依据已知证据作出决定”的特点。在口腔医学中存在着大量可靠证据可以利用的问题。因此，需要在口腔医生中发展 EBD 技能，获取更可靠的证据并用于临床实践。

What is EBD?

EBD has been defined as a “process that restructures the way in which we think about clinical problems” and is characterized by “making decisions based on known evidence”(Richards and Lawrence 1995). There is a problem in dentistry with the amount of reliable evidence available. There is therefore a need to develop the skills of EBD amongst dentists and to gather more reliable evidence on which to base clinical practice.

三、什么是循证预防牙医学？ What is the evidence-based preventive dentistry?

循证预防牙医学是通过审慎地确定，评价与应用最相关的信息，即把证据用于口腔预防决策的实践。循证预防牙医学的基本内容是口腔公共卫生工作者的工作能力，确信的证据以及个人认可的自我价值。证据基础意味着有一种或多种理由相信某件事是真的或者不是真的。一名口腔公共卫生工作者必须能够做到产生适当的证据，并且能够评价充分循证的文献。充分的证据可以来自实验检测，动物试验，人体试验以及临床或者现场试验，预防牙医学有各种干预的方式，如氟化物，控制糖消耗，抗生素，诊断试验，健康教育，行为改变，创建一个支持环境。口腔预防的实际价值只有通过对人群中所发生的情况变化作出评价之后才能看到。清楚的证据表明长期暴露于氟化物之中可以导致龋病下降，而同时可以出现一定程度的氟牙症的副作用。有充分的证据证实，氟摄取的水平需要仔细进行监测，不过，仍然认为全身用氟是最重要的公共卫生措施，而副作用的危险很小。

(3) What is evidence-based preventive dentistry, EBPD?

Evidence-based preventive dentistry has been defined as "the practice of making decision of dental prevention through the judicious identification, evaluation and application of the most relevant information, e.g. evidence. The essential components of EBPD are workability of public health dentists, convinced evidence and self-value of individual willing. The evidence base means one or more reasons for believing something true or not true. A public health dentist must be able to produce appropriate evidence and to review sufficient evidence-based literature.

Sufficient evidence is obtained from laboratory tests, animal tests, human tests and clinical or field trials. In preventive dentistry, there are various intervention forms, such as fluorides, controlling sugar consumption, antibiotics, diagnostic tests, health education, behaviour change, new products and creating a supportive environment, so, the true value of dental prevention appreciated only by seeing what happens in a population group. There is a clear evidence indicated that long term exposure to fluoride results in caries reduction, and appears dental fluosis as a side-effect. However, there are sufficient evidences confirmed that levels of intake are carefully monitored, systemic fluoride is still considered to be a most important public health measure with little risk of side-effects.

四、Meta- 分析：预防口腔医学举例 Meta-analysis: examples from preventive dentistry

在口腔卫生领域内仅有少数 Meta- 分析。有五种系统评价的实例，用来显示系统评价与 Meta- 分析在口腔疾病预防与健康促进活动中的结果。

①与窝沟封闭的效果有关的因素

②用氯甲苯胺兰监测口腔癌

③局部与全身用氟

④口腔健康教育是否有效？

⑤最新机械性口腔卫生实践：疾病预防的循证推荐

Meta-analysis: examples from preventive dentistry

Only a limited number of meta-analysis have focused on oral health. Five of these systematic reviews are discussed below. These five were chosen to illustrate the application of systematic review and meta-analysis to oral disease prevention and health promotion activities.

① Factors associated with the effectiveness of dental sealants

② Screening for oral cancer using tolonium chloride

③ Use of topical and systemic fluorides

④ Is dental health education effective?

⑤ Mechanical oral hygiene practices: evidence-based recommendation for disease prevention

1. 窝沟封闭的效果 Effectiveness of dental sealants

Liodra 等发表了一项 meta- 分析研究文章，评估窝沟封闭的防效果，确定可能影响其效果的因素。通过计算机检索与手工评阅所选杂志的摘要，作者确定 17 种为自凝封闭剂，18 种为光敏封闭剂，作者报告评估每一篇选定的文章质量用 Mantel-Haenszel 法合并结果。

Meta- 分析探索了许多因素对封闭效果的影响，表15-8显示可能影响窝沟封闭剂防龋效果的因素。

Meta- 分析的主要结论是（a）封闭剂防龋是有效果的；（b）自凝封闭剂的效果比光敏剂更好；（c）封闭剂的效果随着时间而下降；（d）封闭剂与氟化有肯定的联系；（e）1976年以前，或期间的报告显示，封闭剂使龋病下降的效果比 1976 年以后开始的研究要更大，作者的结论是操作人员对窝沟封闭剂效果的影响需另作研究。

Effectiveness of dental sealants

Llodra et al. (53) recently published a meta-analysis of studies to assess the effectiveness of dental sealants in preventing dental caries. In particular, the authors sought to estimate the potential effectiveness of dental sealants (measured as the percentage of dental caries prevented) and to identify potential actors that may influence the effectiveness of sealants. Through a computer search and hand review of abstracts from selected journals, the authors identified 17 studies on autopolymerizing dental sealants and 18 studies on dental sealants polymerized via ultraviolet light. The authors reported that the quality of each identified article was assessed and the results were combined using the Mantel Haenszel method.

The meta-analysis explored the influence of a number of factors on the effectiveness of dental sealants. These are shown in Table II. The main conclusions of the meta-analysis were that (a) fissure sealants were effective in preventing dental caries, (b) autopolymerizing dental sealants were more effective than light-cured dental sealants, (c) the effectiveness of dental sealants declined over time, (d) there was a positive association between dental sealants and fluoridation, and (e) studies of dental sealants begun before or during 1976 tended to report a greater reduction in dental caries than studies begun after 1976. The authors concluded that additional studies are needed to asses the influence of the operator on the effectiveness of dental sealants.

表 15-8 Effectiveness of fissure sealants according to factors that may influence effectiveness

factor	Number of studies	% prevented fraction	95% confidence interval
	Type of polymerization		
Auto	44	71.36	69.69-72.94
Ultraviolet light	31	45.92	43.50-48.24
	Length of followup for permanent first molars*		
1-12 months	13	77369	73.29-81.37
13-24 months	11	78.64	75.87-81.09
25-36 months	7	69.79	65.72-73.38
37-48 months	4	68.93	64.57-72.76
>48 months	7	57.36	52.86-61.43
overall	42	71.22	69.55-72.80
	Fluoridation status of drinking water*		
Fluoridated	7	82.69	78.82-85.84
Nonfluoridated	12	71.28	68.51-73.80
Not reported	25	67.79	65.24-70.16
		Operator*	
Dentist alone	25	73.13	70.41-75.61
Dentist plus assistant	12	72.99	70.46-75.31
Dental hygienist alone	2	63.03	53.75-70.44
Dental student plus assistant	5	65.40	60.88-69.69.39
	Beginning date of study*		
Before or during 1976	38	72.04	70.25-73.74
After 1976	6	65.80	61.01-70.00

*data for autopolymerizing fissure sealants only

Reprinted with permission from: Llodra JC, Bravo M, Delgado-Rodriquez M, Baca P & Galvez R. Factors influencing the effectiveness of sealants-a meta-analysis. Community Dent Oral Epidemiol 1993: 21: 261-8. Copyright 1993. Munksgaard International Publishers Ltd., Copenhagen, Denmark

除了评价对效果的影响因素之外，还调查了可能存在的发表偏倚，作者用Vandenbroucke提出的方法，确定了本研究中可能存在的发表偏倚。影响系统评价结果的可能偏倚是只包括了显示有防龋作用的文章。如果能包括很少有或者没有作用而未发表的文章，可能会看到更真实的效果。

In addition to assessing the relative influence of a number of factors on the effectiveness of sealants, the authors also investigated potential publication bias. Using methods suggested by Vandenbroucke (56), the authors did identify the potential for publication bias in their study. This potentialbias may affect the results of the systematic review in that only articles demonstrating a beneficial effect for dental sealants were included. By including articles that show little or no effect, a more accurate picture of the true effectiveness of dental sealants would be obtained.

当作者合并研究结果时，通过检测同质性假设，提出了异质性的影响，作者确定是否研究结果的任何差异可归因于随机变异。结果发现，几乎所有的情况异质性的影响在统计学上都有显著性，（即，在各项研究之间封闭剂效果的可变性预期的随机变异。）按照Dickersin等人的看法，重要的是要提出问题，如meta-分析所提出的一种单一摘要的测量是否真有价值。如果各项研究明显地不同，那么，把研究结果合并成一种单一的测量可能会造成不适当。正如Greenland所指出的，当统计学检验出足够大的异质性时，探讨异质性的来源很重要。Llodra等人完成的多因素线性回归分析，调查是否可以确定变异的来源。结果发现有二个变量可以解释1/3的可变性：在对照组的氟化状态与龋发病率有关。与封闭剂效果有关的其他变量也可能存在，但在meta-分析中没有肯定。

In Llodra et al.'s review (53), the heterogeneity of effects was also addressed by testing the hypothesis of homogeneity when the authors combined the results of the studies. That is, the authors determined whether any differences in the results of the studies were attributable to random variation. They found that, in almost all instances, the heterogeneity of effect was statistically significant (i.e., the variability in effectiveness of dental sealants among studies was greater than would be expected due to random variation).

在明显的存在着变异的情况下，系统评价的优点之一是研究者可以提出问题。一种暴露无遗（或治疗）与一种疾病（或健康状态）在单项研究中观察到的联系是否有可能取决于研究中的人群组成，研究人群的暴露无遗水平，研究所用的疾病定义或者任何一种研究方法质量的测量。

未来关于封闭剂效果的研究设计应以这些发现作为指导，变量的影响，如氟化状况，龋发病率应在分析结果与解释结果中加以考虑。

According to Dickersin and Berlin (17), in instances such as this, "it is important to ask whether a single summary measure, such as is provided by meta-analysis, is indeed valuable"(17:160) . If the studies are sufficiently different, combining study results into a single measure may be misleading and inappropriate. As noted by Greenland (57), exploration of the sources of heterogeneity becomes of great importance when heterogeneity is large enough to be detected by a statistical test. Llodra et al. Performed a multivariate linear regression analysis to investigate whether sources of the variation could be identified. Two variables that explained one-third of the variability were found: fluoridation status and incidence of dental caries in the control group. Other variables associated with the effectiveness of dental sealants also may have been present but were not identified in the meta-analysis.

One of the advantages of systematic reviews in instances of significant variation is that researchers may ask "whether the association between an exposure (or treatment) and a disease (or health state) observed in a single study may depend on the composition of the population under study, the level of exposure in the study population, the definition of disease employed in the study, or any of a number of measures of the methodological quality of the study".

The design of future studies on the effectiveness of dental sealant should be guided by these findings, and the impact of variables such as fluoridation status and incidence rates for caries should be considered in analyzing and interpreting the results.

2. 氯甲苯胺兰用于口腔癌监测 Tolonium chloride and oral cancer screening

Rosenberg等人用Meta-分析评估氯甲苯胺兰（TCI）监测口腔癌的效果，作者确定1964～1986年间16项研究，用TCI评价怀疑为口腔癌的病损，按具体入选标准，从Meta-分析的16项中排除4项。包括的12项中逐项确定其敏感性（检测为阳性的概率）与特异性（检测阴性的概率）。敏感性范围为86%至100%，平均为96.7%。特异性为70%至100%，平均为90.8%。Meta-分析报告的12项研究中的口腔癌患病率范围从8%至100%。12项原始研究数据用4种方式归纳：（a）所有12项数据；（b）从12项研究中排除1项最大的样本量（1,190受试者与第2最大项研究的490比较）；（c）排除由于确定为炎症病损的假阳性研究（n=6）；（d）排除由于确定为炎症病损的假阳性研究和最大的样本量研究。

用12项研究数据计算TCI的敏感性与特异性低于这些研究的平均值。然而，排除较多的组，敏感性与特异性均有改进，尤其是排除了最大样本量研究的影响。因为最大样本量研究中的敏感性与特异性是所有研究中最低的。

通过Meta-分析，Rosenberg等作出以下评价：各组中以TCI确定为口腔癌有着十分不同的疾病水平，而在单一研究中看不到。受监测的人群中口腔癌患病率增加，TCI的阳性预测值增加（检测为阳性而实际发病的概率）。在整个报告的患病率范围中，阴性预测值（检测阴性而没有病的）非常高。根据Meta-分析提出，TCI监测对提高患病检出率有作用，因此监测项目针对高危人群最有价值。

Tolonium chloride and oral cancer screening

Rosenberg and cretin (46) conducted a meta-analysis to assess the efficacy of screening for oral cancer with tolonium chloride (TCl). The authors identified 16 studies conducted between 1964 and 1986 that used TCl in evaluating suspected oral cancer lesions. Based on the inclusion criteria specified, 4 of the 16 studies were excluded from the meta-analysis. The sensitivity the probability that screening with TCl would indicate oral cancer (positive test) when, in fact, oral cancer was present and the specificity the probability that screening with TCl would indicate no oral cancer negative test when, in fact, no oral cancer was present were determined for each of the 12 studies included. Sensitivity ranged from 86 percent to 100 percent, with a mean of 96.7 percent. Specificities varied from 70 percent to 100 percent, with a mean of 90.8 percent. The reported prevalence of oral cancer among the 12 studies included in the meta-analysis ranged from 8 percent to 100 percent.

To determine the overall sensitivity and specificity of TCl, raw data from the 12 studies were aggregated in four ways: (a) for all 12 studies; (b) for all studies except the largest study, which was significantly larger than the other 11 studies (1,190 subjects compared with 490 subjects in the second largest study); (c) for only studies in which false-positive results due to inflammatory lesions were identified (n= 6; and) (d) for only studies in which false-positive results due to inflammatory lesions were identified except the largest study. The results of the meta-analysis are shown in Table15-9.

Using data from all 12 studies, the calculated sensitivity and specificity of TCl were lower than the mean values for the studies considered separately. However, the sensitivity and specificity improved as more subgroups were excluded. In particular, the change illustrated the impact of the largest study.

When the largest study was excluded from the analysis, both the sensitivity and specificity of TCl increased because the reported sensitivity and specificity in the largest study was lowest of all studies included in the analysis.

By conducting this meta-analysis, Rosenberg and Cretin (46) were able to evaluate the performance of TCl in identifying oral cancer lesions among groups with widely different levels of disease, which a single study would be unable to do. The authors (46) found that "as the prevalence of oral cancer in the screened population increases, the positive predictive value the probability that a person with a positive test actually has the disease of TCl improves"(46:625) . Further, the authors (46) reported that, over the entire range of reported prevalence, the negtive predictive value (the likelihood that a person with a negative test does not have the disease was extremely high. As suggested by the meta-analysis, since the performance of TCl screening improves with increasing prevalence, screening programmes targeted toward high risk groups would be most valuable.

表 15-9 Results of Meta-analysis of tolonium chloride and oral cancer screening

subgroup	Individual studies				Combined results	
	Sensitivity %		Specificity %		Sensitivity %	Specificity %
	mean	range	mean	range	mean	range
All studies	96.7	86 ~ 100	90.8	70 ~ 100	93.5	73.3
Exclude large study	97.7	90 ~ 100	92.1	70 ~ 100	97.8	90.1
Exclude inflammatory lesions	96.6	86 ~ 100	85.7	70 ~ 96	93.4	84.2
Exclude inflammatory lesions and large study	98.7	96 ~ 100	87.6	70 ~ 96	97.8	92.2

Reprinted with permission from: Rosenberg D & Cretin S. Use of meta-analysis to evaluate tolonium chloride in oral cancer screening. Oral Surg Oral Med Oral Path 1989;67:621-7. Copyright 1989.Mosby-Year Book Inc., St. Louis, Missouri, USA.

3. 估计防龋制剂的效果 Estimating the effectiveness of caries preventive agents

Clark 等针对口腔健康最早完成的 Meta- 分析之一是估计防龋制剂的效果。根据入选标准，选择评价文献。为了估计一项特殊干预措施的效果，每一项研究结果以总方差反推法加权。然后根据加权估计的标准误计算 95% 可信区限。每项干预的文章数与分析结果见表 15-10。

表 15-10 Results of Meta-analysis of caries-preventive agents

Preventive agent	Number of articles identified in search	Number of studies*	DMFS reduction in individual studies		Estimated DMFS reduction by study results	
			Mean %	Range %	Mean %	95%confidence interval %
Fluoride supplements-permanent dentition	8	11	32	14 ~ 82	41.9	30.8 ~ 52.4
Fluoride supplements-primary dentition	5	10	58.5	0 ~ 80	53	38 ~ 65
APF gels	6	6	22.5	17 ~ 41	26	19 ~ 33
APF solutions	7	7	41	(-1.6) ~ 70	38	20 ~ 57
Fluoride varnishes	3	3	45.6	37.8 ~ 77.5	53	29 ~ 77

DMFS = decayed, missing, and filled tooth surfaces, APF = acidulated phosphate fluoride.

*Some articles included more than one study.

Reprinted with permission from: Clark DC, Hanley JA, Stamm JW& Weinstein PL. An empirically based system to estimate the effectiveness of caries-preventive agents. Caries Res 1985:19:83-95. Copyright 1985.S. Karger AG, Basel, Switzerland.

5种防龋制剂，效果范围很大。以DMFS的减少作测量，其中有一组，对照的DMFS低于干预组，产生负 DMFS 减少。这样，决策者必须决定是否应采纳每一种干预的效果。

本研究中，每项研究每种干预的平均龋减少值并不反映每种研究中样本量或方差的差异。一项恒牙列研究估计氟补充的效果包括545名对照组受试者与450名干预组受试者。另一项评价相同干预的研究对照组仅 16 人，干预组 35 人，很明显，这些研究结果并不给予同等加权。

本研究为初期 Meta- 分析，未对研究质量作评价，而每种研究的质量评价是任何 Meta- 分析的基本内容。虽然观察周期的范围从 1 年到 17 年，只用方差加权结果取代随访周期不同的差异。在Meta-分析中，另一个重要问题是：如何选择参与每项研究的受试者？是否随机化／双盲法？用氟剂量？给氟次数？怎样确定顺从性？在 Meta- 分析评价中均未讨论。

In one of theearliest meta-analyses performed on a topic in oral health, Clark et al. (45) developed and tested an empirically based system for estimating the effectiveness of caries-preventive agents. This effort was an attempt to help decision makers reconcile and combine the numerous, commonly cited estimates of caries-preventive agents' effectiveness. After specifying the criteria for including published articles in the study, the authors reviewed the literature and identified studies that satisfied these criteria. To estimate the effectiveness of a particular intervention, they weighted the results of each study by the inverse of the total variance for that intervention and then estimated the standard error of the weighted estimate to calculate a 95 percent confidence interval. The number of articles for each intervention and the results of the analyses are shown in Table 10.

For each of the five caries-preventive agents in the table, there was a wide range of effectiveness, as measured by a reduction in decayed, missing, and filled tooth surfaces (DMFS). In one instance, the caries rte in the control group was less than that of the intervention group, yielding a negative reduction in DMFS. Yet, the decision maker or policy analyst must determine the effectiveness of each intervention and whether it should be adopted. In this study, the average of the mean values for caries reduction in each study for each intervention does not reflect differences in sample sizes or variances within each study. That is, one study assessing the effectiveness of fluoride supplements in permanent dentition included 545 subjects in the control group and 450 subjects in the intervention group. Clearly, the results of these studies should not be given equal weight.

Since this initial meta-analysis of caries-preventive agents was published, standard criteria for what should and should not be included in a meta-analysis have become more accepted. For example, while this study did not evaluate the quality of studies included in the review, assessment of the quality of each study? Were the subjects randomized? Were the subjects and the researchers blinded to the interventions? What doses of fluoride were used in the studies? How frequently were the fluoride supplements administered how was compliance determined? In the meta-analysis reviewed here, these were not discussed.

4. 口腔健康教育（Oral health education）是否有效

系统评价现有证据　Kay EJ 等作者检索了 1982 ~ 1994 年发表的 143 篇关于口腔健康教育作为一项干预措施效果的系统评价。由2名研究人员独立进行。入选标准最高分值为20，入选评价的有效分值为 12，分值达到 15 或 15 以上的作 meta- 分析，确保只能随机对照设计的研究入选，排除报告不适当的 RCT's。每项研究作二种评价：(a) 每项研究目标的定量评价；(b) 干预的性质评价（参与者种类，人数，干预结果），计算加权的平均基线分值和干预的作用。

结果为共搜集 143 篇文章，排除 72 篇，有效记分：37 篇为 12 分及 12 分以上。7 项研究作正式 meta- 分析，3 项研究用菌斑指数作 meta- 分析，共 161 名干预者，247 名对照，分析显示使菌斑沉积减少。尽管少，证据的平均干预作用为-0.37（95%CI, -0.29, -0.59）。这类干预证实使菌斑指数降低 30%。另外 4 项研究干预组 99 人，对照组 98 人，用牙面菌斑百分比作为测量结果，meta- 分析显示的干预作用为 -11.28（95%CI:-6.68, -15.53）。针对控制菌斑的 DHE 人数牙面菌斑比社区一般人群减少 10%。(Table 11, 12)。

结果表明：

① DHE 教育干预对牙菌斑沉积有部分肯定而暂的作用约 30%；

②对龋病增加无明显下降作用；

③对知识水平提高一致肯定有作用；

④应进一步综合 DHE 信息，用系统方法，严格标准，作出研究评价。

Is dental health education effective? A systematic review of current evidence

In order that health service resources are allocated in the way which most benefits the population, systematic review of the available evidence regarding the effectiveness of programmes and interventions are required. This study examined papers relating to dental health education interventions, which were published between 1982 and 1994 (n=143). Each was scored by two independent researchers according to twenty predetermined validity criteria. For each paper which achieved a validity score of more than 12 (n=37), data concerning the objectives of the intervention, the types and numbers of participants, and the outcomes, were extracted from the article. Where sufficient data were provided in a paper which met more than 15 of the validity criteria quantitative meta-analysis was carried out i.e. the results of the studies were pooled in order to calculate an overall intervention effect with confidence intervals. This combination of qualitative and quantitative review techniques showed that dental health interventions have: a small positive, but temporary effect on plaque accumulation (reduction in plaque index=0.37 95% CI -0.29-0.59); no discernible effect on caries increment and a consistent positive effect on knowledge levels. The results of this analysis suggest that further efforts to synthesise current information about dental health education, in a systematic way, are required, along with maintenance of rigorous scientific standards in evaluation research.

表 15-11 Mean validity scores of subcategories reviewed

Category	Included in qualitative analysis		Included in qualitative analysis	
	n	MVS*	n	MVS
Plaque/gingival health	15	15.8	7	16.4
Caries	4	12.75	0	–
Dietary change knowledge and attitudes	4	12.75	0	–
Knowledge and attitudes	14	15.69	0	–

表 15-12 Mean validity scores of subcategories reviewed

Author	subjects control	Intervention	Outcome measure	Weighted average baseline measurement	Intervention	Follow-up (longest)	× − × + 95%CI
Schou L. 1985	44	45	Plaque index	1.15	Active involvement programme	4 years	−0.43(0.455−0.405)
Stewart et al. 1991	25	25	Plaque index	0.84	Cognitive behaviour programme	5 weeks	−0.28(0.303−0.258)
Rayner 1992	62	58	Plaque index	1.63	Brushing and home visits	1year	−0.42(0.79−0.048)
Glavind et al. 1981	12	12	% surfaces with plaque	63.8	Hygienist OHI	6 months	−0.71(−21.2−7.0)

续表

Author	subjects control	Intervention	Outcome measure	Weighted average baseline measurement	Intervention	Follow-up (longest)	× − × + 95%CI
Hetland et al. 1981	25	23	% surfaces with plaque	81.6	Scaling and OHI	6 months	−37.0(−47.5−26.5)
Soderholm et al. 1982	23	23	% surfaces with plaque	64.2	Scaling and 5 visit programme	6 weeks	−37.5(−46.4−28.63)
Glavind and Zeuner 1985	12	12	% surfaces with plaque	60.0	Scaling and TV	2 month	−2.0(−15+11,2)

5. 最新机械性口腔卫生实践，疾病预防的循证推荐 An update of mechanical oral hygiene practices: evidence-based recommendations for disease prevention

Douglass J. Brothwell 等检索了 1984 ～ 1995Medline 数据库，用疾病结果测量从 106 篇文章中选择适当的研究，依据证据概念的水平作出选择，根据入选与排除标准，只选入机械性口腔卫生干预，不包括化学药物性干预。

表 15-13 推荐摘要：个人机械性口腔卫生实践 - 刷牙

实践	效果	证据水平	推荐
① 刷牙	用含氟牙膏每天刷牙 2 次，防龋与控制龈炎	1(11, 14,17 ～ 20)	有很好的证据推荐每天用含氟牙膏刷牙 2 次防龋与控制龈炎（A）*
② 手动牙刷 尼龙牙刷	可利用任何软毛刷控制龈炎	1(1,22 ～ 27)	中等证据推荐用任何软毛牙刷（B）
海绵状泡沫牙刷	在控制龈炎方面不如传统牙刷有效	128	中等证据不推荐泡沫牙刷控制龈炎（D）
③ 电动牙刷 振动 / 旋转或反转动作电动牙刷	控制龈炎比手动牙刷更有效	1(32 ～ 37)	有很多的证据推荐用振动 / 旋转或反转电动牙刷控制龈炎（A） 推荐给手灵巧性受限、或戴固定矫正器的病人

续表

实践	效果	证据水平	推荐
④ 旋转，颤动或声动作电动牙刷	在控制龈炎方面不比手动牙刷更有效	1(29, 38 ～ 49)	中等证据不向大多数成人推荐应用旋转，颤动或声动作的电动牙刷（D）

* 龋病下降大多是由于氟化物的作用

表 15-14　推荐摘要：个人机械性口腔卫生实践 - 辅助方法

实践	效果	证据水平	推荐
① 牙间隙卫生 i 牙线	在控制成人龈炎方面比只刷牙更有效	1, (46,47,49)	有很好的证据推荐成人用牙线洁牙作为刷牙的辅助方法控制龈炎 (A)
	预防儿童龈炎无作用	151	中等证据不推荐儿童用牙线洁牙控制龈炎（B）
	控制牙周炎比只刷牙更有效	11, (11,48)	中等证据推荐一种牙间卫生方法控制牙周炎（B）
ii 木制牙签	控制成人龈炎比只刷牙更有效	11, (11,48)	中等证据推荐用木制牙签控制成人龈炎（B）
iii 邻间刷	对减少龈炎并不比只刷牙更有效	11, (11,48)	中等证据不推荐用邻间刷（D）

表 15-15　推荐摘要：个人机械性口腔卫生实践 - 辅助方法

② 其他 i 联束（unituft）或端束（end-tuft）牙刷	辅助刷牙控制成人龈炎有效	162	中等证据推荐用联束或端束牙刷控制成人龈炎，不作牙间卫生用（B）
ii 牙龈按摩	与只刷牙比较在控制龈炎方面并无更多效果	1(11,48)	中等证据不推荐用橡胶刺激作为控制龈炎的辅助方法（D）
iii 龈上冲选	比只刷牙比较在控制龈炎方面并无更多效果	11(59,63)	有很好的证据推荐龈上冲洗控制口腔卫生差的成人或戴矫正器的病人（A）
iv 龈下冲洗	作为一种辅助刷牙的方法，尚未做评价	–	无证据推荐（NR）
v 舌刷或刮舌板	控制龈炎无效	169	中等证据不推荐舌刷控制龈炎（D）

结论是：

1. 刷牙

刷牙仍是最普遍的口腔清洁手段　刷牙也是提供局部氟化物于牙面的载体，70年代的以来在发达国家表明是龋病下降的重要原因。含氟牙膏的抗龋效果已很肯定，但单独刷牙的效果不肯定，用含氟牙膏刷牙对龋病与牙周病均有作用

a. 刷牙次数：提倡每天刷牙2次有利于去除牙菌斑及牙龈健康，无充分证据表明刷牙有降

低龋发病率的效果。刷牙质量比次数更重要，每天用含氟牙膏刷牙2次比不常刷牙的防龋效果更好。不论是刷牙，还是增加刷牙次数都对防龋无作用。虽然研究提出增加刷牙次数有益牙周健康，但并没有确定理想的次数，推荐每天刷牙 2 次与牙周健康及减少龋发生率是一致的。

b. 刷牙方法：虽然旋转法对去除牙菌斑效果最小，各种刷牙方法之间在临床上均无显著性差异。1986 年以来，发表的文献并未推荐一种具体的方法。不论用何种方法，应避免刷牙用力过大。

c. 牙刷设计：

- 大部分软毛刷对预防口腔疾病都有效
- 泡沫刷（海绵状）对减少牙周炎的严重程度比传统牙刷的效果差
- 电动牙刷：其作用并没有大于手动牙刷，有些设计的电动牙刷对预防或减少牙龈炎的严重程度比手动牙刷更有效，而且较少伤及牙龈。振动／旋转动作与反转动作的电动牙刷对控制龈炎比手动牙刷更有效。这些对特需病人更好，如正畸病人。其他各种电动牙刷如垂直、旋转或声控均无优点，由于成本高，不推荐。

2. 辅助口腔卫生法

刷牙一般达不到的部位有必要，但非每个人需要。

a. 牙间隙卫生

牙线：刷牙加牙线洁牙对成人牙龈健康比只刷牙好，用牙线的理想次数并没有确定。由于邻间退缩，间隙增加，认识到牙线的作用已逐渐减少，不同的牙线的作用并没有明显的差异。牙线用具与传统用牙线比较无额外效益，儿童用牙线比只刷牙，对牙龈健康并不产生额外效果。没有推荐用牙线的适当年龄，无证据能养成习惯

木制牙签：刷牙，并用牙签辅助，比单独刷牙对减少牙龈出血有效大作用。没有报告用木制牙签有有害作用。

邻间刷：当有足够的间隙允许使用时，是好的邻间清洁工具。然而并没有证实其作用优于其他邻间工具或单纯刷牙。

b. 联束或端束刷：刷头小，与传统牙刷比较，对减少成人龈炎有辅助作用，建议应由专业人员监督。然而由于力量集中能引起龈创伤。

c. 牙龈按摩：用橡皮端刺激器对减少龈炎并没有任何超过刷牙的辅加效益，很少有临床意义。

d. 龈上冲洗：已有减少龈炎的报告。有水冲洗的有害作用很小。专家意见，有细菌性心内膜炎危险的人应避免冲洗。在任何口腔外科手术后所有的病人应推迟一个月冲洗。

e. 龈下冲洗：虽然对改善牙周健康可能有作用，但尚未作过评价。

f. 舌刷或刮舌板：作为刷牙的一种辅助，并不有助于减少龈炎。

小结 Summary

循证医学概念新，其内涵外延日益丰富。现在已广泛用于临床和公共卫生诸方面。但是尚在发展和完善之中，有争议，困难与挑战。尽管如此，循证思想可贵。它以最小危险，最少花费，获得最大健康效益，增进全民健康。

Good decisions about health care rely on more than good reviews of the results of research, reliable evidence about the effects of specific elements of health care, although essential for improving decisions about health care and research, is only part of what is needed for better decision making.

In making decisions about the oral care of individuals and groups, the results of the reviews must be integrated with oral care professional's expertise, which has been acquired through experience and practice.

The evidence will help those who can best benefit from it.

思考题 Review questions

1. what is the concept of evidence-based medicine?
2. describe the definition of a randomized controlled trial
3. what is the systematic review?
4. what is the meta-analysis?
5. describe the basic qualifications possessed in the validity of the results of studies
6. discuss the levels of evidence and its recommendations
7. what is evidence-based preventive dentistry?
8. take one example to describe the basic steps of a meta-analysis

参考文献 References

1. Kay E J, et al. Is dental health education effective? A systemic review of current evidence. Community dentistry and oral Epidemiology, 1996; 24: 231-5
2. Brothwell, Douglas J. et al. an update of mechanical oral hygiene practices: evidence-based recommendations for disease prevention J. candion dental association, 1998 vol 64, No. 4: 295-306
3. 王家良. 循证医学. 人民卫生出版社, 2001
4. Trisha Greenhalgh, et al. evidence based health care workbook: understanding research. BMJ Books, 2000
5. The Cochrane Collaboration. Oral health review group journal hand searchers' manual, revised. January, 2002
6. Blanaid Daly, et al. essential dental public health Oxford University Press, 2002
7. Cohen Lois K, et al. Disease Prevention and oral health promotion Munksgaard, 1995

（卞金有）